Introduction to Health Care

Joyce Mitchell, RN, MSN, MBA

Lee Haroun, MA Education, MBA, EdD (candidate), Education Specialist

\\cypress\Allied Health Share

103

DELMAR

THOMSON LEARNING ™

Australia Canada Mexico Singapore Spain United Kingdom United States

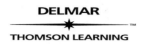

DELMAR

THOMSON LEARNING

Introduction to Health Care
by Joyce Mitchell and Lee Haroun

Health Care Publishing Director:
William Brottmiller

Executive Editor:
Cathy L. Esperti

Acquisitions Editor:
Sherry Gomoll

Developmental Editor:
Marah Bellegarde

Executive Marketing Manager:
Dawn F. Gerrain

Project Editor:
Maureen M. E. Grealish

Production Coordinator:
John Mickelbank

Art/Design Coordinator:
Jay Purcell

Technology Project Manager:
Laurie Davis

Library of Congress Cataloging-in-Publication Data
Mitchell, Joyce.
Introduction to healthcare / Joyce Mitchell, Lee Haroun.
p. cm.
Includes bibliographical references and index.
ISBN 0-7668-1440-8 (alk. paper)
1. Medical care. 2. Medical care—Study and teaching. 3. Medicine—Study and teaching.
4. Medicine—Vocational guidance.
I. Haroun, Lee. II. Title.
R838 .M55 2001
362.1—dc21

2001028197

NOTICE TO THE READER

CONTENTS

Unit 1: Health Care Today

Unit 2: The Language of Health Care

PREFACE

Introduction to Health Care is designed as an introductory text for students entering a variety of college-level health care programs or for those who believe they may have an interest in pursuing a career in health care. The fundamentals that are common to all health care occupations are presented in this full color text to create a foundation on which students can build when they take their specific occupational courses. The topics included are appropriate for occupations that involve direct patient care, such as nursing and dental assisting, as well as those that provide support services, such as health information technology and pharmacy technician. The goal of the text is to present a broad base of health care essentials. Therefore, skills and procedures that apply only to specific occupations are not included.

The text is written in easy-to-understand language. A variety of learning exercises are included in each chapter. These exercises are designed to appeal to the different ways that students learn, including visual, auditory, and kinesthetic. The text can be used by students as a reference book after completion of their introductory courses.

Content for Today's Health Care Worker

Introduction to Health Care includes topics essential for today's student and tomorrow's health care worker. The basic concepts that create the foundation for health care education have been expanded beyond those usually included in an introductory text. The following topics have been added in response to the current needs of health care educators and employers.

- Thinking skills
- Learning styles and study techniques
- Complementary therapies
- Prevention and wellness strategies
- Lifelong learning and continuing education
- Documentation
- Cost-control measures
- Performance improvement
- Personal efficiency
- Customer service

Emphasis on Thinking Skills

The dramatic growth of the health care industry promises to provide increasing numbers of employment opportunities for graduates of health care programs. At the same time, today's graduates face new challenges. Changes in health care are rapid and continuous. Workers at all levels are being given additional responsibilities. Efficiency and flexibility, combined with competency, are vital to workplace success. To be competent and successful in this ever-changing environment, health care workers must be able to think for themselves and adapt as necessary to meet current employment demands.

The authors recognize the need of health care educators for materials that can assist them in preparing students to assess new situations, determine appropriate action, and apply on the job what they learned in the classroom. This text is designed to help meet this need. Students are introduced to the concept of thinking like a health care worker in Chapter 1. The specific skills that make up applied thinking are explained in everyday language. A five-step problem-solving model is clearly described to help students systematically approach new situations. Every chapter includes exercises called "Thinking It Through" that require students to apply the concepts presented in the text to typical on-the-job scenarios. Each chapter then concludes with two application exercises that provide opportunities to summarize and apply chapter content.

Organization of the Text

Introduction to Health Care is divided into nine units that contain between two and five chapters of related topics. The following overview highlights many of the major concepts included in the text:

Unit 1: Health Care Today

- Characteristics and trends of modern health care, including managed care and complementary therapies
- Descriptions of many health occupations, organized by type of work performed
- Explanation of how to think like a health care worker

- Legal and ethical responsibilities required of all health care workers

Unit 2: The Language of Health Care

- Introduction to basic concepts of medical terminology
- Examples of common word elements
- Suggested ways to approach the study of terminology and learn it systematically
- Review of math skills necessary for health care applications
- Tips for dealing with math anxiety

Unit 3: The Human Body

- Brief overview of the basic organization, structure, and functions of the body systems, intended as an introduction rather than a complete A & P course
- Examples of diseases and conditions related to each system
- Preventive measures for each system, including lifestyle management tips
- Physical and mental milestones of growth and development over the life span and the implications when providing health care

Unit 4: Personal and Workplace Safety

- Basic skills and habits needed to protect both health care workers and patients
- Emphasis on body mechanics and infection control
- Hands-on skills, such as using a fire extinguisher

Unit 5: Behaviors for Success

- Self-care practices important for health care workers, including dealing with stress
- Characteristics of professionalism essential for career success
- Lifelong learning and continuing education strategies

Unit 6: Communication in the Health Care Setting

- Patients as individuals
- Basic human needs
- Acknowledging diversity while avoiding cultural stereotypes
- Using questions and observations to assess specific patient needs
- Basic oral and written communication techniques

- Overview of computer applications in health care
- Basics of health care documentation

Unit 7: Health Care Skills

- Basic assessment skills
- Hands-on skills such as taking vital signs and measuring height and weight
- Normal ranges and significant changes
- Step-by-step instructions for performing basic emergency procedures (CPR is not included because certification is frequently required of health care students and the course is taught by certified instructors who use annually updated written materials instead of a textbook.)

Unit 8: Business of Caring

- Health care as a business
- Improving care while controlling costs
- Working efficiently

Unit 9: Securing and Maintaining Employment

- Application of job search skills to health care employment
- Tips for remaining successfully employed
- Behaviors for job success, including teamwork and leadership skills
- Employment legalities

Instructional Supplements

Instructor's Manual

The instructor's manual includes the following items to help instructors use the text most effectively in planning and teaching an introductory course:

- Answers to review questions found at the end of each chapter in the student text
- Suggested answers to "Thinking it Through" and "Application Exercises" found in the student text
- Procedure check-off forms for evaluating student skills
- Suggestions for class activities
- Teaching thinking skills
- Transparency masters

Computerized Test Bank

The testbank is on CD and contains approximately 1,000 test questions. These include true/false, multiple choice, matching, short answer, and essay questions. Users can add their own questions. This software allows the user to create tests in less than 5 minutes with the ability to print them out in a variety of layouts. It also has electronic "take-home testing" (put test on disk) and Internet-based testing capabilities. Additionally, the software allows the user to include multimedia in the electronic tests (video, audio).

About the Authors

Joyce Mitchell has a Master's of Science Degree in Nursing from the University of California, San Francisco and a Master's in Business Administration Degree from the University of Santa Clara. The combination of the two degrees provides a framework for understanding and functioning within the current and rapidly evolving world of health care today.

Joyce has 25 years of experience in health care, including education, management and curriculum consultation. Besides many years in classroom and clinical teaching, she has developed and implemented unique and innovative health care programs at both the vocational and associate's degree levels.

Lee Haroun has a Master's of Art Degree in Education from Portland State University (Oregon) and a Master's in Business Administration Degree from National University in San Diego. Her doctoral studies include creating ways to help new college faculty increase their instructional effectiveness.

Lee has 30 years of experience in teaching and educational administration. She has developed health care curriculum for a variety of postsecondary programs, including occupational therapy assistant, health information technician insurance coder, and patient care technician. She has a special interest in working with students to help them reach their maximum potential in both school and career.

DEDICATION

To my parents, for encouraging and supporting my pursuit of a health care education. And to my brother, Gary Moberly, and his wife, Arlene, who provided a safe haven in which to write this book.

–Joyce Mitchell

To Dad, Bob, and David, for their support, encouragement, and never wavering belief that I could do this.

–Lee Haroun

HOW TO USE

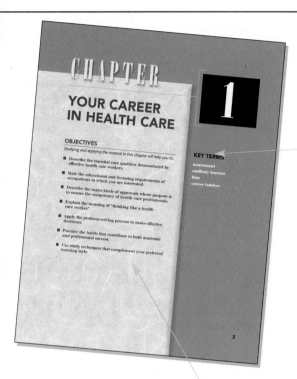

Key Terms: List of important vocabulary and key concepts. Understanding vocabulary is critical to understanding the concepts presented in the chapter. Key terms are bolded and defined the first time they appear in the chapter. There is also a comprehensive glossary in the back of the book.

Objectives: Overview of chapter content and goals for learning. Review these before beginning to read the chapter and use the objectives to check your progress after completing the chapter.

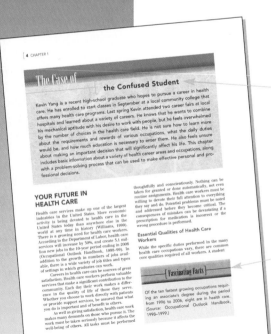

The Case of . . . : These health care scenarios introduce chapter content and show why the material in the chapter is important for the competent health care worker. An application exercise at the end of the chapter refers back to the case.

Fascinating Facts: Interesting information that is related to the chapter topics.

Tables: These provide summaries of related facts. Use them as study aids and for quick reference.

Thinking It Through: These are exercises located throughout the chapter. They are a very important part of this text. The health care scenarios require you to think about the concepts presented in the chapter and use them to resolve typical problems encountered by health care workers. Use the exercises to develop the thinking skills necessary to be a successful health care worker.

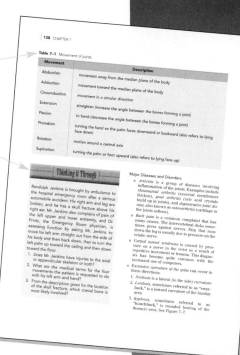

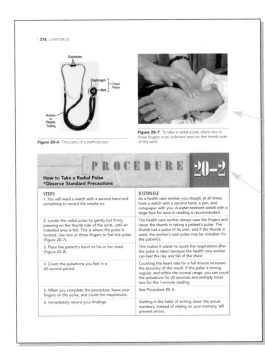

Colored photos and illustrations: These reinforce important concepts and complex topics. Use them to increase your understanding of the material.

Procedures: A step-by-step format helps you master basic hands-on skills. Pay special attention to the rationales that explain the reasons for the actions.

Suggested Learning Activities: Try these interesting projects that include doing research on the Internet, reporting on observations from daily life, and visiting health care facilities.

Application Exercises: Opportunities to apply the chapter's major concepts to typical health care situations. Use these exercises to practice using your knowledge in ways similar to those you may encounter on the job.

Suggested Readings and Resources: Learn more about topics of interest from the books, articles, and Web sites listed in this section.

Review Questions: The questions are keyed to the chapter objectives to ensure your mastery of the chapter content. Use them to check your learning and identify areas that need more study.

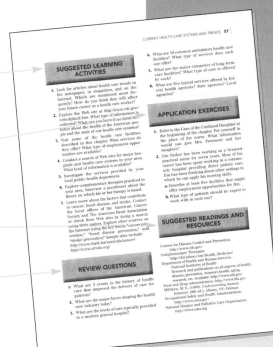

ACKNOWLEDGMENTS

The authors wish to acknowledge the help, support, and continual good humor of Marah Bellegarde, Developmental Editor at Delmar. A special thank you to all the reviewers who offered many wonderful suggestions.

Susan L. Berridge, BSN, MA
Instructor, Health Occupations
Jackson Area Career Center
Jackson, MI

Sue Ellen Bice, MS, RRA
Associate Professor, HITIMR Program Director
Mohawk Valley Community College
Utica, NY

Patti Biro, BS, M.Ed.
Director of Health Care Programs
Del Mar College
Corpus Christi, TX

Maxine Burley, RN, BSN, MA
Instructor
Gateway Community College
Phoenix, AZ

Marilyn Collins, RN
Director of Health Occupations
Citrus College
Glendora, CA

Teresa England-Lewis, MSN, RN
Health Occupations Instructor
North Montco Technical Career Center
Lansdale, PA

Marie Fenske, EdD, R.R.T.
Chair, Health Science
Gateway Community College
Phoenix, AZ

Sally Flesch, PhD, RN
Chair, Allied Health Department
Black Hawk College
Moline, IL

Melanie King Gulliver, RN, MS
Coordinator/ Adjunct Instructor
Broward Community College
Coconut Creek, FL

Sharon Luczu, RN, BS, MA, MBA
Program Director of the Health Services
Management Program
Gateway Community College
Phoenix, AZ

Sheila McNulty, PT
Faculty, Academic Coordinator of Clinical
Education
Del Mar College
Corpus Christi, TX

Ann Sims, RN
Program Director, Nursing Assistant Programs
Albuquerque Technical Vocational Institute
Albuquerque, NM

Julie Slack
Dixie State College
St. George, UT

Susan Wallace, M.Ed, RRA
Chair, Health Science Division
Garland County Community College
Hot Springs, AR

UNIT

1

HEALTH CARE
TODAY

CHAPTER

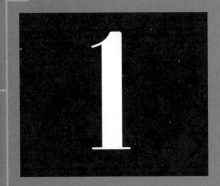

YOUR CAREER
IN HEALTH CARE

OBJECTIVES

Studying and applying the material in this chapter will help you to:

■ Describe the essential core qualities demonstrated by effective health care workers.

■ State the educational and licensing requirements of occupations in which you are interested.

■ Describe the major kinds of approvals whose purpose is to ensure the competency of health care professionals.

■ Explain the meaning of "thinking like a health care worker."

■ Apply the problem-solving process to make effective decisions.

■ Practice the habits that contribute to both academic and professional success.

■ Use study techniques that complement your preferred learning style.

KEY TERMS

assessment
auditory learner
bias
career ladders
certification
kinesthetic learner
learning style
licensure
manual dexterity
objective data
opinion
problem-solving process
registration
reliable
scope of practice
signs
subjective data
symptoms
visual learner

The Case of

the Confused Student

Kevin Yang is a recent high-school graduate who hopes to pursue a career in health care. He has enrolled to start classes in September at a local community college that offers many health care programs. Last spring Kevin attended two career fairs at local hospitals and learned about a variety of careers. He knows that he wants to combine his mechanical aptitude with his desire to work with people, but he feels overwhelmed by the number of choices in the health care field. He is not sure how to learn more about the requirements and rewards of various occupations, what the daily duties would be, and how much education is necessary to enter them. He also feels unsure about making an important decision that will significantly affect his life. This chapter includes basic information about a variety of health career areas and occupations, along with a problem-solving process that can be used to make effective personal and professional decisions.

YOUR FUTURE IN HEALTH CARE

Health care services make up one of the largest industries in the United States. More economic activity is being devoted to health care in the United States today than anywhere else in the world at any time in history (Williams, 1999). There is a growing need for health care workers. According to the Department of Labor, health care services will increase by 30%, and create 3.1 million new jobs in the 10-year period ending in 2006 (Occupational Outlook Handbook, 1998–99). In addition to the growth in numbers of jobs available, there is a wide variety of job titles and types of settings in which graduates can work.

Careers in health care can be sources of great satisfaction. Health care workers perform valuable services that make a significant contribution to the community. Each day their work makes a difference in the quality of life of those they serve. Whether you choose to work directly with patients or provide support services, be assured that what you do is important and of benefit to others.

As well as giving satisfaction, health care work makes many demands on those who pursue it. The work must be taken seriously because it affects the well-being of others. All tasks must be performed thoughtfully and conscientiously. Nothing can be taken for granted or done automatically, not even routine assignments. Health care workers must be willing to devote their full attention to everything they say and do. Potential problems must be noted and addressed before they become critical. The consequences of mistakes can be devastating if a prescription for medication is incorrect or the wrong procedure is performed.

Essential Qualities of Health Care Workers

While the specific duties performed in the many health care occupations vary, there are common core qualities required of all workers. A student

[Fascinating Facts]

Of the ten fastest growing occupations requiring an associate's degree during the period from 1996 to 2006, eight are in health care. (Source: Occupational Outlook Handbook, 1998–1999.)

whose goal is to become an effective health care worker must:

- Care about others: Apply knowledge and skills to decrease suffering and increase the well-being of others. When necessary, be willing to put the needs of patients ahead of one's own. Have respect for all people and help them regardless of their race, nationality, economic status, religion, age, or lifestyle preferences.

- Have integrity: Be honest at all times. Respect the privacy of others. Be loyal to the employer. Never take supplies that belong to the facility home for personal use.

- Be dependable: Be at work on time and as scheduled. Follow through and finish all assigned tasks. Perform work accurately and completely. Work without constant supervision and reminders.

- Work well with others: Strive to understand the feelings and needs of others. Be courteous and considerate. Practice good communication skills. Be a good team member by cooperating and contributing to the achievement of group goals. Take directions willingly from your supervisor. See Figure 1–1.

- Be flexible: Be willing to adapt to changing conditions and emergencies. Do what is needed to carry out tasks. Acquire knowledge and skills necessary to keep up with advances in technology and changes in the way health care is delivered.

- Be willing to learn: Work hard to keep skills up to date. Ask questions, attend workshops, and continue to acquire new skills.

- Strive to be cost conscious: Look for ways to improve patient care while maintaining or lowering expenses.

OCCUPATIONAL PROFILES

There are hundreds of job titles in health care and the number continues to grow. They require a wide range of skills and abilities. Each occupational area, such as radiology and physical therapy, has positions that require different amounts of education and training. These levels are known as **career ladders**.

Students pursuing occupations in health care should learn as much as possible about the requirements and conditions of their areas of interest. This knowledge will enable them to make

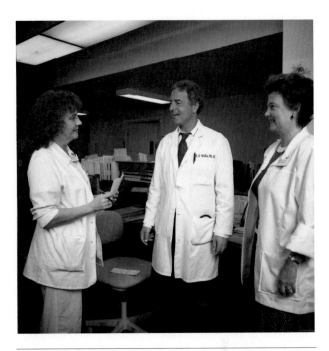

Figure 1–1 Successful health care workers must be able to work well with others.

good career choices that match their preferences and abilities. For example, some individuals interested in health care would find the emergency medical technician's (EMT) job to be interesting and exciting. EMTs have opportunities to apply their skills to help others in significant ways, sometimes even saving lives. At the same time, the work is physically and emotionally demanding. It is often performed under difficult circumstances. Emergencies do not happen at convenient times and places. The schedules for EMTs include nights, weekends, and holidays, and they are called out to work in all types of weather conditions. All aspects of an occupation must be considered to increase the chances of choosing a career that will provide long-term satisfaction.

Students who explore and learn more about career areas that interest them will have a better chance of finding an occupation that matches their abilities and preferences. When choosing an occupation, they should carefully consider the following factors about themselves:

- How much time they are willing to dedicate to their education

- Natural abilities

- What type of activities they most enjoy

- Educational background

- Their preferences for workplace environment and conditions

The occupations described in this section are organized into four categories:

1. Therapeutic and Treatment
2. Diagnostic
3. Information
4. Environmental

Occupational titles are further organized by specific career areas, such as mental health and dental. The educational and licensing requirements for various occupational levels are presented in Tables 1–1 through 1–17. (Note that the abbreviations given in the tables for job titles assume that the individual has achieved the required approval, such as certification.) Following each table, occupations that generally require associate degrees or specific vocational training are described in additional detail.

It is important for students to keep in mind that the information in this chapter provides brief overviews and contains only the most common job titles. In fact, some occupational areas have dozens of job titles for which graduates might qualify. For example, the authors of a book about health information careers identified over 358 different job titles for work in various aspects of medical record-keeping and information management (Anderson and Smith, 1997).

It is also important to note that there are more rungs on the career ladders than appear in the tables. For example, there are many nurse specialties that may be pursued: nurse anesthetist, clinical nurse specialists, as well as doctoral degrees in nursing. Many occupational and physical therapists earn advanced degrees. Students should use the tables as a starting point and then thoroughly investigate all the career options in their areas of interest.

On-the-job training, in which workers learn necessary job skills after being employed, is being replaced in many occupations by formal training. Those at the aide levels of employment are being assigned more responsible tasks, and classroom training is becoming more desirable. Today's health care facilities need workers who have current skills, are able to think for themselves, and can start immediately as contributing members of the health care team.

Therapeutic and Treatment Occupations

Occupations in this category provide services that assist patients to regain or attain maximum wellness. They may involve direct patient care, such as nursing, or provide services that contribute to the patient's recovery, such as the pharmacy professions. The majority of health care occupations fall into this category.

Dental Occupations

Dental workers treat diseases and conditions of the teeth and soft tissues of the mouth. They perform preventive measures, restore missing and defective teeth, diagnose and treat diseases of the gums, and provide patient education. See Table 1–1 and Figure 1–2.

Table 1–1 Dental Occupations

Career	Education	Testing and Approval
Dentist (D.D.S. or D.M.D.)	2–4 years college predental preparation 4 years dental school 2–4 years additional education if seek specialty	Licensed by states: 1. Graduate from accredited dental school 2. Pass written and practical exams
Dental Hygienist (LDH)	Associate's or bachelor's degree 2–4 years depending on program requirements	Licensed by states: 1. Graduate from accredited dental hygiene school 2. Pass national board exams administered by American Dental Association Joint Commission on National Dental Examinations

(continues)

Table 1–1 (continued)

Career	Education	Testing and Approval
Dental Laboratory Technician	On-the-job training or 2-year associate's degree program	Optional certification by National Association of Dental Laboratories
Dental Assistant (CDA or RDA)	1–2 year vocational program or on-the-job training	Optional certification by Dental Assisting National Board

Dental Hygienist

The principal responsibility of dental hygienists is to provide preventive dental care. This is accomplished by cleaning the teeth with special instruments and equipment, examining the mouth and taking x-rays, and providing patient education about dental care. While hygienists perform their work independently, they are under the supervision of a dentist. Work schedules are often flexible, and many hygienists work part-time and/or for more than one dentist. The work involves prolonged patient contact, standing, and reaching, and requires the ability to get along well with others. Good **manual dexterity** (skill working with the hands) and hand-eye coordination are essential. This is one of the 20 fastest growing occupations, with some parts of the country reporting a significant shortage of hygienists.

Dental Assistant

Dental assistants are trained to perform a variety of duties in the dental office. They may work closely with the dentist by preparing patients for treatment, passing instruments, and suctioning the mouth during procedures performed by the dentist. Laboratory duties may include sterilizing and preparing instruments, creating casts of the teeth, and making temporary crowns. Administrative dental assistants greet patients, schedule appointments, keep patient records, send bills, and perform other clerical duties as needed. Dental assistants must have good manual dexterity, the ability and willingness to follow directions, and good interpersonal skills. This occupation is experiencing rapid growth and good job opportunities.

Dental Laboratory Technician

Dental laboratory technicians make the items used by dentists to replace and restore teeth, such as crowns, bridges, and dentures. These are created using models of the patient's mouth and involve working with plaster, wax, metal, and porcelain. Small hand-held tools, grinding and polishing equipment, and heat sources for melting and baking are used. The work is precise and very delicate. Successful technicians are patient and steady-handed and have good vision, especially the ability to discriminate colors, needed for matching replacements to remaining teeth. Growth in the number of jobs is expected to be lower than average because improved dental care has decreased the need for dentures.

Emergency Medical Occupations

Emergency medical technicians (EMTs) provide quick response service to victims of medical emergencies. All EMTs are qualified to give life support and immediate care such as restoring breathing, controlling bleeding, administering oxygen, bandaging wounds, and treating a person for shock. EMTs transport victims to health care facilities and provide necessary care en route. EMT-intermediates

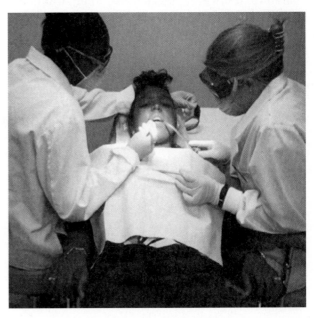

Figure 1–2 Dental assistants prepare instruments and supplies, work closely with the dentist to provide direct patient care, and educate patients about healthy dental habits.

Table 1–2 Emergency Medical Occupations

Career	Education	Testing and Certification
Registered Emergency Medical Technician (EMT) —Paramedic	Completion of EMT basic and intermediate training plus 750 to 2000 additional hours of training	State certification required 1. Complete approved training 2. Pass written and practical exams
Registered EMT— Ambulance/I-Intermediate	EMT-Basic training plus 35 to 55 additional hours of training and internship	State certification required 1. Complete approved training 2. Pass written and practical exams
Basic EMT— Ambulance/A-Basic	110 to 120 hours of classroom training plus 10 hours internship	State certification required 1. Complete approved training 2. Pass written and practical exams

have additional skills that include administering fluids intravenously and using a defibrillator to administer an electrical shock to a person whose heart has stopped. EMT-paramedics are qualified to administer drugs, interpret EKGs (electrocardiograms; measurements of the heart's electrical activity), and perform various invasive procedures (involving puncture or insertion of an instrument or material into the body). EMTs must be emotionally stable, able to deal with stressful situations, physically coordinated, able to move quickly and easily, and able to lift and carry heavy loads. Many EMTs are employed by rescue squads, police departments, and fire departments, and employment is expected to grow rapidly. See Table 1–2.

Medical Office Occupations

Medical offices treat patients who are seeking to maintain or improve their health. They are staffed by a physician, who may be a general practitioner or specialist, and the support staff necessary to assist the physician and perform clinical, laboratory, and administrative duties. See Table 1–3. There are a wide variety of medical specialties as listed in Box 1–1.

Medical Assistant

Medical assistants must be prepared to carry out a wide variety of duties. They may work closely with the physician and perform clinical tasks. Known as "back office assistants," their duties include

Table 1–3 Medical Office Occupations

Career	Education	Testing and Certification
Physician (MD)	4 years college premedical preparation 4 years medical school 1 year internship Residency, length varies	Licensed by states 1. Graduate from accredited medical school 2. Complete internship and residency 3. Pass written examination
Physician's Assistant (PA)	Varies. 2–4 years college + 2-year PA program	Requirements vary by state. Most require passing the exam administered by the National Commission on Certification of Physician's Assistants

(continues)

Table 1–3 (continued)

Career	Education	Testing and Approval
Medical Assistant Administrative and/or Clinical (MA, CMA, RMA) CMA = Certified Medical Assistant RMA = Registered Medical Assistant	Certificate program, usually 8 or 9 months OR associate's degree	Specific tasks, such as giving injections, regulated by some states Optional certification through exam administered by American Association of Medical Assistants Optional registration through exam administered by American Medical Technologists

preparing patients, taking vital signs, helping the physician with exams and procedures, and performing a variety of tests and procedures on patients. Medical assistants may also choose to concentrate on "front office tasks," which include receiving patients, answering the telephone, maintaining patient records, and handling insurance and billing duties. In small offices, the medical assistant may have both front and back office assignments. Medical assistants must be able to follow directions, work accurately, get along well with others, and have good manual dexterity. The occupation is expected to be one of the ten fastest growing through the year 2006.

BOX 1–1 Medical Specialties

Anesthesiologist	Administration of medication to cause loss of sensation or feeling during surgery	Internist	Diseases of the internal organs (lungs, heart, glands, intestines, kidneys)
Cardiologist	Diseases of the heart and blood vessels	Neurologist	Disorders of the brain and nervous system
Dermatologist	Diseases of the skin	Obstetrician	Pregnancy and childbirth
Emergency Physician	Acute illness or injury	Oncologist	Diagnosis and treatment of tumors (cancer)
Endocrinologist	Diseases of the endocrine glands	Ophthalmologist	Diseases and disorders of the eye
Family Physician/ Practice	Promote wellness, treat illness or injury in all age groups	Orthopedist	Diseases and disorders of muscles and bones
Gastroenterologist	Diseases of the stomach and intestines	Otolaryngologist	Diseases of the ear, nose, and throat
Gerontologist	Diseases of elderly individuals	Pathologist	Diagnose disease by studying changes in organs, tissues, and cells
Gynecologist	Diseases of the female reproductive organs	Pediatrician	Diseases and disorders of children

(continues)

BOX 1-1 (continued)

Physiatrist	Physical medicine and rehabilitation	Sports Medicine	Prevention and treatment of injuries sustained in athletic events
Plastic Surgeon	Corrective surgery to repair injured or malformed body parts	Surgeon	Surgery to correct deformities or treat injuries or disease
Proctologist	Diseases of the lower part of the large intestine	Thoracic Surgeon	Surgery of the lungs, heart, or chest cavity
Psychiatrist	Diseases and disorders of the mind	Urologist	Diseases of the kidney, bladder, or urinary system
Radiologist	Use of x-rays and radiation to diagnose and treat disease		

(Source: Simmers, L. (2001). Diversified health occupations (5th ed.). Albany, NY: Delmar.)

Mental Health Occupations

Mental health workers provide care, treatment, counseling, and activities for patients with mental, emotional and/or psychosocial (combination of mental and social) problems. There are a wide variety of settings that provide services for these patients, including medical offices dedicated to the practice of psychiatry, psychiatric hospitals, halfway houses, hospitals and clinics dedicated to treating substance abuse problems, group homes, and prisons. Diagnoses encountered range from mild anxiety disorders, in which patients experience temporary feelings of distress, to serious conditions that result in behaviors that are unsafe for both the patient and the public. See Table 1–4.

Table 1–4 Mental Health Occupations

Career	Education	Testing and Certification
Psychiatrist (MD)	4 years college premedical preparation 4 years medical school 1 year internship Residency, length varies	Licensed by states 1. Graduate from accredited medical school 2. Complete specialized studies, internship, and residency 3. Pass written exam
Clinical Psychologist (Ph.D.)	4 years college 2–3 years graduate school (master's degree) 2–4 years (doctorate)	Licensed by states 1. Pass written exam
Psychiatric Clinical Nurse Specialist	Licensure as a RN 2–3 years graduate school (master's degree)	

(continues)

Table 1–4 (continued)

Career	Education	Testing and Certification
Mental Health Technician	Certificate or associate's degree in human services or mental health	Licensed by some states Certification from National Commission for Human Service Workers
Psychiatric Aide	Some states require formal training program	

Mental Health Technician

Mental health technicians work with patients under the direction of a psychiatrist, psychologist, or registered nurse. They carry out care plans, assist with group activities, listen to patients and provide encouragement, and note behavior. The work requires a strong desire to help others, patience, understanding, excellent oral communication skills, and emotional stability. Employment growth is expected to be average.

Psychiatric Aide

Psychiatric aides assist other health care workers and provide help with the physical needs of patients, such as hygiene and feeding. They provide companionship for patients and may help with escorting patients within or outside the care facility. Aides must be patient, caring, and responsible. Average growth in job opportunities is expected for this occupation.

Nursing Occupations

Nurses promote health and provide care and treatment for patients with all types of health problems. Nursing care is carried out through the application of a structured process to determine each patient's needs, develop individual care plans, implement the plans, and then evaluate their effectiveness. An important responsibility of the nurse is to provide education to patients and their families regarding self-care and health maintenance. See Table 1–5.

Registered Nurse

Registered nurses provide a wide variety of patient care services. They provide direct patient care or supervise other personnel who do so, serve as patient advocates (support the interests of patients), and provide patient education. They frequently are the professionals who coordinate the overall care of patients by interacting with all other health care workers involved. Registered nurses may achieve many educational levels and pursue a great number of specialties. Responsibilities range from direct patient care to management of a hospital department. Specific day-to-day activities are determined by the work setting, which may be a hospital, clinic, long-term care facility, school, prison, or patients' homes. Registered nurses must be caring and responsible, have excellent assessment and communication skills, and be emotionally stable and able to both follow orders and supervise others. Registered nursing is one of the most versatile careers in any field. It is one of the five occupations projected to have the largest number of new jobs.

Licensed Practical/Vocational Nurse

Licensed practical nurses (known as licensed vocational nurses in California and Texas) provide basic patient care under the direction of physicians and registered nurses. Most practical nurses carry out bedside tasks that include taking vital signs, administering medications, applying dressings and hot and cold packs, treating bedsores, and giving various comfort measures. They are also responsible for recording patient information. Practical nurses must be caring, responsible, emotionally stable, and able to follow directions and work under close supervision. Job opportunities vary by region. Most new jobs are in extended-care facilities.

Nursing Assistant/Aide

Nursing assistants and aides work under the supervision of nursing staff to help care for patients' basic needs. They may take vital signs, assist patients with hygiene and feeding, give comfort measures, change bedding, and help transport patients. The variety

Table 1–5 Nursing Occupations

Career	Education	Testing and Certification
Nurse Practitioner (CRNP)	Be a registered nurse Complete additional educational and clinical practice requirements. Most are master's degree programs.	Licensed by states National certification exam
Registered Nurse (RN)	2-year (associate) OR 4-year (bachelor) college degree	Licensed by states 1. Graduate from approved program 2. National Council Licensing Examination for Nurses (N-CLEX)
Licensed Practical or Licensed Vocational Nurse (LPN/LVN)	1–2 year state-approved certificate or diploma program.	Licensed by states 1. Graduate from approved program 2. Pass state licensing exam
Nursing Assistant, Aide (CNA)	States have various training requirements for classroom and clinical experience. Programs must meet specific federal minimum standards.	All states require certification for work in long-term care facilities. Requirements are guided by federal regulations established by the Omnibus Budget Reconciliation Act of 1987 (OBRA). Certification requirements vary for other work environments.
Home Health Aide	States have various training requirements for classroom and clinical experience.	Approval requirements vary by state under the guidance of OBRA.

and level of duties depend on state laws, the amount of training, and the needs of the facility. Assistants and aides must be patient, caring, dependable, and able to follow directions. This is a fast-growing occupation, especially for individuals who are also qualified to work as home health aides.

Occupational Therapy Occupations

The purpose of occupational therapy is to help individuals attain the highest level of self-sufficiency possible. Difficulties in performing the activities of daily living can be the result of physical, mental, or emotional problems caused by disease, injury, or congenital (present at birth) conditions. Occupational therapists evaluate patients, set goals to increase their function and lessen their limitations, and create treat-

ment plans to achieve these goals. Treatment may involve individual or group activities, exercise, providing adaptive equipment such as splints and special tools, and teaching patients new ways to perform daily tasks. See Table 1–6.

Occupational Therapy Assistant

Occupational therapy assistants work under the supervision of occupational therapists. They carry out rehabilitative activities and exercises prescribed by treatment plans. Other important duties include patient education, monitoring patient progress, and preparing reports for the therapist. Typical tasks include teaching a patient to use special devices that enable the performance of everyday tasks such as reaching, dressing, and

Table 1–6 Occupational Therapy Occupations

Career	Education	Testing and Licensure
Occupational Therapist (OTR)	4-year college degree	Licensed in 48 states National registration: 1. Graduate from program accredited by the American Occupational Therapy Association (AOTA) 2. Pass national exam administered by the National Board of Certification for Occupational Therapy (NBCOT)
Occupational Therapy Assistant (COTA)	2-year college degree	Licensure or certification required in most states. National certification: 1. Graduate from a program accredited by the AOTA 2. Pass national exam administered by NBCOT
Occupational Therapy Aide	Certificate program or on-the-job training	None

cooking; assisting with a stretching exercise; or making a hand splint. Occupational therapy assistants must have good communication skills, be patient and caring, and be sensitive to the needs of people who suffer from a variety of disabilities. The number of new positions is not expected to grow rapidly.

Occupational Therapy Aide

Aides help therapists and assistants by perfoming supportive duties such as preparing supplies for activities, assisting with patient transfers, helping with patient treatment and activities, and cleaning activity areas. Some aides are cross-trained to assist other rehabilitation professionals such as physical therapists. Rehabilitation skills may be combined with nursing assistance training and certification. Aides must be responsible and able to follow directions. For workers who are also certified nursing assistants, the number of positions is expected to grow rapidly.

Pharmacy Occupations

Pharmacy workers prepare and dispense medications to promote patient wellness and recovery. Important duties also include educating patients about the proper use of medications and ensuring that patients are not given drugs that will cause harm because of allergic reactions or negative interactions with other drugs. See Table 1–7.

Pharmacy Technician

Pharmacy technicians work under the supervision of a licensed pharmacist. They fill orders for drugs, stock medication carts, record and store incoming drug supplies, and reorder inventory as needed. They also assist in maintaining paperwork and records required for controlled drugs. Pharmacy technicians must be responsible, detail-oriented, and able to follow directions exactly. The number of positions in the field is expected to grow at an average rate.

Table 1–7 Pharmacy Occupations

Career	Education	Testing and Licensure
Pharmacist (R.Ph.)	5-year bachelor's degree OR 6-year Doctor of Pharmacy (Pharm.D.) degree	Licensed by states: 1. Graduate from a college of pharmacy accredited by the American Council on Pharmaceutical Education 2. Pass a state examination 3. Serve an internship
Pharmacy Technician	Up to one year on-the-job-training OR 1–2 year college certificate program OR associate's degree	A few states require licensure, certification, or registration. Voluntary national certification available through examination administered by the Pharmacy Technician Certification Board.
Pharmacy Aide/Helper/ Clerk	On-the-job-training OR vocational training program	None

Physical Therapy Occupations

The purpose of physical therapy is to help patients improve their physical functions by increasing muscle strength, range of motion and movement, and decreasing pain. This is accomplished through assessment and the creation and implementation of treatment programs that may include exercise, massage, and the use of modalities such as heat, cold, and electrical stimulation. Patients are taught to perform exercises and use equipment such as canes and crutches. See Table 1–8.

Physical Therapist Assistant

Assistants work with patients under the supervision of a physical therapist to carry out treatment plans. They teach and supervise exercises, apply - modalities, perform massages, assist patients with ambulatory devices such as walkers and braces, and document progress. Physical therapy assistants must be patient and encouraging and have the physical strength to assist patients with exercises. This occupation is projected to be one of the fastest growing in all industries.

Physical Therapist Aide

Aides support the work of therapists and assistants by preparing and cleaning equipment and therapy areas, assisting with treatments, transporting patients, and ordering and maintaining supplies. Aides must be responsible and able to follow directions.

Respiratory Therapy Occupations

Respiratory therapy involves evaluating, treating, and caring for patients with breathing disorders. Those in respiratory therapy assist patients who cannot breathe on their own because of conditions such as heart disease, acute diseases (lasting a short period of time but relatively severe) such as pneumonia, or chronic diseases (lasting a long period of time) such as emphysema. See Table 1–9 and Figure 1–3.

Respiratory Therapist

Respiratory therapists perform a variety of tasks to assist patients with breathing. These include using special instruments to measure lung capacity and drawing blood samples to test for levels of oxygen and other components. Therapists provide patients with oxygen and connect those who cannot breathe on their own to ventilators. The monitoring and maintenance of equipment are important duties. Therapists also administer aerosol medications and perform chest physiotherapy, which involves thumping and vibrating the patient's chest cavity to remove mucus from the lungs. Respiratory therapists must have good technical aptitude and be attentive to detail and able to work under stress. Jobs are expected to grow somewhat faster than average.

Table 1–8 Physical Therapy Occupations

Career	Education	Testing and Licensure
Physical Therapist (PT)	Master's degree (starting in 2002)	Licensed by states 1. Graduate from program accredited by the Commission on Accreditation in Physical Therapy Education (APTE) 2. Pass exam administered by national certification board
Physical Therapist Assistant (PTA)	Associate's degree	Licensed by most states: 1. Graduate from program accredited by the Commission on Accreditation in Physical Therapy Education (APTE) 2. Pass exam administered by national certification board
Physical Therapist Aide	On-the-job-training OR vocational training program	None

Table 1–9 Respiratory Therapy Occupations

Career	Education	Testing and Licensure
Respiratory Therapist (RRT)	Associate's degree	Licensed in most states 1. Graduate from a program accredited by the Commission on Accreditation of Allied Health Education Programs (CAAHEP) 2. Pass exam administered by the National Board for Respiratory Care
Respiratory Therapy Technician	1–2 year certificate or diploma program	Licensed in most states 1. Graduate from a program accredited by the Commission on Accreditation of Allied Health Education Programs (CAAHEP) 2. Pass exam administered by the National Board for Respiratory Care
Respiratory Aide	No formal training	None

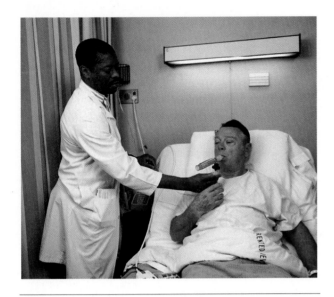

Figure 1–3 Respiratory therapists administer medications and treatments to patients with heart and lung disorders.

Respiratory Therapy Technician

Technicians perform many of the tasks performed by therapists under the direction of the therapist.

They may also carry out supportive duties such as cleaning equipment, stocking supplies, and performing clerical tasks. The personal requirements and job projections are the same as for therapists.

Surgical Occupations

Surgical procedures vary from minor to extremely complex and from emergency to elective. The types of surgery available, and their complexity, are growing at a fast rate. Many people are alive today as a result of modern surgery. Surgical occupations involve the care of the patient before, during, and after surgery. See Table 1–10 and Figure 1–4.

Surgical Technician/Operating Room Technician/Surgical Technologist

The health care workers who are trained to perform important functions in the operating room may work under a variety of job titles. Duties include sterilizing and setting up instruments, preparing equipment and linens in the operating room, and preparing patients for surgery and transporting them to the operating room. During surgery, technicians may perform a variety of tasks: pass instruments to the surgeon, hold retractors (instruments that open or draw back tissue,

Table 1–10 Surgical Occupations

Career	Education	Testing and Licensure
Surgeon (MD or DO)	4 years college premedical preparation 4 years medical school 1 year internship Residency, length varies	Licensed by states 1. Graduate from accredited medical school 2. Complete specialized studies, internship, and residency 3. Pass written exam
Surgeon's Assistant (SA)	Varies. 2–4 years college + 2-year PA program + 2-year surgical assistant associate's degree program	Requirements vary by state. Most require passing the exam administered by the National Commission on Certification of Physician's Assistants.
Certified Surgical Technician (CST), Operating Room Technician (ORT), Surgical Technologist	9-month to 2-year program leading to certificate or associate's degree Clinical experience	Optional certification by passing exam administered by Liaison Council on Certification affiliated with the Association of Surgical Technologists, Inc.

bone, etc.), cut sutures, operate lights and equipment, and assist with the preparation of specimens. Work in surgery requires excellent manual dexterity, attention to detail, the stamina to stand for long hours, and the ability to respond quickly. It is expected that there will be an increased demand for this occupation.

Vision Care Occupations

Vision care workers perform important work in assisting the over 50% of Americans who wear glasses or contact lenses (McCutcheon, 1998). In addition to working to correct vision problems, they identify and treat diseases of the eye, provide education and care to maintain good vision and eye health, and make eyeglasses. See Table 1–11.

Ophthalmic Technician/Assistant

Ophthalmic technicians assist ophthalmologists in their work with patients. They care for equipment, record patient histories, perform eye tests, assist with surgery, and carry out office maintenance duties. Good manual dexterity, observation skills, and attention to detail are important characteristics for success in this occupation. Job growth is expected to be at least average.

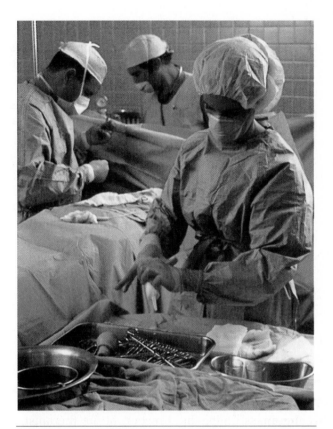

Figure 1–4 Surgical technologists prepare patients for surgery, set up instruments and supplies, and assist during surgery by passing instruments and supplies.

Table 1–11 Vision Care Occupations

Career	Education	Testing and Licensure
Ophthalmologist (MD)	4 years college premedical preparation 4 years medical school 1 year internship Residency, length varies	Licensed by states 1. Graduate from accredited medical school 2. Complete specialized studies, internship, and residency 3. Pass written exam
Optometrist (OD)	3–4 years college 4 years college of optometry 2+ years of residency required to specialize in specific types of optometry	Licensed by states 1. Graduate from accredited optometry school 2. Pass written and clinical state board exams OR exam administered by National Board of Examiners of Optometry (requirement varies by state) (continues)

Table 1-11 (continued)

Career	Education	Testing and Licensure
Optician	On-the-job training OR 2–4 year apprenticeship OR vocational or associate's degree program (apprenticeship means formal on-the-job training with specific conditions and goals)	Licensed or certified in states Certification available through American Board of Opticianry and National Contact Lens Examiners
Ophthalmic Technician	On-the-job training OR associate's degree	Optional Certification: 1. Complete educational program 2. Clinical experience 3. Pass national exam administered by Joint Commission on Allied Health Personnel in Ophthalmology (JCAHPO)
Ophthalmic Laboratory Technician	On-the-job training OR 6–12 month vocational training program	None
Optometric Assistant/ Technician	On-the-job training	None

Ophthalmic Laboratory Technician

Ophthalmic laboratory technicians make eyeglass lenses following prescriptions prepared by ophthalmologists and optometrists. They use special equipment to cut, grind, edge, and finish eyeglass lenses. Lenses must then be checked for accuracy. The job sometimes includes inserting lenses into frames. Technicians must have good manual dexterity, attention to detail, and the ability to follow directions. Job growth is expected to be low because the occupation is small.

Diagnostic Occupations

Those in occupations in this category help determine the causes of diseases and extent of injuries so that proper treatment can be planned. They also monitor patient progress over time to determine if treatment is effective. Occupations may involve working directly with patients to perform tests and collect specimens, operating complex equipment, and carrying out tests in a laboratory setting.

Biometrics Occupations

Biometric workers perform tests that measure the function of the heart, blood vessels, brain, and nerves. The work involves direct patient contact and the use of specialized medical equipment. Electrocardiography (EKG or ECG) records the electrical action of the heart. Technicians attach electrodes to the patient and manipulate switches on a machine that traces the activity on graph paper. Echocardiography (ECHO-C) is use of ultrasound (echoes from sound waves) to form images of the heart and circulatory system. See Table 1–12.

Cardiovascular Technologist

Cardiovascular technologists assist physicians in the diagnosis and treatment of cardiac and vascular problems. In addition to performing the tests described above, they are also qualified to assist with invasive procedures, such as cardiac catheterization, which is the insertion of a small tube though the blood vessels to the heart. Technologists prepare patients for procedures and monitor them throughout. They must work accurately, handle stress well, and have high technical aptitude. Employment growth is expected to be average, but the number of positions is not high because the occupation is small.

Table 1–12 Biometrics Occupations

Career	Education	Testing and Licensure
Cardiologist (MD)	4 years college premedical preparation 4 years medical school 1 year internship Residency, length varies	Licensed by states 1. Graduate from accredited medical school 2. Complete specialized studies, internship, and residency 3. Pass written exam
Cardiovascular Technologist	Associate's OR bachelor's degree	Voluntary registration available with the American Registry of Diagnostic Medical Sonographers (ARDMS) 1. Graduate from an approved program 2. Pass written exam OR Cardiovascular Credential International
Echocardiographic Technician	On-the-job training OR vocational training program OR associate's degree	Voluntary registration available with ARDMS
Electrocardiograph (EKG) Technician	On-the-job training OR 6–12 month vocational education program	Voluntary certification available from National Board of Cardiovascular Testing

Echocardiograph Technician

Echocardiograph technicians use medical sonography equipment to view the structures of the heart. (See Chapter 18 for more information.) In addition to good technical aptitude, technicians must have good communication skills to explain procedures to patients and put them at ease.

Electrocardiograph Technician

EKG technicians perform electrocardiographs. This skill is often included in the training of other patient care occupations, such as medical assisting. The number of jobs for EKG technicians who are not trained to perform other tasks, in addition to this specialty, is expected to grow at a slower-than-average rate.

Medical Laboratory Occupations

Work in medical laboratory occupations involves the collection and study of specimens from the human body. These include blood, tissue, and cells.

Many kinds of tests are performed to detect the presence of disease and determine its cause. These require the use of equipment and various chemicals. See Table 1–13 and Figure 1–5.

Medical Laboratory Technician

Laboratory technicians perform routine tests, which may require preparing slides, counting cells, and using sophisticated equipment. The work may involve the care and cleaning of the equipment, maintaining supplies, and keeping records. Laboratory technicians must have good manual dexterity, great attention to detail and accuracy, and good observation skills. Employment projection is expected to be average, with increasing competition for available jobs.

Medical Laboratory Assistant

Laboratory assistants perform routine tests and tasks that are less complex than those for which the technician is qualified. The necessary qualities and job outlook are similar to those of the technician.

Table 1–13 Medical Laboratory Occupations

Career	Education	Testing and Licensure
Pathologist (MD)	4 years college premedical preparation 4 years medical school 1 year internship Residency, length varies	Licensed by states 1. Graduate from accredited medical school 2. Complete specialized studies, internship, and residency 3. Pass written exam
Medical Laboratory Technologist (MT)	Bachelor's or master's degree	Licensed or registered in some states. Certification available from: 1. American Medical Technologists 2. American Society for Clinical Laboratory Science 3. Credentialing Commission of the International Society for Clinical Laboratory Technology
Laboratory Technician	Completion of certificate program OR associate's degree	Licensing or registration required in some states Certification available from: 1. American Medical Technologists 2. American Society for Clinical Laboratory Science
Laboratory Assistant	1 to 2 year training program	Voluntary certification from Board of Certified Laboratory Assistants
Phlebotomist	On-the-job training OR formal training program	Voluntary certification through American Phlebotomy Society

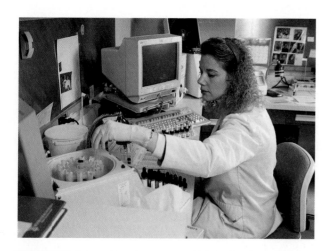

Figure 1–5 Medical laboratory workers perform manual and computerized tests to detect the presence of disease.

Radiology Occupations

Radiology allows the viewing of structures and functions inside the body. Diseases and injuries can be diagnosed without carrying out invasive procedures. Equipment is used that employs x-rays, sound waves, magnetic fields, and radioactive substances. (See Chapter 18 for more information.) The ongoing development of noninvasive diagnostic methods has resulted in new specialties and occupational areas, such as magnetic resonance imager (MRI) technologist. See Table 1–14.

Radiographer/Radiologic Technologist

Radiographers perform x-ray procedures. They explain procedures to patients, position them properly, provide shielding against excessive exposure to x-rays, operate equipment, and develop film.

Table 1–14 Radiology Occupations

Career	Education	Testing and Licensure
Radiologist (MD or OD)	4 years college premedical preparation 4 years medical school 1 year internship Residency, length varies	Licensed by states 1. Graduate from accredited medical school 2. Complete specialized studies, internship, and residency 3. Pass written exam
Radiographer/Radiologic Technologist (RT)	Associate's or bachelor's degree	Licensed in most states Voluntary registration from the American Registry of Radiologic Technologists (ARRT): 1. Graduate from accredited program OR meet other specified requirements 2. Pass certification exam
Diagnostic Medical Sonographer	Certificate program or associate's degree	Voluntary certification available from American Registry of Diagnostic Medical Sonographers (ARDMS): 1. Graduate from accredited program OR meet other requirements 2. Pass national exam
Radiologic Technician	Certificate program	Certification and title of position vary by state. Some require specific education from an accredited program and passing an exam.
Computed Tomography Technologist	2 years college and on-the-job training OR training from manufacturer	Same as radiographer
Magnetic Resonance Imager Technologist	2 years college and on-the-job training OR training from manufacturer	Same as radiographer
Positron Emission Tomograph Technologist	2 years college and on-the-job training OR training from manufacturer	Same as radiographer

This work requires great attention to safety factors, a high degree of technical aptitude, the ability to communicate well with patients, the stamina to stand for long periods of time, and the ability to work under emergency conditions. Average to above average growth is expected. Radiographers who learn a variety of specialties, such as skull x-rays and mammography, will have the best chances for employment.

Diagnostic Medical Sonographer

Sonographers operate equipment that uses sound waves (ultrasound) to produce images of soft tissue.

The technology allows the movement of internal structures to be viewed on a screen as well as the creation of images on film. Sonographers can specialize in cardiac, vascular, or abdominal areas. A common use of ultrasound, because of its safety, is to observe the developing fetus. Sonographers must have good math and technical aptitude, the ability to communicate with patients, and accurate work habits. Employment growth is expected to range from average to above average.

Radiologic Technician

Radiologic technicians are licensed personnel whose duties are similar to those of a radiologic technologist but are more limited in scope. This position does not exist in all states and may have another title such as "radiographic assistant."

Health Information Management Occupations

Occupations in this category gather, analyze, organize, store, and document patient information. Medical information careers are among the fastest-growing occupations in health care. Consistent patient care, as well as regulatory compliance, depend on complete and accurate records. The increasing emphasis on monitoring the cost of health care delivery and the outcomes of patients who undergo treatment has increased the need for high-quality medical recordkeeping. See Table 1–15.

Table 1–15 Health Information Management Occupations

Career	Education	Testing and Licensure
Registered Health Information Administrator (RHIA) (formerly Registered Record Administrator)	Bachelor's degree in health information administration OR bachelor's degree AND certificate in HIA	Voluntary registration available from American Health Information Management Association (AHIMA): 1. Complete an approved educational program 2. Pass a national exam administered by AHIMA
Registered Health Information Technician (RHIT) (formerly Medical Records Technician)	Associate's degree in health information technology	Voluntary registration available from American Health Information Management Association (AHIMA): 1. Complete an educational program accredited by AHIMA 2. Pass a national exam administered by AHIMA
Medical Transcriptionist (MT)	Certificate program or associate's degree	Voluntary certification available from American Association for Medical Transcription: 1. Pass written exam 2. Pass practical exam
Coding Specialist (CCS)	On-the-job training OR coding seminars OR college program	Voluntary certification (Certified Coding Specialist—CCS) available from AHIMA: 1. High-school diploma 2. Written exam
Medical Records Clerk	On-the-job training	None

Registered Health Information Technician

Health information technicians perform a variety of tasks related to the collection and organization of patient data. They organize patient records, perform coding (the assignment of predetermined numbers that designate specific diagnoses and procedures), enter data from paper records into computerized recordkeeping systems, and compile data for reports. Good organizational skills, a high degree of accuracy with details, and good computer aptitude are necessary for success in this field. This is one of the fastest growing occupations in numbers of anticipated openings.

Medical Transcriptionist

Transcriptionists type medical reports from data dictated by physicians. A variety of reports are used in health care to describe all types of findings and procedures. They include topics that range from descriptions of surgeries to autopsies (examination of organs and tissues performed after death to determine cause of death). Transcriptionists must sit and concentrate for long periods of time, be able to hear and interpret spoken language that includes medical terms, have excellent grammar and spelling skills, and produce perfectly accurate work.

Coding Specialist

Medical coders specialize in classifying medical data from patient records. Codes are assigned from the two major coding systems, the ICD-9-CM (diagnoses) and CPT (procedures). A high level of accuracy and attention to detail is necessary for success as a coder. Job growth is expected to be high.

Environmental Occupations

Those in occupations in this category develop and maintain therapeutic environments necessary to support patient care. Responsibilities include the provision of food services, cleaning and maintenance of facilities and equipment, resource management, and the creation of pleasant surroundings.

Dietary Service Occupations

Dietary service workers support patients by planning and providing nutritious foods that are essential to the healing process. Therapeutic diets are sometimes prescribed by physicians for patients with specific health problems and conditions such as high blood pressure and diabetes, and following abdominal surgery. See Table 1–16.

Table 1–16 Dietary Service Occupations

Career	Education	Testing and Licensure
Dietitian (RD)	Bachelor's degree in dietetics, foods and nutrition, food service systems management, or a related area	Licensure, certification, or registration required in most states. Registration available from the American Dietetic Association: 1. Complete academic program 2. Complete supervised experience 3. Pass certification exam
Dietetic Technician (DTR)	Associate's degree	Voluntary registration available from the Commission on Dietetic Registration
Dietetic Assistant	Certificate program in food services or on-the-job training	None

Dietetic Technician

Dietetic technicians work under the supervision of dietitians and perform tasks related to all aspects of food planning and preparation. They assist with creating menus, testing recipes, ordering food and supplies, and preparing meals. Some technicians work with patients to learn their food preferences and design special diets as ordered by a physician. Dietetic technicians must have good communication skills and be attentive to detail and able to follow specific directions. The projected employment rate is expected to be average.

Biomedical Engineering

The application of engineering has resulted in the creation of sophisticated medical equipment that helps in diagnosing, treating, and monitoring patient conditions. Life-enhancing and life-saving inventions resulting from biomedical engineering include the heart-lung machine, cardiac pacemakers, surgical lasers, and ultrasound technology. All engineering specialties, including electrical, mechanical, computer, and chemical, have been applied to seeking improvements in health care. See Table 1–17.

Biomedical Equipment Technician

These specially trained technicians work on medical equipment that requires continual and competent maintenance in order to provide accurate diagnoses and reliable service to treat and monitor patients. Duties of the technician include the installation, testing, servicing, and repair of all types of equipment. Technicians may specialize in one area such as radiology or clinical laboratory equipment. Work in this area requires excellent manual dexterity, hand-eye coordination, mechanical aptitude, and interest in technology. Projected employment is expected to be above average.

Table 1–17 Biomedical Engineering Occupations

Career	Education	Testing and Licensure
Biomedical Engineer	Bachelor's degree or higher in biomedical or other engineering specialty	Licensed for some employment positions. Certification available from the International Certification Commission for Clinical Engineering and Biomedical Technology (ICC) 1. Complete a degree in engineering 2. Have at least 3 years experience as a hospital clinical engineer 3. Pass both written and oral exams
Biomedical Equipment Technician Four levels ranging from I to IV that require increasing levels of education and amounts of experience	Associate's degree	Voluntary certification available by the ICC: 1. Associate's degree in biomedical engineering or specific combinations of training and experience 2. Pass written exam (Various advanced certifications are available for different levels and types of experience.)

STANDARDS FOR HEALTH CARE WORKERS

Standards for health care workers have been established to protect the public from potential harm caused by incompetence. Testing, along with various approval and monitoring mechanisms, has been developed to determine whether workers have met specific standards. The purpose of standards is to ensure that workers master at least the minimum knowledge and skills necessary to safely and competently practice their professions.

Standards may be set by state boards or national professional organizations. There are several terms that designate various types of approvals. **Certification** is a general term that means the process of determining whether a person has met predetermined standards. This usually involves meeting certain educational requirements and passing a professional examination. Most health care professionals go through a certification process, although their title may not include the term "certified." Examples of occupations that do include the term in their title are certified occupational therapy assistant, certified medical assistant, and certified nursing assistant.

Some occupations require **registration,** which means being placed on an official list (registry) after meeting the educational and testing requirements for the profession. Professions in this category include registered nurse, registered respiratory therapist, and registered medical assistant.

Licensure is a designation that means the person has been granted permission to legally perform certain acts. Licenses are granted by government agencies, often the state. The specific occupations that require licensure vary from state to state. Some occupations are licensed in most, but not all states. The word "licensed" does not usually appear with the title of licensed professions. For example, in the following list of licensed professions, only one includes the term: dentist, dental hygienist, physician, registered nurse, and licensed practical/vocational nurse.

The various types of approvals can be confusing. Certification and registration are often, but not always, required to work legally. Even when not required by law, they provide credibility and are preferred by many employers when hiring. Medical assisting is an example of an occupation in which voluntary certification or registration enhances the graduate's chances of being hired. Licensure, if required for a profession, is *never* voluntary.

Some professions have more than one form of approval. Medical assistants, for example, can be either certified or registered. Both approvals require meeting specific educational requirements and passing a national exam. The American Association of Medical Assistants grants the title "certified." The American Medical Technologists grant the title "registered."

Another point of confusion is that some professions are licensed but use the title "registered." Nurses take a national exam that, when passed, entitles them to apply for a license in the state where they want to work. They can become licensed in any state as long as they follow the proper application process. In addition, they are listed in a registry. While "registered nurse" is the title for the occupation, it is also a licensed profession.

Study the contents of Tables 1–5 and 1–6. Note the variety of titles and educational levels within the two occupational areas nursing and occupational therapy. As you can see, professional titles and the types of approval granted do not necessarily indicate the level of education achieved. For example, the educational requirements for a *certified* nursing assistant can be less than 200 hours of instruction; a *certified* occupational therapy assistant, however, must earn an associate's degree. The titles given refer to the specific methods chosen by various organizations to ensure that their standards are met, rather than to the educational requirements. Furthermore, some titles may be acquired with varying amounts of education. Using the example of the registered nurse once again, we see that qualifying education can be either an associate's or bachelor's degree.

It is essential that students understand what is necessary for them to work in their chosen occupation. Most examining and licensing boards require attendance at an accredited school and/or program. This means that the school/program meets the standards set by a national professional organization. Accreditation requires a school or program to formally apply for approval. Once the application is accepted, a team from the national organization visits the campus to ensure that all standards are being met. In addition to attending an accredited program, students must meet the following requirements before most professional exams can be taken:

1. High-school diploma or the equivalent
2. Completion of specific courses
3. Successful completion of the clinical portion of the training
4. Not having been convicted of certain crimes

Once obtained, most certifications require specific amounts of continuing education. This is discussed further in Chapter 14. Individuals who fail to maintain the competency and conduct standards for their profession can lose their approval. The purpose of health care regulation is not to provide one-time approval. It is an ongoing effort to ensure that only qualified professionals are serving the public.

GETTING OFF TO A GOOD START

Health care educational programs are designed to prepare students to succeed in the workplace. Instructors dedicate themselves to ensuring that students who put forth the necessary effort will graduate and become employed. Take advantage of the learning opportunities available in your school and commit yourself to doing your best toward becoming a competent, qualified health care worker.

Learning to Think Like a Health Care Worker

A common problem in health care today is that graduates spend months, or even years, accumulating information, but are unable to apply it when it's needed on the job. The lack of effective thinking skills is a primary reason for this unfortunate situation. Regardless of the health care area or occupational level chosen by students, it is essential that they learn to think like health care workers. This type of thinking actually involves many skills and, in this text, has the following meanings:

- Learning for understanding, not simply to accumulate facts

- Applying learned material to new situations

- Having an organized approach to problem-solving

- Basing decisions on facts, rather than on emotional reactions or **biases** (opinions made before facts are known)

- Drawing on many facts and creating relationships between them

- Locating reliable sources of information with which to make decisions

- Basing decisions on ethical principles (Chapter 3)

- Practicing good communication skills when gathering and distributing information (Chapters 16 and 17)

- Understanding exactly what one is legally allowed to do in one's profession, known as **scope of practice**

One of the major goals of this text is to provide students with opportunities to practice thinking like a health care worker. The concept is being introduced at the beginning of the text so that students will have maximum time to apply and practice thinking skills. The "Thinking It Through" and "Application Exercises," which appear in every chapter, encourage students to apply thinking skills to the topics presented.

Thinking proficiently is much more than an academic skill. While it is true that it is achieved through training and practice, its use is not restricted to school and certainly not to textbook exercises. It should be applied to the personal, as well as professional, areas of life. For example, buying a puppy simply because it is cute and seems the most friendly is an emotional decision. An informed, *thinking* decision would involve some research to learn about available breeds, physical and personality characteristics, common health problems, and methods of training. Knowing these facts would help ensure that the puppy selected best fits the new owner's lifestyle and will be a suitable companion. Knowing ahead of time helps prevent future regrets.

Thinking like a health care worker can be described as an "examined process." This means not accepting situations without observing and thinking about the meaning of what is observed. Effective thinkers are *aware* of their thoughts and of why and how they are acting and/or making decisions.

As stated earlier, nothing in health care work can be done routinely and without thinking. Mindless actions occur as the result of not paying attention or basing decisions on ideas that have been accepted "just because." These ideas may come from family members, friends, personal experiences, television, movies, and magazines. Health care workers must learn to think for themselves, gather facts, and use their own observations for making decisions. See Figure 1–6.

Using Questions in Thinking

An effective way to start improving thinking skills is for students to ask themselves questions about what they are learning and/or doing. Questions serve to gather information, expand one's view of a subject, and stimulate the mind. They help ensure that actions are not based on false assumptions or insufficient information.

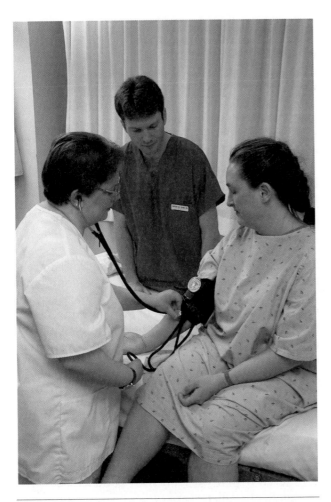

Figure 1–6 Observing carefully, asking questions, and thinking about what you are doing are essential in health care work.

Questions may be asked mentally (to oneself) or of others. Think of the five Ws plus the one H: What, When, Where, Why, Who, and How. The following examples demonstrate the use of questions to promote thinking:

- When learning new information, ask *why* it is true and *how* it relates to what is already known
- When working with patients, ask *what* might work best for them and *when* it should be done
- When sharing important information with a coworker, ask yourself *what* you know about this person that will help you communicate most effectively
- When working in a health care facility, consider *how* your work habits might be changed to improve overall efficiency

Students commonly believe that the role of their instructors is to *tell* them rather than *ask* them. In reality, instructors who continually ask questions that require students to explain their answers and actions are encouraging them to think like health care workers. Some instructors even respond to a student's question with another question. Their intention is to teach students to begin to think for themselves and trust that they are capable of finding the answer. Instructors also use questioning to guide students in pulling known facts together, making connections, and applying what they know to new situations. For example, a respiratory therapy student is working with a hospitalized patient. She has studied the illness presented by the patient and knows how to perform the prescribed breathing treatments. Through questioning, the instructor guides the student to explain why these particular treatments have been prescribed. The student is encouraged to consider the nature of the illness and the properties of the treatments and medications, and draw conclusions about the relationship of one to the other.

Problem-Solving Process

Important applications of thinking skills are problem-solving and decision-making, which are necessary for competency as a health care worker. There are a variety of problem-solving and decision-making models. This book presents a five-step **problem-solving process** to help students approach problem-solving in an organized manner.

Step One—Identify the Problem

Identifying problems is not always as simple as it sounds. Factors that are described as *the problem* are often only *symptoms* of the problem. For example, Jamie, a radiologic technician, does not receive the high scores she had hoped for on her performance review at work. When she receives the rating "poor" in the dependability category, she feels upset and believes that her problem is "receiving a poor evaluation." She believes that her supervisor dislikes her.

Identifying the real nature of problems requires a willingness to observe, pay attention, and confront difficult issues. Problem-solvers must look beyond what seems obvious and use questions effectively to identify the real situation. Denying problems does not make them go away. Problems that are not addressed tend to get worse, because no action is being taken to resolve them. In Jamie's case, she must be willing to speak frankly with her supervisor about her low rating. It turns out that the real problem is actually what *caused* the poor evaluation, not the evaluation itself. In Jamie's case, it is her frequent tardiness.

Thinking it Through

Linda Stevens, LPN, works on a medical floor at the local hospital. One of the patients she has been assigned to take care of is Frank Gibbons, a 72-year-old newly diagnosed diabetic (condition in which body does not produce enough insulin to control blood sugar levels). Part of Linda's process of preparing to care for her patients is to review the patient's chart for any new physician orders. She notes that Dr. Romeros was in the previous evening and ordered the patient's blood sugar to be checked at 8 a.m. According to the results, insulin is to be given. (The higher the level of blood sugar, the greater the amount of insulin that is given, based on a formula defined by the physician.) Linda is a "thinking nurse" and starts to question if this is an appropriate order. She reasons that breakfast trays arrive at 7:30 a.m. on her floor and that Mr. Gibbons will already have eaten when she checks his insulin level at 8 a.m. She knows that after eating, a person's blood sugar normally increases for a few hours. This is why blood sugar tests are usually ordered when the patient has not eaten for a number of hours. Linda reasons that if she calculates the amount of insulin based on the temporarily elevated blood sugar levels, Mr. Gibbons will receive too much insulin and may have a negative reaction. Linda calls Dr. Romeros to clarify the order. Dr. Romeros states that he believed the breakfast trays did not arrive until 8:30 a.m. He thanks Linda for catching the error and changes the order.

- What might have happened if Linda had simply performed the blood sugar test exactly as ordered?
- Do you think Linda should have been considered responsible for the error if she had followed the orders exactly?
- Review the five Ws and How question in relation to this situation. Give examples of questions that Linda may have asked herself.

Jamie's first reaction is, "I can't help it. My car is old and breaks down a lot." When her car won't start, she must rely on family and friends to drop her off at work. Their schedules are not the same as Jamie's, so she often arrives late.

Taking the time to think about what she has said, "I can't help it," Jamie realizes that being at work on time *is* her responsibility and *is* under her control. She is finally able to identify the *real problem*: lack of reliable transportation. This enables her to start seeking effective solutions. Accepting responsibility for a problem makes it possible to start doing something about it.

Step Two—Gather Information

Good problem-solving is based on having accurate and reliable information. Acting on assumptions (untested ideas), **opinions** (beliefs not based on certainty), and emotions, is likely to result in poor decisions. In health care, gathering information is also known as **assessment**. There are many methods for gathering information:

- Review what is already known: What knowledge do I have about the problems or situation? About the causes? About possible solutions?
- Collect **objective data**. What can be observed? Measured? Tested? What are the facts? When working with patients, objective data are called **signs**.
- Collect **subjective data**: How do I feel about a situation? What do I want? What do others want? When working with patients, subjective data refer to what is reported by the patient, such as pain and feeling nauseated. Also known as **symptoms**, they cannot be directly observed or measured by the health care worker.
- Conduct research: What are the facts? Are they from a **reliable** (trustworthy) source? How do I know? Are they scientifically based? (Can they be tested?)
- Ask for help: Who has useful knowledge? Are there experts available who can give me reliable information and provide assistance in finding a solution?

When she starts out, Jamie finds the idea of solving her transportation problem overwhelming. The only solution that makes sense to her is buying a new car, but she knows that she probably cannot afford one at this time. When she puts her fear aside and commits herself to gathering information, she discovers the following:

- Carpools have been organized at the facility where she works.
- The most economical new car for sale in her area costs $12,595.
- *Consumer Reports* magazine has a recent article about purchasing used cars and publishes annual reports on the performance of most auto models manufactured over the past 10 years.
- Her credit union sponsors car sales to help buyers who have limited funds to spend. They also offer low-interest loans to buyers who qualify.
- A cousin has an older car that he wants to sell.
- There is a bus route within a half mile of her apartment.
- A local college offers a workshop that teaches people how to buy a car.
- The local high school has an auto mechanics training program. For a small fee, students will check over used cars before they are purchased.

Step Three—Create Alternatives

The third step is to create a list of alternatives. Generate ideas for solutions and actions based on the information collected. All possibilities should be considered before one is selected. Some alternatives may prove, on further investigation, to be impractical or unworkable. It is essential to think through each one and consider the likely consequences, both positive and negative.

Based on her research, Jamie creates the following list:

1. Take the bus to work. When the weather is nice, walking to the bus stop will be a good form of exercise. In rainy weather, common about 5 months of the year where she lives, getting to the bus stop without getting soaked is not likely. Also, the bus ride takes about 30 minutes longer, each way, than driving to work.
2. Take the workshop on how to buy a car, then purchase a used one through the credit union. The monthly car payments and higher insurance rates will result in having to budget carefully to meet all expenses. Chances of buying a "lemon" can be reduced by using the service offered at the high school.

3. Continue to rely on friends for rides to work. (Non-action is also an alternative.)
4. Ask her father for a loan to buy a new car. While Jamie would like to have a shiny new car, she has been financially independent for several years and prefers to remain that way.

Some potential alternatives do not appear on the above list because of information acquired during step two:

1. Carpool participants must have a reliable vehicle of their own. This might be an alternative later, if she purchases a dependable car.
2. Her cousin's car has over 175,000 miles and is not one of the more reliable models, according to the reports she studied.

Step Four—Choose an Alternative and Take Action

Selecting the best alternative should be based on what is known and believed to have the most positive consequences. This is followed by taking the action necessary to implement the alternative. A common difficulty in problem-solving and decision-making is failure to act. Opportunities are missed and accomplishments not realized when there is no follow-through. A benefit of going through the problem-solving process is increased confidence that the right decision has been made.

Jamie decides to combine two alternatives. There are 5 months of dry weather ahead, so she decides to take the bus to work. She will use the extra riding time to read and keep up with advances in radiology. In October, she plans to buy a used car. In the meantime, she will create a personal budget to control expenses, save money, and learn more about how to buy a car and which model is likely to give her the best value.

Step Five—Evaluate and Revise as Needed

Evaluation means reviewing the results of the actions taken. Even well-thought-out plans can prove to be ineffective or have unexpected, negative consequences. And circumstances can change. It is sometimes necessary to make adjustments or choose another alternative. It may even require going back to step two to gather additional information and go through the process again.

Although it is listed as the last step, evaluation should actually be carried on throughout the process. For example, step four, selecting the best alternative, is based on evaluation: each alternative is evaluated to decide which is most appropriate. When applying the process to health care work, it is important to remember that the needs of patients and facilities may change and/or additional information may become available. This can affect the process and force revisions to be made before the entire process has been completed. For example, if the rainy season arrives early or the bus schedules change, Jamie may have to review her alternatives and revise her plans.

Establishing Good Work Habits

Students have many opportunities in school to begin to practice good workplace habits. They should work hard to develop the skills that will make them valuable employees. At the same time, they can be acquiring habits that also contribute to academic success. The qualities essential for health care workers that were listed at the beginning of the chapter can be applied in the classroom, in the lab, and at the clinical site:

■ Care about others: Show respect and consideration for instructors and classmates. Be kind to everyone, regardless of their background. Refrain from talking during lectures. Prepare for classes so the instructor does not need to take time to answer questions about material covered in the reading or study assignments. Practice courtesy in the classroom and throughout the school. Volunteer to help others, as needed.

■ Have integrity: Do your own work. Never copy the homework assignments of others or cheat on exams. Always tell the truth. Never share anything told to you in confidence.

■ Be dependable: Be at school on time and attend all classes. Complete assignments on time. Strive for accuracy in all written and practical assignments. Follow through on all obligations and anything you have volunteered to do.

■ Work well with others: Be understanding of the needs of instructors and classmates. Participate in class. Do your share when working on group assignments.

■ Be flexible: Accept instructional differences, changes in class schedules, and other unexpected occurrences. Be willing to cooperate as needed.

■ Be willing to learn: Take your studies seriously. Make school a high priority. Dedicate sufficient time to studying throughout the length of each course to ensure maximum learning.

Getting the Most From Your Studies

People learn in different ways. One often-used method categorizes these differences by the senses used to receive and process new information. These categories are known as **learning styles**, and they are:

1. **Visual**: Learn best from seeing printed materials, images, colors, drawings, diagrams, maps, and films. Visual learners may find it difficult to follow lectures unless the instructor writes on the board, shows overheads, or demonstrates with models. They learn more easily from reading and studying drawings and charts.

2. **Auditory**: Learn best from hearing lectures, music, tapes, or rhymes. Auditory learners often find it difficult to follow printed material. They learn more easily when new material is explained orally.

3. **Kinesthetic**: Learn best from hands-on activities such as labs, practice, experiments, projects, games, and movement. Kinesthetic learners often do not really understand how to perform a procedure until they have performed it themselves. They even learn theoretical material best when activity is involved.

While no one learns in only one way, each person has a dominant learning style or preference. Students who pay attention to their style can develop study techniques to get the most from their study time. For example, there are a variety of ways to learn the first aid techniques presented in Chapter 21:

■ Visual: Study the illustrations in the text; watch a first aid video; make colored charts describing the procedures; read the chapter silently.

■ Auditory: Listen to taped explanations of the techniques; read the chapter aloud; create rhymes to help remember information.

■ Kinesthetic: Practice performing the techniques; read the chapter while pointing and moving finger down page; write in the book; study while standing up or moving about.

The more senses used in learning, the greater the chance that the information will be understood and remembered. This is why it is important for students to read assignments before class (visual), attend all lectures (auditory), and participate fully in lab sessions (kinesthetic). See Figure 1–7.

Learning for Mastery

Health care workers must know what they are doing. Mistakes on the job can result in serious consequences. It is essential that students commit to learning the material presented in their courses. Learning means more than just memorizing facts. It means striving to understand and remember information so that it can be applied to new situations. This understanding provides a basis for thinking like a health care worker, discussed earlier.

Students who do only the minimum necessary to pass tests may think they are learning. But in reality, they are not likely to have acquired the long-term knowledge necessary to perform on the job. Students who study to understand *and always search out the why of the subject* increase their chances of becoming highly competent health care workers who can think on their feet and meet new challenges as they arise.

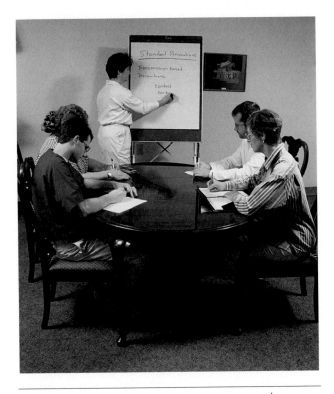

Figure 1–7 Students learn in various ways: by seeing, listening, and doing.

SUGGESTED LEARNING ACTIVITIES

1. Create a personal plan for developing the core qualities demonstrated by health care workers.

2. Seek opportunities to observe health care professionals at work. Report on the qualities that they demonstrate that you believe make them effective.

3. Do research on the occupational area of interest to you: interview a working professional, send for information or visit the Internet site of the appropriate professional organization, request a job description from a local facility, or read the job descriptions in the *Occupational Outlook Handbook*. (See References.)

4. Choose a problem in your life and apply the five steps of the problem-solving process. Report on the results.

5. Identify your preferred learning style and create five study techniques to help you master your class subjects.

REVIEW QUESTIONS

1. Describe the six core qualities that every health care worker should demonstrate.

2. Give examples of behavior that demonstrates each core quality.

3. What are the four major categories of health care occupations? Describe the type of work performed in each.

4. What are the educational and licensing requirements of the health care occupation in which you are most interested?

5. List and describe the three major types of approvals that certify the competency of health care workers.

6. What does it mean to "think like a health care worker"? Give two examples.

7. What are the five steps in the problem-solving process?

8. How can the core health care worker qualities be applied at school?

9. Explain the three learning styles and provide two examples of appropriate learning techniques for each.

APPLICATION EXERCISES

1. Refer back to the Case of the Confused Student at the beginning of the chapter. Using the information in this chapter about specific occupations, list your recommendations for those that Kevin should investigate.

2. Juan has always been interested in helping people. He also likes science and maintained good grades throughout high school in chemistry, biology, and physics. He has enrolled in the local community college and is taking "Introduction to Health Care." Juan thinks that a career in health care might be for him, but he doesn't feel that he knows enough to make a career decision at this time. He's not sure what's out there or what jobs would be appropriate for him.

a. What does Juan need to know in order to conduct an effective career search?

b. Describe how he can use the problem-solving process to help him make a tentative career decision.

c. Explain ways that Juan can research and learn more about different career options.

SUGGESTED READINGS AND RESOURCES

Critical Thinking on the Web: A Directory of Quality Online Resources. Available: http://www.philosophy.unimelb.edu.au/reason/critical/index.html

Deem, S. A. & Deem, J. (1999). *Health care exploration.* Albany, NY: Delmar.

Goleman, Daniel (1994). *Emotional intelligence: Why it can matter more than IQ.* New York, NY: Bantam Books.

Health career information: http://www.learn-jobs-careers.com/health-care

Occupational Outlook Handbook. (2000). Indianapolis: JISTWorks.

CHAPTER

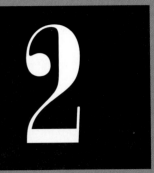

CURRENT HEALTH CARE SYSTEMS AND TRENDS

OBJECTIVES

Studying and applying the material in this chapter will help you to:

- Describe 10 significant events in the history of health care that changed the way care was delivered.

- Describe the major forces in the health care industry today.

- Describe the levels of care offered by the modern hospital.

- List ten ambulatory health care facilities and give examples of the type of services offered by each one.

- Explain the major types of long-term care facilities.

- Provide examples of health care services and care that can be provided in the patient's home.

- Explain the purpose of the hospice movement.

- List typical services offered by federal, state, and local health agencies.

- Explain the concept of "wellness."

- Describe the types of complementary therapies being practiced in the United States today.

- List the challenges facing health care today and explain how the health care worker can contribute to their resolution.

KEY TERMS

assisted living residence

chiropractic

complementary therapies

continuing care community

expanding consciousness

holistic medicine

homeopathy

hospice

inpatient

intermediate care facility (ICF)

massage therapy

osteopathy

outpatient services

psychiatric hospital

psychosomatic

skilled nursing facility (SNF)

vital statistics

wellness

The Case of

the Confused Daughter

Until recently, Dora Freemont, age 87, has lived alone in a small apartment. She recently suffered a slight stroke. After several days in the hospital, she is ready to be discharged. Her daughter, Sally, is very concerned that her widowed mother is no longer capable of living alone and handling all her housekeeping and personal needs. She shares her concern with Angela Cisneros, one of the nurses who cared for her mother during her hospital stay. Sally is frantic and fears she will have to quit work in order to help take care of her mother. Angela knows that there are a variety of long-term care facilities and a number of options available for Mrs. Freemont. She explains these to Sally and then directs her to appropriate sources of information.

The information presented in this chapter will provide health care workers with important information they can use to assist their patients as well as informing workers about the many settings in which they can seek employment.

THE HEALTH CARE INDUSTRY TODAY

The health care industry is the largest service industry in the United States. In 1995, Americans spent $989 billion on health care (Williams and Torrens, 1999). Many factors are shaping the delivery of health care today. It is important for health care workers to understand the characteristics of and forces behind this enormous industry. These will surely influence their working conditions as well as determine what it takes for them to be successful on the job.

Technological Advancements

The long history of health care was marked by gradual change until the beginning of the 20th century. Table 2–1 contains a summary of significant events in the history of medicine. Starting about 100 years ago, the rate of discovery and change increased rapidly so that in the last 20 years, medical technology and diagnostic and treatment methods advanced more than in the previous 100 years. At the beginning of the 1900s, the major killers were infectious diseases. Physicians had a limited number of techniques available. Because of the discovery of penicillin and antibiotics, along with the widespread use of immunizations, these diseases are almost unheard of today.

Modern discoveries and inventions build upon one another, increasing the appearance of new developments. There are now an amazing number of treatments that include organ transplants, microscopic surgery, and gene therapy. Keeping informed about these changes and learning to use and apply new equipment and techniques will be a continual and interesting challenge for the health care worker of the twenty-first century. See Chapter 14.

Specialization

Another significant trend in health care over the last 30 years has been the specialization of medicine (Williams, 2001). This has had several important effects on health care delivery:

- Diagnosis and treatment are improving as physicians and other practitioners concentrate on specific areas of expertise such as endocrinology or cardiology.
- Medical practice is more technical and fragmented, since specialists treat one aspect, rather than the patient as a whole.
- The cost of providing health care has increased.
- Long-term relationships between physicians and their patients are breaking down because one physician no longer provides all or most of the needed care.

Table 2–1 History of Health Care

Timeframe	Event	Impact
Ancient Times (???–400 A.D.)	Study of fossilized bones indicates many modern bone conditions, such as arthritis, tumors of the bone, inflammation of the bone, dental caries (cavities), and infectious bone diseases. Also discovered were numerous healed fractures (broken bones).	Health care problems and diseases have been with us from the beginning of human life.
	Egyptian mummies: Study of preserved bodies indicates additional modern conditions, such as arteriosclerosis, kidney stones, appendicitis, gallstones, pneumonia, pleurisy, sores of the skin, and uterine and intestinal problems.	
	Belief system based on supernatural rather than natural laws. Causes of disease were expected to be supernatural (caused by spirits, ghosts or gods).	Home remedies were used and rituals performed to drive away the evil spirits. Examples of rituals are creating loud noises, beating the ill person, or bloodletting.
		Organic, functional, and mental diseases treated the same way. Procedure called trephining (boring hole through skull) noted but reason unclear. It is suggested it may be related to attempt to relieve headaches or epilepsy, remove evil spirits, or relieve the increased pressure caused by head injury.
		Preventive medicine consisted of wearing amulets and mutilating or painting the body to ward off evil spirits.
	Life span was only 20–35 years.	Chronic illnesses were rare.
	Hippocrates of Cos (460–379 B.C.) was the most famous Greek physician of ancient times. Forty to fifty books are attributed to him (most likely not solely his work). He stressed observation and conservative treatment. Believed that health was the balance of four humors. Stressed ethical ideals and dignity.	Called the "Father of Medicine." His approach was to treat the individual, not the disease, and to treat the entire body, not just a part of it. He believed in the healing power of nature and that the physician's role was to assist nature in the healing process, rather than direct it arbitrarily. Primarily used dietetics as a means of balancing the humors. Only if diet failed would he resort to drugs or surgery.

(continues)

Table 2–1 (continued)

Timeframe	Event	Impact
Medieval Times (400–1350 A.D.)	Two plagues (543 & 568) killed majority of people and lead to breakdown in civilization.	Monks preserved written medical texts and monasteries served as centers of learning to maintain knowledge.
	Christianity became increasing center of power. Believed that disease was punishment for sins, possession by devil, or result of witchcraft.	Christians emphasized saving the soul, not the body. Treatment methods were prayer, penitence, and assistance of saints. Any cure was considered a miracle.
	At the Council of Tours in 1163, the church proclaims that they "do not shed blood." Since most physicians were clergymen, they were no longer able to perform surgery.	Surgery and bloodletting were turned over to barbers. Surgical books disappeared from the libraries at universities.
	The title of Doctor became known and major medical legislation was written in 1140 and 1224 that specified a nine-year curriculum with state examinations and licenses. The regulations also addressed use of pharmaceuticals and control of city hygiene.	Medicine became an official profession although there were not enough physicians for the population. As a result, lower-class citizens still relied on barbers and lay healers.
	Black Plague of 1348 killed large percentage of European population.	Concept of quarantine as preventive measure was recognized. Public health measures were instituted for the first time when the food in markets came under controls. Control of prostitution also was initiated to prevent spread of disease.
	Network of hospitals built.	Marked a new and more humane approach toward the ill. There were not at this time medical institutions as known today. They were primarily a refuge for the sick, old, disabled, or homeless.
Renaissance (1350–1650)	Revival of learning and science. Tremendous growth in inquiry of how the body was structured and how it worked. Numerous dissections performed by Andreas Vesalius and others.	First attempts to connect autopsy results with clinical observations made during life. Accurate anatomical drawings were now available for study.
	Many clinical advances were made.	Bedside teaching of physicans was initiated.

(continues)

Table 2–1 (continued)

Timeframe	Event	Impact
	Despite the new advances, it was still a time of tremendous filth in the cities and its peoples, the spread of disease, and extreme superstitions.	Criticisms of the old ways were frequently met with hatred, such as Pierre Brissot who spoke against bloodletting and died in exile.
	Study of botany (plants) greatly expanded as travel between countries increased.	Plants were the main source of drugs and 500 new plant species were categorized and first modern pharmacopoeia written.
	Girolamo Fracastoro wrote a book in 1546 in which he presented the first theory of contagious diseases.	Not taken seriously and would not be proven for several centuries. High incidence of infections continued as not even handwashing was done between performing autopsies and surgery.
	Efforts made to interpret "miracles" in a rational way.	Insight developed into the role of psychological factors influencing disease.
	Printing press invented.	Allowed for widespread distribution of new information and books.
	Invention of gun powder resulted in numerous gunshot wounds during frequent wars.	Need for surgical treatment of wounds elevated barber-surgeons to a higher status.
17th Century	Increasing interest in experimentation and observation.	Studies in anatomy continued, but the study of physiology (how the body functions) was also now investigated.
	William Harvey, an Englishman, stated that blood circulates throughout the body within a continuous network of vessels. Only the mechanical aspects of the system were addressed.	Vehemently opposed at first, this discovery led to the realization that medications could be injected into the circulatory system and also blood could be transfused. After many failed attempts, it fell out of favor for several centuries.
	Advances in the understanding of other systems were also made (e.g. digestion and respiration).	A greater understanding of how the lungs add oxygen to the blood and how food is digested. But further understanding was limited by lack of advancement in chemistry, which underlies the function of these systems.

(continues)

Table 2–1 (continued)

Timeframe	Event	Impact
	In 1666, Anton van Leeuwenhoek invented the microscope.	Study of microscopic anatomy and visualization of organisms now possible. Germs were only viewed under the microscope; the connection with disease comes several centuries later.
	Quinine imported from Peru as a cure for malaria.	Separated malaria from other types of fevers. Confirmed the idea that specific diseases have specific cures.
	The study of the brain and psychology was of interest. (Prior to this time, a common belief was that the soul resided in the pineal gland and the rest of the body was purely mechanical in nature.)	Nervous system and stimulation of muscles discovered. The long believed theory that mucus from a head cold was produced by the brain was disproved. Thomas Sydenham (1624–1689) reported that 50% of his nonfever patients, male and female, suffered from hysteria (psychosomatic illnesses).
	Medical universities were still teaching straight theory and not clinical skills. Also taught was frequent use of purging and bloodletting.	Great discoveries were made not by the medical universities, but by academies and societies of learned researchers. First medical journal was published by the academies in an attempt to communicate discoveries.
18th Century	Researchers and theorists still struggled with an explanation of how the body functioned.	Three theories were proposed. First, that the body functioned like a hydraulic pump that was run by an undefined fluid flowing through the nervous system. Second, that every disease was the result of overstimulation or inability to respond to stimulation. Treatment was then either a depressant or a stimulant (e.g., opium and alcohol). Third, that direct clinical observation should be used to define and categorize diseases. (This led to the absurd description of 2400 different diseases, as the same disease was listed many times, just because the symptoms varied slightly between cases).

(continues)

Table 2–1 (continued)

Timeframe	Event	Impact
	Surgery became a respected form of treatment in France after the court physician successfully repaired an anal fistula for King Louis XIV.	Surgery was upgraded from a craft to an experimental science. Procedures were developed that could cure problems that were only treatable through surgery.
	In 1761, Giovanni Battista Morgagni of Padua published a comprehensive book titled "On the Sites and Causes of Disease."	Emphasis changed from concentration on general conditions and humors to specific changes in organs.
	Techniques for measuring blood pressure and temperature were developed. Also first recommendations to measure respiration and pulse were described.	Measurements of vital signs were used to monitor patient status.
	Science of chemistry came of age.	Digestion now seen as chemical process, rather than a purely mechanical process or one of putrefication.
	The philosophy of "enlightenment" was developed that stressed the rational approach to problems and dissemination of knowledge for others to read.	Numerous studies and experiments added rapidly to the expanding base of knowledge. Sharing of knowledge with others added to the increasing pace of progress.
	Focus went from belief in the devil and "possession" to recognition of mental illness as a disease. Previously, patients were locked up in filthy conditions as they thought it was due to possession, sin, crime, or vice.	Mentally ill patients were released from their chains and treated in a more humane way. Hypochondria (called neurosis in our time) was recognized as a common psychological problem and was written about by various terms (e.g., melancholy, spinal irritation, neurasthenia, hysteria).
	Preventive health came to the forefront in the form of public health.	Sanitary reform was initiated in hospitals, prisons, and military. Personal hygiene also improved dramatically.
	Interest in child health increased.	Decreased the appalling rate of deaths in infants and children.
	Edward Jenner (1749–1823) demonstrated that vaccination with cowpox provides immunity for smallpox.	Countless lives were saved. It opened the door into investigation for other vaccines to be developed.

(continues)

Table 2–1 (continued)

Timeframe	Event	Impact
19th Century	Industrial Revolution created growth of city population as peasants flooded into the city. Hospitals were built that could hold many patients.	Large hospital populations allowed for the clinical observation of many cases, followed by autopsy when patient died. Previous focus had been on research in libraries, laboratory experiments, or with care of the individual sick person.
	Advances in physiology continued.	Emphasis moved from individual organs to the identification of the more specific tissues. For example, instead of inflammation of the heart, it was now stated as endocarditis, pericarditis, or myocarditis (inflammation of one of the three layers of the heart).
	Tremendous increase in medical knowledge was acquired and documented. Physicians and surgeons were united into one profession.	Many first time surgical operations were performed, such as tracheostomy, removal of thyroid and uterus. Medical profession started to develop specialty areas. For example, pediatrics, psychiatry, dermatology (skin), public health, and preventive medicine.
	Medicine based on observation and autopsies had offered all it could to the field. Further advances would need the study and application of the sciences.	Study shifted from practicing physicians to full-time scientific researchers.
	More powerful microscopes were developed.	Human tissue could now be seen at the cellular level.
	Advances were made in chemistry.	Laboratory tests for diagnostic purposes became common. Metabolism was studied and dietetics came under scientific study. Pharmacology was established as a new science.
	Dentists introduced anesthesia and this practice expanded to major surgical procedures.	Large-scale surgery could now be done. Death rate fell as the anesthesia decreased shock and the need for speed in surgery.
	Vivisection (operation on living animals), was routinely performed in the desire to study more accurate and detailed functions.	Some of the general public and researchers questioned ethics of procedure.

(continues)

Table 2–1 (continued)

Timeframe	Event	Impact
	The first school of nursing was created in 1836 by the German clergyman Theodor Fleidner.	The school served as an inspiration to Florence Nightingale (1823–1910), an English woman whose work in the field hospitals during the Crimean War made her a powerful influence. She opened a school of nursing in 1860.
	Elizabeth Blackwell (1821–1910) was the first woman M.D. in the United States. She opened the first nursing school in the United States in 1860.	Medical education opened for the first time to a female. Nursing is established as a profession in the United States.
	In 1546, Girolamo Fracastoro developed a theory regarding contagious diseases and the microorganisms viewed under the microscope (invented by Anton van Leeuwenhoek in 1666) are finally studied scientifically.	Louis Pasteur (1822–1895), a chemist, proved that specific microorganisms called bacteria are the cause of specific diseases in both humans and animals. The results of his work created the development of the germ theory.
	It was discovered that infectious microorganisms are carried by various means (e.g., humans, animals, mosquitoes, food). Specific identification of microorganisms led to the development of vaccines for prevention.	Revolutionized the ability to prevent, diagnose, and treat infectious diseases Then in 1864, Lord Joseph Lister, M.D. applied the germ theory to his surgical practice by reasoning that microorganisms could also fall into open surgical wounds.
	In 1867, Adolf Kussmaul (1822–1902) used a stomach pump to treat stomach diseases.	Advanced the understanding of digestion in the stomach and led to increased knowledge in dietetics and use of tube feedings.
	Anesthesia, asepsis, and invention of a variety of surgical instruments changed the face of medicine forever.	Previously the public viewed hospitals as a place one went to die. Now there was hope of recovery for the first time. Many more advanced surgeries could be performed (e.g., joints, abdomen, head, spinal column).
	Psychiatry had come to a dead end as it eluded the scientific advances. No satisfactory explanation of mental illness could be given.	Sigmund Freud (1856–1939), an Austrian neurologist, and Joseph Breuer developed the theory of psychoanalysis and presented it to the public in their book on hysteria in 1893. The theory was based on using hypnosis to allow patients to recall prior traumatic and repressed events. Freud later discarded hypnosis and based his new theory on repression of sexual urges as the central theme of psychological illnesses.

(continues)

Table 2–1 (continued)

Timeframe	Event	Impact
	Preventive medicine makes great strides as pasteurization, vaccination, asepsis, and sanitation are implemented.	Life span increased from 40 years in 1850 to 70 years in 1950 due primarily to preventive, not curative measures.
20th Century	In 1921, Karl Landsteiner of Vienna discovered blood groups.	Made transfusion of blood products safe for the first time in history.
	F.G. Banting of Toronto identifies insulin in 1921 for treatment of diabetes.	Diabetes was no longer considered a fatal disease, but can be managed with injection of insulin.
	Large-scale vaccination programs were conducted.	Many commonly feared infectious diseases are eradicated. But the influenza epidemic of 1918 that killed twenty million brought reality back after the euphoria of success.
	New diagnostic and therapeutic techniques are developed. The field of biomedical engineering is made possible with the invention of the computer.	X-rays, electrocardiograph (EKG), electroencephalograph (EEG), ultra sound, pacemakers, dialysis, and tomography provided physicians with more diagnostic and therapeutic tools.
	Vitamins are discovered and the United States took the leadership role in this research.	The belief that all diseases were caused by microbes is disproved when lack of certain vitamins are linked to various diseases (e.g., scurvy, beriberi).
	New synthetic drugs were developed to treat specific problems.	Chemotherapy was used to fight cancer. Antibiotics were developed to fight various infectious caused by bacteria. Medications for treating allergies were developed.
	Life span is 70–80 years.	Geriatrics became a specialty. Chronic illnesses were/are very common.
	Mental illness became an increasing problem in modern society.	Shock treatment and psychosurgery are replaced with new drugs and psychotherapy. Tranquilizers used to calm patients change the approach and assessment of mental patients.

(continues)

Table 2–1 (continued)

Timeframe	Event	Impact
	The end of the 19th and beginning of the 20th centuries were so laboratory and science based with increasing specialization that the patient focus was lost. It has always been known that mental processes can profoundly effect bodily illnesses and symptoms or even cause them, but this is lost in the science of medicine.	Psychosomatic aspects come back into focus where the psychological elements on physical illnesses are considered. But the increasing specialization continues to cloud this issue as specialization breaks the individual into various parts rather than treatment of the patient as a holistic being (i.e., different physicians are seen for cardiac, intestinal, and neurological conditions; one physician may diagnose the problem and another do the surgery).
	Other health care specialties develop and specialize (e.g., physical therapy, occupational therapy, speech therapy) as knowledge base increases.	Increased number of people who come in contact with the patient and who view the concerns from a specialty focus versus holistic perspective.
	Health care costs increase due to increased specialization of knowledge and cost of technological advancements, which makes health care services beyond the reach of many.	This social issue has been present for many centuries, but the increased literacy of people and availability of information from a more global awareness has increased the dissatisfaction of those unable to access health care. The question is raised, "Does everyone have an equal right to health care?"
	Surgical techniques and anesthesia methods make great advancements.	Heart, brain, and prosthetic joint replacements are performed.
	Transplantation of organs is now possible.	Definition of death is changed from cessation of heart & lung function to demonstration of brain death by electroenchephalography (EEG).
	People can be kept alive by mechanical means beyond the point of having any quality of life.	Emphasis placed on people having written Living Wills to specify what they do and do not want done to prolong their lives. In 1975, the New Jersey Supreme Court ruled that the parents of a comatose woman could authorize the removal of life support systems.

(continues)

Table 2–1 (continued)

Timeframe	Event	Impact
	Patients with terminal illnesses wish to die with dignity.	England opens first hospice in 1967. Dr. Jack Kevorkian argues that patients should be allowed to request assistance to end their lives. Between 1990 and 1998, he participated in physician-assisted suicides.
	Development of new and faster machines (e.g., automobiles, airplanes, various recreational vehicles) cause many accidental injuries.	Trauma medicine becomes a specialty.
	Mass media available to public (e.g., television, radio, newspapers, Internet). Medical physicians often seen as cold and uncaring as they focus on trying to find a diagnosis.	Quackery medicine has greater access to public for generation of huge sales of products. Outrageous claims of quick-acting results and complete cures requiring very little effort are a strong draw compared to other forms of health care.
	Scientific approach is used almost exclusively. Traditional medicine primarily based on diagnosis and then treatment with synthetic medications and surgical procedures. Rejection of herbal and alternative therapies by many traditional medical practioners.	Practioners of traditional medicine reject the "old methods" that has been useful in the past, but have not been scientifically proven. People flock to herbalists and alternative therapists in a search for more natural therapies, but lack of regulation in these areas result in many abuses.
	Genetic research into cause of certain diseases and conditions.	Identification of specific genes has been related to certain conditions. But how to alter to prevent condition has not been discovered.
	In 1978, the first "test tube" baby is born in England.	Opens up opportunity for couples previously unable to have children.
	In 1981, Acquired Immune Deficiency Syndrome (AIDS) identified as a disease.	Huge challenge to medical research that has resulted in medications that prolong life, but no cure available.
	First successful cloning of sheep in 1997.	Opens door for human cloning and growth of organs for transplantation.
21st Century and Beyond—What is Possible?	Some of the hopes for the New Millennium: • Vaccine to prevent HIV • Cure for AIDS • Cure for obesity	When health care workers several centuries into the future look back at the 20th century, they will be astounded. This reaction would be similar to when we look back to the previous centuries and are mystified

(continues)

Table 2–1 (continued)

Timeframe	Event	Impact
	• Cloning of organs for transplantation to overcome extreme difficulty in finding suitable organ donors • Cure for heart disease, hypertension and cancer • More effective treatment and cure for mental illnesses • Preventive health and alternative therapies used in complementary way with practice of traditional medicine • Life span of healthy living expanded to 100+ years • Less invasive diagnostic and therapeutic treatments and medications with less harmful side effects will be developed	by the ignorance and resulting unnecessary human suffering.

Specialization has created many employment opportunities for health care workers. At the same time, it has increased the need for caring attitudes and effective communication with patients. Lifelong relationships developed between physicians and their patients are rare today. Much of the care is provided by professionals whom the patient does not know. Health care workers play an important part in helping patients understand and have confidence in the care they are receiving.

Aging Population

Improvements in medical care, especially the development of new drugs and surgical techniques, have lengthened the average life span. Life expectancy for a child born in 1900 was 47 years. This increased dramatically to 76 years for a child born in 1991 (U.S. Census Bureau, 1995).

A second reason for the growing number of seniors is the aging of the group known as the "baby boomers." An unusually large number of births occurred during the years following the end of World War II, starting in 1946 and lasting until 1964. These individuals will be entering their period of heaviest use of the health care system over the next 20 years. See Figure 2–1.

Elderly persons are the heaviest users of health care services. The tremendous growth of this segment of the population is putting increased demands on all types of services, including the following:

▪ Facilities that provide long-term care for elderly persons unable to live in their own homes

▪ Treatment and care devoted to chronic (persisting for a long time, not cured quickly) problems that develop in people who live longer

▪ Home care services ranging from housekeeping duties to high-level nursing care

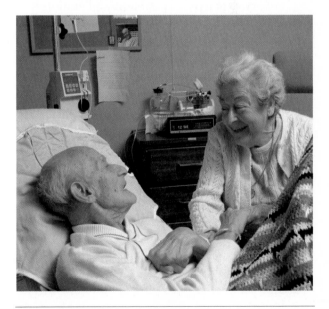

Figure 2–1 Today's growing population of elderly patients is significantly affecting the modern health care system.

Increasing Costs

The cost of providing health care has increased dramatically over the past few decades. While every product and service has steadily increased in price over the years, health care costs have grown at a faster rate than almost anything else. This is due to several factors:

- Technological advances, resulting in the use of very expensive equipment and supplies
- Increased number of elderly citizens, resulting in higher number of patients seeking services
- Rising prices of pharmaceutical products, which make up the most widely used methods of treatment
- Increasing number of diagnostic tests and treatment options available
- Diagnostic tests sometimes being overused to protect physicians against the growing number of malpractice lawsuits
- Lack of competition that will encourage increased efficiency and incentives to lower costs
- Rising expectations of patients that health care should provide more effective solutions
- More effective treatments that encourage increasing numbers of patients to seek medical care
  (Adapted from *Introduction to health services* (5th ed.), by S. J. Williams and P. R. Torrens, 1999, Albany, NY: Delmar.)

In response to skyrocketing health care costs, new methods have been and continue to be developed to deliver and pay for health care. At the same time, efforts are being made to control costs. See Chapter 22.

HEALTH CARE FACILITIES AND SERVICES

There is a wide variety of health care facilities available that offer many services for patients with all types of needs. They range in size from the private physician's office to nationwide healthcare systems that include hospitals, clinics, and long-term facilities. See Figure 2–2. They offer many kinds of services, from preventive care to emergency treatment; from routine physical exams to in-home assistance for dying patients. There are many kinds of employment settings for today's health care worker.

Hospitals

Hospitals are the traditional facilities for the care of the ill and injured. In the past, most patients remained in the hospital for all care needed until they were able to return home. The cost of hospital care has increased so dramatically that other means

[Thinking it Through]

Joseph Appleton's primary care physician has referred him to Dr. Nester, an oncologist (physician who specializes in diagnosis and treatment of cancer). Preliminary tests show that Mr. Appleton may have colon cancer. Mr. Appleton, age 77, is uncomfortable about visiting a specialist he has never met. He is especially distraught about the possibility of having a life-threatening illness and doesn't understand why the doctor he has seen for many years can't take care of the problem. Carmen Rodriguez, Dr. Nester's medical assistant, greets Mr. Appleton on his first visit to the office.

1. Discuss the changes in health care delivery that have lead to the referral of patients to specialists.
2. What do you think Carmen can do to help Mr. Appleton feel more comfortable?

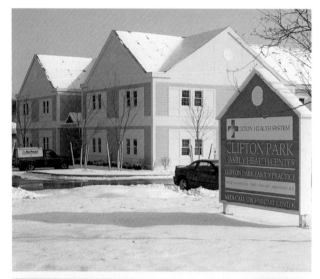

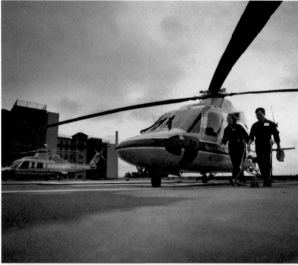

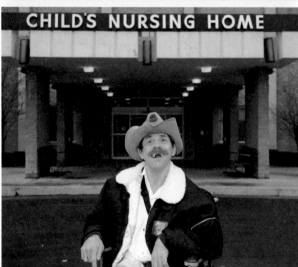

Figure 2–2 Health care workers are employed in a wide variety of settings.

of patient care have been developed to limit the number and length of patient stays. Hospitals are now just one of many facilities that provide patient care.

The trend is for hospitals to be high-tech facilities that specialize in serving patients who need sophisticated treatment and 24-hour nursing care. The various levels of care typically offered by hospitals include the following:

- Emergency room: Treats conditions that occur suddenly and require immediate attention. Examples include serious injuries from accidents and heart attacks.

- Intensive care unit (ICU): Provides specialized equipment and continuous care and monitoring for patients with serious illnesses or injuries.

- Cardiac care unit (CCU): Provides specialized equipment and continuous care and monitoring for patients with serious heart conditions.

- General unit: Provides care for patients who are seriously ill, but do not need a high level of specialized equipment and continuous nursing care.

- Transitional care unit (TCU): Provides lower-level care while patients' needs are assessed and arrangements made to release patients to return home or enter a long-term care facility.

Some hospitals also have rehabilitation units, which provide treatment for musculoskeletal, neurological, and orthopedic conditions. Rehabilitation focuses on assisting patients in regaining as high a level of normal function as possible.

Other hospitals offer specialized care for certain populations, such as children, or specific conditions, such as burns or psychiatric conditions. **Psychiatric hospitals** offer treatment to individuals with psychiatric and behavioral disorders, including assistance with crises, medication management, counseling, and monitoring of activities of daily living. Patients may be treated on an outpatient or **inpatient** (hospitalized) basis, depending on their needs.

The modern hospital faces the challenge of controlling expenses and at the same time, maintaining a certain occupancy rate (number of patients) in order to meet its operating costs. A variety of approaches have been developed to resolve this conflict:

- Diversification of services. Examples include: offering rehabilitation, outpatient surgery, and long-term care in lower-tech wings or separate buildings

■ Elimination of services that duplicate those offered at nearby hospitals

■ Merging with other hospitals to share expenses and avoid duplication of services

■ Joining a large health care system that also operates clinics, nursing homes, diagnostic centers, home health agencies, and so on

■ Being purchased by a national corporation that owns and manages many hospitals

Changes will continue to be made as hospitals seek ways to control costs and at the same time, provide adequate services for the communities they serve. Maintaining quality of care is another concern and many hospitals seek voluntary accreditation from the Joint Commission on the Accreditation of Healthcare Organizations (JCAHO). JCAHO is a private, nonprofit organization whose purpose is to encourage the attainment of high standards of institutional medical care. It establishes guidelines for the operation of hospitals and other facilities and conducts inspections to ensure that standards are being met.

Health care workers who are employed at JCAHO-approved facilities should become familiar with the standards that regulate the duties and areas for which they are responsible.

Ambulatory Services

Ambulatory services refer to those that do not require hospitalization. Also known as **outpatient services**, they include the many diagnostic, treatment, and rehabilitation facilities that account for most patient-care activities. Many procedures that were previously performed in hospitals are now done on an outpatient basis. For example, 60% of surgeries performed today do not require an overnight stay in a facility (Williams, 2001).

The physician's office is the location of the majority of ambulatory services. The average patient visits a medical office 5½ times a year (Williams, 2001). Ambulatory services are also provided by comprehensive facilities that offer a variety of services. A large clinic, for example, may have onsite radiographic and laboratory services. Others facilities are freestanding and offer one type of specialized service, such as an imaging center that only performs x-rays and ultrasound procedures. These facilities accept patients on a referral basis from professionals throughout the area. Table 2–2 lists common ambulatory settings and their services.

Long-Term Care Facilities

Various forms of long-term care are available for people who do not need to be hospitalized, but are unable to live at home. This is one of the fastest growing areas in health care and offers an increasing number of services for patients and employment opportunities for health care workers. There are many categories of long-term care:

■ **Nursing homes**: There are two types of facilities commonly designated as nursing homes:

　■ **Skilled nursing facility (SNF)**: Provides nursing and rehabilitation services on a 24-hour basis. Includes regular medical care for patients with long-term illnesses or those recovering from illness, injury, or surgery.

　■ **Intermediate care facility (ICF)**: Provides personal care, social services, and regular nursing care for individuals who do not require 24-hour nursing, but are unable to care for themselves.

■ **Assisted living residence**: Provides housing, meals, and personal care to individuals who need help with daily living activities, but do not need daily nursing care. The level of assistance provided depends on individual needs. This type of residence is also known by other names. Examples include supportive housing, residential long-term care facilities, adult residential care facilities, board-and-care, and rest homes.

■ **Continuing care community**: Provides a variety of living arrangements that support lifestyles as they change from independent living to the need for regular medical and nursing care. Additional services, such as meals and daily nurse visits, can be contracted for as required.

Providing quality care for an aging population will be one of society's biggest challenges in the coming decades.

Home Health Care Providers

In this area of tremendous growth, various levels of services and care are being provided to patients in their homes. There are several factors that have caused this trend:

■ Shorter hospital stays

■ Increase in the elderly population

Table 2–2 Ambulatory Facilities

Facility	Services Offered
Adult day care	Activities, meals, and supervision for adults who need assistance, such as the elderly and developmentally disabled
Dental offices	Prevention, diagnosis, and treatment of problems with the teeth
Diagnostic centers	Procedures, such as radiography, to determine the cause and nature of diseases and injuries
Emergency and urgent care	Care for conditions that need immediate attention
Health care services in companies, schools, and prisons	Basic and preventive care for employees, students, and prisoners
Laboratories	Clinical labs draw blood and collect urine and other samples. Perform tests that provide information needed to diagnose, treat, or prevent disease. Dental labs make false teeth, crowns, and corrective devices for the mouth.
Rehabilitation centers	Therapies to help patients regain maximum physical and mental function; types include physical, occupational, speech, and hearing. Specialized centers assist patients to overcome problems with substance abuse.
Specialty clinics and offices	Treatment for specific conditions such as cancer and venereal disease; rehabilitative services such as hand therapy, psychological counseling, and many others.
Surgical centers	Outpatient surgeries, which do not require hospitalization
Wellness centers	Routine physicals; preventive measures such as immunizations; educational programs about nutrition, exercise, and so on

■ Advances in equipment that allow more technical procedures to be carried out in the home

A wide range of professionals deliver care to patients in their homes:

■ Registered and practical/licensed vocational nurses: Educate patients about self-care; administer medications, including IV therapy (administered through the veins); check progress; and change dressings, check the healing of wounds, and remove sutures following surgery.

■ Physical therapists and physical therapist assistants: Recommend and teach physical exercises, work to increase physical stamina and movement, monitor progress following injury or surgery.

■ Occupational therapists and occupational therapy assistants: Assist patients in attaining maximum function and perform activities of daily living (ADLs) as independently as possible.

■ Speech therapist: Help patients recover speech and ability to swallow.

■ Medical social workers: assist with financial planning and arranging for in-home help or placement in the appropriate facility.

■ Certified nursing assistant/home health aide: provide personal care such as bathing and grooming, and follow care plans developed and monitored by a registered nurse or other designated professional.

Nonmedical services are also available to help individuals with shopping, cooking, cleaning, and other housekeeping tasks. These are not considered medical in nature and are not usually covered by health insurance plans.

Some of the occupations showing the largest numerical increase in employment involve the provision of health care in the home (Occupational Outlook Handbook, 1998–99). Quality of care becomes a concern when health care providers work in offsite locations without direct supervision. In response to these concerns, states require the licensing of home health agencies. The types of care that may be performed in the home by various health care personnel are strictly regulated, by both state law and insurance reimbursement guidelines. Only services provided by specific personnel are covered in most plans.

Hospice

The hospice movement began in England and is growing in the United States as more people learn about its benefits. **Hospice** refers to palliative (relieves but does not cure) care and support provided to dying patients and their families. It involves a team made up of professionals and volunteers that provides medical, emotional, and spiritual assistance. The emphasis of hospice is to make the patient's last days as pain-free and meaningful as possible. Care may be provided in a special facility, known as a hospice, or in the patient's home. After the patient dies, continuing support is available for the family.

Consolidation of Health Care Services

Mainly due to efforts to control costs, many health care facilities are combining under the same ownership. In this way they enjoy a number of advantages:

- Buy supplies in large quantities, thus negotiating for better prices
- Share expensive equipment
- Avoid duplication of laboratory and diagnostic services
- Share knowledge and management expertise
- Consolidate services

Multiservice systems offer patients more coordinated health care, a sort of "one-stop shopping." For example, following a hospital stay, a patient can be transferred to the system's skilled nursing facility and at the same time, be referred to its rehabilitation services. Some systems include a home health division.

Advantages of consolidation are that patients may experience more consistent care and better follow-through when dealing with one system. A disadvantage to consolidation is that there are fewer choices for health care consumers. There is the danger, too, that the lack of competition will result in higher prices and lower quality. Government regulation and patient demands help prevent these problems and ensure that large health care systems are accountable and maintain good patient care as their first priority.

Government Health Services

Federal, state, and local governments provide a variety of important services to protect the health of the American public. Supported by taxpayers, agencies have been created that concentrate on conducting research, regulatory, and educational activities. The major federal health-related agencies are shown in Table 2–3.

State and local health departments receive monetary and administrative support from the federal government. The following lists include examples of typical services offered:

State Health Departments

- License health care personnel, hospitals, and nursing homes
- Monitor chronic and communicable (contagious) diseases
- Provide laboratory services
- Provide emergency medical services
- Establish health data systems
- Conduct public health planning

Local Health Departments

- Collect **vital statistics** (births and deaths)
- Conduct sanitation inspections
- Provide health education
- Screen for diseases such as cancer and diabetes
- Carry out insect control measures
- Supervise water and sewage systems
- Provide immunizations
- Operate venereal disease clinics (Williams, 2001)

Table 2–3 Health-Related Agencies of the Federal Government

Departments of the U.S. Department of Health and Human Services (DHHS)	
National Institutes of Health (NIH)	**Centers for Disease Control and Prevention (CDC)**
Conduct research on all types of diseases	Research ways to control the spread of diseases that are contagious, caused by conditions, or spread by animals and insects
U.S. Department of Labor Occupational Safety and Health Administration (OSHA)	**Food and Drug Administration (FDA)**
Develops and enforces minimum health and safety standards (that employers must follow) for workers	Ensures that foods are safe, pure and wholesome; therapeutic drugs are safe and effective, and that cosmetics are harmless

Government services provide a variety of employment opportunities for health care workers. Everyone who works in health care, whether public or private, must understand the regulations of these agencies and how they affect their occupation. For example, the CDC has developed standard precautions for the safe handling of body fluids. These are essential for health care workers who have contact with patients. These standards are discussed in Chapter 10.

TRENDS IN HEALTH CARE

Many new approaches to health care are being explored today. This growing interest is due to several factors:

- Access to information about the health care practices of other cultures
- Search for less invasive and less costly alternatives to surgery and drugs
- Growing interest in the use of natural products
- Belief that the mind and body are more closely connected than previously thought
- Interest in preventing rather than simply curing disease
- Increasing number of patients who want to assume more responsibility for their health by participating in preventive and self-care practices

- More patients wanting to conduct their own research and take an active role in making decisions about their treatment and care
- Desire for increased humanization of medicine through touch, massage, and other hands-on methods

Wellness

Wellness is the promotion of health through preventive measures and the practice of good health habits. There are a growing number of people who believe that more emphasis should be placed in health care on the maximization of good health. This is an expansion of the traditional view of health as the absence of disease. Wellness centers have been established to offer services such as routine physicals, immunizations, nutrition and exercise classes, and educational programs on disease prevention.

A part of the concept of wellness is the emphasis on the need for patients to take responsibility for their own health. Encouraging patients and teaching them about the basic principles of health promotion and self-care are increasingly important tasks of today's health care workers. See Chapter 12. Stephen Williams, a professor of public health, states it very well: "We cannot expect to be rescued from every source of morbidity (being diseased) and mortality (death) by the nation's health care system if we do not individually and collectively emphasize prevention of disease and illness in the first place" (Williams 2001).

Some traditional health care providers have become interested in extending the definition of health to mean more than the absence of disease. Margaret Newman, RN, developed a theory she calls **expanding consciousness**. She realized that many of her patients would never be "well" in the traditional sense. They would be living with a non-curable disease or the results of an injury for the rest of their lives. Newman developed a nursing approach to assist patients in making their lives as meaningful as possible by focusing on their possibilities rather than on their limitations (Miller-Keane, 1992).

Complementary Therapies

Complementary therapies are health care practices that have not traditionally been performed in conventional medical offices (Milliken, 1998). Also known as "alternative therapies," they include practices such as the use of herbs and plants to treat symptoms, teaching patients meditation as a way to promote healing, and acknowledging the influence of the mind on physical symptoms. While many health care providers do not accept the claims made for these techniques, a growing number of traditionally trained physicians, nurses, and others are conducting studies and adopting methods that were once considered to be unscientific and ineffective. Many practitioners have documented the successful treatment of patients using these therapies, and therefore the term "complementary" rather than "alternative" is becoming widely accepted.

Complementary therapies are becoming increasingly popular among patients. Health care workers are likely to come into contact with one or more forms of complementary therapy. Patients may ask opinions about something they have

heard about; a friend or family member may seek these services; or their employer may be exploring the use of a complementary method of treatment.

It is important for health care workers to be aware of the various forms of complementary therapies so they can make intelligent decisions and direct patients to reliable sources of information where they can learn more for themselves. It is recommended that they inform themselves through reading, attending workshops and seminars, and asking questions (Milliken, 1998). Milliken also suggests four warning signs that a treatment is likely to be more beneficial for the financial gain of the practitioner than the health of the patient. These occur when the practitioner:

1. Guarantees that the patient will be cured
2. Claims that the treatment is a secret that is not available to other practitioners
3. Demands a large payment before beginning the treatment
4. Refuses to give information about his or her qualifications

Osteopathy and Chiropractic

These health care practices have become so widely accepted that they are no longer generally considered to be alternative. **Osteopathy** is based on the belief that the body can protect itself against disease if the musculoskeletal system, especially the spine, is in good order. The importance of good nutrition and favorable environmental conditions is also emphasized. Osteopathic physicians receive training that is similar to that of traditional doctors of medicine (MDs). They can prescribe drugs, perform surgeries, and have staff privileges at most hospitals. Osteopaths take the same state licensing examinations as MDs.

Chiropractic is based on the belief that pressure on the nerves leaving the spinal column causes pain and/or dysfunction of the body part served by that nerve. Treatment involves manipulation of the spine to correct misalignments. Chiropractors are not allowed to prescribe drugs, but may recommend nutritional and herbal remedies. Every state has licensure requirements for chiropractors.

Homeopathy

Homeopathy is a method of treatment developed by a German physician in the early 1800s based on the idea that "like cures like." Disorders are treated with very small amounts of the natural substances that cause the symptoms of the disorder in healthy people. For example, exposure to onions causes the same runny nose and eyes as are experienced with a head cold. Therefore, very diluted amounts of plants in the onion family are administered to treat cold symptoms (Milliken, 1998). Belladonna, secured from a poisonous European plant, is widely used in homeopathy to treat a variety of symptoms, including pain. It has been used in traditional medicine to dilate the pupils to facilitate examination of the eyes. Homeopathy has been practiced in Europe and India for over 200 years. It is gaining popularity in the United States among people who believe that these remedies are safer than prescription drugs. Some physicians combine homeopathic methods with their traditional medical practice.

Massage Therapy

Massage therapy is widely recognized, when administered by a trained practitioner, as a beneficial health practice. By enabling the muscles to relax, it promotes better blood circulation, faster healing of injuries, and pain relief. It is often recommended to supplement other forms of therapy and as an effective method of stress relief. Many types of formal training programs are available for people who wish to practice massage therapy. Some states and localities require therapists to be licensed.

Holistic Medicine

Holistic medicine is based on the belief that the traditional view of medicine must be expanded. All aspects of the individual–physical, mental, emotional, and spiritual–contribute to states of health and disease. The entire person must be considered when making therapeutic decisions. There is a growing interest in holistic medicine today as evidence mounts that the mind has a powerful effect on physical health. Disorders caused by mental and/or emotional factors are known as **psychosomatic**. Researchers now know that these illnesses are not "all in one's head" but that physical symptoms can be the result of what is happening in the mind. It is believed that as many as 85% of visits to doctor's offices are due to psychosomatic disorders (Milliken, 1998).

All forms of treatment should be considered, both traditional and nontraditional, when treating the patient. Practitioners of holistic medicine also emphasize that:

- Patients must accept responsibility for their own health
- Stress is an important factor in health and should be reduced
- Proper nutrition and exercise are essential

- Attitude has a powerful effect, both positive and negative

Energy Theories

Another area of growing interest concerns the body's energy. Theories have been developed regarding the effects of the fields of energy that surround the body and pathways along which energy flows inside the body. Free flow of this energy, some believe, is necessary to restore and maintain good health. The oldest application of energy theories was probably developed by the Chinese who believe that disease results when the flow of energy is blocked. Acupuncture, the insertion of tiny needles to relieve these blocks, was developed over 5000 years ago. Acupuncture is becoming accepted in this country as people find relief from various health problems. Current theories and techniques based on energy are listed in Table 2–4.

CHALLENGES IN HEALTH CARE TODAY

The tremendous medical progress made during the last century will continue into the new millennium. At the same time, our country faces many challenges in effectively delivering the results of this progress to all who need it. These challenges represent complex problems that affect millions of people. Problems of this size are not easy to solve. Finding solutions that satisfy the needs of everyone is very difficult.

Thinking it Through

Craig Oakley is a physical therapy assistant who does home visits for a rehabilitation service. One of his patients, Mr. Singh, suffers from rheumatoid arthritis and has asked Craig's opinion about taking Chinese herbal remedies that he has read help restore joint health.

1. How should Craig respond?
2. What are resources he can consult in order to find out more about the treatment?
3. What precautions should Craig follow when speaking with Mr. Singh about complementary therapies?

Table 2–4 Therapies Based on Energy Theories

Name of Therapy	Procedure	Developed by:
Acupressure	Pressure points on body	Chinese
Acupuncture	Insertion of small needles	Chinese
Healing Touch	Work with energy field surrounding body	Janet Mentgen, RN
Polarity Therapy	Positioning and moving of hands over the body and touching pressure points	Dr. Randolph Stone
Reflexology	Pressure points on the feet	
Shiatsu	Japanese form of acupressure	Japanese
Therapeutic Touch	Using hands 1–3 inches from body to direct energy flow	Dr. Dolores Krieger

It is important for the health care worker to be aware of major health care issues. They will affect where and how you perform your job as well as influence your relationships with patients and other members of the health care team.

Access to Health Care

Millions of Americans do not have health insurance, do not have the means to pay for needed medical care, or have inadequate insurance coverage. These people belong to three major groups:

■ The unemployed: Group insurance plans provided by employers are the most common source of insurance coverage. The unemployed usually cannot afford to buy private medical insurance and/or do not qualify for Medicaid.

■ The "working poor": These are people who are employed, but do not have the opportunity to participate in group coverage. The employer may not offer health insurance or the employee may work on a part-time or temporary basis and does not qualify. These workers usually do not earn enough to purchase medical insurance on their own.

■ People with preexisting conditions: Many insurance companies will not accept applicants who already have serious health problems.

It is often the case that those who most need health care services are the ones least likely to have access to it. Government-sponsored health care plans have been proposed in an effort to solve this problem, but there are many opponents who fear overregulation and the rationing of services (a system that would predetermine the services to be provided).

Social Conditions

Many current social problems affect the country's health care delivery systems as well as the health of the nation as a whole. An example is the return of tuberculosis as a public health concern. This contagious disease was nearly eliminated by the mid-1900s. Those who are most susceptible to tuberculosis live in crowded, unsanitary conditions and suffer from malnutrition, drug abuse, alcoholism, and general poor health. Unfortunately, these are the conditions in which many Americans live today. The standard treatment for tuberculosis is medication taken over an extended period of time, sometimes up to 1 year. Most patients remain at home during treatment. A problem that has developed is the number of patients who require continual monitoring by social workers or nurses to ensure that they take their medicine as prescribed. This care is provided at public expense, if necessary, because of the highly contagious nature of the disease. Table 2–5 lists a number of social conditions that can produce negative consequences for individual health as well as health care delivery systems.

The sad result of poverty and other social problems is that those who most need health care services are the least able to pay for them. People who cannot afford preventive care are more likely to develop serious conditions. They eventually seek care in emergency rooms, one of the most expensive providers of health care. Preventive care, had it been available, would have spared both patient suffering and the need for expensive emergency care.

Maintaining the Quality of Care

The skyrocketing costs of health care have prompted all levels of government, as well as providers of health care, to initiate cost controls. This has caused widespread concern that quality of care is being sacrificed to cut expenses. For example, patients are given drugs following certain types of surgery to prevent blood clots from forming and moving into vital organs, such as the lungs or brain. A provider may choose to give a drug that has proven to be less effective than another because it costs much less.

A related area of concern is that for-profit insurance and health care organizations emphasize profits more than ensuring high-quality patient care. Some current methods of paying physicians and other providers for their services encourage them to provide less, rather than more care. Reviewers who work on behalf of insurance companies make decisions about patient care. The purpose is to determine whether the proposed procedures are medically necessary and whether lower cost alternatives are available. Permission is required in advance for certain procedures. Nonemergency hospital admissions and surgeries commonly require approval.

Reviewers may or may not have extensive medical training. Their decisions are based on what is known about the "average patient" under the same or similar circumstances. Reviewers can make a variety of decisions. For example, they can:

- Approve the procedure as recommended by the physician
- Deny the procedure
- Require surgery to be performed as an outpatient service (does not occupy a bed in the facility, such as a hospital)

Table 2–5 Social Conditions that Affect Health and Health Care Systems

Condition	Impact on Health Care System
Breakdown of family unit and children born to single women	Poverty among women and children. Lack of access to prenatal care, immunizations for children, and other preventive measures.
Homelessness	Lack of access to medical care. Malnutrition and poor hygiene. Difficult to contact patient for follow-up care.
Violence	Use of emergency and other health care services. Inability of many victims to pay.
Substance abuse	Increased violence and susceptibility to disease. Inability to care for self and family.
Spousal and child abuse	Need for health and protective services. Use of emergency room services for injuries.
Poverty and malnutrition	Poor health and inability to access health care. Lack of prenatal care.
25% of Americans live alone	Need outside assistance when ill or injured. Lack of emotional support.

Adapted from *Essentials of health services*, by S. J. Williams, 2001, Albany, NY: Delmar.

- Approve a different, usually less-costly method
- Approve a limited number of treatments

Many physicians feel they have lost control of the practice of medicine to business interests. Accustomed to having the authority to make decisions about the best care for their patients, they are frustrated by what they see as interference from nonmedical personnel.

Patients, in turn, believe the decisions of their physicians are being questioned and have concerns about the resulting quality of care. They worry that they are being denied needed procedures and treatments and that their health is being sacrificed for the sake of increasing profits.

At the same time, other health care experts point out that the number of unnecessary surgeries and other procedures, especially those used for diagnosis, have decreased. They believe that patient care has not suffered, but has actually been improved by efforts to prevent the overuse of available techniques.

Restoring confidence in the system while controlling costs will be a major challenge to ensuring continued quality of care. As a health care worker, you can help restore this confidence by providing the best care possible and supporting the decisions of the professional for whom you work. See Chapter 23.

Public Health Concerns

The United States faces challenges in its efforts to safeguard the health of the public. Monitoring and research on health issues must be ongoing. For example, while most infectious diseases are under control in this country, the dramatic effect of AIDS on many Americans is a warning that not all threats to public health have been conquered (Williams, 2001). Research must also continue to find effective treatments for diseases such as cancer, which ranks as one of the three top causes of death in the United States.

An important indicator of the effectiveness of a nation's health care system is its infant mortality rate. This is the number of infants who die in the first year of life per 1000 live births. In 1993, the United States ranked 13th in a list of 14 industrialized countries. Compared with Japan's rate of 4.35 deaths per 1000, the U.S. rate was nearly double at 8.37 (Williams, 1999).

This statistic is due to many factors including poverty, unhealthy behaviors such as drug abuse, and lack of access to prenatal care. These factors not only affect infant mortality rates, but also contribute to physical and mental developmental problems in those children who do survive.

Personal Responsibility for Health

The three leading causes of death in the United States–heart disease, cancer, and stroke–are sometimes influenced by lifestyle choices. Individuals have control over the habits that contribute to the state of their health. The following behaviors have been identified as contributing to healthier and longer lives:

- Not smoking
- Getting enough sleep
- Eating moderately and maintaining a balanced diet
- Exercising regularly
- Avoiding alcohol or drinking in moderation
- Practicing preventive measures such as getting immunizations and wearing seat belts
- Using stress reduction techniques

    (Adapted from *Understanding human behavior* (6th ed.), by M.E. Milliken, 1998, Albany, NY: Delmar.)

Individuals must also realize that modern medicine has limitations and that new technological advances do not guarantee that every disease can be cured and every injury repaired. They can gain much by taking positive actions, such as quitting smoking, to promote personal health.

IMPLICATIONS FOR HEALTH CARE WORKERS

Meeting the challenges facing our health care system is the concern of everyone. Health care workers are in the fortunate position of being able to positively influence this important area of life. Some steps that can be taken to help meet these challenges are to:

- Keep informed of important issues by reading, attending workshops, and participating in your professional organization.
- Contribute to the delivery of high-quality service by pledging to perform duties to the best of your ability. Chapter 23 discusses specific ways that health care workers can improve the quality of their performance and give excellent customer service.
- Model good health habits and learn to provide effective patient education (Chapter 12.)

SUGGESTED LEARNING ACTIVITIES

1. Look for articles about health care trends in the newspaper, in magazines, and on the Internet. Which are mentioned most frequently? How do you think they will affect your future career as a health care worker?

2. Explore the Web site at *http://www.cdc.gov/nchs/default.htm* .What type of information is collected? What can you learn from these statistics about the health of the American people and the state of our health care systems?

3. Visit some of the health care facilities described in this chapter. What services do they offer? What type of employment opportunities are available?

4. Conduct a search of Web sites for major hospitals and health care systems in your area. What kind of information is available?

5. Investigate the services provided by your local public health department.

6. Explore complementary therapies practiced in your area. Interview a practitioner about the theory on which his or her therapy is based.

7. Learn more about the factors that contribute to cancer, heart disease, and stroke. Contact the local offices of the American Cancer Society and The American Heart Association or check their Web sites by doing a search using their names. Explore other sources on the Internet using the key words "cancer prevention," "heart disease prevention," and "stroke prevention." Sample sites include: *http://www.hsph.harvard.edu/cancer/* *http://www.stroke.org/*

REVIEW QUESTIONS

1. What are 5 events in the history of health care that improved the delivery of care for patients?

2. What are the major forces shaping the health care industry today?

3. What are the levels of care typically provided in a modern general hospital?

4. What are 10 common ambulatory health care facilities? What type of services does each one offer?

5. What are the major categories of long-term care facilities? What type of care is offered by each?

6. What are five typical services offered by federal health agencies? State agencies? Local agencies?

7. What are the services provided by hospice workers?

8. What is meant by the term "wellness"?

9. Describe five types of complementary therapies being practiced in the United States today.

10. What are the major challenges facing health care today? How can the health care worker contribute to their resolution?

APPLICATION EXERCISES

1. Refer to the Case of the Confused Daughter at the beginning of the chapter. Put yourself in the place of the nurse. What information would you give Mrs. Freemont and her daughter?

2. Jim Parker has been working as a licensed practical nurse for seven years. Most of his career has been spent working in a community hospital providing direct patient care. Jim has been thinking about other settings in which he can apply his nursing skills.

   a. Describe at least five facilities that might offer employment opportunities for Jim.

   b. What type of patients should he expect to work with in each one?

SUGGESTED READINGS AND RESOURCES

Centers for Disease Control and Prevention:
   http://www.cdc.gov
Complementary Therapies:
   http://dir.yahoo.com/Health_Medicine
Department of Health and Human Services
   National Institutes of Health
   Research and publications on all aspects of health:
   disease, prevention, women's health, aging,
   research, etc. Available: http://www.nih.gov

Food and Drug Administration: http://www.fda.gov
Milliken, M. E. (1998). *Understanding human behavior*
   (6th ed.). Albany, NY: Delmar.
Occupational Safety and Health Administration:
   http://www.osha.gov
National Hospice and Palliative Care Organization:
   http://www.nho.org
Williams, S. J. and Torrens, P. R. (1999). *Introduction to
   health services* (5th ed.). Albany, NY: Delmar.

CHAPTER

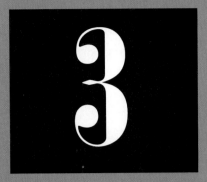

ETHICAL AND LEGAL RESPONSIBILITIES

OBJECTIVES

Studying and applying the material in this chapter will help you to:

■ Explain the meaning of ethics and its importance in the practice of health care.

■ Understand the purpose of professional codes of ethics.

■ Describe the relationship of ethics and law.

■ Explain the eight major ethical principles that apply to health care and describe the laws that support each.

■ Give examples of how the health care worker applies ethics on the job.

KEY TERMS

adult
advance directive
agent
assault
autonomy
battery
breach of contract
code of ethics
confidentiality
consent
contract
damages
defamation of character
discreet
durable power of attorney
emancipated minor
ethical dilemma
ethics
euthanasia
express consent
express contract
false imprisonment
fraud
implied consent
informed consent

continues

KEY TERMS *continued*

implied contract	libel	negligence	slander
invasive procedures	living will	principles	values
justice	malpractice	protocols	
legislation	mercy killing	respondeat superior	

The Case of the Missing Consent Form

Mrs. McChesney is bringing her 3-year-old son, Sammy, to Dr. Michaels for minor surgery to be performed in the physician's office. Medical assistant Gretchen Mills scheduled the surgery in the appointment book. Last night she checked to be sure that the necessary instruments and supplies were prepared and that an appropriate room was ready. When checking Sammy's file on the day of the surgery, she cannot find a consent form, signed by Mrs. McChesney, to authorize the surgery. Proceeding with the procedure without this having been completed could have serious legal implications. Health care workers must understand and help their facilities follow ethical principles and meet legal requirements.

THE PURPOSE OF ETHICS

Over the centuries human beings have struggled to answer questions about the meaning of life and how to properly conduct themselves. **Ethics** is a system of **principles** (fundamental truths) a society develops to guide decision making about what is right and wrong. It helps people deal with difficult and complex problems that lack easy answers.

The ethical principles adopted by a society are influenced by religion, history, and the collective experiences of the people in the group. The United States has one of the most diverse populations of any country on earth, composed of hundreds of cultures. People live by a variety of ethical principles and beliefs that vary about the meaning of right and wrong. This accounts for many of the disagreements that occur when the government tries to pass laws and make policy decisions that affect all citizens. The ongoing debate about abortion is an example of strongly held opposing beliefs in which each side believes it is right.

Even within a single ethical system, following one principle may appear to contradict another. These result in what are known as **ethical dilemmas**, situations in which there are no clear answers. Table 3–1 contains examples of ethical dilemmas faced by Americans today.

Often, there simply is not a clear right answer that will satisfy everyone. Right behavior for some people results in wrong effects for others. Flight (1998), who writes about health care ethics, points out that realizing there may not be a "perfect" answer can prevent some of the agonizing that occurs when trying to make the "correct" decision.

ETHICS AND HEALTH CARE

The importance of ethics in the practice of health care has been recognized for thousands of years. Health care workers have a significant impact on human life. The practice of health care involves life and death issues, which are at the heart of ethical questions.

Table 3–1 Ethical Dilemmas Faced by Americans

Values	Action	Contradiction
1. Criminals should be punished for their crimes. ("An eye for an eye.") 2. "Thou shall not kill."	Capital punishment for convicted murderers	If it is wrong to kill, can society justify killing anyone, even a criminal?
1. Freedom of speech is a human right. 2. All people should be treated equally and be protected under the law.	Speeches on public grounds that contain hate messages directed toward minority groups	Should free speech be allowed if the messages encourage unequal treatment?
1. Citizens should have the right to own guns and protect themselves. 2. Society must protect itself against criminals.	Criminals use guns to harm others.	Should gun sales be controlled if it results in limiting the rights of law-abiding citizens?

Recognition of the important role of health care workers has existed since ancient times. Hippocrates was a Greek physician who lived about 2500 years ago. He was concerned with the ethical considerations of medicine. The Hippocratic Oath, taken by physicians over the centuries, contains issues and ideas that are still being debated today. See Box 3–1 and look for the references to mercy killing and abortion.

Box 3–1   The Oath of Hippocrates

I swear by Apollo Physician and Aesculapius and Hygeia and Panacea and all the gods and goddesses, making them my witness, that I will fulfill according to my ability and judgment this oath and this convenant.

To hold him who has taught me this art as equal to my parents and to live my life in partnership with him, and if he is in need of money to give him a share of mine, and to regard his offspring as equal to my brothers in male lineage and to teach them this art—if they desire to learn it—without fee and covenant; to vie a share of precepts and oral instruction and all the other learning to my sons and to the sons of him who has instructed me and to pupils who have signed the convenant and have taken an oath according to the medical law, but to no one else.

I will apply dietetic measures for the benefit of the sick according to my ability and judgement; I will keep them from harm and injustice.

I will neither give a deadly drug to anybody if asked for it nor will I make a suggestion to this effect. Similarly, I will not give to a woman an abortive remedy. In purity and holiness. I will guard my life and my art.

I will not use the knife, not even on sufferers from stone, but will withdraw in favor of such men as are engaged in this work.

Whatever houses I may visit, I will come for the benefit of the sick, remaining free of all intentional injustice, of all mischief, and in particular of sexual relations with both female and male persons, be they free or slaves.

Source: Lindh, W., Pooler, M., Tamparo, C., & Cerrato, J. (1998). Delmar's comprehensive medical assisting. Albany, NY: Delmar.

[Fascinating Facts]

Regulation of health care for the public good is not a modern idea. Over 4500 years ago, rules for physicians were included in the Code of Hammurabi. It contained a long list of do's and don'ts and penalties for not following the rules. It even included guidelines regarding the fees that physicians could charge.

Health care workers today are confronted by more ethical problems than at any other time in history. Flight (1998) notes that "Technology has progressed beyond society's readiness to deal with the ethical and legal issues it presents" (p. 231). We are able to prevent conception, prolong life, transplant organs, and perform lifesaving procedures to an extent never before imagined. In some cases, cures seem miraculous and add to human happiness. In others, society is confronted with difficult questions like the following:

- Anencephalic babies are born without a brain, only a brain stem. They have no hope for a life other than remaining in a vegetative state. Should these babies be kept alive?
- Should an anencephalic baby be allowed to die so that its organs can be transplanted in babies who have normal brain function, but who need the organs to survive?
- Should life support be withdrawn from patients who are in comas and judged to have no chance of revival? After one year? After five years?
- Should pain killers be given in quantities sufficient to relieve extreme pain even if the patient might become addicted to them?
- If a patient is suffering from a painful form of terminal cancer, should his request to be assisted in dying "in a dignified manner" be honored?
- Should teenagers be given birth control information and products without their parents' knowledge?
- Should anyone be given birth control information and products?

Technological advancements have dramatically increased the price of health care. Spending for specialized training, equipment, and procedures continues to push costs up. As discussed in Chapter 2, this has resulted in efforts to control these costs while attempting to maintain the quality of care provided. Decisions about how to distribute available health care dollars raise serious ethical questions about who receives care. Some argue that health care is a right and should be provided to all Americans regardless of their ability to pay. They propose that a national health care plan be developed to ensure care for everyone. Most industrialized nations have some kind of a national health care program.

Such plans have been rejected in the United States. Many Americans believe that a government-controlled health care system would result in long waits for service and poor care, even for those who can afford to pay for themselves. Working out a solution that ensures adequate care in a timely way for everyone who needs it, is a major challenge facing Americans today.

Professional Codes of Ethics

To help them deal with ethical problems, health care workers are guided by principles outlined in a professional **code of ethics**. These codes have been developed by professional organizations. While they vary in detail, the codes all share the same purpose: to set standards of professional conduct that promote the welfare of patients and ensure a high quality of care. Here are the introductions to three professional codes:

- The purpose of a professional code of ethics is to achieve the high levels of ethical consciousness, decision making, and practice by members of the profession. (Code of Ethics for Dental Hygienists)
- The American Occupational Therapy Association's Code of Ethics is a public statement of the values and principles used in promoting and maintaining high standards of behavior in occupational therapy. (American Occupational Therapy Association Code of Ethics).
- The Code of Ethics of AAMA shall set forth principles of ethical and moral conduct as they relate to the medical profession and the particular practice of medical assisting. (American Association of Medical Assistants)

The "ethical consciousness" mentioned in the Dental Hygiene Code means being aware of, and the need for, standards in health care. You will be confronted by ethical issues throughout your professional life. Ethics is not simply an academic subject to pass in school. It is an essential and ongoing part of your education.

Box 3–2   Code of Ethics

The Code of Ethics of AAMA shall set forth principles of ethical and moral conduct as they relate to the medical profession and the particular practice of medical assisting.

Members of AAMA dedicated to the conscientious pursuit of their profession, and thus desiring to merit the high regard of the entire medical profession and the respect of the general public which they serve, do pledge themselves to strive always to:

A. render service with full respect for the dignity of humanity;
B. respect confidential information obtained through employment unless legally authorized or required by responsible performance of duty to divulge such information;
C. uphold the honor and high principles of the profession and accept its disciplines;
D. seek to continually improve the knowledge and skills of medical assistants for the benefit of patients and professional colleagues;
E. participate in additional service activities aimed toward improving the health and well-being of the community

It is your responsibility to read and understand the full text of the code of ethics for your occupation. You can obtain one by contacting your professional organization (Appendix 1). See Box 3–2 for an example of a complete professional code of ethics.

The ethical problems encountered by health care workers can be confusing and stressful. While there are no simple recipes for handling difficult issues, ethical codes can be of assistance in making important decisions about right conduct.

Personal Values

Values are the standards that provide the foundation for making decisions and guiding behavior. Individuals develop their personal values as they grow. Values are influenced by factors such as family, religious teachings, education, and personal experience. They can be identified by thinking about what is important in life. For example, while one person may place great importance on having material possessions, another believes that enjoying close relationships with friends is more important. The first individual *values* possessions; the second *values* relationships.

Values are not necessarily right or wrong, but it is important to be clear about personal values. They may conflict with situations encountered on the job. Health care workers, however, must support the decisions and practices of the facilities where they work. If this is impossible, it may be best to seek employment elsewhere. It is sometimes necessary to make personal adjustments in order to accommodate strongly held beliefs. The following example illustrates this type of situation:

Hannah is one of eight children in a Catholic family. She attended Catholic elementary and high schools and continues to attend Mass every Sunday. She believes that abortion is wrong and cannot be justified under any circumstances. Hannah recently graduated from a medical assisting program and is ready to seek employment. She realizes that she must be able to support the desires and well-being of her patients and never judge them in any way. Therefore, Hannah has decided not to work in any facility where abortions are performed. In this way, she can avoid ethical conflicts between her personal beliefs and the needs of the patients.

Cultural background and personal values may influence the choice of a specific type of work, as in the following case:

Karen Chin's family emigrated to the United States from China in 1980. Her mother's parents came with the family and have always played an important part in Karen's life. She respects her grandparents' knowledge and experience and often turned to them for advice when she was growing up. Today, in spite of health problems and the inability to handle their daily needs, they remain in the family home, cared for by younger family members.

Inspired by her home experience, Karen decided to do volunteer work in a nursing home. Karen's interest in caring for elderly patients increased. She has decided to specialize in geriatric nursing and devote her career to working with elderly patients. She wants to offer them the care and compassion that she believes the elderly deserve.

ETHICS AND THE LAW

Ethics provides the general principles on which laws are based. Put another way, laws are a means of enforcing ethical principles. For example, if a society agrees that life is precious, its members pass laws that make murder a crime. The American legal system is based on the belief that everyone must take responsibility for his or her actions (Flight, 1998). Its purpose is to require people to act in the best interest of society as a whole. For example, the Occupational Safety and Health Administration (OSHA) was created to protect the health and safety of workers. OSHA regulations provide a way to require employers to follow our society's ethical principle that human life and health are precious and should be safeguarded.

Laws, however, can conflict with the ethical principles held by some members of society. The use of marijuana for medical purposes is an example. It has been found to relieve the nausea experienced by patients undergoing chemotherapy. Its use for this purpose is illegal, however, because many people believe that it encourages inappropriate drug use, an unethical activity. Others believe that it is unethical to allow human suffering when it can be prevented. Both groups believe they are doing the "right thing" for society.

Some well-intentioned laws do not succeed in bringing about justice. Others have harmful consequences that are not recognized until after the laws are in effect. For example, legislation was passed requiring hospital emergency rooms to accept all patients who required care, regardless of their ability to pay. Many hospitals could not afford the financial losses of treating every patient who came for care. This resulted in many emergency rooms closing down, thus denying the community an important health care resource.

The third principle of the American Medical Association Principles of Medical Ethics addresses the issue of problematic laws:

A physician shall respect the law and also recognize a responsibility to seek changes in those requirements which are contrary to the best interests of the patient.

Acting in the best interest of patients is an important responsibility for health care workers. This can present difficulties if workers become aware of laws, regulations, or policies that negatively affect patient welfare. For example, a facility policy may require that patients be given medications that are less effective than more expensive products, in an attempt to control costs.

It is *never* appropriate, however, to undermine a patient's trust in the care being given by discussing what the health care worker believes to be problems with the system. For example, it would be inappropriate for nurses to inform patients about the less effective medications. It *is* proper to listen to patients' concerns and to work to promote positive changes in the system. Professional organizations often provide opportunities to discuss these issues. Many groups represent their members in promoting legislation and policies that are beneficial for both patients and health care workers.

GUIDING PRINCIPLES OF HEALTH CARE ETHICS

There are eight guiding **principles** (fundamental laws) that form the foundation for health care ethics:

1. Preserve life
2. Do good
3. Respect autonomy
4. Uphold justice
5. Be honest
6. Be discreet
7. Keep promises
8. Do no harm

These principles are discussed in the following sections, along with the corresponding laws that were created to support them. Refer to Table 3–2 to see examples of how the health care worker will apply ethical principles on the job.

Thinking it Through

Juan Ruiz is a physical therapy assistant working in a skilled nursing facility. He loves his work and enjoys helping patients regain strength and range of motion through exercise. The amount of rehabilitation that patients may receive is limited by their insurance companies and Medicare. Juan is concerned that patients who could be regaining the full use of their limbs are not being given an adequate number of sessions to reach their wellness potential. One of Juan's patients, on learning that he has only one more session with Juan, asks him if he has received "enough therapy." Juan believes that this person would benefit from at least five more sessions.

1. How should Juan respond?
2. What can he do to help the patient progress toward his full wellness potential?
3. What can Juan do to help increase the funding allocated for rehabilitation services?

Table 3–2 Applying Ethics on the Job

Ethical Principle	Examples of Health Care Worker Responsibilities
Preserve Life	• Provide all patients, including the terminally ill, with caring attention. • Learn about the stages of dying and grieving. See Chapter 8. • Become familiar with your state laws regarding organ donations.
Do Good	• Practice good oral communication skills. See Chapters 15 and 16. • Treat every patient with respect and courtesy. • Serve as a role model and promote healthy living.
Respect Autonomy	• Be sure that patients have consented to all treatment and procedures. • Become familiar with the state laws and facility policies dealing with advance directives.
Uphold Justice	• Treat all patients equally, regardless of economic or social background. • Know the rules for handling all categories of controlled substances. • Learn the state laws and your facility's policies and procedures for handling and reporting suspected abuse. • Follow all safety rules and OSHA guidelines to ensure the safety of yourself and others.
Be Honest	• Admit mistakes promptly. Offer to do whatever is necessary to correct them. • Refuse to participate in any form of fraud. • Document all procedures accurately. Perform coding accurately, if this is part of your responsibilities. • Give an "honest day's work" every day.
Be Discreet	• Never release patient information of any kind unless there is a signed release. • Do not discuss patients with *anyone* who is not professionally involved in their care. • Conduct necessary conversations about patients with other health care workers in private areas. • Keep documentation out of the view of people who are not authorized to see it. • Do not leave records or patient registers on the reception desk in plain sight of anyone who approaches the desk. • Keep phone conversations with or about patients private. • Protect the physical privacy of patients.
Keep Promises	• Be sure that necessary contracts have been completed. • Be very careful about what you say to patients. They may only hear the "good news."
Do No Harm	• Focus on providing excellent customer service. See Chapter 23. • Always work within your scope of practice. Never give information or perform duties you are not qualified to do. • Observe all safety rules and precautions. Keep areas safe from hazards. • Perform procedures according to facility protocols (standard methods for performing tasks). Never take shortcuts. • Ask an appropriate person about anything you are unsure about. • Keep your skills up to date. See Chapter 14 for more information about continuing education. • Keep certifications current (CPR, first aid, professional certifications and/or licenses). • Stay informed about new laws that affect health care.

Preserve Life

The basic guiding principle for health care workers states that life is precious and that all possible means should be taken to preserve it. The Hippocratic Oath, which has influenced medical ethics for over two thousand years, states: "I will neither give a deadly drug to anybody if asked for it, nor will I make a suggestion to this effect."

Difficulties arise when there is disagreement about the definition of "life." Advances in technology have made it possible to maintain life by artificial means, such as respirators and feeding tubes. The argument has been made that patients suffering from terminal diseases and injuries are being forced to exist under cruel and unnatural conditions. Some suggest that a better description would take the quality of life into consideration. Is it worth prolonging a life, they ask, when the patient is:

- In severe pain that cannot be relieved?
- Suffering from a terminal condition?
- In a coma with no reasonable hope of regaining consciousness?
- Without brain function?
- Requesting that treatment be discontinued?
- Asking that life be terminated?

Withdrawing artificial means of supporting life has become widely accepted, as long as this is the desire of the patient or those who are authorized to make this decision. Withholding life support can be justified, it is argued, because it simply allows an existing fatal condition to take its course (Flight, 1998). Artificial support merely delays a death that cannot be avoided.

Euthanasia

Euthanasia, also called **mercy killing**, is performing an action that results in the death of a patient to alleviate suffering or when it is believed that there is no hope for recovery. Most physicians and health care workers believe that this is contrary to their stated professional purpose. Dr. Jack Kevorkian is a Michigan physician who has assisted a number of patients in ending their lives. He believes that helping patients achieve a painless death is the kindest act a physician can perform. He argues that it is wrong to require patients to face lives that they consider unacceptable or to endure unavoidable and painful deaths. The role of the physician, in his opinion, should be to relieve suffering when recovery is impossible.

Most Americans believe that euthanasia is a form of murder. Many also express concern that, if it were legalized, it would be abused. Family members, for example, might authorize the procedure as a means of ending the physical, emotional, and financial responsibilities of caring for an ill relative. Health care providers, in an effort to manage costs, might find it more economical to end lives, than to provide the costly care required to maintain them.

Regardless of their beliefs about euthanasia, it is the duty of health care workers to follow their state laws and dedicate themselves to maintaining as high a quality of life as possible for all patients. Respecting life means giving people attention during every phase of life, even in their final days. Many terminally ill patients report that they believe they receive less attention than those for whom "there is hope." The loneliness experienced in the final days of their lives is worse than the idea of dying (Purtilo, 1990). These patients may want to talk about their lives, fears, and approaching death. Some health care workers find these topics uncomfortable and do not know how to respond. Recognizing death as a natural part of life may help the health care worker listen and react honestly to patients who need consideration and understanding in dealing with their approaching death. Avoiding terminally ill patients or hurrying through their care is unethical.

Organ Transplants

The ability of surgeons to successfully transplant organs has saved the lives of many who, without the procedure, had limited hopes for survival. At the same time, it created an ethical dilemma because not everyone agrees to have their own organs, or those of family members, donated at the time of their death. While the organs harvested from one person can save the lives of as many as eight others, it is illegal to take organs without the prior permission of the patient or, following death, family members. Payment cannot be given to donors or to their survivors. To further prevent abuse, it is illegal for the physician who pronounces the donor's death to participate on the transplant surgical team.

Do Good

Helping and promoting the welfare of others is a basic duty of the health care worker. The needs of patients must be considered before the needs of self. Personal convenience is always secondary to patient welfare.

Working in the best interest of patients requires the following:

- Listening carefully to what they say
- Understanding their cultural backgrounds

Thinking it Through

Dr. C. Everett Koop, formerly Surgeon General of the United States, presents the following situation. It involves a 5-year-old girl who has a type of childhood brain tumor that Dr. Koop has studied for many years. The child's original tumor was removed, but has recurred in spite of all known treatment. Dr. Koop writes: "I know her days are limited and that the longer she lives the more likely she is to have considerable pain. She might also become both blind and deaf." He goes on to explain that the child is severely anemic and this causes her to be unaware of what is happening to her. If he treats the anemia, this may prolong her life. At the same time, it will increase her awareness of pain and ability to understand her situation. Anticancer drugs can be prescribed, but he knows these have no chance of curing the child. Dr. Koop poses the question "Would it be better to let this little girl slip into death quietly . . . or should we prolong her life?"

1. It can be argued that it is Dr. Koop's responsibility as a physician to treat all aspects of the child's condition, including the anemia. Do you agree? Explain your answer.

2. Should anyone else be involved in making the decision about how to treat this child? Explain why.

3. Discuss what you think should be done for this child.

- Carefully assessing their needs
- Being aware of their ethical beliefs
- Explaining what you are doing as you perform tests, treatments, and other procedures
- Providing appropriate instruction

Part of the appeal of health care work is the potential to promote the well-being of the community. Health care workers should serve as role models, in exemplifying healthy living practices. Providing positive examples can have a significant impact. See Chapter 12, "Lifestyle Management."

Health care workers are paid by their employer for their services and should never accept monetary tips from patients. "Doing good" includes the idea of performing one's job without the expectation of receiving anything extra.

Respect Autonomy

Americans value **autonomy**, which means self-determination. Patients have the right to make decisions about their health care. They can choose who, if anyone, will treat them and what treatments they will undergo. As much as possible, based on their physical and mental capabilities and age, they should be involved in their own care.

This right is formalized in the Patient's Bill of Rights, developed in 1992 by the American Hospital Association. The introduction to this important document includes the statement that "Hospitals must ensure a health care ethic that respects the role of patients in decision making about treatment choices and other aspects of their care." See Box 3–3 for the full text.

Consent

Medical treatment cannot be carried out unless the patient gives his or her **consent** (permission). When a procedure has been explained, including possible consequences, the patient's permission is known as **informed consent**. Touching a patient or performing a procedure without his or her permission can result in being charged with the crime of **battery**, which refers to any unauthorized touching of another person. If a patient feels threatened about receiving unwanted treatment, even if it is not performed, this can result in the crime of **assault**. Assault, in this case, is any threatened or implied act, whether carried out or not. (This use of the word should not be confused with an alternate definition of "assault" meaning a violent, physical attack.) It does not matter if the patient benefits from the treatment. The only difference between proper medical treatment and the crimes of assault and battery is whether the patient gives permission. An exception is emergency care administered when the patient is physically unable to give consent. This is discussed in Chapter 21.

Battery can also be charged if patients are handled more roughly than necessary. Flight (1998) describes a case in which a physician spanks a 4-year-old child who refuses to lie still while he is removing her sutures (stitches). The spanking causes bruises that last for three weeks. The mother successfully sues the physician for assault and battery.

Box 3–3   American Hospital Association's Patient's Bill of Rights (1973)

1. The patient has the right to considerate and respectful care.

2. The patient has the right to obtain from his physician complete current information concerning his diagnosis, treatment, and prognosis in terms the patient can be reasonably expected to understand. When it is not medically advisable to give such information to the patient, the information should be made available to an appropriate person in his behalf. He has the right to know by name, the physician responsible for coordinating his care.

3. The patient has the right to receive from his physician information necessary to give informed consent prior to the start of any procedure and/or treatment. Except in emergencies, such information for informed consent should include but not necessarily be limited to the specific procedure and/or treatment, the medically significant risks involved, and the probable duration of incapacitation. Where medically significant alternatives for care or treatment exist, or when the patient requests information concerning medical alternatives, the patient has the right to such information. The patient also has the right to know the name of the person responsible for the procedures and/or treatment.

4. The patient has the right to refuse treatment to the extent permitted by law, and to be informed of the medical consequences of his action.

5. The patient has the right to every consideration of his privacy concerning his own medical care program. Case discussion, consultation, examination, and treatment are confidential and should be conducted discreetly. Those not directly involved in his care must have the permission of the patient to be present.

6. The patient has the right to expect that all communications and records pertaining to his care should be treated as confidential.

7. The patient has the right to expect that within its capacity the hospital must make a reasonable response to the request of a patient for services. The hospital must provide evaluation, service, and/or referral as indicated by the urgency of the case. When medically permissible a patient may be transferred to another facility only after he has received complete information and explanation concerning the needs for and alternatives to such a transfer. The institution to which the patient is to be transferred must first have accepted the patient for transfer.

8. The patient has the right to obtain information as to any relationship of his hospital to other health care and educational institutions insofar as his care is concerned. The patient has the right to obtain information as to the existence of any professional relationship among individuals, by name, who are treating him.

9. The patient has the right to be advised if the hospital proposes to engage in or perform human experimentation affecting his care or treatment. The patient has the right to refuse to participate in such research projects.

10. The patient has the right to expect reasonable continuity of care. He has the right to know in advance what appointment times and physicians are available and where. The patient has the right to expect that the hospital will provide a mechanism whereby he is informed by his physician or delegate of the physician of the patient's continuing health care requirements following discharge.

11. The patient has the right to examine and receive an explanation of his bill regardless of source of payment.

12. The patient has the right to know what hospital rules and regulations apply to his conduct as a patient.

Reprinted with permission of the American Hospital Association.

The patient's full consent must be obtained before performing any procedure. A resisted action, done "for the good of the patient," may be illegal and result in criminal charges or a lawsuit. Particular care should be taken when using any type of restraint, especially with an uncooperative patient. The health care worker must always use proper techniques when moving patients to prevent pulling on limbs or other unintended roughness.

Excessive persuasion is also a form of assault. A patient who feels "talked into" a procedure may charge assault and battery. For example, a woman who believes she was pressured to be sterilized by having her tubes tied, against her true wishes, may successfully sue. Patients who are worried about health problems and/or financial matters often feel afraid and confused. They may accept the advice of a health care provider, only to change their minds later.

There are two types of informed consent: implied and express. **Implied consent** is indicated by the patient's actions: showing up for a medical appointment, opening the mouth for the dentist to administer an injection, or participating in therapeutic exercises. **Express consent** is given in writing and is required for many procedures, especially those that are invasive. **Invasive procedures** involve punctures or incisions of the skin or insertion of instruments or foreign material into the body (Miller-Keane, 1997).

Informed consent (implied or express) clearly advises the patient about the following:

- Procedure or treatment plan
- Possible risks
- Expected results
- Alternative procedures with benefits and risks
- Consequences if procedure is not performed

See Box 3–4 for a model consent form.

The conditions under which a consent form is signed are important. It is not sufficient that patients be given full information. They must understand it as well. If necessary, a translator must be provided. This includes patients and parents giving permission for the treatment of minor children. If they do not understand English or are hearing impaired, means must be arranged to ensure that they completely understand all the required items listed above for informed consent.

A written consent form does not protect the health care provider if the patient claims to have signed under pressure. It is essential that patients understand it is their right to refuse treatment and that signing is completely voluntary. It is legal for patients to refuse treatment, even if doing so may damage their health.

Consent forms can legally be signed by mentally competent adults (who are not impaired by medication). In most states, **adult** is defined as someone over 18 years of age. **Emancipated minors** are individuals under the age of 18 who are financially independent, married, or in the military. They are legally considered to be adults and can sign consent forms on their own behalf for treatment. Individuals under the age of 18 who are not emancipated minors will require a consent form signed by a parent or guardian before a procedure is performed. Many states allow non-emancipated minors as young as 14 to make decisions regarding their health care. Some states do not require parental permission

for minors to receive birth control information, abortions, or drug counseling. It is essential that health care workers learn the laws in the state where they work and keep up with changes to them.

A claim of **false imprisonment** can be charged if patients are held against their will, unless they are mentally incompetent or a danger to themselves. For example, a person cannot be kept in a hospital or clinic "for his own good" because he needs medical attention. Without the patient's consent, release is the only option. Patients may be asked to sign a statement that they are discontinuing care against medical advice.

Box 3–4 Consent for Treatment

Date _____ Time _____

I authorize the performance of the following procedure (s) _____ on _____ (name of patient) _____ to be performed by _____ (name of physician) _____ , MD.

The following have been explained to _____ by Dr. _____ (name of physician) _____ .

Nature of the procedure _____ (describe procedure) _____

For the purpose of _____

The possible alternative methods of treatment are _____

The risks involve the possibility of _____

The possible complications of this procedure are _____

I have been advised of the serious nature of this procedure and have been further advised that if I desire a more detailed explanation of any of the foregoing or further information about the possible risks or complications, it will be given to me.

I do not request a more detailed listing and explanation of the above information.

Signed _____
(Patient/Parent/Guardian)

Witnessed by: _____

This protects the facility and professional staff from liability (blame) if the patient suffers harm as a result of refusing treatment.

Advance Directives

Self-determination is possible for patients who become unable to make decisions about their care through the use of **advance directives**. These are written instructions that outline patients' desires regarding care should they become unable, as the result of illness or injury, to make these decisions. Two major forms of advance directives are described below:

1. **Living will**: This document outlines the patient's wishes regarding the type and extent of care to be given. Specific directions can be included that list whether the patient consents to certain procedures such as cardiac resuscitation, mechanical respiration, and feeding tubes. The request "Do not resuscitate" (DNR) can be included. This means that CPR is not to be administered if the patient stops breathing. Living wills are regulated by state laws. See Figure 3–1 for an example.
2. **Durable power of attorney for health care**: In this document patients designate specific people to act on their behalf if they become unable to make health care decisions. Anyone can be assigned, whether related to the patient or not. Each state has specific requirements for durable powers of attorney. When applied specifically to health care, a durable power of attorney is sometimes known as the *designation of a health care surrogate*. See Figure 3–2 for an example.

The Patient Self-Determination Act passed in 1991 is federal **legislation** (law) that requires hospitals, nursing homes, rehabilitation facilities, and hospices to have written policies about advanced directives and to communicate these policies to patients when they are admitted. While it is not legally required for patients to prepare advance directives, they must be informed of their right to have them.

Problems can arise when patients do not indicate their wishes while they are competent to do so. Family members and physicians may disagree about the proper course of action. In some cases, the courts are called on to make the final decision. A well-publicized case involved Nancy Kruzan, a young woman who was the victim of a car accident. She remained in a coma for many

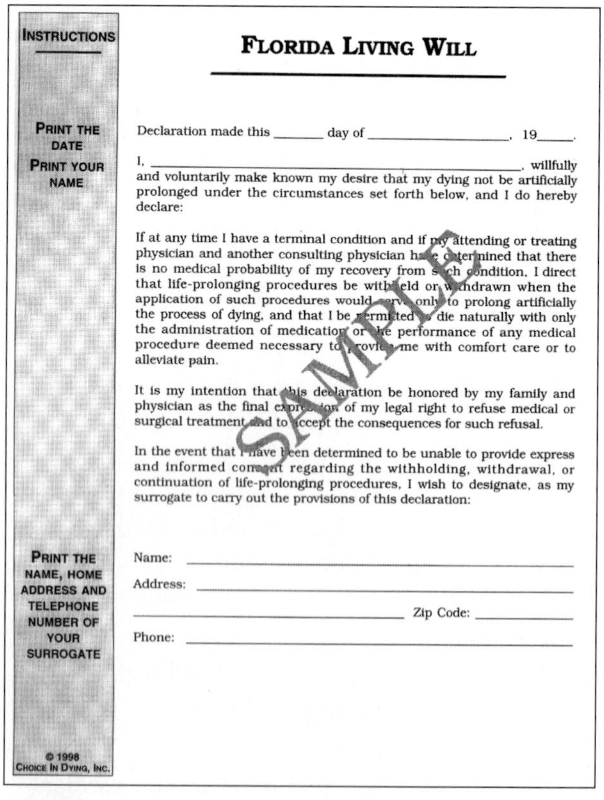

INSTRUCTIONS

FLORIDA LIVING WILL

PRINT THE DATE — Declaration made this ______ day of ________________, 19____.

PRINT YOUR NAME — I, ______________________________, willfully and voluntarily make known my desire that my dying not be artificially prolonged under the circumstances set forth below, and I do hereby declare:

If at any time I have a terminal condition and if my attending or treating physician and another consulting physician have determined that there is no medical probability of my recovery from such condition, I direct that life-prolonging procedures be withheld or withdrawn when the application of such procedures would serve only to prolong artificially the process of dying, and that I be permitted to die naturally with only the administration of medication or the performance of any medical procedure deemed necessary to provide me with comfort care or to alleviate pain.

It is my intention that this declaration be honored by my family and physician as the final expression of my legal right to refuse medical or surgical treatment and to accept the consequences for such refusal.

In the event that I have been determined to be unable to provide express and informed consent regarding the withholding, withdrawal, or continuation of life-prolonging procedures, I wish to designate, as my surrogate to carry out the provisions of this declaration:

PRINT THE NAME, HOME ADDRESS AND TELEPHONE NUMBER OF YOUR SURROGATE

Name: ______________________

Address: ______________________

______________________ Zip Code: ________

Phone: ______________________

SAMPLE

© 1998 CHOICE IN DYING, INC.

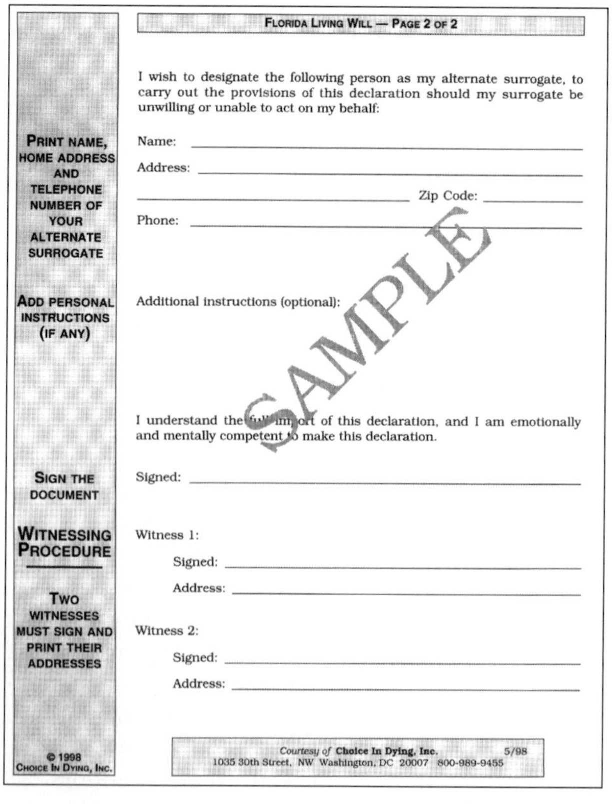

FLORIDA LIVING WILL — PAGE 2 OF 2

I wish to designate the following person as my alternate surrogate, to carry out the provisions of this declaration should my surrogate be unwilling or unable to act on my behalf:

PRINT NAME, HOME ADDRESS AND TELEPHONE NUMBER OF YOUR ALTERNATE SURROGATE

Name: ______________________

Address: ______________________

______________________ Zip Code: ________

Phone: ______________________

ADD PERSONAL INSTRUCTIONS (IF ANY) — Additional instructions (optional):

I understand the full import of this declaration, and I am emotionally and mentally competent to make this declaration.

SIGN THE DOCUMENT — Signed: ______________________

WITNESSING PROCEDURE

TWO WITNESSES MUST SIGN AND PRINT THEIR ADDRESSES

Witness 1:

Signed: ______________________

Address: ______________________

Witness 2:

Signed: ______________________

Address: ______________________

SAMPLE

© 1998 CHOICE IN DYING, INC.

Courtesy of **Choice In Dying, Inc.** 5/98
1035 30th Street, NW Washington, DC 20007 800-989-9455

Figure 3–1 A living will helps ensure that the patient's wishes are carried out. Reprinted by permission of Choice in Dying, Inc., 1035 30th St., N.W., Washington, DC 20007-3823, 1-800-989-WILL.

years, kept alive in a vegetative state by a feeding tube. Her parents wanted the support removed, but the hospital refused, stating that it was not clear that Nancy would have chosen that action. The courts upheld the hospital's decision for many years until finally making the decision to allow life support to be discontinued.

Uphold Justice

Justice refers to fairness. Justice requires that all patients, regardless of race, economic status, religion, nationality, or personal characteristics, receive the same care and consideration.

Illness and injury do not always bring out the best in human nature. Patients may experience fear and anxiety. Health problems shake self-confidence and upset otherwise stable lives. Patients can be unreasonable, unpleasant, and uncooperative. It is these very patients who most need respect and consideration. To disregard or take advantage of them in any way is highly unethical.

The equitable distribution of health care resources is currently an issue of great concern to Americans. The high cost of health care has resulted in restrictions being set by managed care organizations and insurance companies. See Chapter 22.

Health care workers can experience great ethical conflict when confronted with the following:

- Limits on the length of hospital stays
- A prescribed amount of time that the health care provider can spend with each patient
- Substitution of less-expensive medications or limitations on medications allowed
- Limited number of therapy sessions reimbursed for a given health condition
- Restrictions on the number and type of diagnostic tests allowed for a given set of symptoms
- Denial of experimental treatments that might help patients
- Fewer diagnostic tests and less overall care given to patients who do not have medical insurance and are unable to pay themselves than are given to patients who can pay

In spite of current cost-cutting measures, there are still millions of Americans who cannot afford to purchase health insurance. Many fall into the category of the "working poor." These people earn too much to qualify for government assistance, but not enough to purchase insurance. See Chapter 22. Providing health care coverage to all Americans, regardless of their ability to pay, is a major concern that has yet to be resolved.

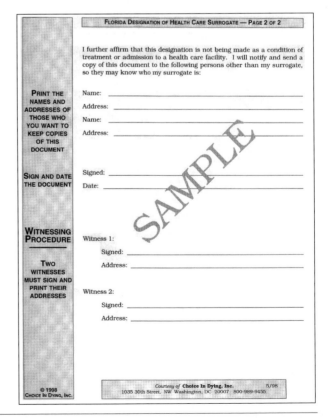

Figure 3–2 A power of attorney designates someone to act on behalf of the patient. Reprinted by permission of Choice in Dying, Inc., 1035 30th St., N.W., Washington, DC 20007-3823, 1-800-989-WILL.

Some states are working to expand the number of people who have access to medical care. For example, the state of Oregon has developed a plan to cover more people under Medicaid. To ensure that the additional costs can be covered, the medical conditions that the state will pay for have been restricted. To determine which would be paid for, the legislature approved the ranking of health care services using the following criteria:

■ Public's perception of value

■ Effectiveness or outcome

■ Cost

Prenatal care was ranked as the most valuable, infertility treatment and cosmetic surgery ranked as the least. Oregonians made the decision that providing basic medical care to everyone was more desirable than providing unlimited services to a smaller number of people (Edge and Groves, 1999).

Organs needed for life-saving transplants are not available to all who need them. How can fair decisions be made about who receives an organ among the many people who need them? Is one patient more "deserving" than another? The American Medical Association has created the following guidelines for making decisions about transplants and the distribution of other limited resources:

■ Decisions must be based on fair and socially acceptable criteria.

■ Priority should be given to the person most likely to receive the greatest long-term benefit.

■ Social prominence and age of the individual cannot be deciding factors.
(Adapted from *Lippincott's textbook for medical assistants*, by J. Hosley, S. Jones, and E. Molle-Matthews, 1997, Philadelphia: Lippincott.)

Reporting Abuse

Justice also refers to the use of authority or power to uphold what is right or lawful. Our society encourages us to protect each other from harm. This principle supports the laws that require health care workers, among others, to report suspected abuse. The Federal Child Abuse Prevention and Treatment Act was passed to require the reporting of physical and mental abuse of children and to protect those who do the reporting. Patient confidentiality does not exist in cases of suspected abuse.

The health care worker must be aware of the signs of possible child abuse and report any suspicions to the supervisor. These signs may be physical or behavioral and include the following:

■ Bruises and welts

■ Burns

■ Lacerations and abrasions

■ Skeletal injuries

■ Head injuries

■ Repeated injuries at a higher rate than normal for a child of the same age

■ Different explanations for the cause of an injury given by the child and the parent

■ Unusually compliant, fearful, or aggressive behavior of the child

With the increasing number of older citizens, elder abuse is a growing problem. The number of reported cases increased 150% between 1986 and 1996 (National Center on Elder Abuse). Estimates are that about 10% of people aged 65 and older are abused or neglected in some way (Tuttle-Yoder and Fraser-Nobbe, 1996). It may be committed by a spouse, other family members, or paid caregivers, and can occur in various forms:

■ Neglect and lack of proper physical care

■ Taking financial and other resources without the permission or understanding of the elder

■ Physical mistreatment

■ Mental and emotional abuse

■ Abandonment

Most states require the reporting of elder abuse. The principal public agencies responsible for investigating elder abuse and providing treatment and protective services are the Adult Protective

Thinking it Through

Oregon's proposed solution to the need for health care coverage has been called a "rationing system" by opponents. They believe that physicians do not have the right to deny coverage of medical treatment of any type.

1. Do you agree or disagree with the concept of basic coverage for everyone, if some treatments and procedures cannot be covered? Explain your reasons.

2. Who should decide which procedures will be paid for and which will not?

3. How would you rank medical procedures? Which ones should never be denied? Are there any that you believe that patients should be required to pay for themselves?

Services, the area agency on aging, or the county department of social services. Most states have an elder abuse hotline. Even if not required by law, it is the ethical duty of health care workers to report suspected cases of elder abuse to their supervisor. Health care facilities have reporting procedures for handling all types of suspected abuse (for example, spousal abuse). Health care workers must be familiar with the reporting procedures for their facility.

Laws That Protect

Americans believe that government has an ethical obligation to protect all citizens. For example, employers may not take advantage of employees by exposing them to dangerous working conditions. The Occupational Safety and Health Act was established in 1970 by the federal government. The act requires employers to accept responsibility for the safety and health of their employees. Health care employers are directed under OSHA to take measures to prevent workers from contracting contagious diseases. Specifically, there must be a written plan that includes waste management procedures, personal protection methods, and employee training programs.

The prevention of behaviors that lead to individual and social harm is another responsibility that the government believes it has an ethical obligation to perform. Drug abuse is an example of a behavior considered to be harmful to not only the individual, but to society as a whole. The Controlled Substances Act is a federal law regulated by the Drug Enforcement Agency (DEA) to help prevent the misuse of addictive substances. Drugs that have addictive potential are classified into five categories. Each group has specific guidelines for medical use, including prescribing and handling. Violations of these laws are criminal acts and can result in fines and imprisonment.

Be Honest

Good health care relies on honesty. Patients' trust in the health care worker is an important factor in their well-being, and trust is built on honesty. Truth-telling is also critical among coworkers and with supervisors. This is not always easy. For example, if you make a mistake in performing a lab test, it is tempting to "forget" to mention it. Mistakes, however, can have serious consequences and must be admitted and corrected as quickly as possible.

Fraud is a form of dishonesty that involves cheating or trickery, and there are several forms that occur in health care:

- Submitting insurance claims for services not performed

- Charging different rates for insured and uninsured patients
- Selling treatments, drugs, and devices that have not been proven effective
- Claiming to have a degree, experience, or credentials that one does not have

Medical fraud can result in severe penalties, ranging from losing the right to bill Medicare to imprisonment.

The health care worker who dedicates time on the job to his or her service of the employer and patients is behaving honestly. Arriving late, using paid time to perform personal tasks, and socializing with coworkers rather than attending to patients are forms of dishonesty. Accepting payment to work in a health care position indicates agreement to do the tasks expected for that occupation. Conducting oneself honestly and ethically on the job means making work a priority and striving to do your best every day.

Be Discreet

Being **discreet** means being careful about what you say, preserving confidences, and respecting privacy. In health care, this is not only one of the most important ethical principles, it is the law. Patients have a legal right to privacy concerning their medical affairs. This is referred to as **confidentiality**. Violating that right, even if well intentioned, can result in a lawsuit.

Patient information cannot be released to anyone without the patient's written approval. See Box 3–5. This includes relatives, friends, insurance companies, and others who may claim to

Thinking it Through

Carin is a medical assistant for Dr. Allen, a dermatologist who has been in practice for many years. During his first 20 years in practice, Dr. Allen had a registered nurse assisting him in the office. When speaking with patients, he often refers to Carin as "my nurse."

1. Do you believe that Dr. Allen is misleading his patients?
2. Why or why not?
3. What could be the consequences?
4. How should Carin handle this situation?

have the "right to know." The only exceptions are disclosures and reports allowed or required by law such as births, deaths, certain infectious and communicable diseases, abuse, and life-threatening injuries caused by violence. The exact requirements and methods for reporting vary by location.

Box 3–5   Authorization to Release Health Care Information

Patient _____ Date of Birth _____

SSN _____ Previous name _____

I request and authorize _____ to release health care information of the patient named above to:

Name _____

Address _____

This request and authorization applies to: (Please initial the appropriate box)

____Health care information **EXCLUDING** specific information relating to sexually transmitted diseases (including HIV/AIDS), alcohol or drug use, or visits related to psychiatric disorders or mental health.

____All health care information **INCLUDING** specific information relating to sexually transmitted diseases (including HIV/AIDS), alcohol or drug use, or visits related to psychiatric disorders or mental health.

____Other:_____

I understand that my express consent is required to release any health care information relating to testing, diagnosis, and/or treatment of HIV (AIDS virus), sexually-transmitted diseases, psychiatric disorders/mental health, or drug and/or alcohol use. If I have been tested, diagnosed, or treated for HIV (AIDS virus), sexually-transmitted diseases, psychiatric disorders/mental health, or drug and/or alcohol use, you are specifically authorized to release all health care information relating to such diagnosis, testing, or treatment.

_____ / _____

Signature of patient or   Relationship
patient's authorized   to patient
representative

_____

Date

Health care workers should not talk about patients with coworkers where they might be overheard by other people. They must remember that hospital cafeterias and clinic elevators are used by the public and are inappropriate locations for such discussions. Reports to friends and family about your work that include the mention of patients must be avoided. Even without giving the names of patients, there may be enough details revealed so that others can guess their identities.

Individual rights to privacy sometimes conflict with the public's right to be informed about matters concerning its safety. An incident in Baltimore illustrates this dilemma. Fire fighters assisted an injured woman and took her to the hospital. The hospital staff was aware that the woman had AIDS, but was forbidden by doctor-patient confidentiality laws to inform the fire fighters that they had been exposed to the virus (Flight, 1998).

Another difficult situation occurs when patients tell health care workers in confidence information that, if not revealed, may result in harm to the patients themselves or to others. For example, if a patient discloses that she plans to use prescription drugs to end her life after her release from the hospital, the health care worker has a duty to inform the patient's physician. Health care workers must tell their supervisors of patient confidences if they believe that harm may result if they do not reveal certain information.

Disclosing unauthorized information can result in being charged with harming the reputation of another. This is known as **defamation of character**. In written form it is called **libel**. In spoken form it is called **slander**. These are serious charges and can result from innocent, but careless behavior. For example, reporting a patient's AIDS test results within the hearing of others could result in charges of slander.

Take care when working with patients to protect their physical privacy. Shut the doors of occupied examination rooms, close curtains around hospital beds when performing procedures, and drape patients properly to ensure that there is no more exposure than necessary. If patients must move from one area to another, be sure they are covered properly and do not pass through a public area.

Keep Promises

In everyday life, promises are an important part of our relationships with others. **Contracts** are formalized promises that are enforceable by law. They contain the agreements of people to do certain specified things. For example, a contract is formed

Thinking it Through

A nurse who worked at the Baltimore hospital in the fire-fighter example decided to tell the fire fighters that they had been exposed to AIDS.

1. Do you believe that she did the right thing? Explain your answer.

2. Do you think that breaking the rules of confidentiality was justified in this case?

3. Do you think this nurse should be fired for her actions?

4. Did the nurse commit slander against the woman?

5. What might you do in a similar situation?

6. What consequences would you be willing to accept in order to carry out your ethical responsibilities?

when an orthopedic surgeon agrees to perform a knee replacement and the patient agrees to pay for the procedure. If one of the parties fails to fulfill his or her part of the agreement, this can result in a **breach of contract**. If this failure results in a loss for the other party, a court may award money to make up for this loss.

In order for a contract to be enforceable, it must contain three components:

1. *Offer*: This is the action that starts the process of forming a contract. Examples:

   - Mr. Nguyen visits the dentist because of a toothache. His attendance is considered a request for the dentist to enter into a contract to provide treatment.

   - Marcia Parsons is referred to a physical therapist. By making an appointment with the therapist, she initiates a contract.

2. *Acceptance*: This means that both parties–the patient and the health care provider–agree to enter into the contract. They each agree to do something. Examples:

   - The dentist agrees to treat Mr. Nguyen.

   - The physical therapist sets a time to see Ms. Parsons.

3. *Consideration*: Something of value must be exchanged by the parties. In health care this generally means that the professional provides

a service and the patient pays for the service. Examples:

- The dentist examines Mr. Nguyen, takes x-rays, and fills a cavity. The patient pays for the service before leaving the office.

- The physical therapist teaches Ms. Parsons to perform a series of leg-strengthening exercises. The patient provides information about her medical insurance coverage and also agrees to pay for any portion not covered by the insurance plan.

In order for a contract to be enforceable, the people who enter it must be competent. The law defines competency by age and mental condition, as it does with consent. State laws govern who may legally enter into a contract. In addition, the actions agreed to must be legal. Suppose that a patient requests his physician to assist him in ending his life (committing suicide). In spite of the action being illegal, the physician agrees. If the drug given does not end the life of the patient as promised, he cannot legally sue the physician for breach of contract because the action agreed to was illegal. (The physician might be charged with a criminal action, however.)

Most contracts between health care providers and patients are **implied contracts**. This means that the actions of the parties create the contract. In the dental example above, the actions of visiting the dentist, filling the tooth, and paying for the service fulfill the requirements of an implied contract. Giving emergency treatment is also a form of implied contract.

An **express contract** is created when the parties discuss and agree on specific terms and conditions. The contract can be either written or oral. It is important for the health care worker to avoid making statements that might be interpreted as a contract. While it is natural to want to reassure and encourage patients, this should never be confused with giving what might be understood as a guarantee or false hope. Being "too nice" as the result of good intentions can cause legal difficulties, as illustrated in the following example:

A middle-aged man was worried after a consultation with a surgeon. "Looks like I'll have to have a heart bypass," the patient remarked to the assistant at the front desk.

"Don't worry," she assured him, "the doctor is very good at that procedure. You won't have any trouble. I can promise you that."

There were several complications during the surgery, and the patient died several weeks later. His family successfully sued the surgeon on the grounds that his assistant had made a promise that amounted to a warranty (Flight, 1998, p. 82).

The surgeon in this case was sued because the assistant was acting as his **agent**. An agent is someone who has the authority to represent another person. Health care workers are generally considered to be agents of the licensed professionals for whom they work. Employers are held liable (legally responsible) for the behavior and actions of their employees. This concept is known as **respondeat superior**, which means "let the master answer." The following examples illustrate this concept:

- A physician could be held liable for the consequences of a medical assistant administering the wrong medication.
- A patient suffering injuries from a fall caused by the incompetence of a physical therapist assistant could be awarded **damages** (money to compensate for an injury or loss). The supervising therapist could be financially responsible.

Do No Harm

An essential responsibility of health care workers is to *do no harm*. They must work within their scope of practice, performing only those duties that they have been trained to do. It is critical that safety rules be followed and that medical advice never be given by a person who is not qualified to do so.

Harm can result from **negligence**. This is failure to meet the standard of care that can be reasonably expected from a person with certain training and experience. Negligence can result from an action performed incorrectly or from the failure to take a necessary action. People who are trained in health care are expected to have special knowledge and skills. Thus, they are held to a higher standard of care than those who are untrained. There are various levels of standards within the health care professions:

- A physical therapist (PT) is held to a higher standard of care than a physical therapist assistant (PTA).
- The PTA is held to a higher standard than the PT aide.
- The PT aide is held to a higher standard than an untrained person.

Malpractice is the term for professional negligence. Malpractice lawsuits are filed by patients who believe they have received improper care. It is important to understand, however, that not all lawsuits are the result of actual malpractice. Leading causes of lawsuits are patient anger and the lack of a satisfactory personal relationship with the health care provider. Good interpersonal relationships are a key factor in preventing malpractice lawsuits. Most patients understand that positive treatment results cannot be guaranteed. But they want to be treated with dignity and to feel that everything possible has been done to help them. Patients who perceive a lack of attention, care, and respect are much more likely to sue than those who feel positive about their care. As Flight (1998) describes it, ". . . anger is the thread running through the entire malpractice saga" (p. 114). Communicating well and treating patients with kindness and respect are the most effective ways to reduce the risk of being sued. See Figure 3–3. See Chapter 23 for more information about providing good customer service.

Good Samaritan Laws

Good Samaritan Laws have been passed by states to protect health care workers from liability when they give care in emergency situations. In order to be held liable, further injury must be caused intentionally or from extreme carelessness. Even in an emergency, it is important for health care workers not to offer aid beyond their scope of training. Good Samaritan Laws are discussed further in Chapter 21.

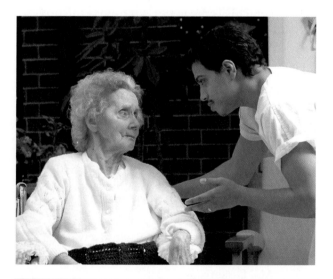

Figure 3–3 Communicating a sincere, caring attitude toward patients is the best defense against malpractice lawsuits.

Thinking it Through

A report was issued in February 2000, indicating that 98,000 people die annually as a result of medical errors. President Clinton requested a law to require the public reporting of these errors. He believes that this will improve the overall quality of medical care. Some health care providers argue that this will result in an increase in failures to report errors and a lack of follow-up to correct them.

1. Do you believe that medical errors should be reported publicly? Explain your answer.
2. How serious should errors be to report them within the organization? Outside the organization?
3. Who should be responsible for tracking and handling medical errors?
4. What do you think might be the consequences if this law is passed?

HANDLING ETHICAL DILEMMAS

The first consideration of the ethical health care worker is the well-being of patients. Illegal and unethical behavior can endanger patient welfare and cannot be tolerated. Observations of this behavior in others must not be ignored. While it is difficult to confront a wrong-doer or "tell on" a coworker, doing what is right must override short-term discomfort. Accepting responsibility for making difficult decisions is part of health care work.

If the behavior observed in a coworker is illegal, it should be reported to the supervisor. For example, if a nurse observes a coworker using an illegal substance at the workplace, it should be reported immediately to the supervisor. If the behavior involves legal, but ethically questionable behavior, such as "badmouthing" an employer, it is best to speak directly to the coworker.

WHO DECIDES?

When an individual or an organization is faced with a case that presents special ethical difficulties, there are several sources of help:

- The American Medical Association Council on Ethical and Judicial Affairs reviews situations and publishes their opinions about current issues to provide guidelines for physicians.
- Hospitals and other large health care facilities have ethics committees composed of health care professionals and members of the community. These committees review individual cases and make recommendations.
- Clergy and counselors provide assistance to health care professionals in making decisions and dealing with personal feelings when coping with difficult situations.
- Conferences are held among the health care team members, the patient, and family members to explore possible actions.
- Many universities and medical colleges study ethical issues and share their findings.
- Hospitals and clinics may have a risk management department. Lawyers and specially trained health care professionals are charged with making ethical and legal decisions on behalf of the organization.

SUGGESTED LEARNING ACTIVITIES

1. Locate and read articles in the newspaper and news magazines about ethical issues. Do you agree with the points of view presented?
2. Secure a copy of the code of ethics for your occupational area of interest. Can you find statements that correspond to the ethical principles presented in this chapter?
3. Explore your personal beliefs about ethical issues such as abortion, euthanasia, and individual privacy versus the public's right to know.
4. Contact the Child Protective Unit of your state's Department of Social Services for information about reporting child abuse.
5. Request information about elder abuse from the American Council on Aging or your state's department on aging, located in the state department of human services. You can also learn more from the National Center on Elder Abuse's web site at http://www.gwjapan.com/ncea/. This site includes a list of elder abuse hotlines.

6. Contact a local health care facility and ask for a copy of their patient consent form.

REVIEW QUESTIONS

1. What is the purpose of ethics?
2. What is the purpose of a professional code of ethics?
3. How are ethics and laws related?
4. For each of the following ethical principles, explain its application to health care and describe the laws that support it.
   - Preserve life
   - Do good
   - Respect autonomy
   - Uphold justice
   - Be honest
   - Be discreet
   - Keep promises
   - Do no harm

APPLICATION EXERCISES

1. Refer to the Case of the Missing Consent Form at the beginning of this chapter. Put together a list of the legal implications that might have resulted if the consent form was not signed.

2. You are working as a licensed practical nurse in a small urgent care center. You love the work. The physicians are excellent, and you have the opportunity to work with a wide variety of patients. You have become good friends with your coworkers and enjoy an especially close relationship with the administrative medical assistant, Amy. One day you observe Amy removing medication from the drug cabinet. You find this to be unusual because the administrative staff do not normally work with medications. While performing a routine inventory check later that day, you discover a shortage of a drug that is classified as a controlled substance. Explain what you would do in this situation.

SUGGESTED READINGS AND RESOURCES

Death and Dying, euthanasia:
http://dying.about.com/msub18.htm

Edge, R. S. and Groves, J. R. (1999). *Ethics of health care: A guide for clinical practice.* Albany, NY: Delmar.

Flight, M. (1998). *Law, liability, and ethics for health care professionals* (3rd ed.). Albany, NY: Delmar.

Hosley, J., Jones, S., and Molle-Matthews, E. (1997). *Lippincott's textbook for medical assistants.* Philadelphia: Lippincott.

Purtilo, R. and Haddad, A. (1996). *Health care professionals and patient interaction* (5th ed.). Philadelphia: W. B. Sanders Company.

UNIT

THE LANGUAGE OF HEALTH CARE

2

CHAPTER

MEDICAL TERMINOLOGY

OBJECTIVES

Studying and applying the material in this chapter will help you to:

- Understand the importance of being able to write, read, and communicate using medical terminology.

- Identify common roots and combining forms, suffixes, and prefixes.

- Break down medical terms into their component parts and interpret the terms correctly.

- Use the spelling and pronunciation guidelines for medical terms derived from Greek and Latin.

- Define common abbreviations and interpret common symbols.

- Evaluate the features of a medical dictionary to determine its value as a reference for your specialty area.

- Approach the learning of medical terminology by using a variety of study techniques.

KEY TERMS

combining form
combining vowel
consonant
medical terminology
prefix
root
suffix

The Case of

"Where Is the Pain?"

Dr. Chen states that Ms. Mitchell called yesterday complaining of *epigastric* (ep ih GAS trick) pain and requests that LaTonya, the medical receptionist, call her to follow up and find out if she is feeling any better. LaTonya calls Ms. Mitchell and says, "Dr. Chen has asked me to call and ask how the epigastric pain is today." Ms. Mitchell is confused and says, "I'm not sure what you mean. What is epigastric?" LaTonya doesn't know what "epigastric" means, and this has prevented LaTonya from restating the question in terms that the patient can understand.

Health care workers must know medical terminology, such as this term (which means "over the stomach"). Failure to learn medical language prevents them from communicating effectively with other health care professionals and with patients. This chapter will help students start learning this new language.

IMPORTANCE OF MEDICAL TERMINOLOGY

Understanding and correctly using **medical terminology** is essential to your career in health care. The study of medical terminology includes not only learning medical terms, but also the associated abbreviations and symbols. Medical terminology is used during conversations with other health professionals, in medical charting and documentation, and in professional journals and texts. It adds necessary preciseness to professional communications. For example, when directions for procedures are described using exact language, there is less chance for confusion and error.

Patients can receive ineffective or even harmful treatment if words or abbreviations are misunderstood. For example, if the physician orders eye drops to be instilled in one of the eyes and the order reads "O.D.," a medication error will result if the health care worker interprets this to mean left eye, rather than right.

It is not always appropriate to use medical language. Most patients find the use of technical words confusing. They may be intimidated and will hesitate to ask for an explanation. When communicating with patients it is essential to first determine their level of understanding. Appropriate language can then be chosen to ensure clear communication.

Patients cannot benefit from, and may even be harmed by, information they do not understand.

THE BUILDING BLOCKS OF MEDICAL LANGUAGE

Medical terms are composed of several parts, referred to as "elements." Each element has its own meaning and location in the term. Like building blocks, they can be combined to create thousands of different words. Learning the meaning of commonly used word elements and applying this knowledge to decipher medical terms is much more efficient than trying to memorize each new word as it is encountered.

The three principle elements that make up medical terms are roots, prefixes, and suffixes.

Roots and Combining Forms

The **root** is the part of the medical term that gives the main meaning. It usually, but not always, refers to the structure and function of the body. All medical terms have at least one root. The following are examples of roots:

- gastr–stomach
- enter–small intestine
- cardi–heart

Combining forms consist of roots plus a vowel, usually the letter "o," separated from the root with a slash mark:

- gastr/o
- enter/o
- cardi/o

The letter "o" is called the **combining vowel**. It links the root to the next element in the term, known as the suffix, if the suffix begins with a **consonant** (any letter *except* a, e, i, o, u). (Suffixes are explained in the next section.) The combining form is always used when linking two roots, even if the second one starts with a vowel. For example, *gastr/o* and *enter/o* are often combined when referring to both the stomach and the intestines. The combining form *gastr/o* is used even though *enter/o* begins with a vowel to form the word *gastroenterology* which means "the study of the stomach and intestines." Note the root *enter* is used because the next element, *ology*, starts with a vowel. Medical roots, when listed in the dictionary, appear in their combining forms, and it is recommended that students learn them this way.

The vocabulary used by health care professionals differs from everyday language because, like the language of other sciences, many medical words have their origins in Greek and Latin. Table 4–1 contains several examples.

There are thousands of roots and combining forms that make up medical language. The complete list of combining forms each student must learn depends on their chosen occupation. Table 4–2 contains a list of commonly used combining forms that refer to the parts of the body.

Diagrams can be helpful when learning a new language. Many students find that illustrations provide visual clues for remembering new terms. Figure 4–1 illustrates some of the terms contained in Table 4–2.

Suffixes

Suffixes are word elements that are attached to the end of roots and combining forms to add to or change their meaning. All medical terms have a suffix. Some common meanings of suffixes include:

- Pathological (disease) conditions
- Diagnostic procedures
- Surgical procedures
- Pertaining to
- Produced by
- Resembling

Recall that the combining form is used when the suffix begins with a consonant, as in the following example:

cardi/o + megaly = cardiomegaly
heart + enlarged = enlarged heart

Notice that the slash mark is dropped when the suffix is attached to the combining form.

When the suffix begins with a vowel, it is attached to the root word, as in the following example:

gastr + itis = gastritis
stomach + inflammation = inflammation of the stomach

Table 4–1 Origins of Medical Root Words

Original Word	Meaning	Modern Medical Combining Form
kardia (Greek)	heart	cardi/o
derm (Greek)	skin	derm/o
enteron (Greek)	small intestines	enter/o
bucca (Latin)	cheek	bucc/o
lumbus (Latin)	loin (lower part of the back)	lumb/o
vivere (Latin)	life	viv/o

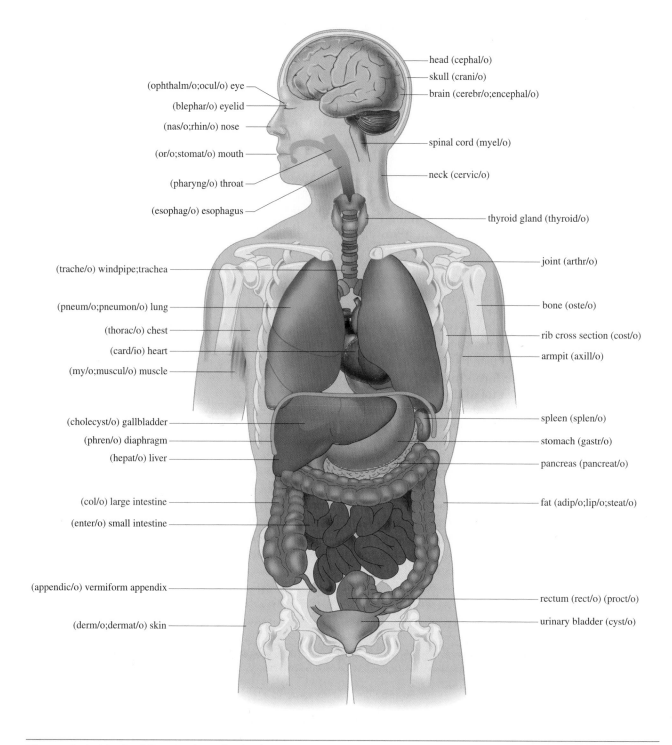

Figure 4–1 Medical Terminology for Body Parts

Table 4–2 Common Root Words that Refer to Body Parts

Combining Form	Meaning	Combining Form	Meaning
adip/o; lip/o; steat/o	fat	ren/o; nephr/o	kidneys
arteri/o	artery	lapar/o	abdominal wall
arthr/o	joint	larygn/o	voice box, larynx
axill/o	armpit	myel/o	spinal cord
blephar/o	eyelid	my/o; mucul/o	muscle
cardi/o	heart	nas/o; rhin/o	nose
cephal/o	head	neur/o	nerve
cerebr/o; encephal/o	brain	ophthalm/o; ocul/o	eye
cervic/o	neck	or/o; stomat/o	mouth
cholecyst/o	gallbladder	oste/o	bone
col/o	large intestine	ot/o	ear
cost/o	rib	pancreat/o	pancreas
crani/o	skull	pharyng/o	throat
cyst/o	urinary bladder	pneum/o; pneumon/o	lung
cyt/o	cell	splen/o	spleen
derm/o; dermat/o	skin	thorac/o	chest
enter/o	small intestine	thyroid/o	thyroid gland
esophag/o	esophagus	trache/o	windpipe, trachea
gastr/o	stomach	ven/o; phleb/o	vein
hem/o; hemat/o	blood	vertebr/o	vertebra
hepat/o	liver		

Each suffix can be added to many roots. Knowing that *-itis* means "inflammation" enables the student to know that the following words all indicate an inflammation of the body part indicated in the root:

1. Appendicitis: Inflammation of the appendix
2. Arthritis: Inflammation of the joint
3. Gastritis: Inflammation of the stomach

Another common suffix is *-ectomy*, which means "surgical removal." Like *-itis*, it can be combined with many root words. In each case, it means removal of the part indicated by the root word:

1. Appendectomy: Removal of the appendix

2. Gastrectomy: Removal of all or part of the stomach
3. Lumpectomy: Removal of a lump

When suffixes are listed in medical dictionaries and word lists, they are positioned alphabetically with other entries, preceded by a dash, and identified as a word element. Dictionary entries typically include the language of origin, as in the following sample dictionary entries:

- *–megaly* word element (Gr.) enlargement
- *–itis* word element (Gr.) inflammation
- *–ectomy* word element (Gr.) surgical removal

See Table 4–3 for a list of commonly used suffixes.

Table 4–3 Common Suffixes

Suffix	Meaning	Term	Meaning
–ac, –al, –ar, –ary, –eal, –iac, –ic, –ical, –ose, –ous, –tic	All of these mean "pertaining to"	cardiac cellular psychotic	pertaining to the heart pertaining to the cell pertaining to psychosis
–algia	pain	Neuralgia (new RAL jee ah)	pain along a nerve
–centesis	surgical puncture to remove fluid	Amniocentesis (am nee oh sin TEE sis)	insertion of needle to withdraw sample of amniotic fluid
–cide	to kill, destroy	Germicide (JER mih side)	a chemical substance that kills germs
–cyte	cell	Leukocyte (LOO koh cite)	white blood cell
–ectomy	removal of	Gastrectomy (gas TREK toh me)	removal of part or all of the stomach
–emia	blood	Bacteremia (back ter EE mee ah)	bacteria in the blood
–gram	record	Electrocardiogram (ee lek troh KAR dee oh gram)	record of the electrical activity of the heart
–graph	an instrument used to record	Electrocardiograph (ee lek troh KAR dee ah graf)	instrument that records electrical variations in cardiac muscle activity
–graphy	process of recording	Electrocardiography (ee lek troh KAR dee ah graf ee)	the making and study of electrocardiograms
			(continues)

Table 4–3 (continued)

Suffix	Meaning	Term	Meaning
–ia	condition, esp. an abnormal state	Tachycardia (tak ee KAR dee ah)	condition of abnormal rapid heart rate
–ism	condition	Hypothyroidism (high poh THIGH roid izm)	condition created by less than normal levels of thyroid hormones
–itis	inflammation of	Carditis (kar DYE tis)	inflammation of the heart
–lithiasis	presence of or formation of stones	Cholelithiasis (koh lee lih THIGH ah sis)	presence of stones in the gallbladder
–logy	study of	Cardiology (kar dee OL oh jee)	study of the heart
–megaly	enlargement	Hepatomegaly (hep ah toh MEG ah lee)	enlargement of the liver
–oid	resembling	Rheumatoid (ROO mah toyd)	resembling rheumatism
–oma	tumor	Myoma (my OH mah)	tumor containing muscle tissue
–otomy	surgical incision	Tracheotomy (tray kee OT oh mee)	incision into trachea
–pathy	disease	Encephalopathy (en sef ah LOP ah thee)	a disorder (disease) of the brain
–plasty	surgical repair	Rhinoplasty (RYE no plas tee)	plastic surgery of the nose
–plegia	paralysis	Hemiplegia (hem ee PLEE jee ah)	paralysis of one side (half) of the body
–pnea	breathing, respiration	Apnea (ap NEE ah)	temporary cessation of breathing
–rrhea	drainage, flow	Rhinorrhea (rye no REE ah)	drainage from the nose
–scope	examination, instrument	Otoscope (OH toh skope)	instrument used to examine the ear
–scopy	examination using a scope	Sigmoidoscopy (sig moy DOS koh pee)	examination of the sigmoid colon using a scope
–stasis	stoppage	Venostasis (vee no STAY sis)	stoppage of blood in an extremity
–stomy	surgically create an artificial mouth or stoma (opening)	Colostomy (koh LOSS toh me)	surgical opening into the colon to create a stoma

Prefixes

Prefixes are word elements that are attached to the beginning of roots and combining forms to add to or change their meaning. Many, but not all, medical terms have a prefix. Some common meanings of prefixes include:

- Location
- Position
- Direction
- Time
- Number
- Negation, absence of
- Color

Just as with suffixes, the same prefixes can be attached to many root words, resulting in thousands of variations. Knowing that the prefix *hyper–* means "abnormally increased" or "excessive" gives a clue to the meaning of the hundreds of words that contain this element, including the following examples:

1. Hyperacid: Abnormally or excessively acidic
2. Hyperactive: Exhibiting abnormally increased activity
3. Hypertension: Persistently high blood pressure

In the same way, knowing that *poly–* means "many" or "much" helps decipher the following examples:

1. Polyatomic: Made up of many atoms
2. Polyglandular: Pertaining to or affecting many glands
3. Polyphobia: Irrational fear of many things

Prefixes can dramatically change the meaning of a word. For example, *systole* (SIS toh lee) means "contraction of the heart." The addition of the one-letter prefix *a*, which means "without," creates the word *asystole* (a SIS toh lee) meaning without contractions. This is a very different condition! Careful spelling is critical when using medical language.

When prefixes are listed in medical dictionaries and word lists, they are located alphabetically, followed by a dash, and identified as a word element, as in the following sample dictionary entries:

- *epi–* word element (Gr.) over
- *hyper–* word element (Gr.) abnormally increased; excessive
- *poly–* word element (Gr.) many; much

See Table 4–4 for a list of commonly used prefixes.

Table 4–4 Common Prefixes

Prefix	Meaning	Term	Meaning
a–/an–	without, not	**Anuria** (an YOU ree ah)	absence of urine formation
anti–	against	**Antibiotic** (an tie buy AHT ick)	substance that inhibits growth of or destroys microorganisms
auto–	self	**Auto**immune (aw toh ih MYOON)	disease that results in immune response to one's own body
bi–	two, double	**Bifurcate** (BUY fur kate)	having two branches or divisions
brady–	slow	**Brady**cardia (brad ee KAR dee ah)	slow heart rate
dys–	bad, difficult, painful	**Dys**pnea (disp NEE ah)	difficulty breathing
epi–	over	**Epi**gastric (ep ih GAS trik)	over the stomach
eu–	good, normal	**Eupnea** (oop NEE ah)	normal breathing

(continues)

Table 4–4 (continued)

Prefix	Meaning	Term	Meaning
hemi–	half	**Hemi**plegia (hem ee PLEE jee ah)	paralysis of one side or half of the body
hyper–	above, excessive	**Hyper**tension (high per TEN shun)	high blood pressure
hypo–	less than, under	**Hypo**tension (high poh TEN shun)	low blood pressure
inter–	between	**Inter**costal (in ter COS tahl)	between the ribs
intra–	within	**Intra**venous (in trah VEE nus)	within a vein
multi–	many	**Multi**nodal (mul tih NO dahl)	having many nodes or knots
non–	not	**Non**toxic (non TOK sik)	not poisonous
peri–	around	**Peri**anal (per ee A nal)	around the anus
poly–	many, much	**Poly**uria (pol ee YOU ree ah)	excretion of large amounts of urine
post–	after, behind	**Post**operative (post OP er ah tiv)	following a surgical procedure
pre–	before, in front	**Pre**operative (pree OP er ah tiv)	before a surgical procedure
pseudo–	false	**Pseudo**hematuria (sue doh hee mah TOO ree ah)	a red pigment in the urine that makes the urine "falsely" appear to have blood in it
quadri–	four	**Quadri**plegia (kwad rih PLEE jee ah)	paralysis of all four extremities
semi–	half	**Semi**permeable (sem ee PER mee ah bull)	half permeable—a membrane that allows fluids but not the dissolved substance to pass through
sub–	under, below	**Sub**sternal (sub STIR nall)	below the sternum
supra–	above, over	**Supra**pubic (sue prah PEW bik)	above the pubic area
tachy–	fast, rapid	**Tachy**cardia (tak ee KAR dee ah)	rapid heart rate
tri–	three	**Tri**chotomy (try COT oh me)	division into three parts

DECIPHERING MEDICAL TERMS

Learning the meanings of commonly used word elements and understanding how they combine enable the health care worker to decipher thousands of medical terms. When confronted with a new term, start at the far right, with the suffix. Think of each word as a combination of building blocks, fitted together to create a precise meaning. See Figure 4–2. Work from right to left, identifying and defining each element, as in the following examples:

Example # 1 cardiology

1. Starting from the right, find element –*ology*
2. Determine meaning: study of
3. Moving left, find element *cardi*
4. Determine meaning: heart
5. Combine elements: study of the heart

Example # 2 polyarthritis

1. Starting from the right, find element –*itis*
2. Determine meaning: inflammation
3. Moving left, find element *arthr*
4. Determine meaning: joint
5. Moving left, find element *poly*
6. Determine meaning: many, much
7. Combine elements: inflammation of many joints

Example # 3 echocardiogram

1. Starting from the right, find element –*gram*
2. Determine meaning: written, record
3. Moving left, find element *cardi/o*
4. Determine meaning: heart
5. Moving left, find element *echo*
6. Determine meaning: echo (reflections of sounds)
7. Combine elements: recording of the heart using echoes (to determine position and motion)

SPELLING AND PRONUNCIATION

Accurate spelling is critical when using medical language. Some words look and/or sound similar and can be easily confused. It is important to pay attention to the context (the surrounding words and facts)

to determine the correct meaning. The following examples contain words that are often confused:

1. Ilium (ILL ee um): Part of the hipbone
   Ileum (ILL ee um): Part of the intestine
2. Alveoli (al VEE oh lie): Tiny air sacs in the lungs
   Areola (ah RE oh lah): Brown pigmented area around the nipple

As with nontechnical English words, which have their origins in many different languages, some medical terms are spelled differently from the way they are pronounced. Table 4–5 contains common examples. Many of the guidelines apply to familiar words as well and are taken for granted in everyday speech. For example, "ph" used as "f" in the words, "philosophy", "Philadelphia", and "Phoenix."

The plural forms of many medical words are created with the original Greek and Latin endings, instead of the familiar "s" used for many English words. Table 4–6 contains guidelines for creating the plural forms of many medical terms.

Misspelled words can lead to treatment and medication errors. When learning new word elements, take the time to learn the correct spelling. Health care workers cannot take the chance that others will guess correctly what they intended to write.

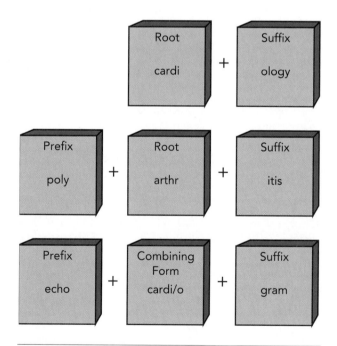

Figure 4–2 Think of the elements of medical terms as building blocks that can be used to construct new words.

TABLE 4–5 Spelling and Pronunciation Guidelines

Letter	Sounds Like	Examples
c when followed by e, i, or y	s	cell, circulatory, cyst
ch	k	chronic
g when followed by e, i, or y	j	genetic, gingivitis, gyration
i when used to create plural	eye	bacilli
ph	f	pharmacist
pn	n	pneumonia
ps	s	psychiatrist
x	z	Xylocaine (Pronounced ZIE loh cane, this is an anestethic applied to the skin)

TABLE 4–6 Guidelines to Plural Forms

Guideline	Singular	Plural
1. If the term ends in **a**, the plural is usually formed by adding an **e**.	bursa vertebra	bursae vertabrae
2. If the term ends in **ex** or **ix**, the plural is usually formed by changing the **ex** or **ix** to **ices**.	appendix index	appendices indices
3. If the term ends in **is**, the plural is usually formed by changing the **is** to **es**.	diagnosis metastasis	diagnoses metastases
4. If the term ends in **itis**, the plural is usually formed by changing the **is** to **ides**.	arthritis meningitis	arthritides meningitides
5. If the term ends in **nx**, the plural is usually formed by changing the **x** to **ges**.	phalanx meninx	phalanges meninges
6. If the term ends in **on**, the plural is usually formed by changing the **on** to **a**.	criterion ganglion	criteria ganglia
7. If the term ends in **um**, the plural usually is formed by changing the **um** to **a**.	diverticulum ovum	diverticula ova
8. If the term ends in **us**, the plural is usually formed by changing the **us** to **i**.	alveolus malleolus	alveoli malleoli

*If you are in doubt as to how a plural is formed, **look it up** in a medical dictionary!*

From *Medical terminology for health professions* (3rd ed.), by A. Ehrlich, 2001, Albany, NY: Delmar.

MEDICAL ABBREVIATIONS AND SYMBOLS

Medical abbreviations and symbols are the shorthand of medical language. Many of them have been standardized and are universally accepted. In addition, each health care profession, agency, and facility has its own list of approved abbreviations and symbols. It is important that the health care worker ask for a copy of and become familiar with the list. *Never* substitute personal versions of abbreviations and symbols for those on the list when preparing any type of written documentation that will be used by the facility. Using abbreviations and/or symbols not on the approved list is against state and federal regulatory guidelines. If misuse is discovered during an accreditation or licensing survey visit, the agency or facility can be cited for not following the guidelines. If there are common abbreviations or symbols missing from the list, the worker should notify the supervisor.

Refer to Tables 4–7 and 4–8 for a list of medical abbreviations and symbols. These are not complete lists, but include examples of those that are frequently encountered in health care. Additional abbreviations and symbols will be encountered as students take health care specialty courses. For example, a dental assistant will learn the standardized numbering system used for identifying each tooth.

Table 4–7 Abbreviations

ad lib.	Freely; at will	O.U.	Each eye
a.c.	Before a meal	$\bar{p}$	After
b.i.d.	Twice a day	P	Pulse
BM	Bowel movement	p.c.	After meals
BP	Blood pressure	P.O.	by mouth
$\bar{c}$	With	p.r.n.	as needed
CDC	Centers for Disease Control and Prevention	q.d.	Daily
c/o	Complains of	q.h.	Every hour
d/c	Discontinue	q.i.d.	Four times a day
h.	Hour	R	Respiration
H_2O	Water	$\bar{s}$	Without
h.s.	at night; at bedtime	stat.	Immediately
I&O	Intake and output	T	Temperature
lab.	Laboratory	t.i.d.	Three times a day
n.p.o.	Nothing by mouth	TPR	Temperature, pulse, and respiration
n&v	Nausea and vomiting	TX	Traction or treatment
O_2	Oxygen	VS	Vital signs
O.D.	Right eye	Wt.	Weight
O.S.	left eye	x	Multiplied by

Table 4–8 Symbols

>	Greater than
<	Less than
↑	Higher, elevate, or up
↓	Lower or down
#	Pound or number
'	Foot or minute
"	Inch or second
°	Degree
♀	Female
♂	Male
Δ	Change

Thinking it Through

Charles Grant, LVN, is given Mr. Grover's chart and asked to take the BP and P Stat. Charles reviews the notes and sees that Mr. Grover has hypertension and tachycardia and that the physician has ordered he be n.p.o. The chart also states that he has polyuria, rhinorrhea, eupnea, and a history of cholelithiasis. When Charles greets Mr. Grover and informs him that he is going to take his BP and P, he requests a drink of water first, as he is feeling quite thirsty.

1. What is BP and P? Is there any urgency in doing these?
2. Noting that he has hypertension and tachycardia, do you expect the readings to be too high, normal, or too low? Explain.
3. What do polyuria, rhinorrhea, eupnea, and cholelithiasis mean?
4. Is it appropriate to give Mr. Grover a glass of water? Why or why not?

Thinking it Through

Mr. Fiacco is complaining of pain and itching in his right eye. You know that Mr. Fiacco has conjunctivitis (inflammation of the conjunctiva of the eye) of both eyes and that the physician has ordered antibiotic drops to be given b.i.d. in O.U. for 10 days. The left eye appears normal, but the right eye is red and irritated. You check the instructions on the prescription packaging and it says to place the drops in the left eye twice a day.

1. Is the patient taking the eye drops correctly?
2. Is there a reason for the lack of improvement in the right eye?
3. What does b.i.d. mean?
4. What do O.U., O.S., and O.D. refer to?
5. What should you do to correct the problem?

MEDICAL DICTIONARY

Students are encouraged to purchase a medical and/or specialty dictionary. It is a valuable resource not only when taking health care courses but also as a handy reference in the work setting. The following features should be considered when selecting a dictionary:

- Clear, easy-to-understand definitions
- Explanations of medical procedures, conditions, disorders, and diseases
- Pronunciation hints
- Abbreviations and symbols
- Reference tables containing information such as laboratory values, units of measurement with conversion values, nutritional values of foods, and emergency resources
- Useful diagrams, charts, and tables
- Expanded explanations of topics of interest to the student
- Application of information to patient care
- Extent of vocabulary coverage specific to student's occupational area

It is very important to check the coverage of terms in the student's specialty area. Some dictionaries are more inclusive than others.

MASTERING MEDICAL TERMINOLOGY

Learning to use medical language is challenging for many students. Many words come from languages, such as Latin, that are no longer spoken. The words look and sound strange and seem long and complex. Medical terminology, however, can be mastered. The keys are *study* and *practice*. The following suggestions have helped many students:

- Study a few words each day. Avoid having to learn entire lists at the last minute just before test time.

- As word parts are learned, practice using them in new combinations.
- Use study techniques that correspond to individual learning styles, as discussed in Chapter 1. See the list of ideas in Table 4–9.
- Practice both the written and spoken forms as much as possible and in as many settings as possible.
- Learn new medical terms as they appear in this and other textbooks.
- Use a medical dictionary when unsure about how to spell or pronounce a word correctly.
- When working in a health care environment, accept help as needed from coworkers and supervisors to correct pronunciation and usage.

Table 4–9 Suggested Study Techniques

Learning Style	Suggestions
Visual	Visual Learners • Write down medical terms that you hear during lectures. • Ask the instructor to write words on the board. • Create cartoons using medical terms. • Prepare flashcards with a word or picture on one side and the definition on the back. • Study roots that refer to the body by studying drawings of the body parts. • Write words many times, using colored ink. • Visualize familiar images along with the new terms. For example, visualize the Queen of hearts playing card for "cardio–"
Auditory	• Concentrate on terms when you hear them presented in lectures. • Read medical terms aloud to yourself. • Use commercially prepared tapes or make your own. • Take turns quizzing each other with another student. • Create verbal rhythms; try setting them to music. • Create audio, "sounds-like" cues to remember definitions.
Kinesthetic	• Draw images, and even color them. • Create flashcards with the medical term on one card and the definition on the other. Then lay them out on a large table and move them around until you have them all matched correctly. • Touch the part of your body referred to in the term or point to where it is located if it's not on the surface • Study the models of the body systems or build them from kits.

Having a strong understanding of the key concepts presented in this chapter will serve as a foundation for learning the material in subsequent chapters and throughout the entire health care educational program. The following are just a few of the subjects that depend heavily on knowledge of medical terminology:

- Anatomy (structure of the body)
- Physiology (function of the body)
- Pathophysiology (study of diseases and abnormal conditions)
- Medical insurance coding (assigning standardized codes to specific diagnoses and procedures)
- Pharmacology (therapeutic drugs)

The time initially spent learning the correct meaning, spelling, and pronunciation of medical word elements will save time later and prevent frustration when learning future subjects. Being proficient in the use of medical terminology is a mark of a competent health care professional.

SUGGESTED LEARNING ACTIVITIES

1. Start a list of new medical terms, with their definitions, as you encounter them. This can be a written list in your notebook or one on your computer.

2. Watch television programs that portray medical settings, such as "Chicago Hope" and "ER," and listen for medical terms. Do the professionals on these programs use a different level of language when speaking among themselves than when speaking with patients? Do you recognize any of the terms used?

3. Watch and listen for "medical" prefixes and suffixes that are also used in everyday English (or Spanish)!

4. Using the examples of terms provided in the boxes in Figure 4–3, create a few medical terms for the other body parts. Use the charts in this chapter and a medical dictionary.

REVIEW QUESTIONS

1. Why is it important to know medical terminology?

2. What do the following terms mean: "roots," "combining forms," "suffixes," and "prefixes"?

3. What are the steps that should be followed to break medical terms into their component parts in order to interpret them correctly?

4. Provide five examples of medical terms that include a prefix and suffix. Give their meanings.

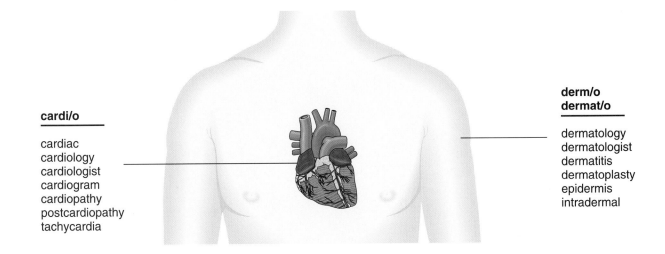

cardi/o

cardiac
cardiology
cardiologist
cardiogram
cardiopathy
postcardiopathy
tachycardia

derm/o
dermat/o

dermatology
dermatologist
dermatitis
dermatoplasty
epidermis
intradermal

Figure 4–3 The root word for each body part is the basis for many terms.

5. What are the guidelines for medical terms when the pronunciation differs from the spelling?

6. Provide five examples of abbreviations and five of symbols. Give their meanings.

7. What are the features of a medical dictionary? How do you determine which one will be the best for your specialty area?

8. What are eight study suggestions for mastering medical terminology?

APPLICATION EXERCISES

1. Refer back to The Case of "Where Is the Pain?" presented at beginning of Chapter. What does epigastric mean? How would you respond to Ms. Mitchell's question "What is epigastric"?

2. Kelly Cordeiro is a recent medical assisting graduate who is hired by a prominent ophthalmologist. She is excited about having the opportunity to work in this area. However, Kelly quickly discovers that there are many terms related to the anatomy of the eye, special procedures, eye surgery, and medications that she is not familiar with. She feels a little lost and is concerned about her ability to communicate effectively with the physician and maintain patient records appropriately.

   a. What references would you suggest for Kelly to learn the vocabulary she needs?

   b. Describe the techniques she can use to quickly learn the new vocabulary.

SUGGESTED READINGS AND RESOURCES

DeSousa, L. R. (1995). *Common medical abbreviations*. Albany, NY: Delmar.

Dorland's Illustrated Medical Dictionary, 29th ed. Philadelphia: W. B. Saunders Company.

Ehrlich, A. (1997). *Medical terminology for health professions* (3rd ed.). Albany, NY: Delmar.

Miller-Keane Encyclopedia & Dictionary of Medicine, Nursing, & Allied Health, 6th ed. (1997). Philadelphia: W. B. Saunders Company.

Stedman's Medical Dictionary, 27th ed. (1995). Baltimore: Williams & Wilkins.

Taber's Cyclopedic Medical Dictionary, 19th ed. (2001). Philadelphia: F. A. Davis.

CHAPTER

MEDICAL MATH

OBJECTIVES

Studying and applying the material in this chapter will help you to:

- Understand how math anxiety prevents comfort and competence with calculations.

- Perform basic math calculations on whole numbers, decimals, fractions, percentages, and ratios.

- Convert between the following numerical forms: decimals, fractions, percentages, and ratios.

- Round off numbers correctly.

- Solve mathematical equivalency problems with proportions.

- Express time using the 24-hour clock (military time).

- Express numbers using Roman numerals.

- Estimate angles from a reference plane.

- Use household, metric, and apothecary units to express length, volume, and weight.

- Know equivalencies for converting between the household, metric, and apothecary systems of measurement.

- Convert between the Fahrenheit and Celsius temperature scales.

KEY TERMS

angles
apothecary system
centigrade
decimal
degrees
estimating
Fahrenheit
fraction
household system
improper fraction
math anxiety
metric system
military time
nomenclature
percentages
proportion
ratios
reciprocal
reference plane
Roman numerals
rounding numbers
whole numbers

The Case of

"Exactly How Much Does My Baby Weigh?"

During a well baby checkup, Jamie Brown weighs Jessica Munoz and reports to the mother that her baby weighs 10 kilograms. The mother states her daughter weighed 20 pounds on the last visit and asks how much 10 kilograms is in pounds. Jamie explains that 10 kilograms is the same as 22 pounds, so there has been a 2-pound increase in weight.

Not knowing how to convert between kilograms and pounds would have prevented Jamie from answering the mother's question. This chapter will cover the math needed by the health care worker, including information about converting between commonly used systems of measurement.

IMPORTANCE OF MATH IN HEALTH CARE

Work in health care requires the use of math skills to measure and perform various types of calculations. There are applications in all types of occupations:

- Calculating medication dosages
- Taking height and weight readings
- Measuring the amount of intake (fluids consumed or infused) and output (e.g., urine, vomit)
- Billing and bookkeeping tasks
- Performing lab tests
- Mixing cleaning solution

Errors in math can have negative effects on patients. For example, administering the wrong dosage of medication is a serious mistake and can harm the patient. Health care workers must strive for 100% accuracy. *If there is any doubt, it is essential to ask your supervisor or a qualified coworker to double-check calculations.*

MATH ANXIETY

Many students suffer from **math anxiety**. Those who do are probably feeling dread at just the thought of reading this chapter. Kogelman and Warren (1978) stated in the introduction to their book *Mind over Math*:

> Many people react to math so strongly that their ability to memorize, concentrate, and pay attention is effectively inhibited. This makes learning impossible. It also makes testing math ability impossible, because often all that can be assessed is the test-taker's math anxiety.

Math anxiety can be overcome. The first step is to recognize that it exists and be willing to do something about it. Many people who think they have a learning disability or just "can never do math" have found that it is the anxiety that causes the mental block and interferes with their ability to learn. Once it's overcome, they are able to learn and perform the math necessary for their work. There are some common myths about math, which, if believed, set up mental blocks to learning. See Table 5–1.

In addition to the common myths about math, there are messages people say to themselves or that others say to them that prevent the mind shift necessary to work successfully with math. See if any of the messages in Table 5–2 look familiar. Replacing negative self-talk with more positive messages ("I can learn math") releases the mental energy needed for mastering new skills. Kogelman (1978) referred to these negative messages as "mind games."

Table 5–1 Twelve Math Myths

Myth	Comments
Men are better in math than women.	Research has proved this to be false.
Math requires logic, not intuition.	Any kind of problem solving requires intuition. This refers to being able to sense the best approach in solving the problem. Some people say that the answer "Just doesn't feel right" when their solution is incorrect.
You must always know how you got the answer.	You may use intuition to solve the problem, but then not be able to logically explain how you did it. Remember that if you get the answer consistently correct, there is no need to explain how.
Math is not creative.	The greatest mathematicians have always been very creative or they would not have been able to create unique insights into how the universe works.
There is a best way to do a math problem.	The best way to do a math problem is the method that works for you.
It's always important to get the answer exactly right.	You need to be accurate when calculating drug doses, but an estimate is adequate when calculating a tip.
It's bad to count on your fingers.	Most people find counting on their fingers helpful, and there is no reason to feel guilty. The Chinese have used an "abacus" for centuries. This is a sophisticated finger-counting machine that is fast and accurate.
Mathematicians do problems quickly, in their heads.	If anyone performs a skill quickly, it is because they have done it many times. Any unfamiliar process takes time and practice.
Math requires a good memory.	Understanding is superior to memorization. If you truly understand something, you will use reason to naturally arrive at the answer.
Math is done by working intensely until the problem is solved.	Learning new skills requires a clear, rested mind. If you feel stuck, stop for a while, do something else or rest, and when you return refreshed you may be amazed at your ability to find the answer. If you say things such as "It's hopeless," "I am too dumb to get this," or "I'm a failure," this approach will not work because you have already defeated yourself. Instead say to yourself, "I'm going to take a break because I cannot get it right now."
Some people have a "math mind" and some don't.	Once you overcome your emotional blocks and develop self-confidence by practice, you will be delighted to find that you also have a "math mind."
There is a magic key to doing math.	There is no magic or any one approach you need to learn to do math well.

Source: From *Mind Over Math* by Stanley Kogelman, Joseph Warren, copyright © 1978 by Stanley Kogelman and Joseph Warren. Used by permission of Doubleday, a division of Random House, Inc.

Table 5–2 Mind Games That Create Blocks

Math Games We Play on Ourselves	Math Games Others Play on Us
"Everybody knows what to do, except me."	"You did it the wrong way."
"I don't do math fast enough."	"You should know that."
"I'm sure I learned it, but I can't remember what to do."	"You will never be able to do math."
"I knew I couldn't do math."	"It's obvious."
"I don't have a math mind."	"That's an easy problem."
"I got the right answer, but I did it the wrong way."	"All you have to do to learn math is to work hard."
"This may be a stupid question, but . . ."	
"It's too simple."	
"Math is unrelated to my life."	

With an awareness of math myths and mind games, students can apply the following ideas to start on the road to math success (Adapted from *Mind over math: Put yourself on the road to success by freeing yourself from math anxiety,* by S. Kogelman and J. Warren, 1997, New York: McGraw Hill.):

■ Overcoming math anxiety calls for experiencing and being aware of emotional responses to math.

■ Anxiety cannot be decreased by fighting it and trying to talk oneself out of it.

■ Everyone needs to learn things they have never learned and relearn what they have forgotten.

■ As long as a student says "I will keep trying" rather than "I can't do it" the mind will work on mastering new material.

■ It is important to assess what is already known and what is not known. This is less overwhelming that simply saying "I can't do math." It provides a starting point for learning.

■ Procrastination increases anxiety.

■ Some topics have to be read, heard, and/or discussed many times before they become clear. There is nothing wrong with this.

■ Very little learning takes place in the face of intense anxiety. It all starts looking like a blur.

■ It is best to take a break when it feels like everything is going in circles and one's thinking is no longer clear.

■ It is hard to concentrate when the worst is expected.

■ Doing math requires confidence and concentration; panic and anxiety make this impossible.

■ There are no secrets to be handed out. What is needed most is participation and engagement in the process.

[Fascinating Facts]

"An adult who has overcome math anxiety can usually master arithmetic in a short time and learn more advanced subjects in about half the time required in high school."
Contrary to what many adult students believe about their inability to learn, the maturity and practical experience acquired over the years actually speed up the learning process.
(Kogelman, 1978.)

Thinking it Through

Ms. Cree is a new graduate and has just been hired as a medical assistant in Dr. Albright's office. She is anxious about learning the new routines and doing a good job. She has always struggled with math calculations, but was able to develop her skills to pass her courses in school. However, when Dr. Albright orders a medication that needs to be calculated, Ms. Cree panics. She is unable to find her calculator, and even though she has been able to manually solve this type of problem in the classroom setting, she now becomes too afraid to trust her own skills and starts to panic. Where *is* that calculator? Ms. Cree is afraid of losing her job if she admits the problem, and yet she knows that if she makes a mistake, she could jeopardize the health of the patient.

1. What job-related factors are contributing to Ms. Cree's anxiety and panic?

2. What suggestions would you recommend to her?

3. What myths and mind games may be adding to the problem?

BASIC CALCULATIONS

The information presented on decimals, percentages, fractions, and ratios is included in this chapter as a review of the basics needed to perform many medical math applications. The purpose is to jog the student's memory: "Yes, that's right, now I remember." For students who cannot easily follow the review or believe they never learned the concepts, a refresher course or more extensive review is recommended. There are many excellent books and computer programs on basic arithmetic. Another option is to find out if your campus has a resource center that offers assistance to students who need to review math.

To work safely in health care, it is essential to be able to add, subtract, multiply, and divide whole numbers, decimals, fractions, and percentages. Students also need to understand equivalents when using decimals, fractions, and percentages. See Figure 5–1.

Many health care workers use small calculators to assist them with calculations. During your health care studies, some instructors will allow the use of calculators, and others will not. It is always best to know how to do the basic functions by "long hand" (without a calculator), because calculators can quit working at any time during a test or at the workplace. Some professional exams required for licensure or certification do not allow the use of calculators.

Whole Numbers

Whole numbers are what we traditionally use to count (1, 2, 3, . . .). They do not contain fractions or decimals. For example, 30 is a whole number, while 30½ and 30.5 are not. Students must be able to accurately add, subtract, multiply, and divide whole numbers.

- Add: $15 + 24 = 39$ (verbal: fifteen plus twenty-four equals thirty-nine)
- Subtract: $54 - 15 = 39$ (verbal: fifty-four minus fifteen equals thirty-nine)
- Multiply: $14 \times 8 = 112$ (verbal: fourteen times eight equals one-hundred and twelve)
- Divide: $60 \div 12 = 5$ (verbal: sixty divided by twelve equals five)

Decimals

Decimals are one way of expressing parts of numbers or anything else that has been divided into parts. The parts are expressed in units of ten. That is, decimals represent the number of tenths, hundredths, thousandths, and so on that are available. For example, 0.7 represents seven of the ten parts into which something has been divided. When

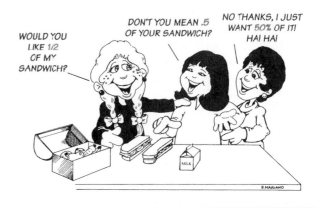

Figure 5–1 An easy way to remember how to convert decimals, percentages, and fractions is to think of this humorous cartoon.

reading decimals verbally, it is necessary to know the placement values for the decimals (digits to the right of the decimal point) and that the decimal point is read as "and." See Figure 5–2. For example:

- 0.5 is read "five tenths"
- 1.5 is read "one and five tenths"
- 1.50 is read "one and fifty hundredths"
- 1.500 is read "one and five hundred thousandths"
- 1.5000 is read "one and five thousand ten thousandths"

Note that a zero is placed to the left of the decimal point if the number begins to the right of the point. This is necessary to prevent errors from occurring if the decimal point is not seen.

Decimals are added, subtracted, multiplied, and divided in the same way as whole numbers.

The most common mistake is incorrect placement of the decimal point. See Table 5–3.

Fractions

Fractions are another way of expressing numbers that represent parts of a whole. A fraction has a numerator (top number) and a denominator (bottom number). An example of a fraction is $\frac{3}{10}$, where the three is the numerator and ten is the denominator. Colbert (1997) described a fraction like this:

> The numerator, or top number, is the actual number of parts of a whole. The denominator, or bottom number, tells how many parts it takes to make a whole.

See Figure 5–3 for an illustration of this concept. The fraction above is read as "three tenths."

Table 5–3 Working with Decimals

Function	Example	Key Points
Add: (+)	1.5 + 2.25 3.75	1. Line up the decimal points. 2. Add the numbers. 3. Bring the decimal point straight down.
Subtract: (−)	3.75 − 1.25 2.50	1. Line up the decimal points. 2. Subtract the numbers. 3. Bring the decimal point straight down.
Multiply: (×)	2.5 × 2.5 125 +50 6.25	1. Multiply the numbers. 2. Count the total number of digits to the right of the decimal points in the numbers you are multiplying. 3. Count the same number of places in your answer. Start to the right of the last digit in your answer and move left that number of places. This is where the decimal point is placed.
Divide: (÷)	2.5$\overline{)50.5}$ 25.$\overline{)505.0}$ $\begin{array}{r}20.2\\25\overline{)505.0}\\\underline{50}\\5\\\underline{0}\\50\\\underline{50}\\0\end{array}$	1. Move the decimal point to the right in the number you are dividing by (to make it a whole number). 2. Move the decimal point the same number of places to the right in the number being divided. Add zeros if necessary. 3. Divide the numbers. 4. Place the decimal point in the answer by moving it straight up from the number that was divided.

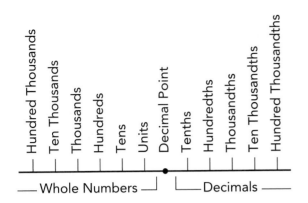

Figure 5–2 The position of the number to the left or the right of the decimal point is its place value. The value of each place *left* of the decimal point is *ten times* that of the place to its right. The value of each place *right* of the decimal point is *one-tenth* the value of the place to its left.

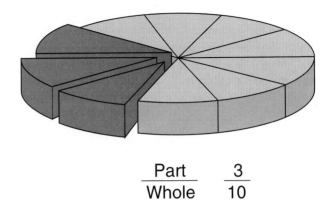

$$\frac{\text{Part}}{\text{Whole}} \quad \frac{3}{10}$$

Figure 5–3 A fraction is a comparison of parts (numerator) to a whole (denominator).

While performing calculations with fractions is not difficult, it does require following a series of steps. These are described in Table 5–4. There are a few special considerations to remember when

Table 5–4 Working with Fractions

Function	Example	Key Points
Add: (+)	$\frac{1}{5} = \frac{6}{30}$ $+\frac{1}{6} = +\frac{5}{30}$ $\frac{11}{30}$	1. If the denominators are not the same, find a number both denominators divide evenly into. 2. Multiply the numerators by the number of times the old denominators divide into the new denominator. 3. Add the numerators. 4. Place the new numerator over the denominator. 5. Reduce the fraction, if necessary.
Subtract: (−)	$\frac{1}{5} = \frac{6}{30}$ $-\frac{1}{6} = \frac{5}{30}$ $\frac{1}{30}$	1. If the denominators are not the same, find a number both denominators divide evenly into. 2. Multiply the numerators by the number of times the old denominators divide into the new denominator. 3. Subtract the numerators. 4. Place the new numerator over the denominator. 5. Reduce the fraction, if necessary.
Multiply: (×)	$\frac{1}{5} \times \frac{1}{6} = \frac{1}{30}$	1. Multiply numerators. 2. Multiply denominators. 3. Reduce the fraction, if necessary.
Divide: (÷)	$\frac{1}{5} \div \frac{1}{6} = \frac{1}{5} \times \frac{6}{1} = \frac{6}{5} = 1\frac{1}{5}$	1. Invert the dividing fraction. 2. Multiply numerators. 3. Multiply denominators. 4. Reduce the fraction, if necessary.

working with fractions. When adding and subtracting fractions, it is necessary to change all the denominators to the same number in order to perform the calculations. This is known as "converting the fractions." To do this, find a number that each denominator can divide into evenly and then adjust the numerators to maintain an equivalent fraction. For example to add $\frac{1}{2} + \frac{1}{3}$ convert both fractions to sixths $= \frac{3}{6} + \frac{2}{6} = \frac{5}{6}$. (The denominators "2" and "3" both divide into 6 evenly; then the numerator is multiplied by the number of times the old denominator divides into the new denominator ("2" divides into 6 three times, so 1×3 then creates the new fraction of $\frac{3}{6}$; "3" divides into 6 two times, so 1×2 then creates the new fraction of $\frac{2}{6}$.

Multiplying fractions is straightforward. First multiply the two numerators and then two denominators. For example, $\frac{1}{2} \times \frac{1}{2}$ is $\frac{1}{4}$ ($1 \times 1 = 1$ and $2 \times 2 = 4$).

Dividing fractions requires the dividing fraction to be inverted (turned upside down). The new, upside-down fraction is called the **reciprocal**. The numerators and denominators are then multiplied to get the answer. For example, $\frac{1}{2} \div \frac{1}{2} = \frac{1}{2} \times \frac{2}{1} = \frac{2}{2}$ or 1.

There are two processes that are frequently used when working with fractions. Reducing the fraction to its lowest terms means finding a number that can be divided evenly into both the numerator and denominator. For example, the fraction $\frac{2}{4}$ can be reduced to the lower equivalent fraction of $\frac{1}{2}$ by dividing both the numerator and denominator by 2 ($2 \div 2 = 1$ and $4 \div 2 = 2$). This process is also known as "simplifying the fraction."

Improper fractions have numerators that are larger than the denominators. To reduce these fractions, divide the denominator into the numerator. The result will be a whole number or a mixed number (whole number and a fraction). For example, the fraction $\frac{12}{4}$ would be reduced to the whole number 3 ($12 \div 4 = 3$) ; the fraction 11/4 would be reduced to the mixed number $2\frac{3}{4}$ ($11 \div 4 = 2\frac{3}{4}$).

Percentages

Percentages are used to express either a whole or part of a whole. The whole is expressed as 100 percent (%). Refer back to Figure 5–3 and imagine this as a hot apple pie sliced into 10 equal pieces. The 10 slices together equal the whole, or 100%, of the pie. One hundred divided by ten equals ten. Therefore, each slice represents 10% of the pie. If each slice is 10%, then three slices represent 30% of the pie.

When working with percentages, it is easier to convert the percentage to a decimal and then perform the addition, subtraction, multiplication, and division. Converting percentages to decimals is explained later in this chapter.

Ratios

Ratios show relationships between numbers or like values: how many of one number or value is present as compared to the other. For example, a bleach and water solution with a 1:2 ratio means that one part of bleach is added for every two parts of water. This relationship applies regardless of the units used:

- 1 cup bleach and 2 cups of water
- 1 quart of bleach and 2 quarts of water
- $\frac{1}{2}$ cup of bleach and 1 cup of water
- $\frac{1}{4}$ cup of bleach and $\frac{1}{2}$ cup of water

The use of ratios to express the strength of a solution is commonly seen in health care. Solution strengths are also frequently expressed as percentages. A 50% bleach solution is the same as the 1:2 ratio. Conversions between ratios and percentages are explained in the next section.

Converting Decimals, Fractions, Percentages, and Ratios

Decimals, fractions, and percentages all express parts of a whole. The cartoon in Figure 5–1 humorously portrayed how they are related: the fraction $\frac{1}{2}$, the decimal 0.5, and the percentage 50% all represent the same amount of the sandwich. The steps involved in converting between these numerical forms are shown in Table 5–5.

Rounding Numbers

Rounding a number means changing it to the nearest ten, hundred, thousand, and so on. Deciding which to use depends on the size of the original number and the degree of accuracy required. Deciding whether to round up or round down depends on the digits (numbers) located to the right of the value chosen for rounding. The following examples illustrate how these rules are applied:

Example 1 When rounding to the nearest 10: look at the digit to the right of the tens place (the ones place). If the number is 5 or above, round up. If it is less than 5, round down.

88 rounds up to 90
83 rounds down to 80

Example 2 When rounding to the nearest 100: look at the digit to the right of the hundreds place (the tens place). If the number is 5 or above, round up. If it is less than 5, round down.

67 rounds up to 100
133 rounds down to 100
668 rounds up to 700
621 rounds down to 600

Table 5–5 Converting Decimals, Fractions, and Percentages

Converting	Example	Key Points
Decimals to fractions	0.75 = 75/100 = 3/4	1. Drop the decimal point. 2. Position the number over its placement value (Figure 5–2). 3. If necessary, reduce the fraction.
Decimals to percentages	5.275 = 5.275 × 100 = 527.5 527.5%	1. Move the decimal point two places to the right because percentages are based on 100. This is the same as multiplying by 100. 2. Add percentage sign.
Fractions to decimals	3/5 = 3 ÷ 5 = 0.6	1. Divide numerator by denominator.
Fractions to percentages	7/8 = 7 ÷ 8 = 0.875 0.875 × 100 = 87.5 87.5%	1. Divide numerator by denominator. 2. Move decimal point two places to the right because percentages are based on 100. This is the same as multiplying by 100. 3. Add percentage sign.
Percentages to decimals	125.5% = 125.5 125.5 ÷ 100 = 1.255	1. Remove percentage sign. 2. Move decimal point two places to the left because percentages are based on 100. This is the same as dividing by 100.
Percentages to fractions	$5\% = 5$ $\dfrac{5}{100} = \dfrac{1}{20}$	1. Remove percentage sign. 2. Place number over 100. 3. If appropriate, simplify fraction to lowest terms.
Percentages to ratios	75% = 75 75:100	1. Remove percentage sign. 2. Create a ratio using the former percentage and the number 100. 3. Insert a colon (:) between the numbers.
Ratios to Percentages	1:2 = 0.5 = 50%	1. Divide number on left of the colon by number on right of ratio sign 2. Move decimal point two places to the right. Add zero(s) if necessary. This is the same as multiplying by 100. 3. Add percentage sign.

Example 3 When rounding to the nearest 1000: look at the digit to the right of the thousands place (the hundreds place). If the number is 5 or above, round up. If it is less than 5, round down.

7777 rounds up to 8000
7355 rounds down to 7000

Numbers of all sizes can be rounded. Review Figure 5–2 and study the examples in Table 5–6.

Table 5–6 Rounding Numbers

Round the Number 1234.5678 to the Nearest:	Result	Comments
Whole number	1235	The digit to the right of the whole number (1234) is five, so you round up one number.
Tens	1230	The digit to the right of the tens place is four, so you round down.
Hundreds	1200	The digit to the right of the hundreds position is three, so you round down.
Thousands	1000	The digit to the right of the thousands position is two, so you round down.
Tenths	1234.6	The digit to the right of the tenths position is six, so you round up.
Hundredths	1234.57	The digit to the right of the hundredths position is seven, so you round up.
Thousandths	1234.568	The digit to the right of the thousandths position is eight, so you round up.
Ten thousandths	1234.5678	No change.

Solving Problems with Proportions

A **proportion** is a statement of equality between two ratios. For example, the proportion 2:6 = 3:9 means that 2 is related to 6 in the same way that 3 is related to 9. It is verbalized as "two is to six as three is to nine."

Proportions are useful for converting from one unit to another when three of the terms in the proportion are known. For example, you need $32.50, but only have quarters. How many quarters are needed? Three of the terms in the proportion are known:

1. $32.50
2. 4 (the number of quarters that are in $1.00)
3. $1.00

The proportion is set up as follows:

$$\frac{4 \text{ quarters}}{\text{x quarters}} = \frac{\$1.00}{\$32.50}$$

The purpose of the proportion is to answer the question: "If four quarters equal one dollar, how many quarters are there in thirty-two dollars and fifty cents?" Or put another way: "4 quarters is to $1.00 as X quarters are to $32.50." *Note that the two unit measurements on each side of the equation are the same* (quarters on the left and dollars on the right). The "X" stands for the number to be calculated.

To solve this problem, follow these steps:

1. Cross multiply:

$$\frac{4 \text{ quarters}}{\text{x quarters}} = \frac{\$1.00}{\$32.50}$$

$$1 \times x = 4 \times 32.50 = 1x = 130$$

2. Divide each side by the number in front of "x" (in this case each number divided by one and this does not alter the number)

3. $1x \div 1 = x$ and $130 \div 1 = 130$

$$x = 130 \text{ quarters}$$

4. 130 quarters are needed to make a payment of $32.50.

5. The completed proportion is:

$$\frac{4 \text{ quarters}}{130 \text{ quarters}} = \frac{\$1.00}{\$32.50}$$

Converting units of measure is another common application of proportions. For example, you want to know how many feet are in 29 inches. Again, three of the terms in the proportion are known:

1. 29 inches

2. 12 (the number of inches in 1 foot)

3. 1 foot

The proportion is set up as follows:

$$\frac{1 \text{ foot}}{x \text{ feet}} = \frac{12 \text{ inches}}{29 \text{ inches}}$$

To solve this problem, follow these steps:

1. Cross multiply:

$$\frac{1 \text{ foot}}{x \text{ feet}} = \frac{12 \text{ inches}}{29 \text{ inches}}$$

$$12 \times x = 1 \times 29 = 12x = 29$$

2. Divide each side by the number in front of "x"

$$12x \div 12 = x \quad \text{and} \quad 29 \div 12 = 2.42$$

$$x = 2.42 \text{ feet (rounded to nearest hundredth)}$$

3. The completed proportion is:

$$\frac{1 \text{ foot}}{2.42 \text{ feet}} = \frac{12 \text{ inches}}{29 \text{ inches}}$$

A common application of proportions in health care is to find the value of an unknown when converting medications from one form to another. For example, a physician orders a patient to have 50 grams of a medication. When the nurse checks, she notes that the medication is only available in 12.5 gram tablets. How many tablets should she give the patient?

$$\frac{1 \text{ tablet}}{x \text{ tablets}} = \frac{12.5 \text{ grams}}{50 \text{ grams}}$$

To solve this problem:

1. Cross multiply:

$$\frac{1 \text{ tablet}}{x \text{ tablets}} = \frac{12.5 \text{ grams}}{50 \text{ grams}}$$

$$12.5 \times x = 1 \times 50 = 12.5x = 50$$

2. Divide each side by the number in front of x

$$12.5x \div 12.5 = x \text{ and } 50 \div 12.5 = 4$$

$$x = 4 \text{ tablets}$$

3. 4 tablets are needed to equal 50 grams

4. The completed proportion is:

$$\frac{1 \text{ tablet}}{4 \text{ tablets}} = \frac{12.5 \text{ grams}}{50 \text{ grams}}$$

ESTIMATING

Health care workers must work carefully and thoughtfully when performing calculations. An important skill to help check work is anticipating the results. This involves **estimating**–calculating the approximate answer–and judging if the calculated results seem reasonable. If calculations are performed without thought and answers simply accepted, errors can go unnoticed. It is easy for mistakes to occur when you're working in a hurry. Numbers can be placed in the wrong order, decimal points misplaced, or operations carried out incorrectly. Knowing when an answer "just doesn't look right" serves as an alert to double-check the results. Working on "automatic pilot" is not acceptable when using math in the workplace.

Learning to estimate and detect incorrect answers takes practice and thought. There are a few guidelines to make estimating useful. First, use rounding to get numbers that are easier to mentally compute. For example, when multiplying 47 times 83, round 47 up to 50 and 83 down to 80. 50 times 80 is much easier to mentally multiply than the original numbers. Second, watch place values carefully. In the 50 times 80 example, if 5 is multiplied times 8, two zeroes must be added to the quick result of 40. Third, look at the size of the answer. Does it make sense? For example, when multiplying whole numbers, the answer should be larger than either of the numbers in the problem. And when dividing, it should be smaller. Fourth, be careful about placing decimal points. Remember that everything to the right of the point is a fraction. Even 0.99999 does not equal 1.0.

MILITARY TIME

Military time is frequently used in healthcare to avoid the confusion created by the AM and PM used in the traditional system to designate the correct time. The problem with the traditional system is that if the AM or PM is omitted or misread, an error of 12 hours is made. Errors in recording times are unacceptable in health care. For example, accuracy is critical when entering data on a patient chart, reporting when medications are given, or signing off physician orders.

When **military time** is the standard used, all time designations are made with the 24-hour clock. The 12th hour is at 12 noon and the 24th hour is at 12 midnight.

See Figure 5–4. When using the 24-hour clock, remember the following key points:

- Time is always expressed using four digits (i.e., 0030, 0200, 1200, 1700)

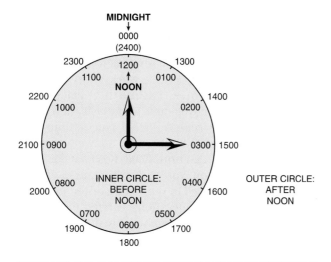

Figure 5–4 The military clock is based on a 24-hour day.

- AM hours are expressed with the same numbers as the traditional clock:

  1 AM: 0100

  5:30 AM: 0530

  10 AM: 1000

- An easy way to convert the PM hours is to add the time to 1200. Examples:

  1 PM: 1200 + 0100 (1:00 PM expressed in four digits) = 1300

  5:30 PM: 1200 + 0530 (5:30 PM expressed in four digits) = 1730

  10 PM: 1200 + 1000 (10:00 PM expressed in four digits) = 2200

- When times are verbalized, there is a specific way in which it is expressed:

  1300 = thirteen hundred hours

  1301 = thirteen oh one

  1730 = seventeen thirty hours

  2200 = twenty-two hundred hours

  Study Table 5–7 to practice converting between traditional and military times.

ROMAN NUMERALS

The traditional numbering system we use every day is referred to as Arabic numerals (1, 2, 3, . . .). In health care, it is necessary to know Roman numerals, because they are used for some medications, solutions, and ordering systems. You may also see some files or materials organized using

Roman numerals. When using Roman numerals, remember the following key points:

- All numbers can be expressed by using seven key numerals:

  I = 1

  V = 5

  X = 10

  L = 50

  C = 100

  D = 500

  M = 1000

- If a smaller numeral is placed in front of a larger numeral, the smaller numeral is *subtracted* from the larger numeral. For example:

  IV = 1 is placed before the 5, so it is subtracted (5 – 1 = 4)

- If a smaller numeral is placed after a larger numeral, the smaller numeral is *added* to the larger numeral. For example:

  VI = 1 is placed after the 5, so it is added (5 + 1 = 6)

- When the same numeral is placed next to itself it is added. For example:

  III = 1 + 1 + 1 = 3

  XX = 10 + 10 = 20

  IXX = this has two of the same numeral preceded by a smaller numeral, but the rules still apply (10 + 10 – 1 = 19 OR 10 – 1 = 9 + 10 = 19)

- The same numeral is not placed next to itself more than three times. For example,

  XXX = 30

  XL = 40 (XXXX is not correct)

  When Roman numerals are used with medication dosages, the lower case (i, v, x, l, c, d, m) may be used rather than uppercase (capital letters). For example, ii = 2, iv = 4, ixx = 19.

  Study Table 5–8 to practice converting between Arabic and Roman numerals.

ANGLES

Angles are used in health care when injecting medications, describing joint movement, and indicating bed positions. **Angles** are always defined by comparison to a **reference plane**, a real or imaginary flat surface from which the angle is measured. The distance between the plane and the line

Table 5–7 Military (24-Hour Clock) and Traditional Time Conversion Chart

Traditional	24-Hour Time	Traditional	24-Hour Time
12:01 AM	0001	12:01 PM	1201
12:30 AM	0030	12:30 PM	1230
1:00 AM	0100	1:00 PM	1300
2:00 AM	0200	2:00 PM	1400
3:00 AM	0300	3:00 PM	1500
4:00 AM	0400	4:00 PM	1600
5:00 AM	0500	5:00 PM	1700
6:00 AM	0600	6:00 PM	1800
7:00 AM	0700	7:00 PM	1900
8:00 AM	0800	8:00 PM	2000
9:00 AM	0900	9:00 PM	2100
10:00 AM	1000	10:00 PM	2200
11:00 AM	1100	11:00 PM	2300
12:00 noon	1200	12:00 midnight	2400

Table 5–8 Arabic and Roman Numeral Conversion Chart

Arabic	Roman	Arabic	Roman
1	I	9	IX
2	II	10	X
3	III	20	XX
4	IV	21	XXI
5	V	22	XXII
6	VI	23	XXIII
7	VII	24	XXIV
8	VIII	25	XXV

(continues)

Table 5–8 (continued)

Arabic	Roman	Arabic	Roman
26	XXVI	40	XL
27	XXVII	50	L
28	XXVIII	100	C
29	XXIX	500	D
30	XXX	1000	M

of the angle is measured in units called **degrees**. For example, if a flat stick is placed on a table (the reference plane), the angle is at 0 degrees. There is no distance between the plane and the stick. If the stick is lifted to stand straight up (perpendicular to the table), there is a 90 degree angle to the table. Moving the stick halfway between these two positions creates a 45 degree angle. Rotating the stick all the way around the arc and returning to the reference point creates a complete circle and represents 360 degrees. See Figure 5–5. The following examples illustrate how angles are used in health care:

Example 1 Angles for injecting needles vary, depending on the type of medication or procedure being performed. See Figure 5–6. Note that in this case the reference plane is the skin surface.

Example 2 When describing the angle of extremities (arms and legs), the body in a full upright position is the reference plane. See Figure 5–7. Each joint (e.g., elbow, knee, hip) in the body has a normal range it is intended to move within. Physicians assess the range of a patient's joint compared to this normal range to chart loss of function or progress of recovery.

Example 3 After surgery on a joint (e.g., hip or knee replacement), the physician will order for that joint not to be moved more than a certain number of degrees to prevent the new joint from "popping" out of place.

Example 4 Sometimes the physician will order to keep the head of the bed elevated by 30–45 degrees at all times. This is usually ordered to aid in respiration or to prevent aspiration (stomach contents entering the lungs). In this situation, the bed in the flat position is the reference plane.

SYSTEMS OF MEASUREMENT

Basic skills in calculation are applied when learning and using the various systems of measurement used in health care. Each system has its own terminology for designating distance (length), capacity (volume) and mass (weight). Converting between these systems requires the use of the skills presented in this chapter. The three systems used in health care are household, metric, and apothecary. Each system has its own **nomenclature** (method of naming).

Household System

The **household system** is probably the method of measurement most familiar to students who are educated in the United States. See Table 5–9. Note that "ounce" is used as both a measurement of capacity/volume and mass/weight. Health care

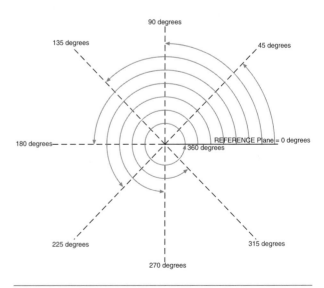

Figure 5–5 All angles are expressed in relation to a real or imaginary reference plane.

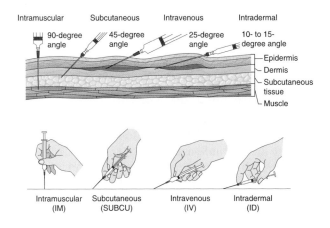

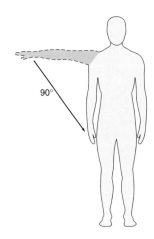

Figure 5–6 The correct angle must be used when inserting needles for administration of injections.

Figure 5–7 Body in full upright position with right arm lifted to 90 degree angle.

workers use both. Liquids, such as an 8-ounce glass of water, are measured in terms of capacity or volume. Determining mass or weight, such as with a 6-pound 12-ounce infant, is done by weighing with a scale. The various units of measurements in the household system relate to each other and can be converted among themselves. For example, volume/capacity is measured in drops, teaspoons, tablespoons, ounces, cups, pints,

quarts, and gallons. Knowing the equivalencies of these units enables you to calculate each one in terms of the others. See Figure 5–8.

When the basic equivalents are known, unknown measurements can be determined using proportions. Suppose that 3 tablespoons of a liquid are needed, but the only measuring device available is a cup marked in ounces (oz). How many

Table 5–9 Household Measurement System

Type of Measurement	Nomenclature	Common Equivalents
Distance/Length	inch (" or in) foot (' or ft) yard (yd) mile (mi)	12 in = 1ft 3 ft = 1 yd 1760 yds = 1 mi
Capacity/Volume	drop (gtt) teaspoon (t or tsp) tablespoon (T or tbsp) ounce (oz) cup (C) pint (pt) quart (qt) gallon (gal)	60 gtts = 1 t 3 t = 1 T 2 T = 1 oz 8 oz = 1 C 2 C = 1 pt 2 pt = 1 qt 4 qt = 1 gal
Mass/Weight	ounce (oz) pound (lb)	16 oz = 1 lb

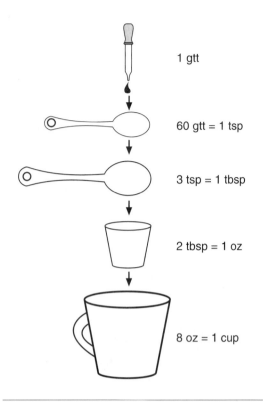

1 gtt

60 gtt = 1 tsp

3 tsp = 1 tbsp

2 tbsp = 1 oz

8 oz = 1 cup

Figure 5–8 Common household measurements used in health care.

ounces are in 3 tablespoons (3T)? Knowing that 2 T = 1 oz, the proportion would be set up as follows:

$$\frac{2\ T}{3\ T} = \frac{1\ oz}{x\ oz}$$

2x = 3 oz
2x ÷ 2 = 3 oz ÷ 2
x = 1.5 oz

The next example involves measurement of height. If a patient is 63 inches tall and asks how many feet that is, the calculation would use the following proportion:

$$\frac{12\ inches}{63\ inches} = \frac{1\ foot}{x\ feet}$$

12x = 63
12x ÷ 12 = 63 ÷ 12
x = 5.25 feet
x = 5.25 feet = 5 feet 3 inches
(0.25 feet × 12 inches = 3 inches)

Metric System

The **metric system** will probably be familiar to students who were educated outside the United States or have taken science classes. It is a more accurate system than the household system and

also is easier to convert between numbers because everything is based on a unit of ten. The nomenclature for the metric units is as follows:

- Distance/length: meter (m)
- Capacity/volume: liter (l or L)
- Mass/weight: gram (g or gm)

The meter, liter, and gram are modified by adding the appropriate prefix to express larger or smaller units (Table 5–10).

Being based on multiples of ten, conversions within the decimal system are calculated by multiplying by 10, 100, 1000, and so on:

- 1 *kilo*liter = 1000 × 1 liter = 1000 liters
- 1 *hecto*liter = 100 × 1 liter = 100 liters
- 1 *deca*liter = 10 × 1 liter = 10 liters
- 1 *deci*liter = 0.1 × 1 liter = 0.1 liter
- 1 *centi*liter = 0.01 × 1 liter = 0.01 liter
- 1 *milli*liter = 0.001 × 1 liter = 0.001 liter

A shortcut for performing these operations is to move the decimal point the number of places indicated by the prefix. Here are three examples:

Example 1 Multiplying 1 by 10 means moving the decimal point one place to the right. This may require adding one or more zeroes.

Example 2 Multiplying 4.2 by 10 = 42

Example 3 Multiplying 4.2 by 100 = 420

Converting units within the metric system is accomplished by moving the decimal point. For example, if the physician orders 2000 milligrams

Thinking it Through

Part of Mrs. Cabinos's job as an admitting assistant in an ambulatory clinic is to ask all patients their height and weight and record it on a graph. When she asks Mr. Summerton, he reports that he is 6 feet tall and weighs 160 lbs and 8 oz. The graph used at this clinic is in inches and pounds.

1. How many inches are in 6 feet?
2. How do you convert 160 lbs and 8 oz to pounds only?

Table 5–10 Common Prefixes of the Metric System

Prefix	Meaning	Examples	Meaning of Examples
kilo	1000 times	kilogram kilometer kiloliter	1000 grams 1000 meters 1000 liters
hecto	100 times	hectogram	100 grams
deca (also "deka")	10 times	decaliter	10 liters
meter, liter, gram	Whole units of measurement		
deci	1/10	decigram	1/10 of a gram
centi	1/100	centimeter	1/100 of a meter
milli	1/1000	milliliter	1/1000 of a liter
micro	1/1,000,000	microgram	1/1,000,000 of a gram

of a medication and this needs to be converted to grams, the conversion is made as follows:

1. Milli is in the third place to the right of gram. Move the decimal point three spaces to the left toward gram: 2000 = 2.000, or 2

2. Change unit name to grams: 2 grams

3. The proper dose would be 2 grams, or two 1 gram tablets

A second example involves converting 1000 centimeters to kilometers:

1. Centi is five decimal places to the right of kilo, so move the decimal point five spaces to the left *toward* kilo. Add zeros as needed: 1000 = 0.01

2. Change unit name to kilometers: 0.01 kilometers.

See Figure 5–9 for a visual representation of decimal placement.

In addition to moving the decimal point the correct number of places, it is critical that it be moved in the correct direction. This can be confusing. The easiest way is to determine if the answer should be a larger or smaller number and then just move the decimal point accordingly:

1. If converting from a larger to a smaller prefix (i.e., kilo to milli), the answer will be larger. It takes more smaller units to make up the larger unit.

2. If converting from a smaller to a larger prefix (i.e. milli to kilo), the answer will be smaller. Many smaller units can be contained in a smaller number of larger units.

PREFIX	KILO-	HECTO-	DEKA-	BASE	DECI-	CENTI-	MILLI-	DECIMILLI-	CENTIMILLI-	MICROMILLI-
Common Units	kilogram			gram liter meter		centimeter	milligram milliliter millimeter			microgram
Value to Base	**1000**	100	10	**1.0**	0.1	**0.01**	**0.001**	0.0001	0.00001	0.000001

Figure 5–9 Comparison of Common Metric Units Used in Health Care.

A common health care application of the metric system is in the measurement of medications. Two units that are often seen and which represent the same amount are milliliters (mL) and cubic centimeters (cc). Both are units that measure volume and they are often interchanged when dispensing liquids. For example, 1 mL = 1 cc, 2mL = 2 cc, etc. It is also worth noting that 1 mL or cc has a weight of 1 gram. See Figure 5–10.

Apothecary System

The **apothecary system** is the oldest and least used of the three systems of measurement presented. Some physicians still write orders using the apothecary system, so it is necessary to be familiar with these units of measurements (Table 5–11). Health care workers must be able to convert within the system as well as to convert to the metric system.

Roman numerals can be used in conjunction with the apothecary system, and may be seen in uppercase or lowercase. If lowercase is used, the Roman numeral for "1" is written with a line and a dot. For example "2" would be written as ii. A commonly used abbreviation that originated with the apothecary system is s̄s̄, which means "half." For example 2½ would be written as iiss.

Converting Systems of Measurement

Health care work sometimes requires that units from one system of measurement are converted to those of another. This requires knowledge of the equivalencies between the units of the systems. There are frequently no exact equivalents, so when converting between systems the answer is considered to be a close approximation. See Table 5–12.

Using the appropriate equivalencies, a proportion is then set up to identify and solve for the

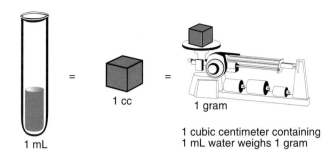

Figure 5–10 The metric units that measure weight and volume are related.

unknown quantity. The following steps are used for performing conversions:

1. Identify an equivalent between the two systems
2. Set up a proportion so unit measurements on each side of the equation are the same
3. Use x for the unknown value being calculated
4. Cross-multiply
5. Solve for x
6. Verify if the answer is reasonable
   a. If converting from a smaller unit to a larger unit, the answer will be smaller. For example, when converting 2 quarters to dollars, the result will be smaller than 2 because a quarter is a smaller unit than a dollar. Because there are 4 quarters in 1 dollar, 2 quarters = 0.5 dollar.
   b. If converting from a larger unit to a smaller unit, the answer will be larger. For example, when converting 2 dollars to quarters, the result will be larger unit than 2 because a dollar is a larger unit than a quarter. Because there is 1 dollar for every 4 quarters, 2 dollars = 8 quarters).

Table 5–11 Apothecary Measurement System

Type of Measurement	Nomenclature	Common Equivalents
Distance/Length	N/A	N/A
Capacity/Volume	minim ♏ fluid dram (fl dr or ƒ ʒ) fluid ounce (fl oz or ƒ ʒ) pint (pt) quart (qt)	1 minim = 1 drop 60 minims = 1 fl dr 8 fl dr = 1 fl oz 16 fl oz = 1 pt 2 pt = 1 qt
Mass/Weight	grain (gr) dram (dr or ʒ) ounce (oz. or ʒ)	60 gr = 1 dr 480 gr = 1 oz

Table 5–12 Approximate Equivalents Between Measuring Systems

Distance/Length	Capacity/Volume	Mass/Weight
1 in = 2.5 cm 39.4 in = 1 m	1 tsp = 5 ml = 5 cc 1 oz = 30 ml = 30 cc 1 qt = 1000 ml = 1000 cc	2.2 lb = 1 kg 1 grain = 60 milligrams 15 grains = 1 gram

The following examples illustrate how to perform conversions:

Example 1 Convert 19 inches to centimeters:

1. Identify equivalency: 1 inch = 2.5 centimeters
2. Set up a proportion with same units on each side of equation. Use x for the unknown.

$$\frac{1 \text{ in}}{19 \text{ in}} = \frac{2.5 \text{ cm}}{x \text{ cm}}$$

3. Cross-multiply:

$$1x = 47.5 \text{ cm}$$

4. Solve for x:

$$1x \div 1 = 47.5 \div 1$$
$$x = 47.5 \text{ cm}$$

5. Verify if answer is reasonable: It takes a larger number of centimeters (2½ times) to measure the same distance as 1 inch. Therefore, it makes sense that the answer is larger than 19.

Example 2 Convert 1.5 meters to inches:

1. Identify equivalency: 39.4 inches = 1 meter
2. Set up a proportion with the same units on each side of equation. Use x for the unknown.

$$\frac{39.4 \text{ in}}{x \text{ in}} = \frac{1 \text{ m}}{1.5 \text{ m}}$$

3. Cross-multiply:

$$1x = 59.1 \text{ inches}$$

4. Solve for x:

$$1x \div 1 = 59.1 \div 1$$
$$x = 59.1 \text{ inches}$$

5. Verify if answer is reasonable: It takes many inches to measure the distance designated by 1 meter. Therefore, the answer 59.1 makes sense.

Example 3 Convert 5 teaspoons to milliliters:

$$\frac{1 \text{ tsp}}{5 \text{ tsp}} = \frac{5 \text{ ml}}{x \text{ ml}}$$
$$x = 25 \text{ ml (25 cc)}$$

Example 4 Convert 75 milliliters to ounces:

$$\frac{1 \text{ oz}}{x \text{ oz}} = \frac{30 \text{ ml}}{75 \text{ ml}}$$

$$30x = 75 \quad \text{(Note that in solving for x, each side is divided by 30)}$$

$$x = 2.5 \text{ oz}$$

Example 5 Convert 120 pounds to kilograms:

$$\frac{2.2 \text{ lb}}{120 \text{ lb}} = \frac{1 \text{ kg}}{x \text{ kg}}$$

$$2.2x = 120 \quad \text{(Note that in solving for x, each side is divided by 2.2)}$$

$$x = 54.5 \text{ kg (rounded to nearest tenth)}$$

Example 6 Convert 60 kilograms to ounces:

$$\frac{2.2 \text{ lb}}{x \text{ oz}} = \frac{1 \text{ kg}}{60 \text{ kg}}$$

This problem cannot be solved using this proportion, because the unit measurements on the left side of the equation are not the same size (pound and ounce). To solve this problem, pounds must first be converted to ounces. Refer back to the household system and Table 5–9: 16 ounces = 1 pound.

$$\frac{16 \text{ oz}}{x} = \frac{1 \text{ lb}}{2.2 \text{ lb}}$$
$$x = 35.2 \text{ oz}$$

Knowing that 2.2 pounds = 35.2 ounces = 1 kilogram allows the appropriate proportion to be set up:

$$\frac{35.2 \text{ oz}}{x \text{ oz}} = \frac{1 \text{ kg}}{60 \text{ kg}}$$
$$x = 2112 \text{ oz}$$

Example 7 Convert 15 gr to milligrams:

$$\frac{1 \text{ gr}}{15 \text{ gr}} = \frac{60 \text{ mg}}{x \text{ mg}}$$
$$x = 900 \text{ mg}$$

Example 8 Convert 2 gm to grains:

$$\frac{15 \text{ gr}}{x \text{ gr}} = \frac{1 \text{ gm}}{2 \text{ gm}}$$
$$x = 30 \text{ gr}$$

TEMPERATURE CONVERSION

Thermometers using **Fahrenheit (F)** as the measuring unit are more familiar to people living in the United States, though the Celsius or **centigrade (C)** system of measurement is frequently seen in medical practice. One way to start understanding the difference between the two systems is to compare how each one expresses the boiling and freezing points of water.

Boiling points: 212°F = 100°C

Freezing points: 32°F = 0°C

See Figure 5–11 for a comparison of Fahrenheit (F) and Centigrade (C) thermometers and Table 5–13 for a conversion chart. Health care workers may have to convert between the F and C systems when a conversion chart is not available. Table 5–14 contains the formulas for conversion. There is a fraction and a decimal approach that give the same results. Deciding which to use depends on whether you have stronger skills working with fractions or decimals. All the formulas include parentheses. These are used to indicate that the enclosed calculation must be

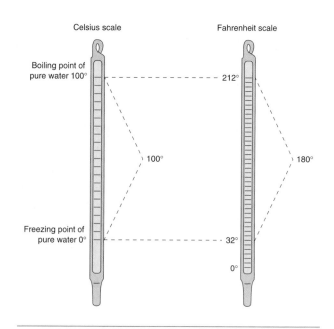

Figure 5–11 Comparison of Fahrenheit and Celsius temperature scales.

performed first. For example the steps to solve the formula (°F − 32) × ⅝ = °C are to first subtract 32 from the value for °F and *then* multiply that value by ⅝.

Table 5–13 Fahrenheit–Centigrade Conversion Chart

Fahrenheit	Centigrade
32 (freezing point)	0 (freezing point)
95	35
96	35.6
97	36.1
97.4	36.3
98	36.7
98.6	37
99	37.2
99.4	37.4
100	37.8
101	38.3
102	38.9
103	39.4
104	40
212 (boiling point)	100 (boiling point)

Table 5–14 Temperature Scale Conversion Formulas

Convert From:	Fraction Formula	Decimal Formula
Centigrade to Fahrenheit	(°C × 9/5) + 32 = °F Example: 37°C (37 × 9/5) + 32 = °F 333/5 + 32 = 98.6° F	(°C × 1.8) + 32 = °F Example: 37°C (37 × 1.8) + 32 = °F 66.6 + 32 = 98.6°F
Fahrenheit to Centigrade	(°F – 32) × 5/9 = °C Example: 101°F (101 – 32) × 5/9 = °C 69 × 5/9 = °C 345/9 = 38.3°C (rounded to nearest tenth)	(°F – 32) ÷ 1.8 = °C Example: 101°F (101 – 32) ÷ 1.8 = °C 69 ÷ 1.8 = 38.3°C (rounded to nearest tenth)

SUGGESTED LEARNING ACTIVITIES

1. Consider the math anxiety section of this chapter. Do you feel you have math anxiety? Identify available resources and create a plan to conquer the problem.

2. Cut a whole pie, cake, or paper plate into slices (you determine how many). Then practice by separating out some of the slices and expressing them as part of the whole in decimals, fractions, percentages, and ratios.

3. If you have a large wall clock, attach numbers cut out of paper to it to indicate military time. Or make a paper clock and put it up where you see it frequently. Practice telling time using the 24-hour format.

4. When you see numbers on street signs, practice converting them to Roman numerals.

5. Stand in front of a mirror and as you move your extremities try to estimate the degree of movement.

6. Practice, practice, practice using the systems of measurement until you can consistently do them accurately:
   - Weigh yourself in pounds and convert to kilograms.
   - Measure your height in inches and convert to meters.
   - Find various household measurement items (teaspoon, tablespoon, measuring cups) and convert them to the metric system.
   - Look at the strength of any medications you currently have in the house and convert it to another system of measurement (i.e., if the Tylenol or aspirin bottle has the strength listed in grains convert to milligrams or if listed as milligrams convert to grains).
   - Take your temperature in Fahrenheit and convert to centigrade.

REVIEW QUESTIONS

1. What is math anxiety, and what are the common myths and games that help create the anxiety?

2. What are the key points to remember when adding, subtracting, multiplying, and dividing decimals and fractions, and when converting decimals, fractions, percentages, and ratios?

3. How does military time differ from the traditional system? What are the advantages?

4. How do Roman numerals differ from the traditional numbering system? What are the key points to remember when using Roman numerals?

5. Give three examples of how angles are used in health care.

6. What are the three systems of measurement currently used in health care? Within each system, what is the nomenclature used for length, volume, and weight?

7. What are the equations for converting between the three systems of measurement?

8. What are the equations for converting Fahrenheit to Celsius? Celsius to Fahrenheit?

APPLICATION EXERCISES

1. Refer back to The Case of Exactly How Much Does My Baby Weigh? at the beginning of this chapter. Jaime explains that the baby also grew 2 inches. How many centimeters would this be?

2. Maria is working in the hospital and when taking vital signs, she discovers that a patient has a temperature of 37.6°C. When she checks the orders, she finds the physician has ordered Tylenol gr x to be given every four hours as needed for a temperature above 101°F. Maria notes it is 4 PM and the last dose was given at 1300 hours. The Tylenol tablets she has available are marked as 525 mg/tablet. She gives the patient two tablets and charts the time given as 1500.

   a. Assuming the last dose was given at 1300 hours, when would the next dose of Tylenol be due? If it is now 4 PM, how much time has elapsed since the medication was given?

   b. Did Maria note the time correctly? If not, how is 4 PM expressed in military time?

   c. What would be the equivalent of 101°F in the Celsius system? Was the temperature elevated high enough to give the Tylenol as ordered?

   d. Was the correct amount of medication given? If not, was too much or too little given?

SUGGESTED READINGS AND RESOURCES

Benjamin-Chung, M. (1999). *Math principles and practices: Preparing for health career success.* Upper Saddle River, NJ: Prentice-Hall.

Kee, J. L. and Marshall, S. M. (1996). *Clinical calculations with applications to general and specialty areas* (3rd ed.). Philadelphia: W. B. Saunders Company.

Kogelman, S. and Warren, J. (1978). *Mind over math: Put yourself on the road to success by freeing yourself from math anxiety.* New York: McGraw Hill.

Math learning resources: http://forum.swathmore.edu/math.topics.html

Richardson, J. K. and Richardson, L. I. (1994) *The mathematics of drugs and solutions with clinical applications* (5th ed.). St. Louis: Mosby Year-Book, Inc.

Simmers, L. (1996). *Practical problems in mathematics for health occupations.* Albany, NY: Delmar.

UNIT

THE HUMAN BODY

3

CHAPTER

ORGANIZATION OF THE HUMAN BODY

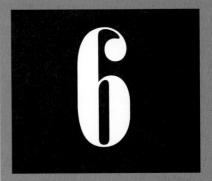

6

OBJECTIVES

Studying and applying the material in this chapter will help you to:

- Explain the meaning of homeostasis.

- Name the levels in the structural organization of the body.

- Name and explain the function of the main cellular components.

- Name and describe the four primary types of tissues.

- Describe the anatomical position.

- Identify and describe the location of the three directional body planes.

- Use directional terms to describe various locations on the body.

- Name the main body cavities and what structures are found in each.

- Identify the abdominal regions and quadrants.

KEY TERMS

abdominal cavity
anatomical position
anterior (ventral)
anterior body cavity
apex
base
body system
caudal
cell
cephalic (cranial)
cranial cavity
deep
distal
frontal plane
homeostasis
inferior
lateral
medial
midsagittal plane
organ
pelvic cavity
peripheral
posterior (dorsal)
posterior body cavity
proximal

continues

KEY TERMS *continued*

spinal cavity	superior	thoracic cavity
superficial	tissue	transverse plane

The Case of
the Exact Location

Paula Holland is seen in the Urgent Care Center with complaints of pain in the left lower arm. Several bruises and cuts are also noted on the upper and lower areas of the same arm. Arlene Dealy is working at the center and charts: "Mrs. Holland has lower arm pain, with multiple bruises and cuts on the arm."

When the patient returns the following week for complaints of pain in both of her arms, Gary Heinz reads the notes made by Arlene and is unable to determine if the original visit was for pain in the left or right arm. He also questions, how many, what size, and exactly where the bruises and cuts were located.

The material in this chapter will give the health care worker a medical language that is used to describe body locations, so other health care workers will know where to check when they see the patient.

THE BASIS OF LIFE

The processes that maintain life are remarkable in their complexity and effectiveness. They can only be truly appreciated by studying all the structures and functions that make up the human body. Sormunen (1995) expresses it well:

> Our bodies are marvelously intricate, delicate, and unique. Each part of the body has a purpose and function that fits into the whole. Cells, tissues, organs, and systems are all part of the human anatomy.

> The body is constantly working to keep itself in what is called a state of homeostasis. **Homeostasis** is the tendency of a cell or the whole organism to maintain a state of balance. To maintain this balance there are numerous tiny adjustments made every second throughout the body. These occur without our conscious awareness.

The structural organization of the body can be described as a series of levels. Organized from the smallest to the largest it can be summarized in the following order:

1. **Cells**: Smallest living structures in the body
2. **Tissues**: Cells with similar function grouped together
3. **Organs**: Two or more types of tissues combined to work together (examples: kidneys, lungs, heart, and liver)
4. **Body** (organ) **systems**: Two or more organs combined to provide a major body function (examples: respiratory, nervous, and urinary systems)
5. Human body as a whole

The cells and tissues will be presented in this chapter and the organs and body systems in the next. (See Figure 6–1.)

Cells

Cells are the smallest structures that carry on all the fundamental functions of life. Many of them perform

LEVEL

EXAMPLES

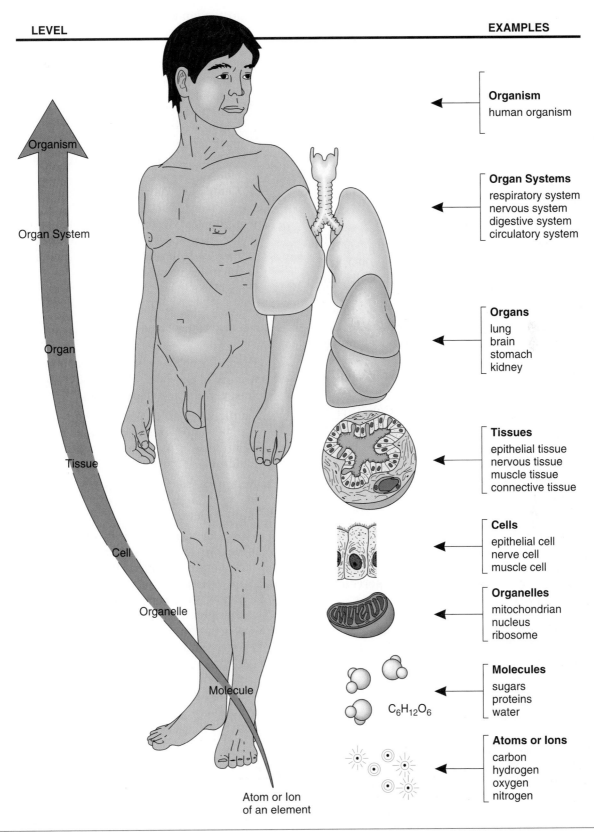

Organism
human organism

Organ Systems
respiratory system
nervous system
digestive system
circulatory system

Organs
lung
brain
stomach
kidney

Tissues
epithelial tissue
nervous tissue
muscle tissue
connective tissue

Cells
epithelial cell
nerve cell
muscle cell

Organelles
mitochondrian
nucleus
ribosome

Molecules
sugars
proteins
water

$C_6H_{12}O_6$

Atoms or Ions
carbon
hydrogen
oxygen
nitrogen

Organism

Organ System

Organ

Tissue

Cell

Organelle

Molecule

Atom or Ion
of an element

Figure 6–1 The structural organization of the body progresses from cells to the body as a whole.

specialized functions, such as support (bone cells), communication (nerve cells), oxygen transportation (red blood cells), movement (muscle cells), and protection (skin cells). See Figure 6–2. Cells can reproduce, grow, and repair themselves. To perform these functions, they take in nutrients (food) and oxygen to create heat and energy. Cells can move, adapt to their environment, and eliminate waste products.

Cells generally contain the following components (Figure 6–3):

1. Cell membrane: The outer covering; it controls which substances enter and leave the cell

2. Cytoplasm (protoplasm): Gel-like liquid inside the cell that consists of water, proteins, carbohydrates, lipids (fats), and salts

3. Organelles: Structures that have specialized functions

   ■ Nucleus: Controls the activity of the cell, including reproduction; contains the 23 (normally) chromosomes that contain the genes that transmit hereditary characteristics

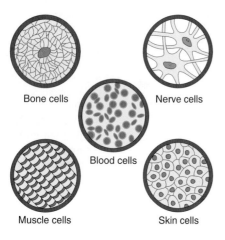

Figure 6–2 Cells vary in size, shape, and function.

■ Mitochondrion: Produce energy used for cellular processes; called the "powerhouse"

■ Lysosome: Contains various enzymes that help to digest (break down) molecules

■ Ribosomes: Produce protein for the cell structures

■ Golgi apparatus: Produces, stores, and packages products for discharge from the cell; (e.g., transports proteins made by the ribosomes)

■ Centrioles: Play a role in the division of the cell (reproduction)

■ Endoplasmic reticulum: Network of tubular structures to facilitate transport of materials in and out of the nucleus

■ Vacuole: Storage unit

Tissues

Tissues are categorized into four primary types (Figure 6–4):

1. Epithelial: Covers the internal and external organs of the body; lines body cavities, vessels, glands, and body organs

2. Connective: Holds parts of the body in place; can be liquid (blood), fibrous (tendons and ligaments), solid (bone), fatty (protective padding), or cartilage (rings of the trachea)

3. Nervous: Transmits impulses throughout the body to activate, coordinate, and control many functions

4. Muscular: Contracts and relaxes to cause or allow movement; the three types are:
   ■ Skeletal: Attached to bone and causes movement of the skeleton
   ■ Smooth (visceral): Found in the walls of the hollow internal organs of the body (e.g., stomach and intestines), blood vessels, and lung airways
   ■ Cardiac: Makes up the muscular wall of the heart

(Adapted from *Delmar's comprehensive medical terminology: A competency-based approach*, by B. D. Jones, 1999, Albany, NY: Delmar.)

DESCRIBING THE BODY

Health care workers need a language to use when speaking or writing about a particular location of a structure or area of the body. This language and special vocabulary describe body planes, directional terms, body cavities, and abdominal regions.

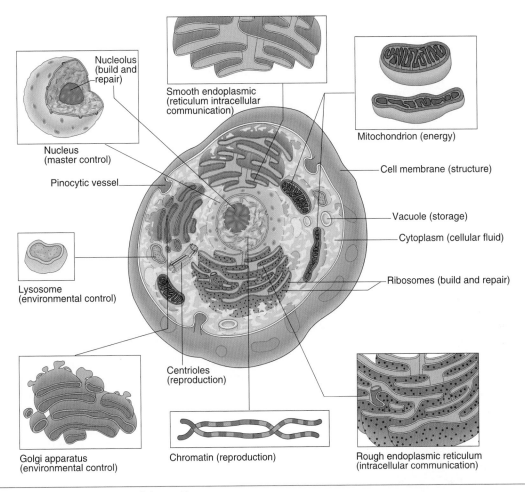

Figure 6–3 Major components of the cell.

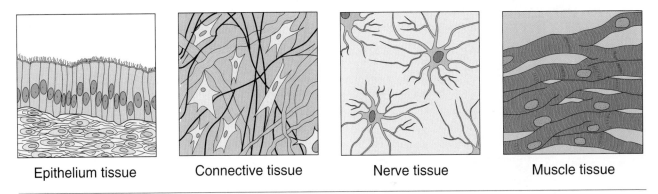

Epithelium tissue   Connective tissue   Nerve tissue   Muscle tissue

Figure 6–4 The four primary types of tissues found in the human body.

A mastery of these terms will allow you to accurately interpret descriptions written by other personnel and also to chart (document in writing) your findings in a way that others can understand.

The descriptive terms refer to the body as viewed in a full upright position (standing), with the arms relaxed at the side of the body, palms facing forward, feet pointed forward, and the eyes directed straight ahead. This is called the **anatomical position** (Figure 6–5).

Body Planes

A body plane is an imaginary flat surface that cuts through the body either horizontally or vertically. Imagine the body divided up by a large pane of window glass. There are three primary planes (Figure 6–6a & b):

1. **Midsagittal** (median or midline) plane: Passes from top to bottom through the center of the body and divides it into equal right and left sides

2. **Frontal plane** (coronal): Divides the body from top to bottom through the center and divides the body into front and back portions

3. **Transverse plane**: Divides the body horizontally (crosswise) into top and bottom portions

Directional Terms

Using east, west, north, and south works well for traditional directions, but would be of no value when referring to the body (have you ever heard of the eastern part of your body?) (Ehrlich, 1997). Directional terms for medical descriptions were created to solve this problem and are listed in Table 6–1. Also refer to Figure 6–6a & b.

The Body Cavities

Within the body there are interior spaces called cavities that contain and protect the internal organs. See Figure 6–7. The **posterior** (dorsal) **body cavity** protects the structures of the nervous system and has two parts (although the space is continuous):

1. **Cranial cavity**: Located in the skull and contains the brain

2. **Spinal cavity**: Located within the spinal column and contains the spinal cord

The **anterior** (ventral) **body cavity** protects the internal organs and has three parts:

1. **Thoracic cavity**: located in the chest and contains the heart, lungs, and major blood vessels; the diaphragm separates this cavity from the abdominal cavity

2. **Abdominal cavity**: located in the abdomen and contains the stomach, intestines, liver, gallbladder, pancreas, and spleen (the kidneys are located behind the abdominal cavity); the abdominal and pelvic cavities are continuous

3. **Pelvic cavity**: located in the lower abdomen and contains the urinary bladder, rectum, and reproductive organs

Smaller cavities include the orbital which contains the eyes and associated muscles, nerves, and ducts; the nasal which contains the structures of the nose; and the buccal, which contains the teeth and tongue.

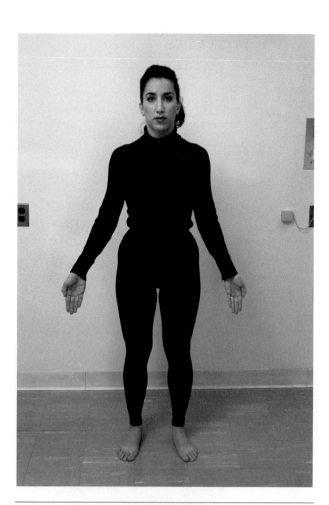

Figure 6–5 The anatomical position.

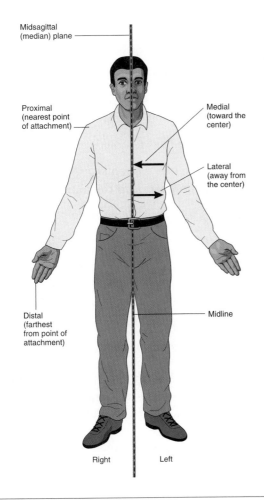

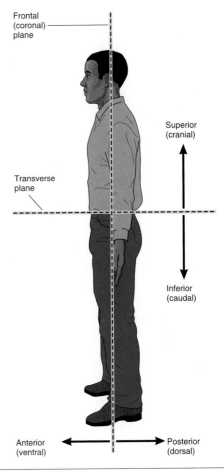

Figure 6–6a Sagittal Plane. The midsagittal (median or midline) plane divides the body from top to bottom into equal left and right halves.

Figure 6–6b Frontal and Transverse Planes. The frontal (coronal) plane divides the body into front (anterior) and back (posterior) portions. It is located at right angles to the sagittal plane. The transverse plane divides the body horizontally into top (superior) and bottom (inferior) portions. This division can be at the waist or any other level across the body.

Table 6–1 Directional Terms

Term	Meaning	Example
Lateral	away from center of body (toward the sides)	The lateral ligament of the knee is located on the outer side of the knee.
Medial	toward midline or center of body	The navel is on the medial line.
Anterior (ventral)	toward the front of body	The breasts are on the anterior surface of the body.
Posterior (dorsal)	toward the back of the body	The buttocks are on the posterior surface of the body.
Inferior	below	The lungs are inferior to the head.

(continues)

Table 6–1 (continued)

Term	Meaning	Example
Superior	above	The nose is superior to the mouth.
Caudal	closer to the coccyx (lower back)	The hips are caudal to the waist.
Cephalic (cranial)	closer to the head	The neck is cephalic to the shoulders.
Deep	farther from the body surface	The accident victim had a deep laceration (wound or irregular tear) that exposed the muscle.
Superficial	near or close to the body surface	There were only superficial scrapes on the skin.
Distal	further from reference base point	The hand is distal to the elbow.
Peripheral	away from the center	The patient had peripheral edema (excess fluid in the extremities—arms and legs).
Proximal	closer to reference point	The shoulder is proximal to the elbow.
Apex	at the top (highest point)	The top of the lung is called the apex.
Base	at the bottom (lowest point)	The bottom of the lung is called the base.

(Martini, 1997)

Abdominal Descriptions

The abdominal area is so large that it has been divided into nine regions so specific areas can be described with greater accuracy. The nine regions include the lower portion of the thoracic cavity and the abdominal and pelvic cavities (Figure 6–8).

These regions are:

- Epigastric ("over the stomach"): Located just below the sternum (breastbone)

- Right and left hypochondriac regions: Located below ribs on either side of the epigastric region

- Umbilical: Located around the umbilicus (navel)

- Right and left lumbar regions: Extend anterior to posterior on either side of the umbilical region (a person will complain of lumbar or back pain)

- Hypogastric ("below the stomach"): Located over the pubic area

- Right and left iliac (hip bone) regions: Located on either side of the hypogastric region (also called right and left inguinal areas)

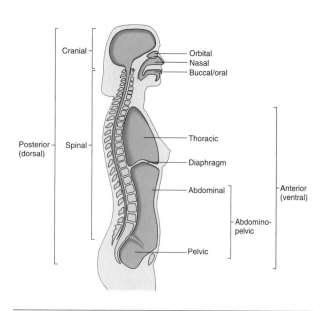

Cranial
Orbital
Nasal
Buccal/oral
Posterior (dorsal)
Spinal
Thoracic
Diaphragm
Abdominal
Anterior (ventral)
Abdomino-pelvic
Pelvic

Figure 6–7 Cavities of the body.

Thinking it Through

A patient arrives at the Urgent Care Center to be seen for a recent laceration (cut) of the arm. Miss Heather Jones, a health care worker at the clinic, examines the arm and describes the injury as to size and location.

1. Examine the diagram below to visualize what Miss Jones observed.
2. Describe the size and location of the injury.

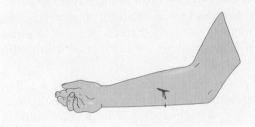

Another approach used in health care for describing the abdomen is quadrants. Imaginary lines are used to create four quadrants (Figure 6–9) that divide the abdominal area. All of the quadrants contain part of the large and small intestines, but some of the other internal organs can be identified within a particular quadrant.

1. Right upper quadrant (RUQ): Liver and gallbladder.
2. Right lower quadrant (RLQ): Appendix and some of the female reproductive organs.

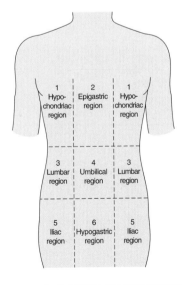

Figure 6–8 Regions of the lower thorax, abdomen, and pelvic cavities.

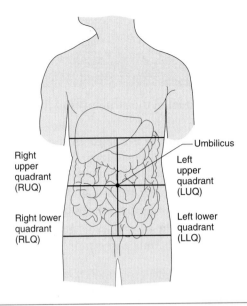

Figure 6–9 The abdomen divided into quadrants

3. Left upper quadrant (LUQ): Pancreas, stomach, and spleen.
4. Left lower quadrant (LLQ): Some of the female reproductive organs.

Thinking it Through

Esteban Valdez is a patient on a medical-surgical floor of a community hospital. He is experiencing some discomfort in the right buttock area and reports it to Martha Duarte, a Licensed Vocational (Practical) Nurse. The patient points to the area of discomfort, and Martha can see a small red dot, but no other abnormalities. Martha notes that the location identified by the patient is on the lateral side of the right buttock and inferior to the waist. She thinks it may be tenderness due to a recent injection (shot) that was given to the patient and checks the medication record. The record shows that Mr. Valdez had an injection into the RUQ of the buttock.

- RUQ, RLQ, LUQ, LLQ does not apply only to the abdomen, but can be used to divide any area into four equal parts. When giving an injection into the buttocks, the only correct sites would be into the upper quadrant of either buttock. Based on the description given, where was the small red dot located?
- Do you agree with Martha's conclusion?

SUGGESTED LEARNING ACTIVITIES

1. Draw and label the structures of the cell from memory.
2. Stand in front of a mirror in the anatomical position and visualize the midsagittal, frontal, and transverse planes of the body.
3. Point to any area of your body and describe its position using the directional terms.
4. Stand in front of a mirror and identify the abdominal regions and quadrants.

REVIEW QUESTIONS

1. What is homeostasis?
2. What are the levels in the structural organization of the body?
3. What are the components of the cell, and what are their functions?
4. What are the four primary types of tissues?
5. What is the anatomical position?
6. What are the three body planes and how do they divide the body?
7. What are the main directional terms used for medical descriptions?
8. What are the primary body cavities and what structures are in each one?
9. What are the two methods used for describing the abdominal area?

APPLICATION EXERCISES

1. Refer back to The Case of the Exact Location. If Arlene had used anatomical descriptions to identify Mrs. Holland's site of original pain and scratches, what words would she have used?
2. A patient comes into the physician's office complaining of a lot of abdominal pain. You ask her to show you where the pain is located. She points to an area between her breasts and to another area to the right of the pelvic area. You then leave to report your findings to the physician.
   a. What abdominal descriptor would you use to describe the first location?
   b. What abdominal descriptor would you use to describe the second location?

CHAPTER

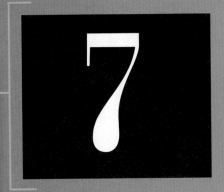

STRUCTURE AND FUNCTION OF THE HUMAN BODY

OBJECTIVES

Studying and applying the material in this chapter will help you to:

■ Understand and explain the difference between anatomy, physiology, and pathophysiology.

■ Define what determines a state of wellness as opposed to illness.

■ Describe the primary anatomical features and physiological actions of the systems for movement and protection of the body.

■ Name and demonstrate the movements made possible by joints.

■ Describe the primary anatomical features and physiological actions of the systems for providing energy and for removing waste from the body.

■ Describe the primary anatomical features and physiological actions of the systems for sensing, and for coordinating and controlling the body.

■ Describe the primary anatomical features and physiological actions of the systems for producing new life.

■ Name common diseases or disorders associated with each system.

■ Describe the behaviors and actions for each body system that promote health and prevent major diseases and disorders.

KEY TERMS

anatomy
diagnosis
diagnostic procedures
diseases
etiology
illness
objective data
pathophysiology
physiology
prevention (of disease)
prognosis
signs and symptoms
subjective data
syndrome
wellness
treatment

131

The Case of
the Unfamiliar Diagnosis

Janet Waring is an x-ray technician who works in a large medical center. Mr. Petersen is admitted with a diagnosis of Red Cedar Disease, and a lung x-ray is ordered. Janet has never heard of this disease and decides to do some independent research. The reference she uses explains why and how this disease damages the lungs, what to watch for when caring for the patient, and what tests may be ordered. By understanding how to properly use reference materials, Janet is able to learn that this condition can occur in loggers and sawmill workers when there is a high concentration of sawdust that is inhaled, causing damage to the lungs. Janet knows the normal structure and function of the lungs and can now apply this new knowledge to determine what consequences the damaged lungs may have for her patient. It also clarifies why the chest x-ray was ordered and what to observe for when caring for the patient. Understanding the material in this chapter will assist the health care worker to understand the normal structure and function of the body.

THE IMPORTANCE OF ANATOMY AND PHYSIOLOGY

The study of anatomy and physiology (A&P) is fundamental to understanding the normal structure and function of the body. **Anatomy** is the study of the *form and structure* of an organism, such as the names and locations of the bones, muscles, and organs. **Physiology** is the study of the *functions* (how and why something works) of these structures. Examples include how bones and muscles produce movement, how organs assist in digestion, and how nerve impulses from the brain trigger the eyelids to blink.

Understanding the normal structure and function of the body provides a base to help the health care worker to recognize abnormal conditions. These abnormal conditions are called **diseases**. When an abnormality occurs it is referred to as pathophysiology (patho = disease). **Pathophysiology** is the study of why diseases occur and how the body changes in function in reaction to the diseases. When studying pathophysiology, there are other terms that are used to describe a complete picture of the disease process and related information. These terms are:

- **Etiology**: Study of the causes of diseases. Diseases have a variety of causes. Examples include bacteria, viruses, hazardous materials, and personal habits.

- **Signs and symptoms**: Signs and symptoms (Sx) are usually used as one phrase, but actually have separate meanings. Signs are **objective** evidence of an illness. This means that they can be observed by the health care worker. Signs include patient behaviors, visible marks on the body, and test results. Symptoms are **subjective**. They cannot be directly observed by the health care worker but are reported by the patient. For example, a patient may report pain (subjective data), which cannot be observed directly. However, a behavior (objective data) such as a facial grimace or limp could be present that is a sign of pain. Another example is a patient who states that he has hypertension. This is subjective data and must be verified by taking the blood pressure to obtain objective data. Signs and symptoms serve as clues to the nature of underlying diseases or **syndromes** (not a precise disease but a group of related signs and symptoms).

- **Diagnostic Procedures**: Tests performed to determine the **diagnosis** (name of the disease or syndrome). To arrive at a diagnosis, the signs and symptoms are evaluated by taking a thorough patient history, doing a physical exam, and ordering laboratory tests, x-rays, or other special tests. An accurate diagnosis is necessary to determine the correct treatment and predict the outcome of the problem.

- **Treatment**: Medications or procedures used to control or cure the disease. Common treatments include surgery, exercise, and special diets.
- **Prognosis**: Prediction of the possible outcome of the disease and potential for recovery
- **Prevention**: Behaviors that promote health and prevent disease

The state of wellness or illness of individuals is directly related to their anatomy, physiology, or underlying pathophysiology. A state of **wellness** is experienced when the body maintains homeostasis. As explained in Chapter 6, homeostasis is the tendency of a cell or the whole organism to maintain a state of balance. A state of **illness** occurs when one or more of the body's control systems loses the ability to maintain homeostasis. All the cells of the body suffer when this occurs. A moderate dysfunction causes illness, and a severe dysfunction can lead to death.

There is increasing focus on preventive measures as researchers learn more about the causes of diseases and injuries. Prevention is organized into three levels:

1. Primary: Prevent the initial occurrence of the disease or injury by maintaining homeostasis. Practicing good lifestyle habits (Chapter 12) and avoiding exposure to bacteria and viruses (Chapter 10) are examples of preventive measures.
2. Secondary: Treat conditions that do occur as quickly as possible to prevent further damage.
3. Tertiary: Rehabilitate to allow the person to regain as much function as possible and prevent further disability.

THE SYSTEMS OF THE BODY

Chapter 6 included a discussion about the function of cells and how cells that perform a similar function group together to form tissues. Recall that when two or more of the four primary types of tissues (epithelial, connective, nervous, and muscular) combine to work together, they form organs. When two or more organs combine to perform a major body function, it is called a body system. Examples of body systems include respiratory, nervous, and urinary.

The systems work together in a very complex manner to maintain the body in a state of homeostasis or wellness. They are all interrelated and changes in one will affect others. A good practice when studying each system is to ask, "How does the function of this system affect all the other systems?" Some systems have a wide range of functions, and there are organs that actually belong to several systems and have more than one role.

Systems for Movement and Protection

The skeletal, muscular, and integumentary (skin) systems provide support, allow movement, and protect the body. Without bones and muscles, the body would be like an empty sack of skin without shape or the ability to move. The skin plays a critical role because it protects the body from hazards, prevents fluid loss, and helps control temperature.

Skeletal

The *skeletal system* is composed of the bones that provide a framework that:

- Gives shape to the body
- Provides places to which muscles can attach to produce movement
- Protects the internal organs
- Stores minerals
- Manufactures blood cells

Newborns have 270 bones (Keir, Wise, and Krebs, 1998). But as children grow, some of the bones fuse together so adults only have about 206 bones. (The number of bones in the hands and feet can vary among individuals.)

Bones vary in shape and are classified as follows (Figure 7–1):

- Long bones: Longer than they are wide (arms: humerus, radius, ulna; legs: femur, tibia, fibula; fingers and toes: metacarpals, metatarsals, phalanges)
- Short bones: Similar in length and width (bones of the wrist and ankles, which are called carpals and tarsals, respectively)
- Flat bones: Two layers with space between them (cranium, ribs, shoulder blade–scapula, breastbone–sternum, pelvis)
- Irregular bones: Those that do not fit into the other categories (spinal column–vertebrae, facial bones, patella)

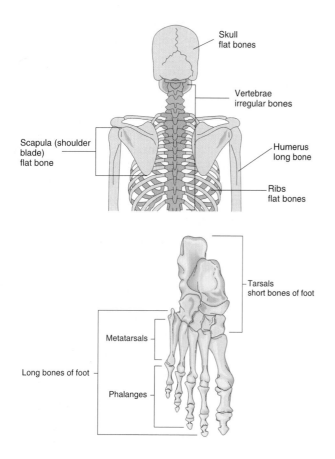

Figure 7–1 Bone shapes.

Bone Structure

It may be difficult to think of bones as organs, but they take in nutrients and oxygen and perform functions just like other organs. Bones do not consist of solid material, but contain layers that have different functions. The long bones have the following structure (Figure 7–2):

- Medullary canal: Center cavity containing *yellow marrow* (primarily fat cells); covered by a layer called *endosteum*

- Diaphysis: Portion that runs between the ends of the bone; also called the "shaft"

- Epiphyses: Ends of bone (proximal and distal)

- Periosteum: White, fibrous layer that covers the outside of bone; contains blood and lymph vessels, and nerves. Bone growth, repair, and nutrition occur in the periosteum. It is also serves as an attachment for muscles, tendons, and ligaments.

- Red marrow: Manufactures the red blood cells (RBCs), which carry oxygen and the white blood cells (WBCs), which protect the body from infections. Red bone marrow is

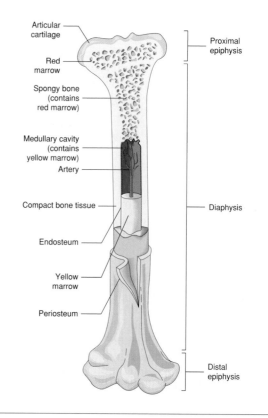

Figure 7–2 Structures of a long bone.

also found in other types of bones such as ribs (flat) and vertebrae (irregular).

- Cartilage: Elastic connective tissue that covers the end of the bones and functions as a cushion between bones. Cartilage also covers the surface of joints and forms the flexible parts of the skeleton such as the ear lobes and the tip of the nose.

The skeletal system is divided into two major parts known as the axial and the appendicular skeleton. The *axial skeleton* includes the bones of the:

- Skull
- Inner ear
- Hyoid (U-shaped bone lying at base of tongue)
- Spinal column
- Ribs
- Sternum (breastbone)

The *appendicular skeleton* includes the bones of the:

- Shoulders
- Arms
- Hands
- Pelvis

- Legs
- Feet

See Figure 7–3.

The 206 bones in the adult can be divided as follows:

Axial Skeleton:

- Head: 29 bones (22 in the cranium, 3 in each inner ear, and 1 hyoid)
- Trunk: 51 bones (26 vertebrae in spine, 24 ribs, and 1 sternum)

Appendicular Skeleton:

- Upper extremities: 64 bones in shoulders, arms, wrists, and hands
- Lower extremities: 62 bones in pelvis, legs, ankle, and feet

The Axial Skeleton

The *cranium* is composed of the skull and facial bones (Figure 7–4). The skull may feel smooth to the touch like one continuous bone, but it actually consists of eight bones:

- Temporal (2): shapes area around ears
- Occipital (1): shapes the base and back of the head

- Parietal (2): shapes the top and sides of head
- Frontal (1): shapes the forehead
- Sphenoid (1): a "bat shaped" bone that forms part of the cranial floor that acts as a bridge between the cranial and facial bones, and braces the sides of the skull
- Ethmoid (1): located between the eyes and anterior to the sphenoid bone that forms part of the cranial floor, medial surface of the orbit of eyes and the roof and sides of the nasal cavity

The face consists of 14 bones:

- Nasal (5): Shapes the nose
- Lacrimal (2): Located in the inner corner of the eye (tear duct)
- Maxilla (2): Shapes the upper jaw
- Zygomatic (2): Shapes the cheeks
- Mandible (1): Shapes the lower jaw (only movable bone in the face)
- Palatine (2): Shapes the hard palate of the mouth

Other structures that are related to the cranium include:

- Suture lines: Areas where the cranial bones have joined together (e.g., lambdoidal, squamous, and coronal). This joining does not occur

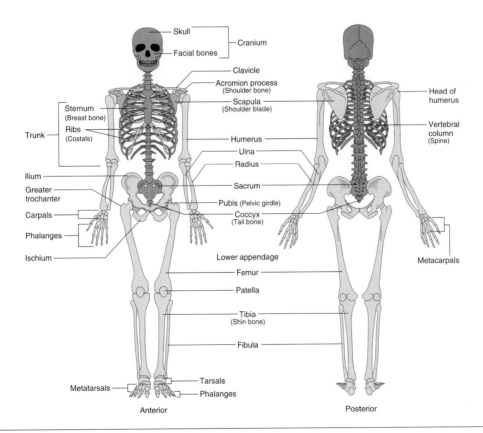

Figure 7–3 Bones of the skeleton (axial in red, appendicular in blue).

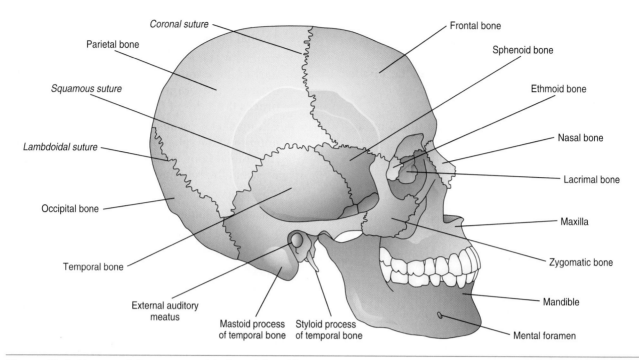

Figure 7–4 Bones of the cranium (skull and facial bones).

until after birth, usually by the end of the second year. Called fontanelles, or "soft spots," they allow the skull to expand and accommodate the growing brain.

- Sinus: Air cavity within a bone that acts as a resonating chamber for voice quality
- Foramina: An opening in the bone for blood vessels and nerves to pass through (e.g., mental foramen)

The spinal column consists of 26 *vertebrae* that serve to protect the spinal cord, support the head, and give shape to the back. The vertebrae are separated from each other and cushioned by *intervertebral disks* that are made of cartilage. See Figure 7–5.

There are 12 pairs of *ribs* that give shape to the chest wall and protect the internal organs. The first seven pairs of ribs are called "true ribs" because they attach to the sternum (breastbone) in the front of the body. The next five pairs are called "false ribs." The first three pairs of false ribs attach to the cartilage of the rib above. The last two pairs are called "floating ribs" because they do not attach to the front of the body. The small piece of cartilage at the bottom edge of the sternum is called the *xiphoid* process. Health care workers become very familiar with the xiphoid process when they learn to perform CPR.

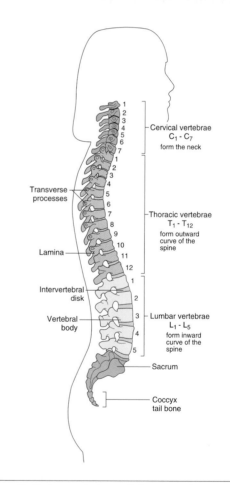

Figure 7–5 Lateral view of the spinal column.

The Appendicular Skeleton

The upper extremities include the shoulder girdle, arms, wrists, and hands:

- Shoulder girdle: Two curved *clavicles* (shoulder bones) and the two triangular *scapulae* (shoulder blades)

- Arm: Long bone of the upper arm is the *humerus* which is connected to the scapula by muscles and ligaments. The two long bones of the forearm are the *radius* (runs up thumb side) and *ulna* (proximal end forms the elbow that connects to the humerus).

- Wrist and hand: Eight bones in the wrist (*carpals*) form two rows of bones. The hands have five *metacarpal* bones (palm), and the five fingers have fourteen *phalanges* (each finger has three except for the thumb, which has two). The hand, with its many bones, is truly an engineering marvel.

The lower extremities include the pelvic (hip) girdle, legs, ankles, and feet:

- Pelvic girdle: Serves as an area of attachment for the leg and to protect the internal organs of the lower abdomen. The girdle starts out as three bones *(ilium, ischium, and pubis)*, which allows for growth. In adulthood these fuse to form the girdle. The bones fuse on the posterior side with the sacrum and in front by forming the *symphysis pubis*. The pelvis and pelvic inlet of the female are wider than that of the male to allow for childbirth.

- Leg: Long bone of the upper leg (thigh) is the *femur*; the femur is the longest bone in the body and fits into a cavity of the ilium known as the *acetabulum*. The two long bones of the calf are the *fibula* and *tibia*. The *patella* (kneecap) is found in front of the knee joint.

- Ankle and foot: Seven bones in the ankle (*tarsals*) provide a connection between the foot and leg bones. The foot has five *metatarsal* bones (forming the arch of foot) and the five toes have fourteen *phalanges* (each toe has three except for the big toe which has two).

Joints

A joint (articulation) is the connection between bones that allows for movement. Joints are covered by a synovial membrane that produces a lubricating fluid called *synovial fluid*. This enables them to move freely and without discomfort. *Ligaments* are fibrous connective tissue that connect one bone to another and create the stability of the joint. Another structure that some joints (elbow, knee, and shoulder) have is a *bursa*, a small fluid-filled sac or cavity. A bursa serves as a cushion and prevents friction between moving parts, such as tendons and bones.

Joint types that enable a wide range of mobility are ball-and-socket (shoulder and hip) and hinge (elbow and knee). Not all joints have the structures that allow a lot of movement. For example, vertebrae move only slightly, and the bones of the cranium do not move at all, with the exception of the mandible (jaw), which is a hinge joint. Common movements made possible by joints are described in Table 7–2 and Figure 7–6.

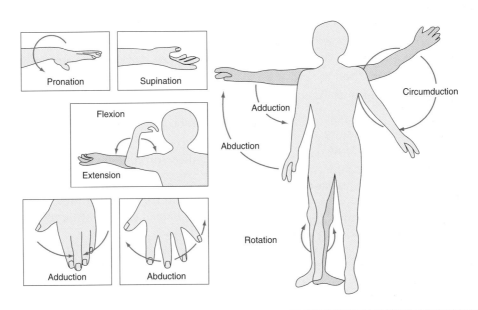

Figure 7–6 Movements of joints.

Table 7–1 Movement of joints

Movement	Description
Abduction	movement away from the median plane of the body
Adduction	movement toward the median plane of the body
Circumduction	movement in a circular direction
Extension	straighten (increase the angle between the bones forming a joint)
Flexion	to bend (decrease the angle between the bones forming a joint)
Pronation	turning the hand so the palm faces downward or backward (also refers to lying face down)
Rotation	motion around a central axis
Supination	turning the palm or foot upward (also refers to lying face up)

Thinking it Through

Randolph Jenkins is brought by ambulance to the hospital emergency room after a serious automobile accident. His right arm and leg are broken, and he has a skull fracture above his right ear. Mr. Jenkins also complains of pain of the left upper and lower extremity, and Dr. Printz, the Emergency Room physician, is assessing function by asking Mr. Jenkins to move his left arm straight out from the side of his body and then back down, then to turn the left palm up toward the ceiling and then down toward the floor.

1. Does Mr. Jenkins have injuries to the axial or appendicular skeleton or both?
2. What are the medical terms for the four movements the patient is requested to do with his left arm and hand?
3. From the description given for the location of the skull fracture, which cranial bone is most likely involved?

Major Diseases and Disorders

- *Arthritis* is a group of diseases involving inflammation of the joints. Examples include *rheumatoid arthritis* (synovial membranes thicken), *gout arthritis* (uric acid crystals build up in joints), and *degenerative joint disease,* also known as *osteoarthritis* (cartilage in the joints softens).

- *Back pain* is a common complaint that has many causes. The intervertebral disks sometimes press against nerves. Pain that runs down the leg is usually due to pressure on the sciatic nerve.

- *Carpal tunnel syndrome* is caused by pressure on a nerve in the wrist as a result of repetitive movement or trauma. This diagnosis has become quite common with the increased use of computers.

- Excessive *curvature of the spine* can occur in three directions.

  1. *Scoliosis* is a lateral (to the side) curvature
  2. *Lordosis,* sometimes referred to as "swayback," is a inward curvature of the lumbar area
  3. *Kyphosis,* sometimes referred to as "hunchback," is rounded bowing of the thoracic area. See Figure 7–7.

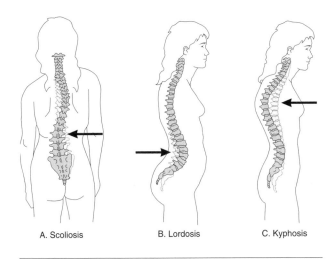

Figure 7–7 Abnormal curvatures of the spinal column.

- *Fractures* (broken bones) usually occur from some external injury to the body, but can also occur without injury if the bone is thin and brittle as a result of a disease (e.g. osteoporosis, Paget's Disease). The fracture may be closed (skin not broken) or open (bone breaks through skin). The different types of fractures are shown in Figure 7–8.
- *Osteomyelitis* is an infection of the bone.
- *Osteoporosis* is a weakening of the bones caused by the loss of calcium in the bones.

Preventive Measures

- Get adequate exercise, especially weightbearing activities such as walking.
- Avoid overextension of joints.
- Eat properly and intake sufficient calcium and vitamin C.
- Do stretching exercises, especially before participating in other forms of physical activity.
- Maintain good posture (Chapter 9).
- Position body properly when using a computer and other types of equipment (Chapter 9).
- Use proper lifting techniques (Chapter 9).
- Use protective equipment, such as seat belts and helmets, when cycling and skiing.

Age Related Changes—Skeletal System

- Decreased: Height, bone mass, flexibility
- Increased: Joint & cartilage erosion, thinning of vertebrae, demineralization of bones (Stence and Kegler, 1995)

Muscular

The *muscular system* (Figure 7–9) consists of over 600 muscles that produce movement, provide support, and produce heat to maintain body temperature. There are different types of muscles:

- Cardiac (heart): Located only in the heart. The pumping contractions and relaxations of the muscle occur with no conscious effort on the part of the individual (involuntary control).
- Skeletal: Attached to the bones, these require conscious effort to function (voluntary control). They are referred to as striated because they have alternating light and dark bands circling the muscle fibers. Any movement

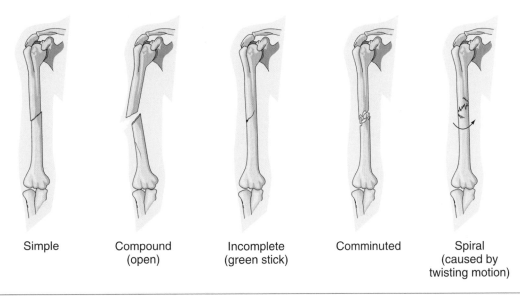

Simple   Compound (open)   Incomplete (green stick)   Comminuted   Spiral (caused by twisting motion)

Figure 7–8 Types of fractures.

that is self-generated involves skeletal muscles (walking, chewing, talking).

- Smooth (visceral): Located in the walls of internal organs (e.g., stomach, intestines, uterus, and blood vessels). It is involuntary, nonstriated (no markings) and controlled by the autonomic (automatic) nervous system.

- Sphincter (dilator): This is a circular muscle that controls the opening and closing of a passageway, such as in the digestive (food passing into and out of the stomach) and urinary (urine passing out of the bladder) systems.

All muscles have the following four characteristics:

- Contractibility: Tightening of a muscle, which makes it shorter and thicker

- Excitability (irritability): Readiness to respond to various types of stimuli

- Extensibility: Ability to be stretched

- Elasticity: Ability to return to its original length when relaxing
(Scott, 1998.)

Skeletal muscles are attached to the bones by bands of strong, tough connective tissue known as *tendons* (do not confuse these with ligaments, which connect bone to bone) or by a sheet-like membrane that covers, supports, and separates the muscles known as *fascia*. Skeletal muscles are attached to bones at two points: the *origin* and the *insertion*. The origin is the less movable bone; the insertion is attached to a more movable bone that will be affected by the action of the muscle. For example, the origin of the triceps muscle is towards the shoulder and the insertion is by the elbow. The *belly* is the central part of the muscle, seen most easily in the "bulges" developed by weightlifters.

Skeletal muscles work in pairs. The *prime mover* produces movement in one direction, and the *antagonist* produces movement in the opposite direction. The antagonist is the muscle on the opposite side of the joint and must relax to allow the prime mover to contract. Bend your elbow and you can feel the biceps contract (top of upper arm) and the triceps (back of upper arm) relax. Now extend your forearm and feel the biceps relax and the triceps contract. To demonstrate the need for opposing pairs of muscles, extend your arm partway, contract both the biceps and the triceps, and you will discover that movement is no longer possible.

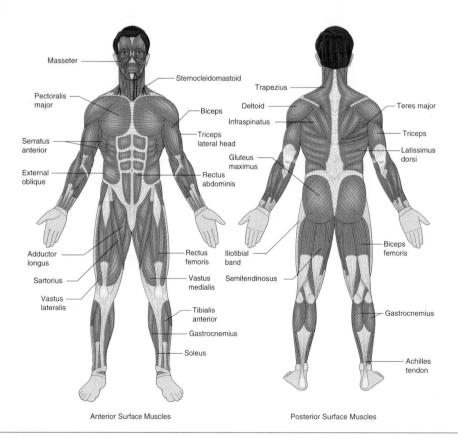

Anterior Surface Muscles

Posterior Surface Muscles

Figure 7–9 Muscles of the body.

Muscle tone is a muscle's normal resistance to stretching caused by muscles always being in a state of slight contraction. Loss of muscle tone can occur from illness, injury, or from lack of use. Too much tone is called *spasticity*. This, too, can be caused by illness or injury. Spastic muscles are too tight to move smoothly.

When the muscles are not used, they can *atrophy* (shrink in size and become weak) and appear floppy. Lack of use can also result in a *contracture*, in which a shortened muscle holds the joint in a flexed position.

Major Diseases and Disorders

- *Contractures* occur when the muscle stays in a shortened position. If the joint is not moved regularly, it will lose its flexibility as ligaments and tendons shorten.
- *Gangrene* is caused by Clostridium bacteria, which kills muscle tissue.
- *Muscle spasms* (cramps) are sudden and painful involuntary muscle contractions.
- *Muscle sprain* is a traumatic injury to the muscle, ligaments, or tendons of a joint. *Muscle strain* is torn or stretched tendons and muscle.
- *Muscular dystrophy* is an inherited disease that causes progressive deterioration of the muscles.
- *Myasthenia gravis* is a chronic neuromuscular disease that causes gradually increasing muscle weakness.

Preventive Measures

- Perform warm-up exercises before engaging in physical activity.
- Remain active, engaging in walking or exercise every day.
- Receive therapeutic massage to relax stiff muscles.
- Practice relaxation exercises to relieve muscle tension (Chapter 12).
- Use proper lifting techniques.
- Do muscle-strengthening exercises, such as weightlifting.
- Eat adequate amounts of protein.

Age Related Changes—Muscular System

- Decreased: Muscle mass, tone, and strength
- Increased: Risk of falls
  (Stence & Kegler, 1995)

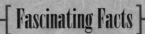

Fascinating Facts

Muscles make up about half the weight of your entire body (Colbert, 1997).

Integumentary

The skin is the largest organ of the body and accounts for about 15% of total body weight. The skin provides protection from environmental hazards such as sunrays and bacteria. The nerve endings located in the skin are another protective feature. They respond to touch, heat, cold, pain, and pressure (Figure 7–10). Without this warning system, individuals would not know when to move away from hazards. The skin participates in controlling body temperature through sweating and by widening and narrowing the blood vessels to control the entry and escape of heat. Finally, the skin acts as a waterproofing membrane. Without it, death would occur within minutes from *dehydration* (loss of water).

The *integumentary system* includes the skin and its appendages (Figure 7–11). The *appendages* include hair, nails, and the sweat and oil glands.

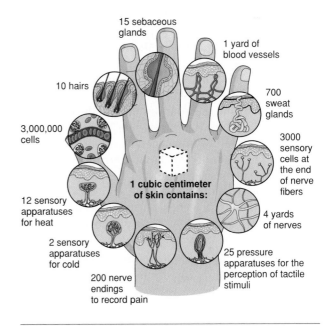

Figure 7–10 What is in the skin?

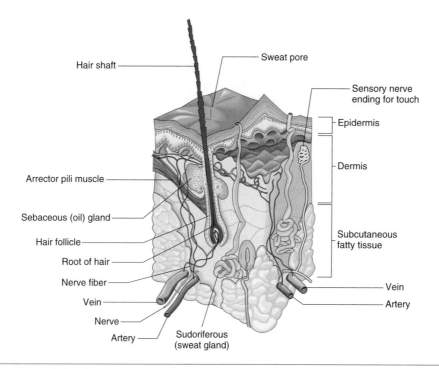

Figure 7–11 Structures of the skin.

Layers of the Skin:

- Epidermis: This outer layer of the skin, consisting of five or six layers, contains no blood supply or nerves. The outermost layer is composed of cells (squamous) that have died from environmental exposure and are shed daily. These lost cells are then replaced with cells produced in the lower layers, a process that continues throughout the lifetime. About 500 million squamous cells are lost every day as we bathe, dry, dress and move within our environment (Colbert, 1997). Skin pigmentation is determined by the melanocytes that produce the pigment *melanin.* Melanin can be black, be brown, or have a yellow tint, depending upon racial origin. The amount of melanin (and other skin pigments such as carotene and hemoglobin) in the melanocytes determines the various shades of human skin. Patches of melanin are called freckles or "age spots." An albino is a person who has no skin pigmentation.

- Dermis: This is the second layer of skin which contains involuntary muscles (arrector pili muscles cause "goose bumps"), blood vessels, nerves, hair follicles, sudoriferous (sweat) glands, and sebaceous (oil) glands.

- Subcutaneous tissue: This is the innermost layer of the skin containing fatty and connective tissue, which fastens the skin to the underlying muscles.

The Appendages:

- Hair: Each hair is encased within a hair follicle and ends in a root where new hair growth occurs. Hair is composed of a fibrous protein called keratin, which is a nonliving cell (good thing or haircuts would be very painful).

- Nails: Fingernails and toenails are also composed of keratin. The growth of the nail occurs at the base of the nail under the half-moon-shaped area. The function of the nails is to protect the fingers and toes.

- Sudoriferous (sweat) glands: During perspiration, water mixed with salt and waste products are excreted through the sweat glands. The function of the sweat glands is to excrete excess water and to assist the cooling of the body by the evaporation of water from the skin.

- Sebaceous (oil) glands: These excrete an oily substance (sebum) to lubricate and protect the skin. Sebum is slightly acid so it discourages the growth of bacteria.

Major Diseases And Disorders

- *Athlete's foot* is an infection of the skin caused by a fungus.

- *Boils (furuncle)* are a bacterial infection of the hair follicles or sebaceous glands.

- *Cancer of the skin* has three forms: basal cell, squamous cell, and melanoma. Basal cell is the most common and easiest to treat; squamous cell is more serious; melanoma the most serious and can be life-threatening.
- *Cellulitis* is a bacterial infection of the dermis and subcutaneous layers of the skin.
- *Decubitus ulcers* (bed or pressure sores) are areas of skin breakdown that occur over a bony prominence due to excessive and prolonged pressure that prevents adequate circulation to the tissues.
- *Dermatitis* is a general name for inflammation of the skin. *Contact dermatitis* is an allergic reaction to a substance that makes contact with the skin. *Eczema* is a generalized skin irritation usually caused by an irritant that appears as reddened areas on the surface of the skin.
- *Psoriasis* is a chronic, noncontagious, inherited skin disease in which too many epithelial cells are produced.
- *Warts* are caused by a viral infection of the skin.

Preventive Measures

- Practice good hygiene and keep the skin clean.
- Do not break open pimples or other growths on the skin.
- Do not scratch insect bites or other irritations.
- Avoid excessive exposure to the sun.
- Use sunscreen and wear a hat when in the sun.
- Have skin changes checked immediately.
- Protect skin from poisonous plants and insect bites.
- Get adequate amounts of vitamins A and C and niacin.

Age Related Changes—Integumentary System

- Decreased: Elasticity of the skin, subcutaneous fat (insulation), and hair (head, face)
- Increased: Dryness, wrinkles, skin pigmentation, and susceptibility to irritation (Stence and Kegler, 1995)

Systems for Providing Energy and Removing Waste

These systems work together to provide energy for the body and to remove the products of waste. The circulatory system includes two powerful transportation systems–cardiovascular and lymphatic–that reach every area of the body and work closely together to maintain fluid balance and prevent infections and disease.

The respiratory system supplies oxygen, and the digestive system turns food into the fuel needed for energy and for the growth and repair of cells. This fuel is then delivered to the body cells via the cardiovascular system. The digestive and urinary systems excrete the waste by-products and help maintain fluid balance.

Circulatory

The cardiovascular and lymphatic systems are the two great transportation (circulatory) systems of the body. In the cardiovascular system, the heart pumps blood that circulates throughout the body and then back to the heart through a network of blood vessels. The lymphatic system does not have a central pumping station, but it does have an extensive network of lymphatic vessels similar in design to blood vessels. The two systems are in constant physical contact and work together to transport fluids, dispose of waste products, and fight infection.

Cardiovascular System

The cardiovascular system transports blood cells and dissolved materials, including nutrients and oxygen, to all areas of the body. The other important function of this system is temperature regulation. Human beings are warm-blooded animals and require a fairly narrow temperature range to maintain homeostasis. This temperature range is maintained by circulating the warmer blood from the center of the body to the surface of the skin where it is cooled. Regulation takes place by the blood vessels dilating to increase heat loss or contracting to reduce heat loss. On hot days the skin is pinker and warmer because the blood vessels are dilated to release heat. The opposite occurs when the outer temperature is cold because the blood flow is restricted. The skin appears pale and feels cool.

[Fascinating Facts]

Your fingerprints will grow in size during your lifetime, but unless your fingers are injured, the patterns of your fingerprints will remain the same. Those patterns are unique to you (this is also true of your voice) (Colbert, 1997).

The cardiovascular system consists of the heart and blood vessels. The blood vessels that carry blood away from the heart are called *arteries* and the blood vessels that return blood to the heart are *veins*. Both arteries and veins are like branches on a tree, becoming narrower at each branching. The smallest of the branches are called *capillaries* and are not even as large as the period at the end of this sentence.

The heart is a strong pump composed of cardiac muscles. Its main function is to pump enough blood at a high enough pressure to supply every part of the body. A fully developed heart is about the size of an adult fist. It is located in the chest cavity, between the lungs, where it is protected by the ribs and sternum. The components of the heart include:

- Endocardium: A smooth layer that lines the inside of the heart

- Myocardium: Thick layer of muscle tissue that performs the pumping action

- Pericardium: Sac-like membrane that surrounds the heart

- Four chambers: Two for receiving blood (*atria*) and two for moving it out of the heart (*ventricles*). When blood is pumped out of the chambers, valves snap shut with a "thump-thump" (frequently referred to as "lub-dub"), which is the sound heard when listening to the heart. The valves prevent backflow of blood.

The blood arriving at the heart from the body takes the following path:

1. Arrives via the *inferior* and *superior vena cavae*
2. Enters the *right atrium* of the heart
3. Passes through a valve to the *right ventricle*
4. Passes through another valve into the right and left *pulmonary arteries*
5. Travels to the *lungs* to pick up fresh oxygen and drop off carbon dioxide
6. Returns to the heart by the *pulmonary veins* to the *left atrium*
7. Passes through another valve to reach the *left ventricle*
8. Leaves the *left ventricle* via the *aorta* to once again circulate throughout the body

Note: The pulmonary artery carries oxygen-poor blood to the lungs. The pulmonary vein carries oxygen-rich blood to the heart. In the rest of the circulatory system, arteries carry oxygen-rich blood to the body. Veins return oxygen-poor blood to the heart. See Figure 7–12.

The average adult heart rate is between 60–80 beats per minute. It is higher in children, gradually decreasing from its highest rate at birth until reaching its adult rate. Athletes generally have lower rates because their heart muscle is stronger and pumps more blood with each beat. The heart rate varies to accommodate the body's

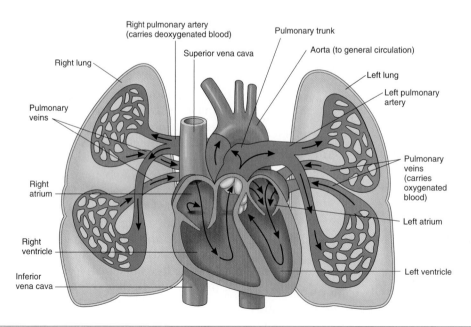

Figure 7–12 Cardiopulmonary circulation.

needs. It speeds up during exercise to increase the flow of blood to skeletal muscles, after a meal to send extra blood to the digestive system, and during a fever so more blood flows to the surface of the body to release heat.

The heart has its own blood supply that wraps around its surface to provide it with nourishment and remove wastes. These are called the coronary arteries and veins. It is the blockage of coronary arteries that causes heart attacks. See Figure 7–13.

The heart also has its own electrical system that stimulates the cardiac muscle to contract and act as a pump. The electrical impulses, like the blood, follow their own set path through the heart:

1. An impulse originates at a cluster of nerve cells located in the upper right wall of the right atrium, called the *sinoatrial node (SA node)*. This is the natural pacemaker of the heart, functioning to originate and regulate the heart beat.

2. The SA node sends the impulse through a network of nerves that reaches all areas of both atriums.

3. The right and left atria respond to the impulse by contracting and forcing the blood into the ventricles.

4. The impulse reaches another node, called the *atrioventricular node (AV node),* that is located between the atrium and ventricle.

5. The AV node sends the impulse through a network of nerve fibers called the *Bundle of His*

that splits into the *right and left bundle fibers* and then terminates in a diffuse network of nerve branches called the *Purkinje fibers.*

6. The right and left ventricles contract.

It is this electrical pattern that is measured during an electrocardiogram (ECG or EKG). The pattern gives information that is helpful in diagnosing heart problems (Figure 7–14).

Blood is carried throughout the body by means of a vast system of vessels, channels that carry fluid. There are three types of blood vessels: arteries, veins, and capillaries.

1. Arteries carry oxygenated blood away from the heart and out to all areas of the body (the pulmonary artery is the only artery that carries oxygen-poor blood, or what is called deoxygenated blood). The aorta, which receives blood pumped from the left ventricle, is the largest artery. On leaving the heart, it immediately begins to branch into smaller and smaller arteries. The smallest arteries are called *arterioles*. Arteries are muscular and elastic in order to handle the force of pumped blood. See Figure 7–15.

2. Veins carry deoxygenated blood back to the heart from all areas of the body (the pulmonary vein is the only vein that carries oxygenated blood). The furthest veins from the heart, *venules*, are also the smallest. The veins increase in size as they approach the

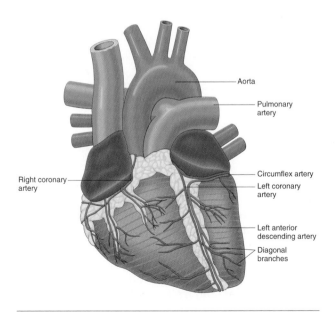

Figure 7–13 The coronary arteries.

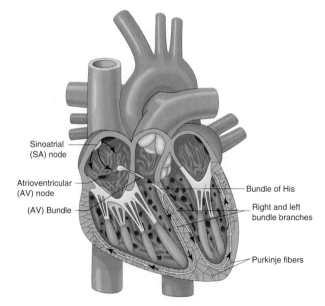

Figure 7–14 The electrical system of the heart.

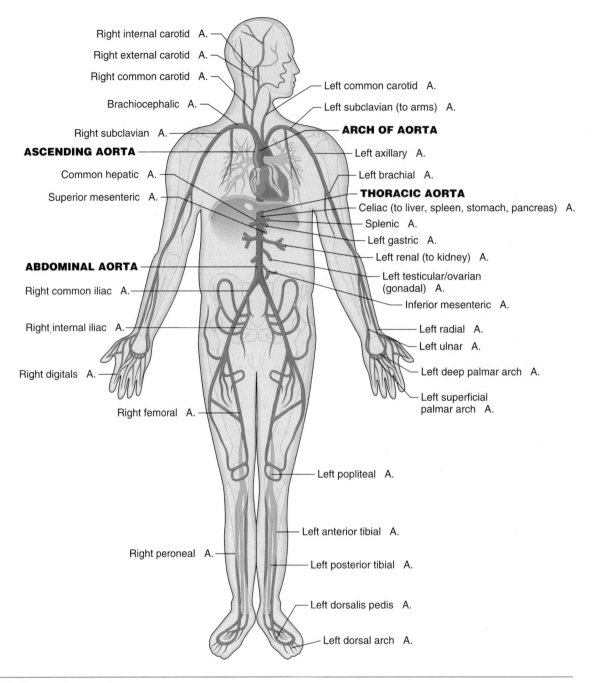

Right internal carotid A.
Right external carotid A.
Right common carotid A.
Brachiocephalic A.
Right subclavian A.
ASCENDING AORTA
Common hepatic A.
Superior mesenteric A.
ABDOMINAL AORTA
Right common iliac A.
Right internal iliac A.
Right digitals A.
Right femoral A.
Right peroneal A.

Left common carotid A.
Left subclavian (to arms) A.
ARCH OF AORTA
Left axillary A.
Left brachial A.
THORACIC AORTA
Celiac (to liver, spleen, stomach, pancreas) A.
Splenic A.
Left gastric A.
Left renal (to kidney) A.
Left testicular/ovarian (gonadal) A.
Inferior mesenteric A.
Left radial A.
Left ulnar A.
Left deep palmar arch A.
Left superficial palmar arch A.
Left popliteal A.
Left anterior tibial A.
Left posterior tibial A.
Left dorsalis pedis A.
Left dorsal arch A.

Figure 7–15 The major arteries.

heart. The largest veins are the *inferior* (carrying blood from lower body) and *superior* (carrying blood from upper body) vena cavae. These deliver the blood to the right atrium. Veins have one-way valves that prevent the blood from flowing in a backward direction and are thinner and less muscular than arteries. See Figure 7–16.

3. Capillaries are the smallest blood vessels. They connect the arterioles with the venules. Their one-cell thick walls allow substances to exit and enter the bloodstream. Nutrients and oxygen move from the blood into surrounding tissues. Waste materials and carbon dioxide are picked up for transport to the lungs and kidneys for removal from the body. See Figure 7–17.

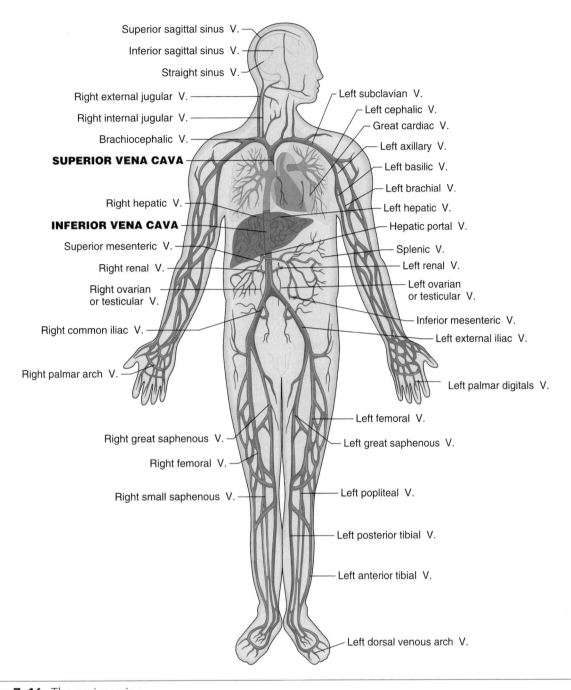

Figure 7–16 The major veins.

The blood consists of red blood cells (RBCs), white blood cells (WBCs), platelets, and plasma:

- *Red blood cells* carry oxygen to the body cells. They pick up oxygen in the lungs and bind it to a substance called hemoglobin, then give up the oxygen when they reach the capillaries. An adequate intake of iron in the diet is essential for the production of hemoglobin to carry oxygen. RBCs have no nucleus so they cannot reproduce themselves. They

are primarily manufactured in the red bone marrow.

- *White blood cells* fight infections. They pass through the blood vessels to work in the tissues as needed. They function as scavenger cells that engulf, ingest, and destroy infection cells (*phagocytosis*) and then remove wastes and dead cells. WBCs are manufactured in the bone marrow and the lymph system and can be produced on demand as needed by the body.

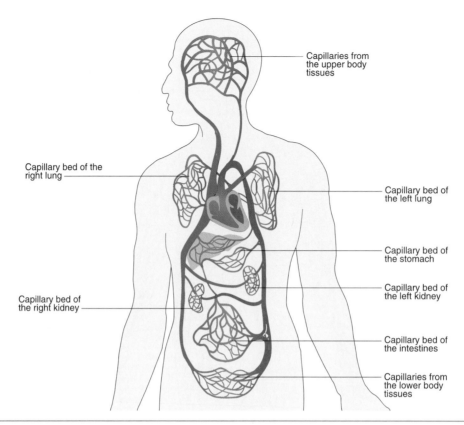

Figure 7–17 Examples of capillary beds.

- *Platelets* clump together to form clots when a blood vessel is damaged. These aid in preventing loss of blood. Platelets are manufactured in the bone marrow.

- *Plasma* is the liquid part of the blood, consisting mostly of water. Its purpose is to transport the other blood cells along with other nutrients and hormones. It also supplies the fluid needed inside and around the body cells.

Lymphatic System

The second essential transportation system of the body is the *lymphatic system*. This network of fluid, called lymph, serves to defend against infection, maintain fluid balance, and remove waste products. Lymph is a straw-colored fluid that consists of water, waste products, digested nutrients, hormones, salts, and lymphocytes (special type of WBC). Lymph travels through vessels that are similar to blood vessels. Lymphatic capillaries combine to form increasingly larger vessels that eventually empty into two *lymphatic ducts*. The ducts, which are walled passageways, then empty into the superior vena cava, and the lymph joins the blood as it enters the right atrium.

As the lymph passes through the lymphatic vessels, it is filtered by oval-shaped *lymph nodes* made of specialized tissue. This tissue has the ability to remove substances, such as cancer cells, disease-causing organisms, and dead blood cells found in the blood. See Figure 7–18.

Lymphoid tissue is also found in the tonsils, adenoids, and the spleen. The spleen is located in

[Fascinating Facts]

The body has about 25,000,000,000,000 (25 trillion) red blood cells circulating in the blood, and the average life span of a RBC is 120 days. This means that the body must produce 3 million new RBCs every second! In times of crisis (heavy blood loss), the body can step up production by 10 times and convert some of the fatty yellow bone marrow to red marrow (Colbert, 1997).

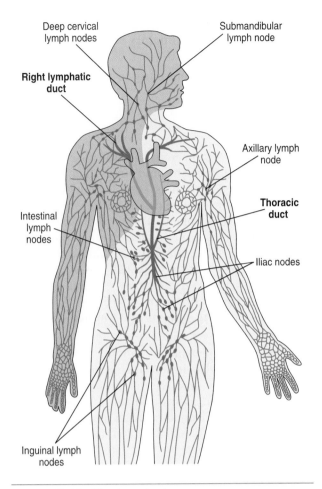

Figure 7–18 The lymphatic system.

the upper-left area of the abdomen just under the diaphragm. It filters blood instead of lymph fluid and has the following functions:

- Removes old, worn-out RBCs
- Removes iron from hemoglobin for reuse by the bone marrow
- Creates RBCs prior to birth (this function stops shortly after birth)
- Produces lymphocytes and antibodies to help the body fight infection
- Acts as a filter for foreign bodies
- Serves as a reservoir for blood that can be added to the cardiovascular system as needed (Adapted from *An integrated approach to health sciences: Anatomy and physiology, math, physics, and chemistry,* by B. J. Colbert, J. Ankney, J. Wilson, and J. Havrilla, 1997, Albany, NY: Delmar.)

The lymphatic system also has a role in the immune response. The *immune response* occurs when something enters the body that it does not identify as its own tissue. Foreign substances are

known as *antigens.* Examples include microorganisms, splinters, and poison. The body responds by producing antibodies to attack the antigen. The lymphatic system produces antibodies and lymphocytes. Signs that the immune system is fighting infection include fever, inflammation, and pus.

Major Diseases and Disorders
Cardiovascular:

- *Anemia* results when the blood has an inadequate amount of hemoglobin, red blood cells, or both. There are many different types of anemia, including *pernicious anemia* (red blood cells not developed due to poor absorption of vitamin B_{12}), *iron-deficiency anemia* (inadequate hemoglobin due to iron shortage), and *aplastic anemia* (bone marrow destroyed by chemicals, radiation, or medications). There are also two genetic forms of anemia called *sickle cell anemia,* most common in people of African origin, and *thalassemia,* most often seen in people of Mediterranean origin.
- *Aneurysm* is a ballooning out of the arterial wall that weakens the wall and disrupts blood flow.
- *Angina pectoris* is heart pain caused by an inadequate supply of oxygen to the heart by the coronary arteries. If this condition is severe enough, part of the heart tissue will die, resulting in a *myocardial infarction* (MI; heart attack). A common misconception is that men are more prone to heart disease than women, but it is the number one cause of death of women.
- *Arteriosclerosis* is a hardening or thickening of the arterial walls, resulting in loss of elasticity and contractility.
- *Atherosclerosis* occurs when fatty plaques are deposited on the walls of the arteries and narrows the lumen (opening). The narrowing decreases or prevents blood flow.
- *Congestive heart failure* is a condition in which the heart fails as a pump.
- *Hypertension* is high blood pressure.
- *Inflammation of the heart* can occur at any of the three layers of the heart: *endocarditis* affects the inner lining of the heart and heart valves; *myocarditis* affects the cardiac muscle; *pericarditis* affects the sac that surrounds the heart.
- *Leukemia* (blood cancer) is an abnormal increase in white blood cells that are immature and less effective than mature cells in fighting infections. These immature cells become so prevalent that they replace the red blood cells and cause anemia.

- *Septicemia* (blood poisoning) occurs when an infection enters the blood vessels.

- *Thrombosis* is a blood clot that forms in a blood vessel. If it breaks loose and travels through the body, it is called an *embolus*.

- *Varicose veins* are dilated veins filled with blood. Veins that lose their elasticity allow the blood to pool (stasis), and the result is decreased blood flow.

Lymphatic:

- *Acquired immunodeficiency syndrome (AIDS)* is caused by a virus and results in failure of the body's immune system.

- *Autoimmune diseases* occur when the body does not recognize its own tissue and initiates an immune response to destroy the tissue. Examples are *systemic lupus erythematosus* which affects connective tissue, and *Hashimoto's disease,* which destroys the thyroid gland.

- *Hodgkin's disease* is a form of cancer that affects the lymph nodes.

- *Tonsillitis* is an infection of the tonsils caused by the large number of microorganisms they are filtering through their lymph tissues.

Preventive Measures

- Practice good nutrition.
- Avoid being overweight.
- Get adequate exercise.
- Check blood pressure regularly (hypertension does not have symptoms).
- Treat cuts in the skin promptly to prevent infection.
- Do not smoke.
- Do not cross the legs for long periods of time.
- Develop coping skills for handling stress (Chapter 12).
- Practice safe sex habits.
- Follow Standard Precautions, specific techniques and practices to prevent the transmission of disease. Chapter 10 contains a detailed explanation of Standard Precautions.

Age Related Changes

Cardiovascular System:

- Decreased: Arterial elasticity, efficiency of heart valves, cardiac contractility, cardiac output

- Increased: Narrowing of the arteries due to plaque buildup

Lymphatic System:

- Decreased: Inflammatory response; effectiveness of vaccines

- Increased: Susceptibility to viral and bacterial infections
  (Stence, 1995)

Respiratory

The *respiratory system* consists of the nose, pharynx, larynx, trachea, bronchi, and lungs (Figure 7–19). The main function of the system is to deliver air to sites where gas exchange can occur between the air and the circulating blood. The cardiovascular and respiratory systems function together and are sometimes referred to as the *cardiopulmonary system.* The lymphatic system also works closely with the respiratory system to transport excess fluid from the tissues and to destroy any particles that have escaped the filtering systems and traveled deep into the lungs.

- Nose: The sensory organ for smell (olfactory), it is also important in the respiratory system. The nose is the first filter for the incoming air. Hairs and bony ridges in the nasal cavity trap the larger particles, while the nasal cavity has a *mucous* membrane that produces *mucus* to trap smaller particles.

[Fascinating Facts]

Cardiovascular—If you don't think your heart is a hard worker, just try this—let your hand imitate the squeezing action of your heart by fully opening and fully closing your hand at the same rate that your heart beats. Do this for 5 minutes without stopping. How do the muscles of your hand and forearm feel after 5 minutes? If your heart rate is 80 beats-per-minute, your heart beats over 115,000 times each day! If your hand got tired, you could always switch to the other hand, but you only have one heart, so take good care of it (Colbert, 1997).

Lymphatic—Lymph nodes are usually found in groupings throughout the body. The number of lymph nodes per group can range from 2 to more than 100 (Colbert, 1997).

(Note that mucous and mucus sound the same, but are spelled differently). The nose also humidifies and warms the air as it passes through with moisture from the mucus, sinuses, and tear ducts. *Sinuses* are cavities filled with air that are located around the eyes and nose. Lined with mucous membrane, they also create a resonance to the voice. (The change in the voice during a nasal cold is due to the blockage of sinuses.)

- Pharynx: The throat. Located behind the nasal cavities, it is the passageway for food and liquids, along with air. To prevent swallowed items from entering the passageway to the lungs, there is a flap-like structure called the *epiglottis* that closes off the larynx automatically during swallowing. The soft palate, at the upper rear of the roof of the mouth, blocks food and liquid from entering the nose.

- Larynx: The voicebox containing the vocal cords. These are usually relaxed and open. Sounds, such as speech and singing, are produced when the cords are tightened at the same time that air is passed out of the lungs.

- Trachea: The windpipe which serves as a passageway for air. At its distal end, it splits to form the right and left bronchi.

- Bronchi: The right and left bronchi continue to branch into smaller and smaller airways until they become the thin-walled *bronchioles*. The bronchioles terminate into tiny, sac-like structures called *alveoli*. It is through the walls of the alveoli that the exchange of oxygen and carbon dioxide takes place.

- Lungs: The right lung has three lobes and the left has two lobes, each containing a branch of the bronchi with its system of airways. The lungs are soft, elastic, spongy, and very light. Each is surrounded with an airtight covering called the pleura. Lungs have no muscles of their own and depend on the muscles around the chest cavity to do their work.

- Diaphragm: A sheet of muscle that separates the chest from the abdomen and stretches from the spine to the front of the rib cage. It provides a movable floor for the lungs. As the diaphragm contracts, it moves downward. This causes the air pressure in the lungs to decrease and this pulls air into the lungs (called inhalation). As the diaphragm relaxes, it moves up, raising air pressure in the lungs and forcing air out (called exhalation). The diaphragm is the major muscle involved in respiration, but there are also some small muscles between the ribs that sometimes help, especially when taking a deep breath.

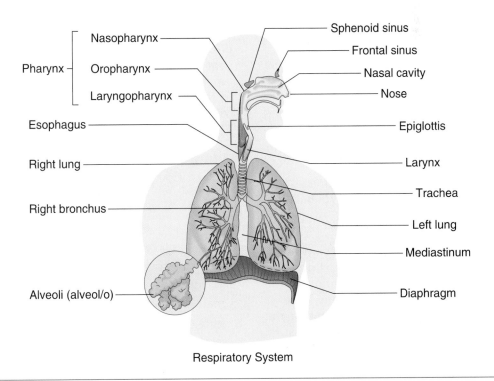

Respiratory System

Figure 7–19 Structures of the respiratory system.

Important protective structures built into the respiratory system in addition to the mucous membranes are the small, hair-like structures called *cilia*. They sweep mucus upward toward the nose and mouth so that trapped debris can be swallowed, coughed up, and sneezed or blown out. Coughing removes harmful particles that irritate the lining of the throat, trachea, or bronchial passages. Sneezing removes particles from the nasal cavity.

Major Diseases and Disorders

- *Atelectasis* occurs when the alveoli are either partially or totally collapsed. Common causes are blockage in the lung, not breathing deeply due to pain or injury, and inability to cough up secretions.

- *Chronic obstructive pulmonary disease (COPD)* is a general term that refers to chronic diseases that obstruct air flow. For example, *asthma* causes the bronchial tube walls to spasm that narrows the passageway for air flow. The narrowing prevents an easy exhalation of air and the patient experiences a sense of suffocation. *Chronic bronchitis* is an inflammation of the bronchi and bronchial tubes. *Emphysema* causes the alveoli to become stretched out which prevents them from efficiently exchanging oxygen and carbon dioxide.

- *Lung cancer* is the growth of tissues in the lung that destroys or blocks the flow of oxygen to the healthy lung tissue. This results in the entire body being deprived of oxygen.

- *Pneumonia* is an inflammation of the lungs that can be caused by bacteria, viruses, or fungi.

- *Pneumothorax* is the collapse of a lung due to air in the chest cavity. The lung can develop an internal leak or air can enter through a hole from the outside, such as a gunshot or stab wound.

- *Tuberculosis* is a disease that damages the lungs and is caused by the Tubercle bacillus. It is transmitted from person to person through the air.

- *Upper respiratory infection (URI)* is any infection of the upper respiratory structures. For example, *rhinitis* is an inflammation of the nasal mucosa resulting in a runny nose or congestion; *sinusitis* is an inflammation in the sinuses and can cause headache or pressure, congestion, discharge, and change in voice quality; *pharyngitis* (pharynx) causes a sore throat; *laryngitis* (larynx) is inflammation of the vocal cords and can result in hoarseness or loss of voice; *tonsillitis* is a painful inflammation of the lymph nodes. A URI includes the symptoms usually referred to as a common cold.

Preventive Measures

- Do not smoke.

- Use a protective mask when working around dust, toxic fumes, paints, cleaners, and so on.

- Maintain good posture.

- Take deep breaths occasionally.

Age Related Changes—Respiratory (Pulmonary) System

- Decreased: Lung elasticity, lung expansion, functional alveoli, vital capacity, ciliary action, sense of smell

- Increased: Respiratory rate, diameter of chest (barrel chest), rigidity of lungs (Stence and Kegler, 1995)

Digestive

The *digestive system* provides energy for the body by processing food. All the cells require nutrients to do the work of building, repairing, and controlling body systems. Carbohydrates, proteins, and fats are taken in and converted into glucose, amino acids, and fatty acids that are distributed throughout the body through the capillaries. Minerals and vitamins do not require digestion, but can be absorbed directly by the capillaries. The body requires adequate amounts of water to maintain and support functions. Undigested food products are eliminated by the digestive system. The entire digestive system consists of a long tube called the alimentary canal. This canal is about 30 feet long and extends from the

[**Fascinating Facts**]

Your lungs produce about a quart of mucus every 24 hours, and the cilia (microscopic hairs) in your airways move it at a rate of approximately 2 cm/min up to your larynx. When it gets to your larynx, what happens to the mucus if you don't cough it out? You swallow it! You do this every day (Colbert, 1997).

mouth, where food is taken in, to the anus, where waste products are eliminated.

The digestive system uses both mechanical and chemical means to process food. Mechanically the food is chopped, massed, and mixed. Chemically, food is broken down by digestive enzymes that are produced within the system or added by other organs. Enzymes break down food into absorbable nutrients.

The digestive system is frequently referred to as the *gastrointestinal system*. The main structures that participate in the digestion of food include the mouth, esophagus, stomach, small intestines, and large intestines (Figure 7–20).

- Mouth: Food enters the mouth, where its taste triggers the saliva glands to produce digestive enzymes, which begin the breakdown of carbohydrates. The teeth chop and grind and the tongue mashes the food against the hard palate, mixing it with saliva. The mouth cools or warms the food to body temperature. The tongue moves the food to the back of the throat to be swallowed.

- Esophagus: A strong, muscular tube that connects the pharynx to the stomach. It lies behind the trachea and in front of the spinal column. It is composed of layers of muscle that contract to move the food. This action, called *peristalsis*, is controlled by the autonomic nervous system. Food passes into the stomach through the *cardiac sphincter* which prevents the acidic content of the stomach from backflowing into the esophagus.

- Stomach: A muscular, elastic bag that fits under the diaphragm on the left side of the abdomen and is protected by the lower ribs. Food usually remains in the stomach for 2 to 4 hours while its muscles contract to mix it well with digestive juices. The glands in the stomach release hydrochloric acid to kill bacteria, pepsin to break down protein, and mucus to protect the stomach wall from the acidic gastric juices. When the partially digested food leaves the stomach, it goes through the pyloric sphincter and enters the small intestine.

- Small intestines: Also known as the small bowel, it consists of three parts: duodenum, jejunum, and ileum. Once the food passes into the small intestine, additional intestinal juices are added, including bile from the liver and pancreatic juice from the pancreas. Digestion continues, but absorption also begins to occur through a network of small,

finger-like projections called *villi* that line the small intestine. Each villus contains a network of blood and lymph capillaries; the lymph system absorbs the fatty acids and the blood capillaries absorb the amino acids and simple sugars. Vitamins and minerals pass unchanged from the small intestine into the blood and lymph. The material leaving the small intestine normally consists only of indigestible substances, waste material, and excess water. This passes through the *ileocecal valve* into the large intestine.

- Large intestines: Also known as the large bowel. Nutrients and water not absorbed in the small intestine are absorbed here. The large intestine contains bacteria that works on the undigested substances and synthesizes vitamin K (essential for blood clotting) as well as some of the B-complex vitamins (promote various body functions). The *appendix*, located just below the *ileocecal valve* in the lower right quadrant of the abdomen, has no known function. The last portion of the digestive system serves as a storage and elimination structure for indigestible substances.

Accessory Organs:

- Liver: Located in the upper right quadrant under the diaphragm; produces a thick, green liquid, called bile, that breaks down lipids (fat) into fatty acids for absorption. The liver has many other vital functions: maintaining blood sugar levels; filtering out and destroying old red blood cells, saving the iron to be used again; storing vitamins; producing prothrombin, necessary for blood clotting; and filtering out harmful toxins (poisons) that have been swallowed, including alcohol and many drugs.

- Gallbladder: Small green organ located on the inferior side of the liver; stores bile made by the liver until it is needed for the digestion of fats.

- Pancreas: Located posterior to the stomach; excretes pancreatic digestive enzymes into the duodenum of the small intestine. These enzymes help digest proteins and fat. The pancreas also functions as an endocrine gland, which will be discussed under the endocrine system presented later in the chapter.

Major Diseases and Disorders

- *Appendicitis* is an inflammation of the appendix from unknown causes. The only treatment is surgical removal (appendectomy).

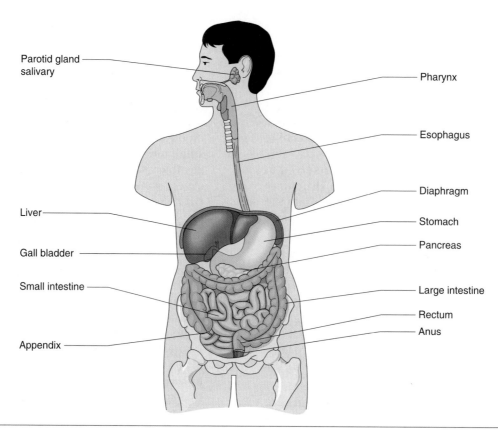

Figure 7–20 Structures of the digestive system.

- *Ascites* is not a disease, but a general term used to describe the abnormal accumulation of fluid in the peritoneal cavity (space between the layers of the membrane that lines the abdominal and pelvic cavities). Cirrhosis, cancer, and advanced congestive heart failure can cause this condition.

- *Cirrhosis* is a group of chronic diseases that involve scarring of liver tissue, which decreases the ability of the liver to perform its functions.

- *Cholelithiasis* is the presence of stones in the gallbladder. *Cholecystitis* is an inflammation of the gallbladder.

- *Colon cancer* involves an abnormal growth in the large intestines that damages tissue and can cause a blockage of the digestive system.

- *Constipation* is the inability to pass feces, the body's waste that is passed through the anus. The most common causes are lack of dietary fiber, inadequate fluids, certain medications, and lack of exercise. It causes abdominal distention and discomfort.

- *Diarrhea* is the passage of frequent and watery stools. It can be caused by certain diseases, stress, medications, and diet.

- *Diverticulosis* is the weakening of the colon wall leading to an out pouching in the wall (diverticula). These diverticula can trap digestive material and become infected. *Diverticulitis* is an inflammation of the diverticula.

- *Gastroenteritis* is an inflammation of the mucous membranes that line the stomach and intestines. Causes include food poisoning, infection, and toxins. *Gastritis* is when the lining of the stomach becomes inflamed and can be caused by spicy foods and certain medications.

- *Heartburn* occurs when the gastric juices back up through the cardiac sphincter and irritate the lower end of the esophagus (the esophagus does not have a protective mucous membrane like the stomach does to protect it against the acidic juices).

- *Hemorrhoids* are painful, dilated veins in the lower rectum or anus.

- *Hepatitis* is an inflammation of the liver caused by a virus or poison.

[Fascinating Facts]

If you possess an average appetite, you will consume at least 35 tons of food in your lifetime (Colbert, 1997).

- *Pancreatitis* is an inflammation of the pancreas that can be caused by a variety of factors.

- *Peritonitis* is a condition in which the lining (peritoneum) of the abdominal cavity becomes inflamed.

- An *ulcer* is an open sore in the lining of the digestive system. Pain occurs when the protective lining is damaged and the acidic juices come into contact with the delicate tissues underneath. A *Peptic ulcer* can occur in the stomach or duodenum. Stomach ulcers are also called *gastric ulcers*. *Ulcerative colitis* is a severe inflammation of the colon with the formation of ulcers and abscesses (collection of pus in a cavity).

Age Related Changes—Digestive (Gastrointestinal) System

- Decreased: Peristalsis, control of external sphincter, taste, saliva production, liver size, weight, and efficiency; gastric acid secretion; intestinal movement; appetite

- Increased: gum disease, constipation, indigestion
  (Stence and Kegler, 1995)

Preventive Measures

- Eat an adequate amount of fiber.

- Drink plenty of water.

- Avoid excessive alcohol.

- Follow Standard Precautions (Chapter 10).

- Avoid large amounts of high-fat foods.

- Avoid fad diets and other extreme eating habits.

- Avoid pushing hard during bowel movements (avoid constipation).

- Do not rely on the regular use of laxatives.

- Make routine dental appointments for examination and cleaning of teeth.

- Have colonoscopy performed at the age and frequency recommended by your health care provider.

Urinary

The *urinary system* eliminates excess water, salts, and waste products from the body. It consists of the kidneys, ureters, urinary bladder, and urethra. See Figure 7–21 a–b.

- Kidneys (2): Located behind the peritoneum (lining of the abdominal cavity) and on either side of the spinal column, below the diaphragm, the kidneys clean the blood and regulate the amount of water in the body. The artery that enters the kidney divides into a network of blood vessels that terminate in a grouping of capillaries called a *glomerulus*. Each glomerulus is surrounded by a kidney tube that forms a capsule called *Bowman's capsule*. This intertwining of the blood capillaries and the kidney tubules is called a *nephron* and is where the real work of the kidney occurs: retaining waste products while returning most of the water, glucose, amino acids, and salts to the body. The nephrons, numbering over 1 million per kidney, are located in the cortex (outer layer) of the kidney. The waste products flow into the *medulla* (inner layer) of the kidney, where water is returned to the body. The average daily fluid output of urine is about 1500 cc (1½ quarts), but varies with fluid intake.

- Ureters (2): The ureters connect the kidneys with the bladder, forming passageways for the urine.

- Urinary bladder: Stores urine, expanding and contracting its smooth-muscle walls as needed. When the bladder wall is stretched by a large amount of urine, the nerves in the wall send a message to the brain conveying the need to urinate. The opening to the urethra is kept closed by two sphincter muscles, one of which is under voluntary control.

- Urethra: The tube through which urine is passed to the outside of the body. Passage requires relaxation of the voluntary sphincter.

Major Diseases and Disorders

- *Edema* is not a disease, but a general term used to describe the abnormal accumulation of fluid in the tissues. Kidney failure, congestive heart failure, and many other conditions can cause edema.

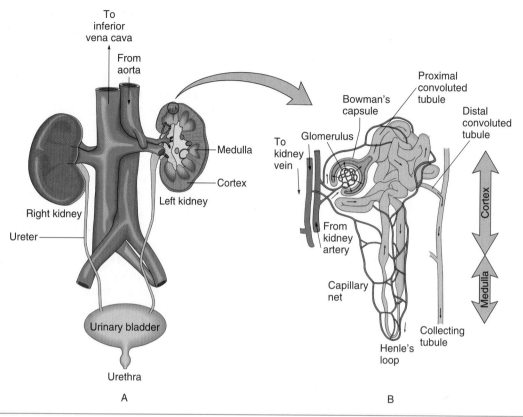

Figure 7–21a Structures of the urinary system.

Figure 7–21b Nephron and related structures.

- *Kidney (renal) failure* occurs when the nephrons are unable to filter liquid waste from the blood. The buildup of waste products in the blood is called *uremia*. To sustain life, toxins are removed by regular *dialysis* treatments. Hemodialysis is a procedure in which the blood is passed through a device that functions as an artificial kidney.

- *Kidney (renal) calculi* are kidney stones and are usually composed of uric acid or calcium crystals.

- *Urinary incontinence* is the inability to control urination. *Urinary retention* is the inability to urinate when the urge is felt or the bladder is full. These conditions have many causes.

- *Urinary tract infection (UTI)* is an infection of the lower urinary structures. *Urethritis* is an inflammation of the urethra and *cystitis* is an inflammation of the bladder.

- *Kidney infections* include *nephritis* or *glomerulonephritis,* which refers to an inflammation of the glomerulus (nephrons). *Pyelonephritis* is an inflammation of the kidney tissue and renal pelvis (collecting part of kidney that narrows into the ureter).

Preventive Measures

- Drink adequate amounts of water (eight glasses per day).

- Use proper toilet hygiene to prevent bladder infections.

- If you have hypertension or diabetes, manage them closely because they are primary contributors to renal failure.

- Be aware of and take cautiously, any medications that can damage the kidneys. Never take illegal drugs.

- When taking antibiotics increase your intake of water to prevent crystals from forming in the kidneys.

Age Related Changes—Urinary System

- Decreased: Glomerular filtration rate; renal blood flow; renal mass; functional nephron units; bladder capacity; sphincter muscle control

- Increased: Frequency and urgency of urination; nocturia (need to urinate during the night) (Stence and Kegler, 1995)

Systems for Sensing, Coordinating, and Controlling

The five senses (seeing, hearing, smelling, tasting, and touching) provide the brain with input from the external environment. The nervous system, in turn, interprets this input into sights, sounds, odors, flavors, or sensations of touch.

Eyes and Ears

The *eye* is frequently compared to a camera. It receives visual information from light rays through a transparent layer called the *cornea*. The light then enters an opening called the *pupil*, the round, black center of the eye. The *lens* projects the light rays on the *retina*, the innermost layer of the eye (Figure 7–22). An upside-down image is produced which is then converted to electrical signals and transmitted by the *optic nerve* to the brain, which "sees" it as right side up. A series of muscles attached to the eye coordinate movement so the eyes can focus.

The eye has three layers, the sclera, the choroid, and the retina (Figure 7–23 a–b):

- Sclera: The "white of the eye" is tough, fibrous tissue that serves as a protective shield. It contains the *cornea.*
- Choroid: Containing many blood vessels to nourish the eye, it includes the iris, pupil, and lens. The *iris* is the colored part, usually shades of blue, brown, or green and what people refer to when they say you have blue, brown, or hazel eyes. It is a sphincter muscle that controls the size of the pupil opening. In low light the iris relaxes, allowing the pupil to dilate and more light rays to enter for a better image. In bright light it contracts to protect the eye from too much light. Behind the pupil is the *lens* that is attached by ligaments to the *ciliary muscles*, which adjust the shape of the lens to ensure that a sharp image is projected on the retina.

- Retina: Thin membrane attached to the back of the eye on which images are projected. It contains two types of light-sensing receptors called *rods* and *cones.* The rods are responsible for seeing in dim light and the cones for seeing colors and in bright light.

There are a number of structures that provide protection for the eye:

- Orbit: Skull bones that form a protective cavity for the eye
- Eyelids, eyelashes, and eyebrows: Eyelids help distribute moisture over the eye and remove small particles that get into the eye. They also automatically close when an object suddenly comes toward the eye. The eyebrows and eyelashes catch moisture and particles to prevent them from falling into the eye.

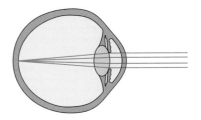

Normal eye
Light rays focus on the retina

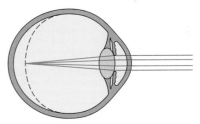

Myopia (nearsightedness)
Light rays focus in front
of the retina

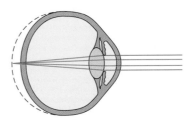

Hyperopia (farsightedness)
Light rays focus beyond
the retina

Figure 7–22 Normal vision occurs when the light rays are focused on the retina. An eyeball that is too long or too short prevents the proper focus.

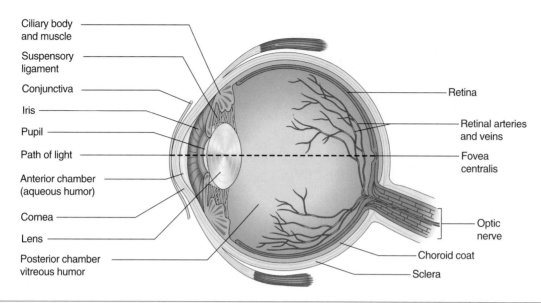

Figure 7–23a Internal view of the eye.

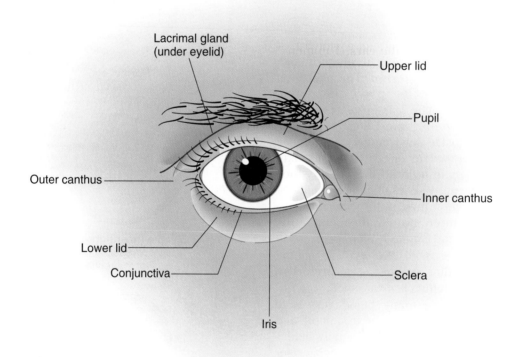

Figure 7–23b External view of the eye.

- Conjunctiva: Membrane that lines the underside of each eyelid and extends to the cornea on the surface of the eye

- Lacrimal glands: Produce tears for cleaning and moisturizing the eye

- Aqueous humor: A clear, watery fluid in the anterior chamber of the eye that bathes the iris, pupil, and lens

- Vitreous humor: A clear, jelly-like fluid in the posterior chamber that maintains the shape of the eyeball and bends light rays

The *ears* have both auditory (hearing) and balance organs. The outer ear collects sounds waves which are directed through a canal to the *eardrum.* When sound waves hit the eardrum, they set up a vibration that travels through the middle and inner ear chambers. From the *inner ear,* the vibration is converted to electrical signals and transmitted by the *auditory nerve* to the brain, which "hears" it as sounds such as words and music.

The ear can be divided into three areas: the external (outer) ear, middle ear, and internal (inner) ear. Each has its own structures and functions. (Figure 7–24):

Outer Ear:

- Pinna and auricle: The outer, visible projection of the ear. Designed to direct sound waves into the ear canal.

- External auditory canal: The canal that extends from the outside to the eardrum. Earwax (cerumen) is produced by ceruminous glands to prevent foreign bodies from entering the ear.

- Eardrum (tympanic membrane): Located at the end of the external auditory canal, it separates the outer and middle ears. The membrane vibrates when hit by sound waves which are then transmitted to the middle ear.

Middle Ear:

- Ossicles: Three tiny, delicate bones that form a chain to carry and amplify (make louder) sound vibrations from the eardrum. Because of their shapes, these bones are called the *hammer (malleus),* the *anvil (incus),* and the *stirrup (stapes).* The malleus connects to the eardrum on one side and the incus on the other; the incus then connects to the stapes, which is attached to the *oval window* on its other side. The oval window separates the middle and inner ears

- Eustachian tubes: Connect the nose and throat to the middle ear to equalize pressure. The uncomfortable sensations sometimes experienced in airplanes and under water are caused by sudden pressure changes. Chewing gum is recommended in airplanes because it helps open the tubes so that pressure is equalized.

Inner Ear:

- Cochlea: A spiral-shaped, bony structure filled with fluid. The vibrations amplified in the middle ear set the fluid in motion. This then starts a wave-like motion in tiny, hair-like receptors, signals that the auditory nerve sends to the brain.

- Semicircular canals: These are the organs of balance (equilibrium). They contain receptor cells that report movements of the head. There are three canals: one is parallel to the ground; a second parallel to the side of the head; a third is parallel to the face. Dizziness experienced after spinning around rapidly is caused by movement of the fluid in these canals.

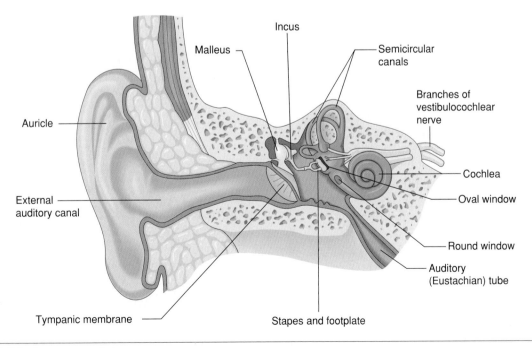

Figure 7–24 Structures of the ear.

Major Diseases and Disorders

Eyes:

- *Cataract* is the condition in which the lens of the eye loses its transparency, preventing light from reaching the inner eye.
- *Conjunctivitis* is an inflammation of the eyelid lining caused by bacteria or irritation from a particle of debris in the eye. Sometimes referred to as "pink eye."
- *Glaucoma* occurs when the pressure within the eye increases. This pressure can cause deterioration of the optic nerve.
- *Macular degeneration* is a disorder of the retina that results in dimming and/or distortion of vision.
- *Visual impairments* include a number of very common problems that require corrective lenses. For example, *myopia* (nearsightedness) occurs when the eyeball is longer than normal and cannot focus clearly on faraway objects. *Hyperopia* (farsightedness) occurs when the eyeball is shorter than normal and results in the inability to focus clearly on nearby objects. *Astigmatism* is an imperfect curvature of the cornea that results in blurred vision. *Presbyopia* is farsightedness caused by the loss of lens elasticity that occurs as part of the normal aging process. This is why a lot of people over forty need to wear "reading" glasses.

Ears:

- *Hearing loss* is classified as either conductive or sensory. *Conductive hearing loss* occurs when the sound waves do not reach the inner ear (e.g., wax plug, ruptured eardrum, infection, or obstruction in ear). *Sensory hearing loss* results from damage to the inner ear or auditory nerve. Many cases of hearing loss can be treated with amplification devices (hearing aids, corrective surgery, and cochlear implants (a device that does not restore normal hearing, but allows the individual to hear sounds that can be interpreted for meaning).
- *Labyrinthitis* is an inflammation of the inner ear.
- *Otitis externa* is an inflammation of the external auditory canal. For example, *swimmer's ear* occurs in this part of the ear.
- *Otitis media* is an infection of the middle ear.
- *Ruptured eardrum* can occur as a result of infection, a sudden blow to the ear, a violent change in air pressure such as occurs with an explosion, or from an object placed in the ear. Ruptures usually heal without treatment, but massive or repeated injury can form scar tissue and impair hearing.
- *Tinnitus* is not a disease, but a medical term for ringing in the ears. It can only be heard by the patient (subjective) and can occur when there is wax buildup in the ear or an ear infection, or as a result of an overdose of certain drugs (e.g., quinine or aspirin).

Preventive Measures

- Protect the ears from loud noises.
- Do not insert objects into the auditory canal.
- Use earplugs when swimming.
- Wear UV protective sunglasses when in the sun.
- Wear and clean contact lenses only as instructed.
- Get regular eye tests for glaucoma.
- Use eye protective devices around machinery and other hazards.

Age Related Changes—Sensory System

Eyes

- Decreased: Peripheral (side) vision, night vision
- Increased: Difficulty in reading small print and seeing objects at a distance, time to adjust from light to dark, sensitivity to glare

Ears

- Decreased: Ability to hear high-frequency sounds (e.g., telephone ringing, doorbell)
- Increased: Difficulty hearing when there is background noise (e.g., music or other people talking)
(Stence and Kegler, 1995)

[**Fascinating Facts**]

EYE—The human eye can see about 7 million shades of color (Colbert, 1997).

EAR—The three smallest bones in your body exist in your ears and take up an area about the size of a child's thumb nail (Colbert, 1997).

Nervous

The *nervous system* consists of the brain, spinal cord, and nerves. It detects sensations from all parts of the body and controls all the body's actions. It is also responsible for thoughts, emotions, and memories. A complex network of nerves constantly collects information from both inside and outside the body. This information is then transmitted by electrical stimuli through the spinal cord to the brain for interpretation. The information is stored, and if any response is required, such as pulling the hand away from a hot stove, direction is immediate and usually accomplished by coordinating the activities of other organ systems. In the case of the hot stove, communication would be with the muscles.

As students read this paragraph, their nervous systems are performing numerous functions:

1. Directing the eyes to move across the page
2. Recognizing the images as letters and combining them to form words and sentences
3. Storing some of the ideas as memories
4. Recalling previous memories to help in understanding the new information
5. Directing skeletal muscles to maintain a sitting position
6. Causing the eyes to automatically blink to stay moist and clean
7. Controlling the heart rate, blood pressure, and respiration to keep fresh oxygen supplied to the brain to keep them alert
8. Sending sensations of tiredness or hunger after a few hours of studying

These eight examples are just a small fraction of what the nervous system is actually doing at any given moment. It is amazing how complex this system actually is and how well it works.

The brain only makes up about 2% of the body's weight but uses 20% of the energy produced. It requires a constant supply of glucose (sugar) and oxygen to function. Low blood sugar causes the brain to partly shut down, resulting in feelings that begin as hunger and irritability and then progress to a weak, faint feeling. The brain is even more sensitive to the lack of oxygen and brain cells begin to die within five minutes when they are deprived of oxygen.

Central Nervous System

The *central nervous system (CNS)* includes the brain and the spinal cord. The brain consists of the cerebrum, cerebellum, diencephalon, and the brain stem (Figure 7–25).

- Cerebrum: Two large hemispheres that control the higher brain functions. Their many folds *(convolutions)* greatly increase the brain's surface area and thus the storage capacity of the brain. The hemispheres are joined by bands of nerve fibers, including the *corpus callosum* that helps the hemispheres communicate. Each hemisphere has a core of white matter that is surrounded by a layer of gray matter called the *cerebral cortex.* The cerebral cortex controls the voluntary actions, including physical action (running, walking, and chewing), mental activity (learning, judgment, decision-making, and creativity), conscious body sensations (sense of pleasure to what we see or how we are touched), and some emotions (Figure 7–26). It is surprising to note that one hemisphere of the cortex controls the opposite side of the body. That is, the right hemisphere controls the left side of the body and vice versa. For example, a stroke that occurs on the right side of the brain can cause paralysis of the left arm and leg. The left hemisphere is generally responsible for learning academic subjects such as speech, reading, writing , math, and logic. The right hemisphere generally affects how an individual learns and the learning of the arts (enjoyment of music, artistic ability, creativity) and how an individual experiences emotions. When people refer to themselves as either right-brained or left-brained, they are describing their interests and abilities in these areas.

- Cerebellum: Located in back of the brain between the cerebrum and brain stem. Working in conjunction with the cerebrum by fine-tuning and coordinating messages for muscular movement, it is also involved in balance, posture, and muscle tone.

- Diencephalon: Contains the *thalamus* and *hypothalamus.* The thalamus relays sensory stimuli to the cerebral cortex. The hypothalamus initiates and controls many involuntary body functions necessary for living such as water balance and body temperature.

- Brain stem: Consists of the midbrain, pons, and medulla oblongata. It serves as a pathway between the spinal cord and brain and regulates respiration, blood pressure, and heart rate.

The *spinal cord* carries messages between the brain and other parts of the body. It is attached

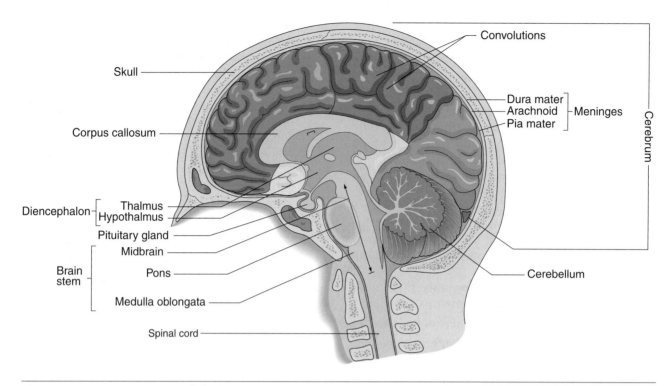

Figure 7–25 Cross-section of the brain.

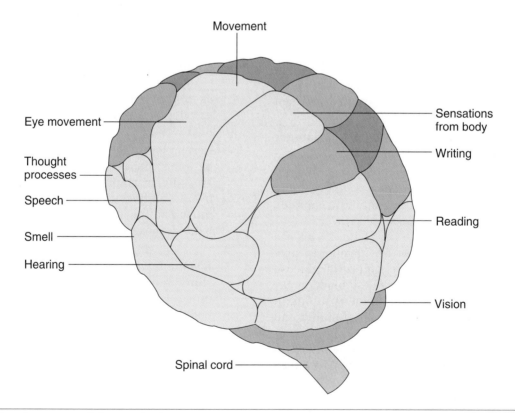

Figure 7–26 Functions of the cerebral cortex.

to the brain and is encased in the spinal column. Thirty-two pairs of nerves branch out from the cord and pass between each vertebrae and extend to the various parts of the body. Once the nerves branch off from the spinal cord, they are part of the peripheral nervous system.

Besides carrying messages to and from the brain, the spinal cord also serves as a reflex center. Reflexes are automatic responses that do not require any communication with the brain. For example, when the jerking that occurs when the doctor taps the knee, elbow, or wrist during a physical exam is an automatic reflex action. Also, when a finger touches a hot surface, a reflex occurs to pull it away. The reason pain is not felt until after the finger is removed from the hot surface is that the sensation must travel through the spinal cord to the brain for interpretation as pain.

The brain and spinal cord are not only protected by bone (skull and vertebrae), but also by membranes and a fluid cushion. Wrapped around the brain and spinal cord are three layers of protective membranes called *meninges*. The two innermost meningeal layers form a space where *cerebrospinal fluid (CSF)* flows around the brain and spinal cord.

Peripheral Nervous System

The *peripheral nervous system* consists of the nerves that emerge from the brain (*cranial nerves*) and spinal cord (*spinal nerves*). These nerves have both a voluntary and an involuntary component. The peripheral nerves contain two types of fibers, one for carrying messages to the central nervous system (sensory fibers) and another for carrying messages from the central nervous system to the skeletal muscles (motor fibers). See Figure 7–27.

The *involuntary nerves* of the peripheral nervous system contain fibers leading to and from the internal organs. These nerves belong to the *autonomic nervous system*, which means the individual has no voluntary control. For example, the body cannot be told when and how to digest food, when and how much urine to produce, or where and how much blood to circulate. It is a good thing the body's internal processes are automated or it would be necessary to continually think about taking the next breath or telling the heart to beat.

The autonomic nervous system can be divided into the sympathetic and the parasympathetic systems. The *sympathetic system* is activated in times of stress when the body senses the need to get away from a perceived threat or danger, commonly referred to as the "fight or flight" reaction. The sympathetic nervous system can make the difference between life and death. For example, in a crisis this system has enabled people to perform amazing feats of strength to perform rescues. But the body cannot tolerate prolonged stress without suffering physical or mental harm. The *parasympathetic system* maintains normal function on a day-to-day basis. See Table 7–2.

The autonomic nervous system works closely with the hormones produced by the hypothalamus. This will be discussed in the section on the endocrine system.

Neurons

There are billions of *neurons* (nerve cells) in the body, the majority of them located in the brain. Neurons grow rapidly before birth, then stop reproducing after birth. When a person learns a new skill, new brain cells are not being produced. Rather, the neurons are trained to connect in a new way. New ideas come from new connections between neurons. When people who have brain damage are relearning to speak or walk, they are working to establish new connections between the neurons they had at birth. Damaged cells may be able to repair themselves, but dead ones cannot be replaced.

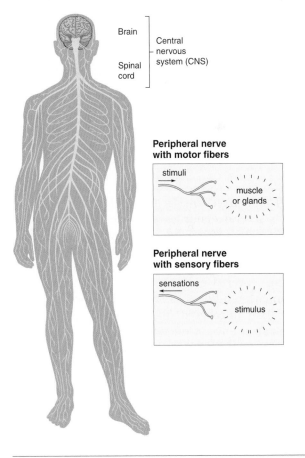

Figure 7–27 The peripheral nervous system connects the CNS to the structures of the body. When the peripheral nerve contains both motor and sensory fibers, it is called a mixed nerve.

Table 7–2 Actions of the Sympathetic and Parasympathetic Nervous Systems

System or Organ	Sympathetic System (to cope with emergencies)	Parasympathetic System (normal daily functions)
Heart	increases rate and force of contraction	decreases rate and force of contraction
Lungs	dilates airways to take in more oxygen for body	constricts air passages
Arteries	constricts arteries, thus raising blood pressure	dilates arteries to lower blood pressure
Gastrointestinal	slows peristalsis and digestive activity to send more blood to the brain and skeletal muscles	speeds peristalsis, increases digestion
Urinary	relaxes bladder	constricts bladder, thus encouraging urination
Eye muscles	dilates pupils, thus allowing more light to enter eyes	constricts pupils
Sweat glands	increases secretion to prevent overheating of body	decreases secretion
Hair muscles	contracts muscles and causes piloerection (goose bumps)	relaxes muscles, causes hair to lie flat

Adapted from *An integrated approach to health sciences: Anatomy and physiology, math, physics, and chemistry* (p. 94), by B. J. Colbert, J. Ankney, J. Wilson, and J. Havrilla, 1997, Albany, NY: Delmar.

The neuron consists of a *cell body*, from which branch several dendrites and one axon. The *dendrites* are short fibers that bring electrical signals to the cell body, and an *axon* is a long fiber that carries the signal away from the cell body. Some of the neurons are covered in a fatty material called *myelin*. Myelin-covered fibers can transmit impulses much faster than uncovered fibers. The myelin gives a white appearance to the neurons. For example, the white matter of the cerebrum is covered with myelin, and the gray matter (cerebral cortex) is not.

The neurons do not actually touch each other when impulses are transmitted. When the axon of one cell reaches a dendrite of another cell they are separated by a gap, called a *synapse*. The electric impulse crosses the synapse with the help of chemicals, called *neurotransmitters* (Figure 7–28). For a summary overview of the nervous system, see Figure 7–29.

Major Diseases and Disorders

- *Cerebral palsy* is caused by brain damage and results in a lack of control over the voluntary muscles.

- A *cerebrovascular accident (CVA)* involves the brain and its blood supply, and is commonly referred to as a "stroke." A CVA can be caused by a block in the blood flow (e.g., emboli) or from a ruptured vessel. The disruption of blood flow to the brain can cause tissue damage or even death. The signs and symptoms will depend on what part of the brain has been damaged. Common results are paralysis of one side of the body (*hemiplegia*), difficulty in or inability to communicate through speech, writing, or signs (*aphasia*). *Transient ischemic attacks* (TIAs), called "little strokes," occur when blood flow is only temporarily impaired. TIAs may be warning signs of a future CVA.

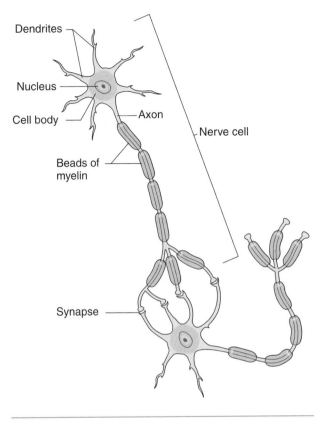

Figure 7–28 The neuron.

- *Dementia* is a loss of memory and impairment of intellectual function. *Alzheimer's disease* is only one of several diseases that cause dementia. *Senile dementia* refers to dementia when it occurs in the elderly.

- *Encephalitis* is an infection of the brain.

- *Epilepsy* is a disorder of the brain resulting from abnormal electrical impulses in the neurons. Seizures can range from very mild (petit mal) to generalized severe seizures (grand mal). Anticonvulsant drugs are very effective in controlling epilepsy.

- *Meningitis* is the inflammation of the protective covering (meninges) of the brain and spinal cord.

- *Multiple sclerosis* is a chronic, progressive, disabling condition resulting from a defect in electrical transmission of the neurons which is caused by degeneration of the myelin sheath.

- *Neuritis* is the inflammation of a nerve. *Neuralgia* is nerve pain.

- *Parkinson's disease* is a chronic, progressive condition involving degeneration of brain cells because of a decrease in a neurotransmitter (dopamine). It is characterized by tremors, shuffling walk, muscle rigidity, and loss of facial expression.

- *Shingles (herpes zoster)* is caused by a virus. Blisters appear on the skin following the nerve pathways. It is very painful and even after the blisters heal, pain can be experienced for years along these nerve pathways.

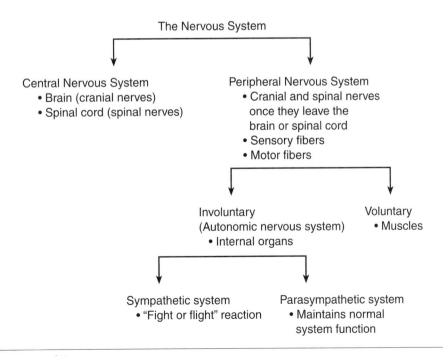

Figure 7–29 Overview of the nervous system.

- *Spinal cord injury* results in a loss of sensation and voluntary movement. The location of the injury determines the amount of impairment. If the injury is in the lower portion of the spinal column, only the lower half of the body is affected. This is called *paraplegia*. If the injury is in the upper portion of the cord, all four extremities can be affected. This is called *quadriplegia*.

Preventive Measures

- Do not use illegal drugs.
- Avoid excessive alcohol.
- Continue learning new things throughout life.
- Use protective devices such as helmets and seat belts.
- Get sufficient sleep.

Age Related Changes—Nervous System

- Decreased: Response and reaction time, number of brain cells, amount of neurotransmitters; ability to sleep, balance and coordination; cerebral blood flow
- Increased: Awakenings during sleep, muscle tremors
  (Stence and Kegler, 1995)

Endocrine

The *endocrine system* consists of glands that manufacture hormones. A *hormone* is a chemical substance secreted by a gland in one part of the body that travels via the bloodstream to direct changes in the activities of other organ systems. There are many different hormones and each has its own function.

The nervous and endocrine systems work closely together to coordinate and control the body's functions. For example, recall that the sympathetic nervous system is stimulated in times of crisis. This is caused by a hormone secreted by the adrenal glands, part of the endocrine system.

There are two types of glands: exocrine and endocrine glands. Exocrine glands do not produce hormones, but rather produce liquids that flow through a duct (small tube) to reach a body cavity or to the surface of the skin. Examples of exocrine secretions are sweat, saliva, mucus, and digestive juices. The pancreas has the unique characteristic of being both an exocrine (see digestive system) and an endocrine gland (produces the hormone insulin).

The hypothalamus is attached to the brain and spinal cord by many nerves. This organ links the autonomic nervous system and endocrine system. It plays an important role in the regulation of most of the involuntary mechanisms of the body and regulates the work of the pituitary gland.

The pituitary gland is frequently called the "master gland" because it secretes hormones that stimulate other endocrine glands to produce their own hormones. An important feature of the endocrine system is the *feedback mechanism*. This mechanism is similar to the thermostat that controls the temperature in a house. The thermostat measures the internal temperature and then turns heat or air conditioning off or on as needed to maintain the desired temperature. In a similar way, the pituitary determines if there is enough of each hormone circulating in the blood stream and turns the stimuli to produce hormones on and off. Study Figure 7–30 and Table 7–3 to learn more about each of the endocrine glands, the hormones they produce, and the action of the hormones. The ovaries and testes are part of the endocrine system, but will be discussed with the female and male reproductive systems.

Major Diseases and Disorders

Adrenal glands:

- *Addison's disease* is caused by inadequate hormone production by the adrenal cortex. It causes excessive skin pigmentation, decreased sugar and salt in the blood, and decreased blood pressure.
- *Cushing's syndrome* is caused by excessive hormone production of the adrenal cortex triggered by oversecretion of ACTH (anterior lobe of pituitary). This results in a redistribution of fat to create a more rounded face (*"moon face"*) and a hump below the back of the neck (*"buffalo hump"*). It also causes increased blood pressure, unusual hair growth called *hirsutism*, and easy bruising.

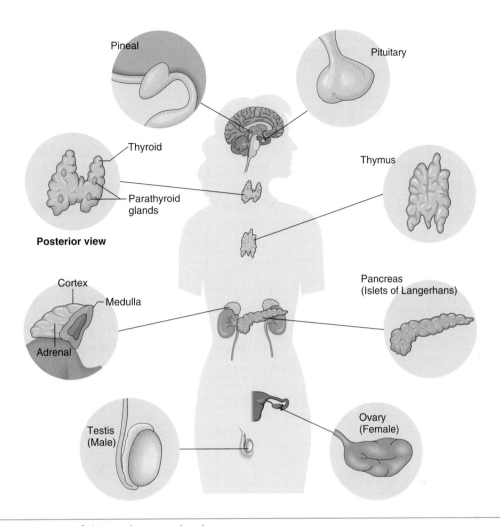

Figure 7–30 Locations of the endocrine glands.

Pancreas:

- *Diabetes mellitus* is caused by inadequate insulin production. This results in *hyperglycemia* (too much glucose in the blood). The signs and symptoms are *polydipsia* (unusual thirst), *polyuria* (increased urine output), and *polyphagia* (unusual hunger).

Parathyroid glands:

- *Hyperparathyroidism* is caused by excessive parathormone that results in an increased calcium blood level. The excessive calcium levels cause stone formation in the urinary system and elsewhere. The bones are also robbed of their calcium and this makes them vulnerable to fractures.

- *Hypoparathyroidism* is caused by inadequate parathormone and results in a decreased calcium blood level that interrupts the normal function of nerves. This causes a condition called *tetany,* convulsive muscle twitching, and can lead to death if the respiratory muscles are affected.

Pituitary gland:

- *Acromegaly* is caused by excessive growth hormone (anterior lobe of pituitary) in adults. It causes an enlargement in the bones of the hands, feet, and jaw.

- *Diabetes insipidus* is caused by a decrease in antidiuretic hormone (posterior lobe of pituitary). It causes an increase in urine production that can lead to dehydration and electrolyte imbalances.

- *Dwarfism* can be caused by inadequate secretion of growth hormone as a child develops. The body does not develop to an average adult size.

- *Gigantism* is caused by excessive secretion of growth hormone as a child develops. This causes elongation of the long bones and results in excessive height.

Table 7–3 Hormones and Their Actions

Gland & Location	Hormone	Actions
Pituitary (cranium) *Anterior lobe:*	GH—growth hormone	Directs normal growth of body tissues
	ACTH—adrenocorticotropic hormone	Stimulates cortex of adrenal gland
	TSH—thyroid stimulating hormone	Stimulates thyroid gland
	MSH—melanocyte stimulating hormone	Stimulates production of melanin, which causes skin pigmentation
	FSH—follicle stimulating hormone	Promotes egg development in the female and sperm production in the male
	LH—luteinizing hormone (or)	Stimulates ovulation and production of female hormones (estrogen and progesterone)
	ICSH—interstitial cell stimulating hormone	Stimulates production of male hormone (testosterone)
	LTH—lactogenic hormone or prolactin	Promotes development of breast tissue and production of milk in females
Posterior lobe:	ADH—antidiuretic hormone, or vasopressin	Acts on kidneys to concentrate urine and conserve fluid in the body; also constricts blood vessels
	Oxytocin (pitocin)	Causes contraction of uterus during childbirth; stimulates milk flow
Pineal (cranium)	melatonin	Controls onset of puberty
Thyroid (neck)	thyroxine (T_4) and triiodothyronine (T_3)	Controls metabolism and stimulates physical and mental growth
	calcitocin	Moves calcium from the blood stream into the bones for storage
Parathyroid (neck)	PTH—parathormone	Promotes absorption of calcium from the intestines, decreases calcium excretion by the kidneys, and moves calcium from the bones to the blood (opposite effect of calcitonin)
Thymus (chest beneath sternum)	thymosin	Stimulates production of antibodies in early life

(continues)

Table 7–3 (continued)

Gland & Location	Hormone	Actions
Adrenals: (one on top of each kidney) *Cortex:*	mineralocorticoids (aldosterone)	Regulates the balance of electrolytes (chemicals which, when dissolved in water, can conduct electrical current) by stimulating the kidneys to retain salt (sodium) and excrete potassium
	glucocorticoids (cortisone)	Aids in metabolism of proteins, fats, and carbohydrates; provides resistance to stress; depresses immune responses (anti-inflammatory)
	gonadocorticoids (androgens)	A sex hormone, produced by both males and females, whose function is unclear
Medulla:	epinephrine (adrenaline) and norepinephrine	Activates sympathetic nervous system in times of stress; increases blood pressure by constricting blood vessels
Pancreas (mid-abdomen under stomach)	insulin	Regulates the transport of glucose (sugar) from the blood into the body cells
	glucagon	Increases the amount of glucose in the blood by stimulating the liver to convert glycogen (stored form of glucose) to glucose (type of sugar that is main source of energy to cells)

Thyroid glands:

- *Hyperthyroidism* is caused by excessive thyroid hormones. It results in nervousness, increased pulse rate, weight loss, irritability, sensitivity to heat, and increased blood sugar.
- *Hypothyroidism* is caused by inadequate thyroid hormones. It results in edema (excessive fluid in tissues), obesity, lethargy (extreme fatigue), decrease in heart rate, decreased mental function, sensitivity to cold, and thinning of the hair.

Preventive Measures

- Maintain healthy weight.
- Avoid excessive refined sugars.
- Take children for checkups to monitor growth and development.
- Avoid the use of steroids unless prescribed (never use for purposes of muscle building during weight training programs).

Age Related Changes—Endocrine System

- Decreased: Thyroid gland function; basal metabolic rate (energy needed to maintain body functions); adrenal gland function; insulin release; ability to breakdown glucose to provide energy for the body
- Increased: Incidence of hyperglycemia (increase in blood sugar) with ingestion of sugars (Stence and Kegler, 1995)

Thinking it Through

Mary Steward recently retired after 40 years of teaching high school. Since her retirement, she has noticed that she is increasingly tired, sleeping much more than usual, and seems to feel cold all the time. She loved her job and at first thought that her tiredness was just part of adjusting to retirement and that feeling cold was from lack of exercise. But the symptoms have become more severe, and she made an appointment with her family physician. After an examination and blood work, Mrs. Steward is informed that she has hypothyroidism.

1. What is the function of the thyroid gland?
2. Based on the symptoms, does Mrs. Steward have too much or too little thyroid function?
3. Is the thyroid an exocrine or endocrine gland? Why?

Systems for Producing New Life

Reproduction is one of the most fundamental functions common to all living organisms. The reproductive system allows the creation of a new human being who is both like and unlike each of the two parents. Reproduction is essential for the continuation of human life on the earth.

Female Reproductive

The *female reproductive system* can be divided into the internal and external reproductive organs (Figure 7–31):

Internal Reproductive Organs:

- Ovaries: There are two ovaries, one on each side of the uterus, which is located in the lower abdomen. They produce the hormones *estrogen* and *progesterone*, which determine the female characteristics (body shape, hair patterns, and breast development) and are necessary for pregnancy and subsequent childbirth to occur. Within each ovary are tiny sacs called *graafian follicles*, each of which contains one *ovum* (egg). The ovum is the female sex cell.

- Fallopian tubes: Arise from the upper portion of the uterus and end in finger-like projections (*fimbriae*) that draw the ovum, released from an ovary, down into the tube. Sperm (male sex cells) travel up into these tubes, which is where fertilization takes place. Once fertilized, the ovum moves down into the uterus.

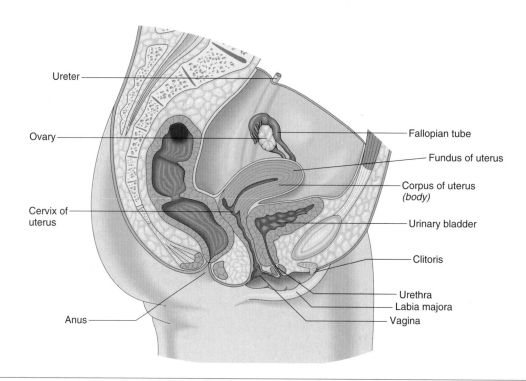

Figure 7–31 Cross-section of the female reproductive organs.

[**Fascinating Facts**]

Females stop growing when they are about 18 years old. Males grow taller for a few years following their eighteenth birthday (Colbert, 1997).

■ Uterus (womb): A muscular, hollow organ located behind the urinary bladder and in front of the rectum. It has three parts: the *fundus* (upper portion where fallopian tubes attach), the *corpus* (body or middle section), and the *cervix* (narrow, bottom area that attaches to the vagina). When the fertilized ovum reaches the uterus it implants itself into the wall and grows and develops into a fetus. If a fertilized ovum is not implanted, then the lining of the uterus is shed and menstruation occurs.

■ Vagina: Opening that connects the outside of the body to the uterus. Made of smooth muscle and lined with a mucus membrane, it is capable of expanding to allow for childbirth and then contracting back to original size.

External Reproductive Organs (*genitalia*):

■ Labia majora: Large fleshy folds of fat tissue that surround and protect the opening of the external female genitalia. They are covered with hair on their outer surfaces.

■ Labia minora: Smaller fleshy folds that lay inside the boundaries of the labia majora for further protection.

■ Clitoris: Located at the top junction of the labia minora, this is a very sensitive organ composed of erectile tissue similar to that of the male penis.

■ Bartholin's glands: Located on each side of the external opening of the vagina, these produce mucus secretions that lubricate the vagina.

The *breasts (mammary glands)* are composed of connective and fatty tissue and contain milk ducts. The female hormones signal when milk production (*lactation*) is needed after childbirth.

Major Diseases and Disorders

■ *Menstrual disorders* can result from hormonal imbalances, structural deformities, excessive exercise or stress, and nutritional imbalances. *Amenorrhea* is the absence of menstruation.

Menorrhagia is excessive bleeding. *Dysmenorrhea* is painful menstrual cramps.

■ *Ectopic pregnancy* occurs when the fertilized ovum becomes implanted outside of the uterus. The most common site is in the fallopian tube. As the embryo develops, pain is caused by the distention of the tube. The tube will eventually rupture which creates a life-threatening situation if excessive internal bleeding occurs.

■ *Endometriosis* is the growth of endometrial tissue (which lines the uterus) outside the uterus. The tissue can be transferred from the uterus by the fallopian tubes, blood, lymph, or during surgery.

■ *Fibroid tumors* are tumors in the uterus. They are usually benign (not cancerous) and often produce no symptoms.

■ *Pelvic inflammatory disease (PID)* is an inflammation of all the pelvic reproductive organs and causes scarring of the fallopian tubes. This can lead to an increased occurrence of ectopic pregnancies and infertility. Sexually transmitted diseases are frequently the cause of PID.

■ *Premenstrual syndrome (PMS)* is a general term for a variety of symptoms that occur prior to the beginning of bleeding (menses). They include irritability, depression, impaired concentration, headache, and edema. PMS may be related to hormonal, biochemical, or nutritional imbalances.

■ *Sexually transmitted disease (STD)* or venereal disease is a general term that refers to any disease transmitted through sexual contact. Examples include gonorrhea, syphilis, chlamydia, scabies, pubic lice, genital herpes, genital warts, trichomonas, and AIDS.

■ *Vaginitis* is a nonspecific infection of the vagina.

Preventive Measures

■ Practice safe sex, if sexually active (Chapter 12).

■ Use good toilet hygiene.

■ If menstrual irregularities occur or PMS is severe, have your health care provider perform an evaluation.

■ Have early and routine examinations during pregnancy.

■ If using contraception, be informed about the effectiveness of the method and any potential complications.

[Fascinating Facts]

Thousands of tiny sacs (graafian follicles) are found in each ovary (Colbert, 1997).

- Do not routinely perform douches.
- Consult a health care provider if sexual intercourse is uncomfortable or painful.
- Do monthly self-examination of the breasts. Report any lumps or irregularities to your health care provider for further evaluation.
- Have pap smears and breast examinations (including mammograms) at the age and frequency recommended by your health care provider.
- Report any sores or growths on labia and any unusual vaginal discharge or itching.

Age Related Changes—Female Reproductive System

- Decreased: Vaginal lubrication
- Increased: Susceptibility to vaginal infections (Stence and Kegler, 1995)

Male Reproductive

Most parts of the male reproductive system are located outside of the body because sperm are heat sensitive and would not survive normal body temperatures (Figure 7–32):

- Testes (testicles): The two testes are encased in a sac-like structure known as the *scrotum* and manufacture *sperm (spermatozoa),* the male sex cell. Once sperm is manufactured it is stored in the *epididymis,* a coiled duct along the back part of the testes. During ejaculation (expulsion of the semen from the body), the sperm travels through a small tube (*vas deferens*) that enters the lower pelvic area, goes around the urinary bladder, and back down to join the urethra. The testes also produce a male hormone called *testosterone* which aids in the maturation of sperm and is responsible for the development of male characteristics (body and facial hair, large muscles, and deep voice).
- Seminal vesicles: These glands join at the final portion of the vas deferens to form the ejaculatory duct. They produce a thick, yellow secretion that nourishes the sperm.
- Prostate gland: Secretes an alkaline fluid into the ejaculatory duct to aid in the movement of sperm (motility) and neutralize the acidity of

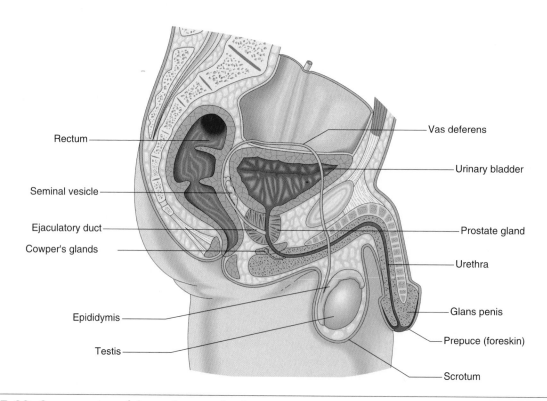

Figure 7–32 Cross-section of the male reproductive organs.

the vagina. It contracts during ejaculation to propel the semen forward and to close off the urethra to prevent urine from passing at the same time.

- Penis: Composed of erectile tissue that when aroused fills with blood and becomes erect. At the distal end of the penis is an enlarged area known as the *glans penis* that is covered with a *prepuce (foreskin)*. The foreskin is sometimes removed in a surgical procedure called *circumcision*.

- Urethra: Connects to the urinary bladder, passes through the penis, and exits at the end of the penis through an external opening called a *meatus*. It serves as a passageway for both urine from the urinary bladder and semen from the reproductive tubes.

- Cowper's (bulbourethral) gland: Produces a thick, white, alkaline secretion to lubricate the urethra and decrease the acidity of urine residue in the urethra.

Major Diseases and Disorders

- *Epididymitis* is an inflammation of the epididymis. It causes intense pain, swelling, and fever.

- *Prostatic hypertrophy* is an enlargement of the prostate that causes symptoms as a result of pressing on the urethra. It can be an age-related condition known as *benign prostatic hypertrophy* (BPH). It can also be caused by an inflammation, change in hormonal activity, benign (noncancerous) tumor, or a malignant (cancerous) tumor.

- *Orchitis* is inflammation of the testes. It causes swelling of the scrotum, pain, and fever. It can lead to atrophy of the testes and cause sterility.

- *Phimosis* refers to a tightness of the foreskin over the end of the penis.

- *Sexually transmitted diseases*—see section under female reproductive diseases and disorders. Some of the diseases listed are asymptomatic (have no symptoms) in males. However, males can be carriers of the disease-causing organism and require treatment to prevent the female from being infected.

Preventive Measures

- Practice safe sex, if sexually active (Chapter 12).

- Use good toilet hygiene.

- Male contraceptive methods may become more common in the future. If contraception is used, be informed about the effectiveness of the method and any potential complications.

- If a decrease in libido or ability to obtain an erection develops, discuss this with the health care provider because there are both physical and emotional factors that can be involved. Medications (e.g., antihypertensives–decrease blood pressure) can also cause this to occur and can be discussed. Do not take medications to increase libido (e.g., Viagra) until there is a thorough examination to detect risk factors and potential complications.

- Consult a health care provider if orgasm or urination is uncomfortable or painful.

- Report any lumps or irregularities of the breasts to your health care provider for further evaluation.

- Have prostate gland examinations performed at the age and frequency recommended by your health care provider.

- Report any discharge from the urethra, and any sores or growths of the genitalia.

Age Related Changes—Male Reproductive System

- Decreased: Production of sperm and seminal fluid, size of testes

- Increased: Size of prostate gland (Simmers, 1998)

Review Table 7–4 for an overview of the organ systems covered in this chapter.

[**Fascinating Facts**]

There are approximately 100 million spermatozoa in every milliliter of seminal fluid. Every time a male ejaculates, he releases on the average 2 to 4 milliliters of semen. (Colbert, 1997).

Table 7–4 Organ Systems of the Body

Organ Systems	Major Functions
Systems for Movement and Protection	
Skeletal system	• Provide framework to support muscles, fat, soft tissues, and skin • Furnish locations for attachment of skeletal muscles • Protect internal organs • Store minerals • Help in formation of red and white blood cells
Muscular	• Enable locomotion (movement) • Give support to body • Produce heat
Integumentary system	• Protect from environmental hazards • Control temperature
Systems for Providing Energy and Removing Waste:	
Circulatory system (cardiovascular and lymphatic)	• Transport cells and dissolved materials, including nutrients, wastes, and gases • Provide defense against infection and disease • Maintain fluid balance • Remove waste products
Respiratory (pulmonary) system	• Deliver air to sites where gas exchange occurs
Digestive (gastrointestinal) system	• Process food and absorb nutrients, minerals, vitamins, and water • Eliminate undigested food from the body
Urinary system	• Eliminate excess water, salts, and waste products

(continues)

Table 7–4 (continued)

Organ Systems	Major Functions
Systems for Sensing, Coordinating, and Controlling	
Sensory systems (eyes, ears)	• Collect visual and auditory information Note that the organs for the other three senses are covered in other systems: • smell (olfactory)—nose discussed in respiratory • taste (gustatory)—tongue discussed in digestive • touch—skin discussed in integumentary
Nervous system	• Direct immediate responses to stimuli, usually by coordinating the activities of other organ systems
Endocrine system	• Direct changes in the activities of other organ systems
Systems for Producing New Life:	
Female Reproductive system	• Produces sex cells and hormones necessary for female characteristics to develop, and for pregnancy, delivery, and breast-feeding to occur.
Male Reproductive system	• Produces sex cells and hormones necessary for male characteristics to develop, and for production of semen for impregnation of female.

Adapted from *Essentials of anatomy and physiology* (p. 5), by F. H. Martini and E. F. Bartholomew, 1997, Upper Saddle River, NJ: Prentice-Hall.

SUGGESTED LEARNING ACTIVITIES

1. Think of the last time you were ill. Identify the system that was involved (e.g., respiratory for head colds, digestive for stomach flu) and review its anatomy and physiology. Identify the pathophysiological changes that occurred with this illness. What was the etiology of the illness? What were your signs and symptoms? Did you have any diagnostic procedures done? What was the treatment for this illness? What was the prognosis? Are there any preventive measures you can take to avoid a reoccurrence of the problem?

2. Think about the physiological changes your parents or grandparents have experienced. Can you describe these changes to them in everyday language?

3. Locate and name as many bones and muscles as you can in your own body by pressing on the outer surface of your skin.

4. Move your extremities to demonstrate the various positions made possible by your joints.

5. If you have a stethoscope, listen to your heartbeat and identify what is happening in the chambers, with the valves, and in the electrical system of the heart when you hear the "thump-thump" or "lub-dub" sounds.

6. Take in a deep breath of fresh air and review the path that will be taken until the oxygen reaches the level of the individual body cell. What physiological actions occur along the way?

7. Next time you have a meal, review the path the solid food and the liquids will take through your body until they are excreted. What physiological actions occur along the way?

8. Change the italicized phrase in the following saying to its correct medical equivalent: "Don't shoot until you see the *whites of their eyes*!"

9. Think of the last time you were very frightened ("fight or flight" reaction) and identify the physiological changes that the sympathetic nervous system would have initiated.

10. Review all the conditions that must be present for pregnancy to occur (remember to include the endocrine system).

REVIEW QUESTIONS

1. What is the difference between the terms "anatomy", "physiology", and "pathophysiology"?

2. What is the key difference between wellness and illness?

3. What are the primary anatomical features and physiological actions of the systems for movement and protection of the body?

4. What are the names of the movements made possible by joints?

5. What are the primary anatomical features and physiological actions of the systems for providing energy and for removing waste from the body?

6. What are the primary anatomical features and physiological actions of the systems for sensing, and for coordinating and controlling the body?

7. What are the primary anatomical features and physiological actions of the systems for producing new life?

8. What are the common diseases or disorders associated with each body system?

9. What are three preventive measures for each body system?

APPLICATION EXERCISES

1. Now that you know the normal anatomy and physiology of the lungs, what signs and symptoms can you anticipate that Mr. Petersen may experience as a result of Red Cedar Disease discussed in The Case of the Unfamiliar Diagnosis?

2. Kelly Alexico comes into the office and states he was recently diagnosed with diabetes. Wanda Hector, the health care worker asks him if he is referring to diabetes mellitus or diabetes insipidus. He responds by saying, "I don't know for sure, all I know is that I was peeing a lot."

a. Is this adequate information to determine if it is diabetes mellitus or diabetes insipidus?

b. What other questions could the health care worker ask him to determine which type of diabetes is most likely the diagnosis?

c. If it is diabetes mellitus what can Wanda tell him about the anatomy and physiology of the related system? What is the pathophysiology of this diagnosis?

d. If it is diabetes insipidus what can Wanda tell him about the anatomy and physiology of the related system? What is the pathophysiology of this diagnosis?

SUGGESTED READINGS AND RESOURCES

American Cancer Society: http://www.cancer.org

American Diabetes Association: http://diabetes.org/default.asp

Arthritis Foundation: http:www.arthritis.org

Borgstadt, M. (1995). *Understanding and caring for human diseases.* Albany, NY: Delmar.

Ehrlich, A. (1997). *Medical terminology for health professions* (3rd ed.). Albany, NY: Delmar.

Elson, L. M. (1993). *Anatomy coloring book.* New York: Addison-Wesley.

Epilepsy Foundation: http://www.epilepsyfoundation.org

Muscular Dystrophy Association: www.mdausa.org

National Kidney Foundation: http://www.kidney.org

National Parkinson Foundation, Inc.: http://www.parkinson.org

Scott, A. S. and Fong, E. (1998). *Body structures and functions* (9th ed.). Albany, NY: Delmar.

Sickle Cell Disease Association of America: http://sicklecelldisease.org

Tamparo, D. D. and Lewis, M. A. (1995). *Diseases of the human body* (2nd ed.). Philadelphia: F. A. Davis Company.

CHAPTER

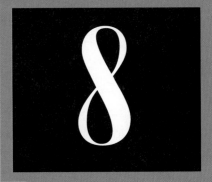

GROWTH AND DEVELOPMENT

OBJECTIVES

Studying and applying the material in this chapter will help you to:

- Explain the difference between "physical," "cognitive," and "psychosocial" as they relate to growth and development.

- Identify the nine life stages and the corresponding age span for each.

- Discuss the physical, cognitive, and psychosocial changes that occur at each life stage.

- Identify the psychosocial developmental tasks to be accomplished according to the theory of Erik Erikson.

- Implement specific approaches to care at each life stage based on a knowledge of growth and development.

- Identify and describe the five stages of the dying process.

KEY TERMS

chronic illness
cognitive
development
Erikson's Stages of
    Psychosocial Development
growth
life review
physical
psychosocial
stages of dying
terminal illness

179

The Case of

the Curious Four-Year-Old

Paul, a four-year-old child, is brought to the physician's office by his mother for a routine examination. Heathrow Wilson, the medical assistant directs them to the room and begins to ask the mother routine questions and to take Paul's vital signs (blood pressure, temperature, heart and respiratory rate). Heathrow finds the tasks impossible to accomplish as the child wiggles, tries to pick up or touch everything, and asks continual questions. The mother becomes increasingly frustrated as she repeatedly tells the child to be quite and sit still.

This may seem like a simple situation that has been observed many times, but there is a deeper dynamic being portrayed. The material in this chapter will help the health care worker to understand that Paul's behavior of tremendous curiosity and activity is normal for his age group. As a result of understanding the stages of growth and development, the health care worker could alter his approach to constructively deal with Paul's behavior by implementing a strategy that will allow the child to participate (e.g., engaging the child by giving him something to do to help, asking questions directly of the child, or first letting Paul listen to his heart with the stethoscope). An age-appropriate response will prevent frustration and allow the child to meet his needs for this stage of development.

KNOWING YOUR PATIENT

From before human beings are born until they die, all individuals go through a series of stages in which they develop physically and mentally. Becoming a person happens over time. The study of growth and development is about these stages in life and what is accomplished in each. **Growth** refers to the physical changes that take place in the body. Examples of physical changes include:

- Increases in height
- Increases in weight
- Motor sensory adaptation
- Development of the sex organs

Development refers to the increase in mental, emotional, and social capabilities of the individual. Examples include increases in:

- Intellectual (cognitive) ability
- Variety in expression of emotions
- Ability to cope with complex situations

- Social and interpersonal skills

The following terms describe key concepts in human growth and development:

- **Physical**: Growth of the body, including motor sensory adaptation. Monitoring growth is an important task in health care. The health care worker may be responsible for measuring and recording height, weight, and head circumference for infants and children. The Learning Activities at the end of this chapter cite the address for the government Web site that publishes the norms for weight, height, body mass, and head circumference according to percentiles. It is important for the physician to be notified if the measurements fall outside the norms because it may be an indication of a problem that can be addressed before it worsens.

- **Psychosocial**: Includes both psychological and social development. Psychological refers to the emotions (love, hate, joy, fear, anxiety), attitudes, and other aspects of the mind. Social refers to an individual's interactions and relationships with other members of society.

- **Cognitive**: This refers to intellectual processes and includes thought, awareness, and the ability to rationally comprehend the world and determine meaning. Seeking new information and applying it to make judgements and solve problems in positive, productive ways helps develop cognitive ability. For example, using the problem-solving model presented in Chapter 1 is a way to work on mental development. The information presented in each chapter of this text and the decision-making applications incorporated into the "Thinking It Through" exercises are designed to develop cognitive ability.

Human needs vary as individuals move through the life span. It is important for health care workers to understand the developmental milestones of each stage of life, because they may provide care to individuals of all ages. The study and application of growth and development along with individual patient assessment will guide the health care worker in age-appropriate communication and care. It is also important to realize that there are always exceptions and that no one follows the stages exactly. Generalizations cannot take the place of considering each patient as a unique individual.

LIFE STAGES

The study of growth and development across the life span has been categorized into time frames. Certain changes and needs characterize each. There are a number of variations of these time frames in terms of the months or years that they cover. The age ranges listed in Table 8–1 are commonly used. They start with conception (when an ovum is fertilized) and proceed through infancy, childhood stages, adolescence, and adulthood. A study of the life span includes the final stage, that of dying.

The psychosocial aspects of each life stage are based on **Erik Erikson's Stages of Psychosocial Development** (Table 8–1). Erikson, an immigrant from Germany who taught at Yale and Harvard, studied the influence of society and culture on human development. He studied human responses to life's events to gain an understanding of how attitudes and behaviors change throughout the life span. He based his stage theory, first published in 1950, on the belief that psychosocial development occurs as the result of resolving specific types of conflicts encountered at each stage. Resolving these conflicts, at least in part, allows the individual to advance successfully to the next stage. Erikson's developmental tasks are explained in the discussions of each stage later in this chapter.

Table 8–1 Life Stages and Erik Erikson's Stages of Psychosocial Development

Stage	Age	Erikson Stage
Prenatal	Conception to birth	
Infancy	Birth to 1 year	Trust vs. Mistrust
Toddler	1 to 3 years	Autonomy vs. Shame/Doubt
Preschooler	3 to 6 years	Initiative vs. Guilt
School-Age Child	6 to 12 years	Industry vs. Inferiority
Adolescence	12 to 20 years	Identity vs. Role Confusion
Young Adulthood	20s and 30s	Intimacy vs. Isolation
Middle Adulthood	40s and 50s	Generativity vs. Stagnation
Later Adulthood	60s to death	Ego Integrity vs. Despair

While failing to complete a stage can delay the psychosocial growth of the individual, it does not necessarily prevent the successful completion of the stage at a later date. It is also important to understand that transitions are gradual between stages: they do not begin and end abruptly at exact ages. When individuals are under stress, such as during an illness, they may regress (return) to the behavior characteristic of a previous stage. Erikson did not assign specific beginning and ending ages to each stage, but he emphasized that they occur in the same order for each individual. Researchers and writers have assigned different age ranges to his stages. The ranges chosen for Table 8–1 are representative of the life span of today's adult.

Prenatal

The *prenatal* period begins with conception (fertilization of an ovum by a sperm) and ends with birth. The cell formed when the two reproductive sex cells join is called a *zygote*. The zygote contains all the genetic information from both parents that will determine gender and physical characteristics, such as eye color, hair color and texture, and skin pigmentation. Many other areas are not completely determined by genetics. For example, personality, intellect, and other mental characteristics are influenced by many other factors, such as:

- Family relationships
- Cultural customs
- Religion
- Education
- Physical health

Physical growth is affected by factors such as adequate supplies of appropriate food, opportunities for exercise, and access to health care. Individuals are not simply combinations of genetic material, but unique combinations of both genetic and environmental influences.

Human growth and development begin the moment that fertilization occurs. The fertilized ovum is implanted into the uterine wall and rapid cell division and multiplication occurs. The time period from the 2nd to the 8th week after fertilization is called the *embryo stage*. At 8 weeks and until birth, the embryo is called a *fetus.*

Rapid prenatal growth and development make the developing human especially vulnerable to environmental factors. Congenital anomalies (birth defects) can occur if the mother inhales toxins or consumes alcohol, drugs, or nicotine. Therapeutic drugs, beneficial for the mother, can cause harmful side effects in the fetus. Therefore, all over-the-counter (OTC) and prescription medications must be reviewed by the physician to determine is they are safe to take during pregnancy.

The speed of prenatal growth is illustrated by the following examples (Guyton and Hall, 1995):

- Within 1–3 weeks after fertilization the heart starts to beat, the central nervous system starts to develop, and all the organs are present.
- By 6 weeks the arms and legs are visible, lungs are formed, and the liver begins to produce blood cells.
- By 20 weeks the fingers and toes are separated, the nose and eyelids are formed, and the mother can feel fetal movement.
- By 28 weeks the eyes open and close, there is thick hair on the head, and also a thick coating of body hair that will later be lost (prior to birth).
- Week 40 signals the completion of fetal development. The fetus is now ready to survive outside the uterus. This is the optimal time for birth. The average weight is 6 to 8 pounds and the length 18 to 22 inches.

Infancy

During the first month of life the newborn is frequently referred to as a *neonate* (Figure 8–1). Then from 1 month to 1 year, the term *infant* is used. In this text, "infant" will be used to describe the time frame from birth to 1 year of age.

This is a period of tremendous physical growth. The birth weight triples or quadruples to 21 to 24 pounds by age one. Length will increase to between 29 to 30 inches. Teeth erupt between age 8 and 12 months.

The muscular and nervous systems develop rapidly. At first, movements are primarily reflexive rather than being purposefully made by the infant. Over time, infants develop the ability to raise their heads, then move on to turning and rolling over. They increase their ability to focus their eyes. By 1 year many infants crawl, stand alone, and walk with assistance.

Cognitively, vocalization progresses to several words. Infants learn by imitation. During the first few months of life, they learn to manipulate objects, recognize familiar objects and persons, and obey simple commands. It has been proven that infants must receive adequate tactile stimulation (e.g., touching, cuddling, and hugging) to have normal physical and mental development.

Erikson's psychosocial stage for the infant is *trust versus mistrust.* Infants are dependent on others

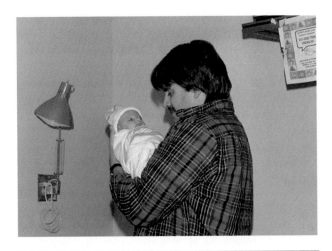

Figure 8–1 It is important that the parents bond with the newborn because this will initiate a loving and trusting relationship.

for their physical and emotional survival. Those who receive consistent loving care that satisfies the need for food, warmth, and other physical comforts will develop trust in their caregivers. Inconsistent and inadequate care leads to mistrust of others.

Toddler

The *toddler* stage is from 1 to 3 years of age (Figure 8–2). Physical changes occur as the body grows and proportions change. The characteristic protruding abdomen is still present, but the head no longer looks as oversized for the body as it does in the infant. By 3 years of age, approximately 20 teeth are present, and many toddlers, especially females, have achieved bowel and bladder control.

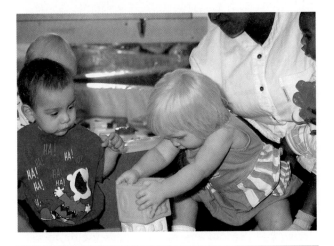

Figure 8–2 These toddlers develop motor sensory and cognitive skills as they manipulate and investigate items in their environment.

The motor sensory ability progresses from walking independently to running, jumping, and climbing. This is a very difficult time for the parents, because the activity of the toddler is directed towards continually investigating and searching out new experiences. Keeping the toddler safe and away from hazards requires "child-proofing" the environment and maintaining constant surveillance of the child, as in the following examples:

- Placing breakable items out of their reach
- Locking cabinets
- Using gates to prevent access to swimming pools and other hazards
- Locking away all poisonous substances
- Ensuring that they cannot leave the house by themselves
- Preventing access to any item that can be used for climbing

Cognitive skills develop rapidly as toddlers acquire language skills and begin to speak in sentences. They can understand simple instructions and requests, but their attention span is very short. Toddlers begin to learn ideas, attitudes, and values, but at the same time, they also believe that their point of view is the only one. This belief, combined with an emerging sense of independence, can lead to temper tantrums.

Erikson's psychosocial stage for the toddler is *autonomy versus shame and doubt.* Toddlers who receive encouragement to explore their environment and learn independent skills such as dressing, feeding, and toilet training will develop confidence in their ability to care for themselves (autonomy). If parents are overly protective or have unrealistic expectations, toddlers may develop doubt and shame. This can lead to a sense of general inadequacy.

Preschooler

The *preschooler* stage ranges from 3 to 6 years of age (Figure 8–3). Physically, preschoolers become taller and thinner than toddlers. Self-care skills increase, and they progress to being able to independently dress themselves.

Continuing motor sensory development leads to an improved sense of balance. This allows toddlers to skip and jump in a coordinated manner and enables them to learn skills such as jumping rope and skating.

Cognitively, they can now speak quite well in sentences. They have also developed an awareness of other people who are not in their immediate

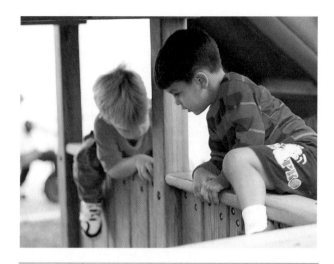

Figure 8–3 Preschoolers develop confidence as they succeed at new activities. Socialization skills are also practiced by interacting with their peers in group events.

environment. They still assume that everyone thinks as they do. They have short attention spans. They are able to count, recite the alphabet, and recall their address and phone number.

Erikson's psychosocial stage for the preschooler is *initiative versus guilt*. Preschoolers can build on the confidence developed as a toddler to initiate their own learning. They seek out new experiences and knowledge and strive to understand new activities. If their parents severely restrict this initiative, criticize, or scold them for their attempts, a sense of guilt will develop. This feeling of guilt will diminish the preschooler's natural enthusiasm for learning new motor and language skills. As a consequence, they can become hesitant to take on new challenges.

School-Age Child

The *school-age child* stages ranges from 6 to 12 years of age (Figure 8–4). The physical growth of the body continues with a more pronounced development between 10 and 12 years with the beginning of puberty (the period in life when boys and girls become functionally capable of reproduction). The permanent teeth also begin to erupt at this stage of growth.

The motor sensory skills become well coordinated, and the child develops grace and agility. School-age children can assist with household duties and show more responsibility in assigned tasks. They have a desire for both quiet time and intense physical activity.

Cognitive development has progressed to logical thinking and the ability to see things from different perspectives. The attention span has increased, and pride is taken in personal accomplishments. Children at this state reason, problem-solve, learn to follow rules, and develop a sense of morality (right and wrong) to guide their behavior.

Erikson's psychosocial stage for the school-age child is *industry versus inferiority*. They experience pleasure from the successful completion of projects and anticipate recognition for their accomplishments. They prefer friends to family and are influenced by the approval of their peers. If the child is not accepted by peers or cannot meet the expectations of family, a sense of inferiority and lack of self-worth may develop.

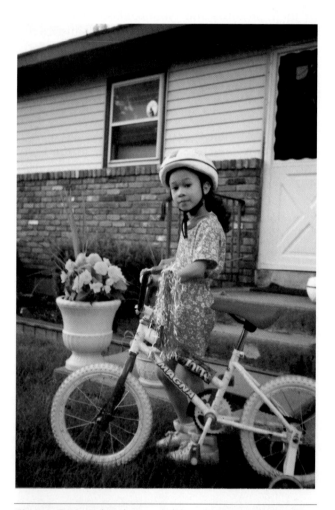

Figure 8–4 School-age children have the motor sensory skills to master activities that require coordination and agility. Protective equipment, such as a helmet, plays an important role in keeping them safe.

Adolescence

Adolescence is the stage ranging from 12 to 20 years of age (Figure 8–5). There are dramatic physical changes as the maturation of the reproductive systems occurs.

The fine motor skills improve, but awkwardness in the gross motor skills is evident. The adolescent may easily become fatigued with activity and requires adequate rest and sleep.

Cognitive abilities greatly increase. Adolescents are able to acquire large quantities of knowledge and are able to use reasoning skills. They have the capacity for introspection and start to develop their philosophy of life and create their future occupational identity. Adolescents are also more prone to stress than those at the other life stages.

Erikson's psychosocial stage for adolescence is *identity versus role confusion.* They are interested in the tremendous changes taking place in their bodies, but are also confused about identities as they move through the transition from child (dependent) to adult (independent). Mood swings are quite common as a result of the hormonal changes. Adolescents may try different roles, including rebellion, in the search for their identity as to who they are and who they will become. They may be critical of parents and resent the advice offered or criticism given. Peers continue to exert a significant influence on their behavior, because of strong concerns about how they are perceived. If adolescents are unable to determine their identity and direction, they will lack a sense of who they are. This is known as "role confusion."

Young Adulthood

Young adulthood includes the 20s and 30s (Figure 8–6). Physical functioning peaks at about 30 and then starts to slowly diminish as aging continues. For example, after 30 the skin begins to lose moisture, gastrointestinal secretions diminish, and problems with weight gain may begin.

Motor sensory skills also peak during this time and then begin to decline. Muscular strength peaks in the 20s and 30s and then begins to decline after the mid-30s. The visual and auditory senses also start to decline.

Young adults experience optimal cognitive functioning. Their problem-solving skills and creativity are excellent. This is a period of maximum potential.

Erikson's psychosocial stage for young adulthood is *intimacy versus isolation.* The task of young adults is to complete the transition from dependency to responsibility, to make commitments to others, and establish themselves in society. The responsibilities of this time are usually great: form an intimate relationship, have and raise children, obtain advanced education, and establish a career. A fear of making commitments to others may result in isolation and loneliness.

Middle Adulthood

Middle adulthood includes the 40s and 50s (Figure 8–7). The physical abilities continue to decline. For example, bone and muscle mass,

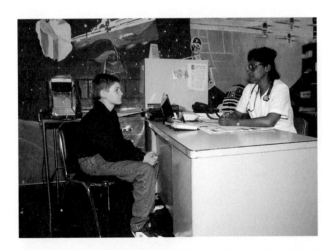

Figure 8–5 Adolescents need adults they can easily talk with to share their concerns and to help them understand how their mental and physical health is affected by the decisions they make.

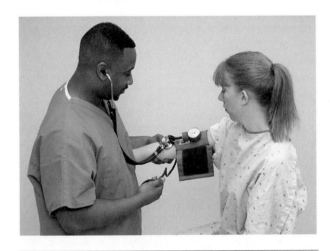

Figure 8–6 Young adults can feel a great deal of stress as they attempt to succeed at the many roles they have at this stage. When caring for young adults, it is important to maintain open communication that allows them to discuss and problem-solve these concerns.

physical strength, and endurance decrease. At the same time, the skin loses some of its elasticity, wrinkles begin to develop, and major body systems begin to decline. Middle adults may begin to have concerns about their physical health. While a **chronic illness** (health problem of long duration in which the disease or condition shows little change or slowly gets progressively worse) may begin at any time, it is during this stage that they are more likely to begin to appear.

The motor sensory skills diminish. The reflexes, muscles, and joints respond more slowly. There is decreased balance and coordination and a more prolonged response to stress. The visual, auditory, and gustatory senses diminish.

The cognitive abilities are still quite strong, although learning may take longer. Problem-solving and memory remain consistent until the late middle years. Creativity may increase during this stage.

Erikson's psychosocial stage for middle adulthood is *generativity versus stagnation.* This is a time of shifting concerns from the self to the next generation as well as towards an increased involvement with friends and community. There is a desire to make a contribution of value. It is a time of self-assessment and evaluation of the accomplishment of goals. There may be many adjustments if children leave home, health issues develop, and concerns arise about retirement. This is the time period when many individuals face what is referred to as a "mid-life crisis." This may be brought on by the recognition of limitations and unmet goals. If individuals are unable to establish their worth or recognize their contribution to the world, stagnation

may occur. This can result in self-absorption and becoming obsessed with health concerns.

Later Adulthood

Later adulthood encompasses the 60s through death (Figure 8–8). Physical decline continues to occur, with loss of muscle and bone and atrophy of the reproductive organs. The cardiac, renal, and immune systems decline. Decreased peripheral (arms and legs) circulation leads to less tolerance for heat and cold.

The motor sensory abilities also continue their decline. The visual, auditory, gustatory, and olfactory senses diminish. The ability to tolerate pain will decrease, physical responses will be slower, and some motor skills will decline.

Erikson's psychosocial stage for later adulthood is *ego integrity versus despair.* The many challenges are a continuation of changes that began in middle adulthood: retirement, loss of spouse and friends, new family roles (children marrying, becoming in-laws and grandparents), and increasing concerns about health. As individuals face their mortality, they review the events of their life and the related successes and failures. If they experience a sense of satisfaction and pleasure from the events of their lives, a sense of ego integrity will be experienced. In contrast, if the review is interpreted as a series of failures and disappointments, there is a sense of sadness and despair.

The life span has increased in the last several decades, and people are living longer than ever before in history. Many older adults maintain active, productive lives. It is no longer uncommon to see adults working into their nineties. Elderly

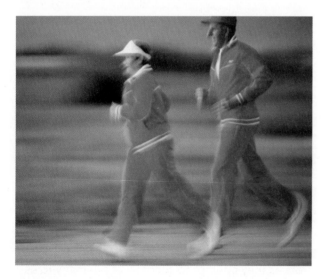

Figure 8–7 Middle adulthood leads to more physical challenges. Keeping active adds to health, vitality, and longevity.

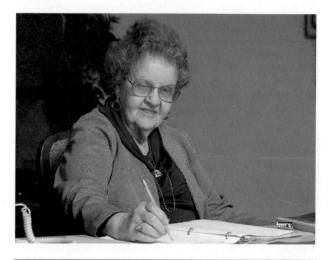

Figure 8–8 Keeping involved and active during later adulthood adds greatly to the enjoyment of life.

Many young people think that creativity and contributions diminish as one ages. Read the following examples, and evaluate this assumption.

- Sarah Bernhardt (1844–1923) was a famous American actress. She lost a leg in her early 70s but continued acting until her death at age 78.

- Mahatma Gandhi (1869–1948) successfully completed negotiations with Britain to grant India's independence at the age of 77.

- Frank Lloyd Wright (1867–1959), America's most famous architect, designed the Guggenheim Museum in New York City at 91.

- Eleanor Roosevelt (1884–1962), the wife of President Franklin D. Roosevelt, and herself very active in social causes, chaired the United Nations Commission on Human Rights from age 62–67. She wrote her autobiography, titled *On My Own* at 74.

- Alfred Hitchcock (1899–1980) directed the movies *Psycho* and *The Birds* in his 60s and *Frenzy* at 73 years of age.

- Nelson Mandela (1918–) was inaugurated as president after South Africa's first free election at the age of 75. This was after he had spent 27 years of his life in prison for his political beliefs.

- George Burns (1896–1996), comic and actor, was still appearing in public and telling jokes with perfect timing when he was 100.

- Grandma Moses (1860–1961), the famous American painter by the name of Anna Mary Robertson, started her career in art when she was in her 70s.

citizens are able to make various kinds of valuable contributions to society. Americans' views of what it means to be "old" will continually adjust as this segment of the population increases.

CARE CONSIDERATIONS

Each life stage is characterized by its own physical, cognitive, and psychosocial challenges. The advantage of studying general categories is that it assists health care workers in their understanding of areas to focus on during patient assessment and for determining age-appropriate approaches to care. The danger of using generalizations is that it is possible to make false assumptions about people and lose sight of the unique individual needs of each patient.

All patients at all times need respectful, compassionate, and empathetic care. Families and friends are also involved in and affected by the health of the patient, so the same consideration must be extended to them. A routine question to always ask is if the family members have any concerns, problems, or questions they would like to discuss. Examples of specific care considerations as they relate to each life stage are presented in Table 8–2. Some considerations apply to most stages such as involving the patient in decisions regarding their care and adapting education and instructions to the learning style of the patient. They are included in the chart when they are considered to be primary considerations for that stage.

DEATH AND DYING

Death is the natural end to life. It is, in a sense, the last stage of human development. Health care workers may work with patients and their families during this last phase of the life process. To help understand dying, many turn to the classic work of Swiss physician, Elisabeth Kübler-Ross. She earned her medical degree at the University of Switzerland in 1957 and her degree in psychiatry from the University of Colorado in 1963. After years of study and research, she published her first book *On Death and Dying* in 1969. She was the

Calvin Bell is a dental hygienist in an urban dental clinic. His patients range in age from toddlers to the very elderly. On one busy day, he saw patients in the following stages: preschooler (3), school-age (9), adolescent (15), young adult (26), and later adulthood (83).

1. Explain how his behavior might change to be most appropriate with each patient.

2. What would be the most likely dental health care concerns for each patient?

3. What might be the most effective patient education techniques to use with each?

Table 8–2 Care Considerations for the Health Care Worker

Life Stages	Care Considerations
Prenatal	• Emphasize care of mother to ensure a normal pregnancy. • Address unhealthy habits. • Assist mother in developing strategies to make healthy changes. • Always ask if any over-the-counter medications or products from health food stores are being used. Commonly used medications and products can have harmful effects on unborn babies. • Inquire about mother's nutrition. • Educate the mother about the need for adequate nutrition and fluids.
Infancy	• Involve parents in care. • Provide for safety. • Do not allow the infant to play with objects that have moving or removable parts. • Cuddle and hug infants. • Obtain height, weight, and head circumference measurements to track growth patterns.
Toddler	• Use a firm, direct approach. • Distract and use a game approach to improve cooperation. • Give only one direction at a time and state it simply. • Involve toddlers in their care by allowing them to make choices when possible. • Prepare them for procedures with simple explanations. • Set limits and maintain safety.
Preschooler	• Explain procedures and unfamiliar objects prior to performing or using them. • Encourage verbalization of skills. • Praise good behavior. • To improve acceptance of painful procedures, allow them to make choices when possible (injection site); give a token of bravery, such as a colored Band-Aid; and use distraction (have them recite alphabet or sing their favorite song).
School-Age Child	• Explain procedures and equipment using correct terminology, but in words they understand. • Provide for privacy and some personal control. • Define and enforce behavior limits. • Encourage independence. • Educate with clear, simple visual aids.
Adolescence	• Give explanations along with the rationale. • Encourage questions. • Involve them in the decision-making process. • Determine how they learn best and adapt an approach for their needs, including visual aids and written materials. • Provide privacy. • Don't talk about them where they can overhear the conversation.

(continues)

Table 8–2 (continued)

Life Stages	Care Considerations
Young Adulthood	• Involve significant other as appropriate. • Watch body language for clues regarding feelings. • Assess the person for stress resulting from the multiple roles and responsibilities of this stage. • Involve the person in the decision-making process. • Provide teaching according to their learning style.
Middle Adulthood	• Involve them in the decision-making process. • Encourage self-care. • Explore their concept of illness as it relates to body image and career. • Provide teaching according to their learning style. • Encourage lifestyle changes such as quitting smoking, improving nutrition, and increasing exercise to help lessen the effects of natural age-related decline.
Later Adulthood	• Explore support systems. • Involve family members in care giving. • Provide a safe, comfortable environment. • Be sensitive to sensory impairments. • Provide care to maintain skin integrity and regular bowel habits. • Be alert to overmedication and sensitivity to medications.

first person to study and write about death in a way that brought it to public attention. Kubler-Ross conducted extensive interviews with people who knew they were going to die and made notes about the process they followed as they struggled to put their lives in perspective. These studies encouraged general discussion of what had previously been a taboo topic. Her research findings and subsequent books have provided the information that health care workers and the general public need to become more informed about this area.

Based on her research, Kubler-Ross developed a model called the "stages of dying" or "stages of grief." According to the model, there are five stages that a dying person goes through when they learn that they have a **terminal illness** (a condition or disease that because of its nature can be expected to cause the patient to die). The five **stages of dying** are summarized below:

■ Denial: When first learning about a terminal illness, the individual may feel numb and in a state of disbelief. The belief is that this cannot be happening or that a mistake has been made. Common reactions are an inability to focus, feeling a sense of it as unreal, hysteria or passivity, or the contemplation of suicide.

■ Anger: Once the reality of death hits, intense anger may be experienced. It is common for the individual to ask, "Why me?" It seems unfair, and there is envy of those with good health. Acute rage is experienced at the prospect of the upcoming loss. This rage may be directed only toward the illness, but it is also frequently directed toward everyone and everything.

■ Bargaining: In this stage the person bargains for the one thing not possible–more time. Dying individuals want time to complete unachieved goals, to see their children reach a certain level of maturity, have grandchildren, or travel to unseen parts of the world. The bargaining is often done with whoever they consider to be the higher being who has authority over life and death. They make promises to be better people, to change bad habits, and to live an exemplary life if only given more time.

■ Depression: This is a profound sadness felt over the prospect of no longer being alive and not being able to change the course of events. There is a turning inward as they consider all the time that was wasted, the things left undone, and the joys that will not be experienced. Younger individuals feel particularly deprived of a long healthy life and feel they should have had the opportunity to live up to their potential.

■ Acceptance: When this stage is reached, there is a dramatic change. Individuals experience a sense of peace with themselves, family, friends, and community. They now accept that they are dying and can now focus on tying up any loose ends they perceive need to be resolved in preparation for death. This is referred to as "completing any unfinished business." For example, they may want to talk to certain friends or family to express their feelings or resolve issues or complete any necessary financial arrangements. Another important component of this stage is the need to do a life review. The **life review** involves telling the events of their lives to those close to them (including health care workers). Part of the process is the desire to put one's life in perspective by performing a self-evaluation. This leads to a sense of closure. During this stage, dying individuals may be very open to talking about their feelings about death. As the time of death approaches, however, withdrawal frequently occurs. It is as if the external world is no longer important. It is also possible that they do not have the energy to try to communicate with others who do not have the same understanding of life as the dying have now achieved.

During the acceptance stage of dying, it was stated that patients often feel the need to do a life review. This same behavior is also frequently noted in the elderly even though no specific terminal illness has been diagnosed. As a health care worker, it is important to take the time to hear (or hear again) these stories because it is a significant step in the patient's developmental process. You may note that some patients will tell their life story with acceptance of past events, others with bitterness, guilt, or anger. Sometimes the events will be told in a glorified manner or it may be merely a dispassionate telling of stories. Another approach is for them to phrase past events in such a way as to pass on their wisdom or cultural heritage. There is no one right way, and the health care worker can be of most help by showing interest and allowing patients to express themselves in the manner most comfortable to them.

Dying patients do not always go through all of these stages, nor do they go through them in an orderly and sequential manner. One of the criticisms

Thinking it Through

Veronica Johnson, age 77, is a home health patient. She lives in her home and is cared for by her husband. Josephine Mitchell, a hospice nurse, visits Mrs. Johnson on a regular basis to determine if the patient's needs are being met, to educate her husband on how to care for his wife, to offer emotional support, and to help resolve any difficulties that may arise. Mrs. Johnson states, "I am dying. I have known this for some time. I know it will not be much longer now, but I have had a full life and I am not afraid." But she also states, "I want to tell my daughter how much I love her, but I don't know how to do this as there seems to be a distance between us. I am also afraid I will begin to cry and not be able to stop." Ms. Mitchell speaks with the daughter and determines that the daughter also wishes to talk with her mother to say goodbye, but is reluctant to because she is also afraid of starting to cry and not being able to stop.

Mrs. Johnson asks Ms. Mitchell to be present when her daughter arrives to visit her. When the daughter arrives, both mother and daughter repeat their concerns about starting to cry and not being able to stop. Ms. Mitchell then says with humor, "Don't worry about it, I will start mopping up if it gets too deep." At that point, the daughter rushes to her mother's bedside, and a very loving conversation takes place.

1. What stage of the dying process is Mrs. Johnson in?
2. Mrs. Johnson is in which life stage? According to Erik Erikson's Stages of Psychosocial Development, what is the conflict to be met at this life stage? Does it sound like she has successfully met this challenge or not, and why?
3. Should the hospice nurse have been present during the meeting between the mother and daughter?
4. Was the humor used by the hospice nurse appropriate?
5. What outcome would you anticipate to occur as a result of the daughter and mother openly sharing their feelings?

of Elisabeth Kübler-Ross's theory is that the stages are too rigid. Theorists who followed her have confirmed these stages, but note that not all people experience all of them, or go through the same sequence, or complete the stages. In addition, tremendous differences are caused by gender, class, and culture.

This model has been presented as it applies to the dying patient, but there is a wider application that will also assist the health care worker. It can be applied to any form of loss. When any loss is perceived, there is suffering and a grieving process is initiated. There are many types of loss:

- Failure to achieve an important goal
- Loss of a job, resulting in a change of social identity
- Divorce
- Death of a pet
- Accident
- Injury
- Upcoming surgery
- Moving away from friends and family
- Grieving about the impending or recent death of a loved one

Helping patients—and others with whom they have contact—handle loss is a valuable skill for health care workers. Providing caring concern in times of need promotes patient welfare, eases the dying process, and helps others come to terms with their losses.

SUGGESTED LEARNING ACTIVITIES

1. Go to the Web site www.cdc.gov/growthcharts/ to find the growth charts published by the government for the purpose of monitoring normal physical growth. Then answer these questions: What is the normal range in inches and centimeters for the head circumference of a 12-month-old girl? What is the normal weight range in pounds and kilograms for a 15-year-old boy?

2. Observe family members and friends who fit into each of the life stages from infancy to later adulthood and relate the information given for each stage. How does it compare? What can you identify in terms of physical, cognitive, or psychosocial behaviors?

3. What life stage are you currently in? Can you relate your current activities and focus to the life stage?

REVIEW QUESTIONS

1. What do the terms "physical," "cognitive," and "psychosocial" mean, as they relate to growth and development?

2. What are the nine life stages? What age group does each stage represent?

3. What are the primary physical changes that occur at each of the life stages?

4. What are the challenges of each stage according to Erik Erikson's Psychosocial Development theory?

5. What specific care considerations would relate to each of the life stages that would address age-appropriate communications and care?

6. List the five stages of grief and give an example of behaviors that may be observed during each stage.

APPLICATION EXERCISES

1. Refer to The Case of the Curious Four-Year-Old. What life stage is Paul in, and what are the unique challenges of this stage? What are the possible psychosocial ramifications if his initiative is restricted, and he is severely criticized and scolded for his attempts to explore and question his environment? What are the potential positive outcomes if the time is taken to answer his questions and engage him in his care?

2. Ed Klein has been diagnosed with terminal cancer. He has elected to stay at home with his wife who is his principal caregiver. They also have regular visits from various hospice health care workers who assist with pain management, bathing, and any problems that arise. The hospice nurse, Sandy Johnson, visits three times a week. She notes that Mr. Klein frequently mentions what he will do as soon as he gets better. Sandy also notices that

Mrs. Klein is reluctant to enter the room when she is working with Mr. Klein. On her third visit, Sandy decides to ask Mrs. Klein to come in and assist her with Mr. Klein's care. During the procedure, he acts very angry with his wife and criticizes everything she does to help.

a. What stage(s) of dying does Mr. Klein demonstrate?

b. Why do you think the wife was reluctant to enter the room?

c. Do you think Mr. Klein truly does not know he has a terminal illness?

d. What type of care assistance do you think this couple needs?

SUGGESTED READINGS AND RESOURCES

DeLaune, S. C. and Ladner, P. K. (1998). *Fundamentals of nursing: Standards and practice.* Albany, NY: Delmar.

Interview with Elisabeth Kübler-Ross "On Death and Dying." Available: http://www.doubleclickd.com/kubler.html

National Council on the Aging: http://www.ncoa.org

National Network for Child Care: http://nncc.org/Child.Dev

Personality Theories–Erik Erikson (1902–1994). Available: http://www.ship.edu/~cgboeree/erikson.html

UNIT

PERSONAL AND WORKPLACE SAFETY

4

CHAPTER

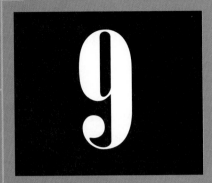

BODY MECHANICS

OBJECTIVES

Studying and applying the material in this chapter will help you to:

- Understand and explain the importance of practicing good body mechanics and ergonomics at all times to prevent injury.

- Explain how repetitive injuries occur and how to prevent them.

- Demonstrate proper methods of sitting when working, to prevent injury.

- Demonstrate proper methods of walking and standing at work, to prevent injury.

- Demonstrate proper methods of lifting, to prevent injury.

- Demonstrate proper methods of working at the computer, to prevent injury.

- Properly use special adaptive devices to reduce the risk of workplace injuries.

KEY TERMS

body mechanics
ergonomics
repetitive motion injury
    (RMI)

195

The Case of

Broken Dreams

Rene Alvarez has dreamed of a career in health care for many years. She is thrilled about graduating next month and anticipates that the large medical center where she has been hired will be the fulfillment of her dreams. She has decided to move into a new apartment that is closer to her new employer and only has the weekend to get everything moved, in addition to studying for an important exam. Rene packs quickly and with the help of family and friends starts to load the truck rented for the move. In her haste, Rene forgets to follow proper body mechanics and lifts a box that is very heavy. She feels a tearing sensation in her back, followed by severe pain. She is rushed to the emergency room and is told that she will need to stay in bed for several weeks and surgery may be required if the bed rest provides her no relief.

This chapter will cover the basic principles of good body mechanics and ergonomics that should be followed at all times to prevent personal injury. Health care workers are particularly at risk for injury because their daily job duties frequently include lifting equipment, supplies, and patients. Other health care workers may not lift as much in their jobs, but may have long periods of sitting, standing, or working with computers and other table-top equipment.

THE IMPORTANCE OF PREVENTION

Health care workers perform a number of mechanical movements with their bodies that can lead to injury. Following safety guidelines reduces the chance of injury and prevents unnecessary pain and suffering. Injuries are usually the result of poor practices over time that involve the repetition of improper movements. In other words, it is not the one-time incident that leads to the greatest number of injuries, but rather the same mistakes repeated over time. As one ages, it is especially important to follow sound practices. As flexibility decreases and recovery time increases, the chance of sustaining injuries is greater.

Certain risk factors increase the likelihood of injury. These include:

- Poor posture
- Poor body mechanics
- Low level of fitness
- Obesity
- Stress, both mechanical and psychological

The best preventive practices are simple and common sense:

- Use good posture during all activities
- Stay fit by exercising regularly
- Maintain flexibility with stretching exercises
- Stay trim by eating correctly
- Reduce mental stress through good lifestyle habits (see Chapter 12)

Most injuries are cumulative and so it is habitual activity repeated over years that determines the future risk of injury. Health care workers should build good habits and safe practices into everyday life. While the focus of this chapter is on workplace injuries and their prevention, the same principles apply to activities at home, at play, and even at rest.

Body mechanics and ergonomics are two terms used when discussing the prevention of injury. **Body mechanics** are the correct positioning of the body for a given task, such as lifting a heavy object or typing. **Ergonomics** is the science of designing and arranging things in the working and living environments for maximum efficiency and maximum health and safety. A good ergonomic environment provides the highest possible comfort level and efficiency while limiting possible exposure to discomfort or potential injury. Developing the habit of following proper body mechanics and working in an ergonomically correct workplace is vital to decreasing the chance of injury to the worker.

GENERAL GUIDELINES

There are numerous activities done every day at work and play that can cause injuries. Workplace examples include:

- Nurses lifting patients
- Insurance coders sitting and working at the computer for long periods of time
- Surgical technicians standing during long operations
- Medical transcriptionists keyboarding for many hours each day
- Laboratory technicians bending over microscopes for prolonged periods

Injuries commonly suffered by health care workers involve the musculoskeletal or nervous systems. Strained back muscles and inflamed tendons are common examples.

Repetitive motion injuries (RMI) encompass many different injuries, but they are all based on the overuse of one part of the body. Motions that are repeated over time eventually put undue stress on tendons, nerves, or joints and cause inflammation, swelling, and pain. Common RMIs suffered

today include carpal tunnel syndrome and tendonitis. See Table 9–1.

The following general principles help prevent injury to the musculoskeletal and nervous systems:

- Practice proper posture by maintaining the three normal curves of the back. See Figure 9–1. (e.g., avoid hunching over the desk or computer).
- Warm up and stretch before and after activities that are repetitive, static (lacking movement), or prolonged.
- Use the largest joints and muscles to do the work (e.g., squat down to lift a box because this uses your legs and not your back).
- Avoid static positions for prolonged periods. Muscles fatigue faster when they are held in one position. Take a break and move around every 20 to 30 minutes when it is necessary to maintain a sustained position. This is also a good time to stretch stiff muscles. Alternately contract and relax muscles to increase blood circulation. See Chapter 12 for muscle relaxation exercises.
- Change positions or stop whenever activities cause pain.
- Use splints and wrist supports only upon recommendation of a physician or therapist. Be sure to follow instructions on the proper use of equipment.
- Seek treatment early if problems arise. Do not delay and simply hope the problem will go away.

Table 9–1 Most Common RMIs

Condition	Etiology (Cause)	Signs and Symptoms
Carpal tunnel syndrome	Repeated hand motions cause inflammation and swelling, which pinches nerves that pass through a tunnel of bones and ligaments in the wrist.	• tingling, numbness, and pain in the hand • inability to make a fist • loss of strength in hand
Thoracic outlet syndrome	Repeated motion causes bones or disks to compress nerves in the neck	• tingling, numbness, and pain in the neck, shoulder, arms or hands • poor blood circulation in the hands and fingers • weakness in arms and hands
Tendonitis	Repeated motion in a joint inflames tendons	• swelling, tenderness, or weakness in the tendons of the shoulders, elbows, or hands

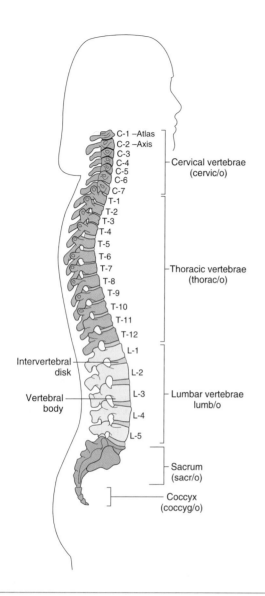

C-1 –Atlas
C-2 –Axis
C-3
C-4
C-5
C-6
C-7

Cervical vertebrae (cervic/o)

T-1
T-2
T-3
T-4
T-5
T-6
T-7
T-8
T-9
T-10
T-11
T-12

Thoracic vertebrae (thorac/o)

Intervertebral disk

Vertebral body

L-1
L-2
L-3
L-4
L-5

Lumbar vertebrae lumb/o

Sacrum (sacr/o)

Coccyx (coccyg/o)

Figure 9–1 Normal curves of the spinal column.

Study Boxes 9–1, 9–2, and 9–3. They include specific information about proper sitting, standing, walking, and lifting.

[**Fascinating Facts**]

In 1997, the Bureau of Labor Statistics reported there were 1,833,380 injuries and illnesses serious enough to require days away from work.

Box 9–1   While sitting:

1. Use a chair that supports the normal curves of the back (use a lumbar support if needed). Avoid sitting on stools. Don't slouch in chairs or on couch.

2. Keep head and shoulders aligned over hips. Avoid bending neck forward for long periods of time.

3. Avoid pressing the back of the knees against the edge of the chair seat.

4. Minimize twisting and bending motions. Position equipment and work so that the body is directly in front of and close to them.

5. When turning is necessary, pivot entire body in unison or use a swivel chair.

6. Change positions frequently. Get up and move around and stretch at regular intervals.

7. Position your chair so work is at eye level and feet are flat on floor or on a footrest.

8. When using the telephone frequently or for extended periods, use a speakerphone or headset.

9. When not using your hands, keep your upper arms close to your body, elbows at a 90–100° angle, forearms neutral (thumbs toward ceiling), and wrists straight.

Box 9–2   While standing and walking:

1. Be aware of your posture. Maintain the three normal curves of the back.

2. Keep your neck in a neutral position (avoid jutting the chin forward or slouching).

3. Wear cushioned shoes with good support if work requires standing or walking a lot.

4. When standing, shift your weight often.

5. If standing in one place for long periods, use a footstool. Alternate placing one foot up on the stool to take the strain off the back.

Box 9–3 While lifting:

1. Move in close to the object to be lifted.

2. Be aware of your posture. Maintain the three normal curves of the back. See Figure 9–2.

3. Increase the base of support by positioning your feet 6 to 8 inches apart. See Figure 9–2 & 9–3.

4. Squat down (bending hips and knees), maintaining normal curves of the back (Figure 9–4). When picking up objects, bend at the knees rather than at the waist.

5. Position your hands underneath the object to be lifted.

6. Take a deep breath and tighten your abdominal muscles prior to lifting. This increases intraabdominal pressure to increase the support for the spine and back muscles.

7. Lift the load with the legs (NOT with the back). Use the large muscles of the legs to lift load (Figure 9–2).

8. Use two hands to lift rather than one, even with light objects (Figure 9–3).

9. Carry objects close to body at waist level (Figure 9–3).

10. When turning, move your entire body in unison (avoid twisting). To change directions, use the feet rather than the back: move and turn the feet instead of twisting the spine while the feet are planted in one position (Figure 9–3).

11. Avoid reaching overhead with heavy loads (use step stools, ladders, etc.)

12. Push rather than pull heavy objects. The exception to this rule is when on ramps, where you would pull from the higher level.

13. Slide or push objects, when possible, instead of lifting them.

14. Use carts and dollies to carry heavy loads. If possible, break up the load into several trips to avoid lifting heavy loads. Or have someone assist with the lifting of heavy objects.

15. Tilt containers or objects to avoid bending the wrist to pick up objects.

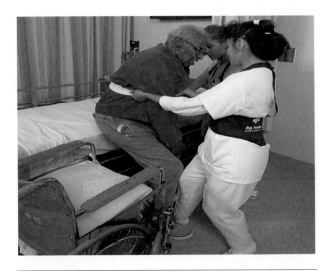

Figure 9–2 When lifting maintain proper posture, position feet for wide base of support, and lift with the leg muscles.

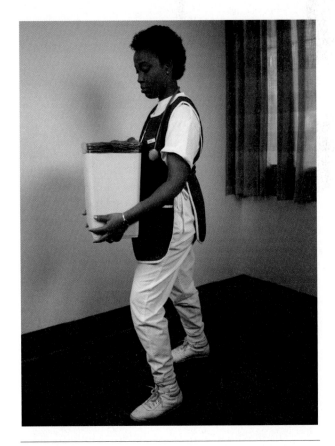

Figure 9–3 When lifting maintain proper posture, position feet for wide base of support, and hold the object close to the body at waist level using both hands.

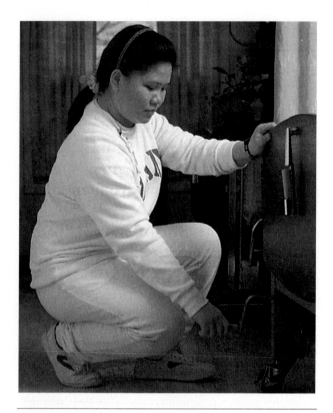

Figure 9–4 Maintain proper posture when bending from the hips and knees.

Back Belts

In addition to applying body mechanics and learning how to lift properly, some facilities and health care workers believe that back belts decrease lower back injuries (Figure 9–5). This is controversial, as demonstrated by the excerpt from an Occupational Safety and Health Administration (OSHA) Standards Interpretation and Compliance Letter. (The purpose and role of OSHA will be discussed in the next chapter.)

> Back belts are not recognized by OSHA as effective engineering controls to prevent back injury. While they may be accepted by individual workers because they feel as if they provide additional support, the effectiveness of back belts in the prevention of low back injuries has not been proven in the work environment.

Those who feel that back belts are helpful, state they increase the intra-abdominal pressure, which creates support for the spine and back muscles when lifting. They also feel that the belts increase the flexibility of the stomach and back muscles by keeping them warm. Finally, it is argued that their presence serves as a reminder to workers to follow proper body mechanics.

Opponents to using back belts state that the belts increase the worker's blood and pelvic pressures, which can lead to cardiac problems. They also believe that the warmth and sweating created by wearing back belts can cause heat rashes, that improper fitting of belts can cause abdominal pain and injuries, and that they can give a false sense of security so that workers may attempt to lift heavier loads than their strength can safely handle. Finally, they suggest that if used, back belts should be tightened only when lifting and left loose the rest of the time.

COMPUTERS AND ERGONOMICS

Although ergonomics is not a new field, the advent of computers has created an increased awareness of the field because of the number of injuries being reported. In the past, keyboarding was done by a small number of employees and the resulting RMIs were limited to a relatively few workers.

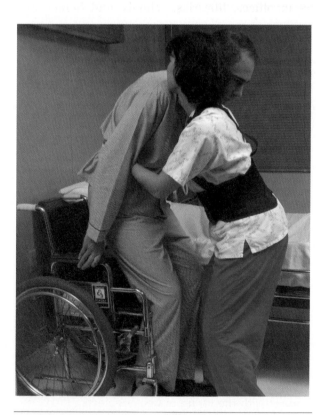

Figure 9–5 This health care worker is wearing a back belt as she helps a patient transfer from the bed to the wheelchair.

Box 9–4   While using the computer:

1. Position the screen at arm's length to reduce eyestrain and head-forward posture.

2. Position the top of the monitor just below eye level directly in front of the body.

3. Place a document holder next to screen rather than working from a document placed flat on desk.

4. Place both feet flat on the floor or footrest to reduce back strain.

5. Keep your back in total contact with back of chair.

6. Position your abdomen close to edge of desk to prevent a forward-leaning posture.

7. Maintain your wrists in a neutral (straight) position when keying or using a pointing device.

8. Position the keyboard so your elbow is at the same height as the keyboard. Slant the keyboard as necessary to maintain your elbows at an angle of 90–100 degrees and a neutral wrist position.

9. Rest your eyes and reduce eyestrain by blinking your eyes rapidly, closing them, or focusing on another object away from the computer screen for 10 seconds every 15 minutes.

10. Stretch frequently (shrug shoulders, arch back, nod head, roll feet in circular motion). See Table 9–2 for computer exercises.

11. Use wrist rests during pauses to help maintain neutral position. They are not meant to be used during active keying.

12. Avoid resting wrists against hard surfaces and sharp edges.

13. Try using an ergonomically-designed keyboard.

The enormous increase in the number of computers in offices, libraries, schools, and homes has resulted in a corresponding increase in injuries. Computers are used not only at the workplace, but also to play games, communicate with others, purchase items, and conduct research. The popularity of computers has grown to the point where many people are now suffering from ailments that are the direct result of the repetitive motion of typing or using a mouse as a pointing device.

All computer users should take steps to protect themselves from potential RMIs. Health care workers such as transcriptionists, insurance coders, information management technicians, admitting clerks, and others who work at computers for several hours each day should be especially careful about setting up work stations that fit their physical needs. Figure 9–6 illustrates proper positioning, and Box 9–4 includes tips for the safe use of the computer.

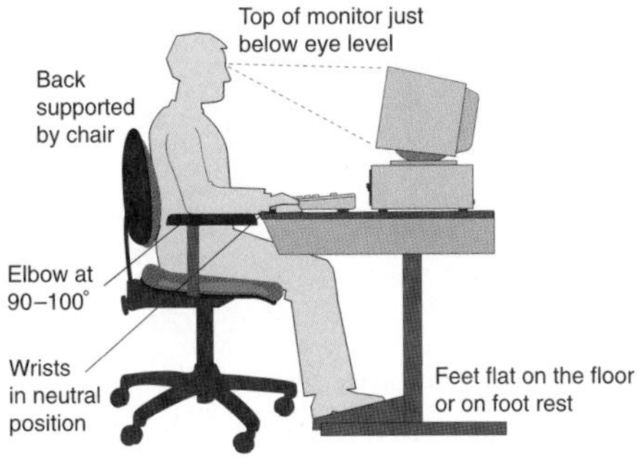

Use of a Mouse as Pointing Device

The extensive use of the mouse as a pointing device when working with a computer has been shown to be a major contributor to RMIs. It is important that the mouse be within easy reach and that the user not stretch to use it. If a mouse is used on a keyboard tray, there needs to be enough room for the mouse so that it is positioned at the same level as the keyboard.

The chance of injury can be lowered by developing the ability to use the mouse with either hand and alternating hands throughout the day. Another preventive measure is to use the keyboard to give common commands. This involves simultaneously pressing the special function keys, such as "ctrl" and "F1" and the lettered keys, or pressing the function keys alone. Examples include the following:

- Crtl + s   saves a document
- Ctrl + p   prints a document
- Alt + F4   closes a program

Some keyboard commands are universal and apply to many software programs. Others are specific to programs such as WordPerfect. Learning the commands for the programs used most often can speed input and help avoid computer injuries.

Top of monitor just below eye level

Back supported by chair

Elbow at 90–100°

Wrists in neutral position

Feet flat on the floor or on foot rest

Figure 9–6 Proper positioning for working at the computer.

Table 9–2 Computer Exercises

Exercise	Description	Benefit
	Make a fist, then open your hands while spreading fingers apart.	relaxes muscles of hands, wrists, and forearms
	Interlace the fingers of both hands, then extend your arms at shoulder level, palms facing away from you.	stretches the muscles of the arms, shoulders, and upper back
	Slowly rotate your head by tilting it to one side, then roll it to a forward position, to other side, and then to the back. Repeat.	stretches the neck muscles and helps relieve tension
	Shrug shoulders up towards the ears, then relax and let them return to their normal position.	decreases tension in neck and shoulder muscles
	Place your left arm on your right shoulder and turn your head to the left. With your right arm, gently push your left arm for increased stretch.	stretches muscles of upper arm and upper back

Visual Problems

Visual discomfort is frequently reported as a result of computer work. Eyestrain and headaches are the most common problems. The eyes tire more quickly when looking at a computer screen than when reading printed materials. This is because of the different characteristics of the type. Printed material has dark, dense, consistent lines that are easy to focus on. Computer screens display

Thinking it Through

Gary Carlson is a nurse who works at an intermediate care facility. During the shift, he frequently needs to lift patients as he cares for or assists them during their activities of daily living. The facility has just implemented a new policy that all health care workers must wear a back belt while lifting or moving patients. Gary attended the inservice on how to properly wear and use the back belt, but has several concerns. He has hypertension (high blood pressure) and fears that the back belt may elevate it further. He has also noticed that the increased perspiration from wearing the belt has caused an uncomfortable rash. He has decided to stop wearing the belt and hopes that his supervisor will not notice.

1. Are Gary's concerns valid?
2. Is Gary's solution to the problem appropriate?
3. Are there other solutions Gary could consider to resolve the problem?

images with a less consistent density, and this results in the eyes having to work much harder to focus. This extra effort can result in eyestrain. See Box 9–5 for guidelines to prevent eyestrain.

People who wear bifocals have an additional challenge to overcome when working on the computer. The lower section of bifocals is used for reading and is adjusted to focus at a closer distance than the typical distance one sits from the computer. Bifocals are also angled downward for reading, so bifocal wearers will typically tilt their heads upward so they can view the screen at this angle. This moves the neck out of the neutral position and can lead to neck problems. One solution is to position the monitor lower than eye level. For the person who does a great deal of computer work, it is preferable to have the ophthalmologist prepare a set of bifocal lenses specifically designed for use at the computer.

Box 9–5 To prevent eyestrain:

- Look away from the computer screen and focus on other objects in the environment at frequent intervals.
- Rest the eyes every 20–30 minutes.
- Adjust the contrast on the computer screen to a comfortable level.
- Keep the computer screen clean.
- Position the screen to avoid glare from surrounding lights and windows.
- Use a paper holder to prevent having to look down to see text.
- Use glare screen on monitor.

SUGGESTED LEARNING ACTIVITIES

1. If you have a computer area or office at your home, evaluate whether any changes to the workstation would improve the ergonomics.
2. Observe health care professionals at work. What measures do they take to avoid workplace injuries?
3. Evaluate your compliance with the guidelines in this chapter. Do you have any "at risk" behaviors? What modifications can you make to decrease the risk of injury?

REVIEW QUESTIONS

1. What do the following terms mean?
   a. Body mechanics
   b. Ergonomics
   c. Repetitive motion injuries
2. What are the three most common RMIs, and why do they occur?
3. How can health care workers protect themselves from injury when sitting, walking, standing, and lifting?
4. What are the characteristics of correct posture?
5. What guidelines should be followed to prevent injury when working at a computer?

6. Why is it important to do stretching exercises when spending extended time working at the computer? Describe exercises that stretch the neck, hands, arms, and upper back.

7. How can you decrease the risk of RMIs when using a mouse as a pointing device?

8. What is the cause of eyestrain when reading from a computer screen? What can you do to prevent this from occurring?

APPLICATION EXERCISES

1. What could Rene, in The Case of Broken Dreams at the beginning of this chapter, have done to help prevent sustaining her injuries?

2. John Jones, a health care student, has been saving for months to purchase a laptop computer to assist him with his classes. He plans to purchase a computer table and chair as soon as he saves the additional money. In the meantime, he will be using the computer on his lap or at the kitchen table.

   a. What possible injuries is John risking by not having an ergonomically sound setup?

   b. What criteria should he consider when purchasing a computer table and chair?

   c. What can he do in the meantime to adapt the kitchen to a safe working environment? Include RMI and eye strain prevention. Describe in detail or prepare a sketch of your suggestions.

SUGGESTED READINGS AND RESOURCES

Information about ergonomics:
   www.ergoweb.com

CHAPTER

INFECTION CONTROL

OBJECTIVES

Studying and applying the material in this chapter will help you to:

- Understand and explain the importance of infection control practices in maintaining the safety of the health care worker, patients, and others.

- List the milestones that led to the development of germ theory and infection control.

- Identify the five types of microbes and give examples of infectious diseases caused by each type.

- Describe the chain of infection and list methods the health care worker can use to break it.

- Give examples of the body's defense mechanisms.

- Describe the CDC and OSHA and explain their roles in health care safety.

- Identify the preventive procedures included in the Standard Precautions.

- Identify situations when handwashing is indicated and demonstrate the technique.

- Identify the three types of transmission-based precautions and when they may be used.

- Explain the differences between antiseptics, disinfectants, and sterilization.

- Identify and describe the three major disease risks for health care workers.

- Describe how pathogens become drug resistant and the impact this has in health care.

- Describe measures that will protect the health care worker and others from bloodborne pathogens.

KEY TERMS

aerobic

AIDS

anaerobic

antibiotic

antiseptics

asepsis or aseptic technique

bacteria

bacteriocidal

bacteriostatic

Centers for Disease Control and Prevention (CDC)

chain of infection

communicable disease

contaminated

disinfectants

fungi (pl. of fungus)

germ theory

hepatitis B

HIV positive

host

immune response

infection control

infectious disease

medical asepsis or clean technique

continues

KEY TERMS *continued*

microbes

microbiology

microorganisms

microscope

normal flora

nosocomial infection

opportunistic
   infections

Occupational Safety
   and Health
   Administration
   (OSHA)

parasite

pathogens

protozoa

rickettsia

standard precautions

sterile field

sterilization

surgical asepsis or
   sterile technique

transmission-based
   precautions

tuberculosis (TB)

The Case of

the Traveling Microorganisms

Ralph Romero, a health care worker at a large metropolitan hospital, awakens in the middle of the night with coughing, sneezing, runny nose, and a temperature of 101°. He is scheduled to work the next day and so takes medications to treat his symptoms and goes back to bed. He awakens still feeling ill and wishes he could stay home, but knows the hospital is always so busy on the weekends and decides to go despite being ill. He works his shift, being careful that when he coughs or sneezes to turn his head away from the patient and uses some handkerchiefs he brought from home to use when coughing, sneezing, or blowing his nose. He also makes sure that he washes his hands when entering each patient's room. In this chapter, health care workers will learn their role in preventing the transmission of microorganisms while performing their duties.

IMPORTANCE OF INFECTION CONTROL IN HEALTH CARE

Before ever entering a health care facility or having contact with a patient, it is essential to have a clear understanding of infection control. The main goal of **infection control** is to prevent the spread of infectious diseases. An **infectious disease** is any disease caused by the growth of **pathogens**, disease-causing microorganisms (germs), in the body.

It is essential that health care workers maintain a safe environment by following specific policies and procedures designed to reduce the risk of transferring infectious diseases. Failure to prevent the spread of an infectious disease can cause unnecessary pain, suffering, and even death. Regulatory standards have been developed to prevent pathogens

from being passed from patient to patient, staff to patient, patient to staff, or staff to staff. Improperly cleaned instruments and equipment are other means of transmitting pathogens. Strict adherence to proper procedures also prevents health care workers and visitors to facilities from spreading pathogens to the community.

It is critical to identify any signs or symptoms of an infection as quickly as possible so an evaluation can be performed and treatment prescribed as indicated. An infection can be *generalized,* or *systemic* (affecting the whole body), or *localized* (affecting one area of the body). For generalized infections, signs and systems commonly experienced are headaches, fever, fatigue, vomiting, diarrhea, and an increase in pulse and respiration. In localized infections, the area will be red, swollen, warm to the touch, and painful. There may also be drainage.

MICROBIOLOGY

Microorganisms are very small, usually one-celled, living plants or animals. They exist everywhere in the environment but can only be seen with the aid of a **microscope** (an instrument fitted with a powerful magnifying lens). It is easy to forget their significance because their presence is not obvious. *But it is critical to remember that the actions of the health care worker can assist destructive microorganisms in their travel, allowing them to infect workers and others.*

The study of microorganisms is called **microbiology** and is derived from the Greek *micros*, meaning small, *bios*, meaning life, and *logy*, meaning the study of. Although the microscope was invented in the 1600s by Anton van Leeuwenhoek, scientists did little more than simply observe microorganisms under the lens. No one questioned their origin or relation to other life forms. It was not until Louis Pasteur's (a French biochemist and physicist) work in the 1800s that the germ theory was developed. The **germ theory** states that specific microorganisms, called bacteria, are the cause of specific diseases in both humans and animals.

Important highlights in the history of infection control include:

- An article written in 1843 by Oliver Wendell Holmes, MD stating that a *contagious disease* or **communicable disease** (a disease that may be transmitted either directly or indirectly from one individual to another) might be spread by the **contaminated** (presence of infectious material) hands of doctors and nurses

- The observation by Ignaz Philipp Semmelweis, MD, a Hungarian obstetrician, that mortality rates were higher when patients were attended by physicians or medical students who came directly from the morgue or autopsy room without first washing their hands

- The development in 1864 of *surgical aseptic technique* to prevent contamination of the wound and operative site by Lord Joseph Lister, MD (Fong, 1994)

Not all microorganisms are harmful. Many commonly reside in a particular environment on or in the body and are known as **normal flora**. The skin, vagina, and intestines are examples of areas that have normal flora.

Some microorganisms are even necessary to maintain normal function. For example, Escherichia coli (E. coli) aids the digestive process in the colon. In this case E. coli is a nonpathogen. E. coli can also be a pathogen and create an infection when it invades an area of the body where it is not a part of the normal flora, such as the blood or urine.

Other microorganisms are part of the normal flora but have no beneficial role. They normally do no harm unless the individual becomes susceptible to an infection due to an alteration in the normal physiological state of the body. This can occur through suppression of the **immune response**, which is a specific defense used by the body to fight infection and disease by producing antibodies (protective proteins that combat pathogens). Also, long-term **antibiotic** (medications capable of inhibiting the growth of or destroying microorganisms) therapy suppresses the normal flora and creates an imbalance that can decrease the body's ability to resist pathogens. When an infection occurs due to the weakened physiological state of the body, it is called an **opportunistic infection**. The ability of the body to resist infection is determined by age, presence of other disease, level of physical health, degree of mental stress, nutritional state, and certain medications.

Microorganisms are either **aerobic** (require oxygen to live) or **anaerobic** (do not require oxygen to live). Many microorganisms prefer a warm, moist, dark environment that provides a source of food. The human body meets these requirements and is thus an ideal environment for microorganisms to flourish.

Some microorganisms derive nutrients for growth and reproduction from nonliving material and others from living organisms or **hosts**. If this relationship is beneficial to the host, it is called

[Fascinating Facts]

Prior to the germ theory, it was believed that microorganisms spontaneously arose from decomposing nonliving matter. The "proof" of this theory was the observation that:

"Decaying meat gave rise to maggots (fly larvae); sweat-laden shirts, stored with wheat in a dark area, gave rise to mice; and hairs from a horse's tail, when placed in water, produced worms!" (Fong, 1994)

symbiosis. If there is no affect on the host, it is called *neutralism.* But if damage is done to the host, the condition is *parasitic.* An organism that nourishes itself at the expense of other living things and causes them damage is called a **parasite**.

Types of Microbes

Microbe is the term used for a microorganism that is pathogenic. Plant and animal microbes are classified as bacteria, viruses, fungi, rickettsia, and protozoa.

Bacteria

Bacteria are one-celled plants and can be either pathogenic or nonpathogenic. Many produce *toxins* (poisonous substances). Most bacteria require oxygen and grow best in moderate temperatures. When a group of bacteria grows in one place it is called a *colony.* Bacteria are categorized according to their shapes: round, rod, and spiral. Each type causes certain diseases and conditions. See Figure 10–1.

Round- or *ovoid-shaped* bacteria are called *cocci.* Cocci can be further defined by a description of their appearance.

- Micrococci: Appear singly
- Diplococci: Appear in pairs
- Staphylococci: Appear as irregular clusters
- Streptococci: Form chains

Micrococci cause a variety of skin and wound infections. Diplococci cause gonorrhea, meningitis, and some types of pneumonia. Staphylococci are pus-producing and can cause abscesses, boils, wound infections, urinary tract infections, and other types of pneumonia. Streptococci can cause rheumatic fever and a severe sore throat referred to as strep throat.

Rod-shaped bacteria are called *bacilli.* Bacilli can also be further defined by a description of their appearance.

- Bacilli: Appear singly
- Coccobacilli: When rods are somewhat oval
- Diplobacilli: Appear in pairs
- Streptobacilli: Attached end to end to form chain

Some common diseases caused by various bacilli are tuberculosis, tetanus, pertussis (whooping cough), botulism (severe form of food poisoning), diphtheria, and typhoid fever.

The third shape bacteria can take is *spiral.* Spiral-shaped bacteria can be further defined by their characteristics or appearance.

- Vibrios: Form curved rods

- Spirilla: Organism is rigid
- Spirochetes: Organism is flexible

Some common diseases caused by spiral-shaped bacteria include syphilis and cholera.

While cocci are incapable of movement, some of the rod- and spiral-shaped bacteria have slender whip-like appendages called *flagella* (sing. flagellum) that give them the power of independent locomotion.

Diagnosing which bacteria is causing an infection is essential for proper treatment. A laboratory method that is often used to identify the general category of microorganism is called *gram staining.* Bacteria are stained with a substance called crystal violet. The type of cell walls of a bacteria determines how it reacts to staining. This is why their reactions are clues to their identity. There are three categories of reactions:

1. Gram-positive: Retains the stain
2. Gram-negative: Loses the stain
3. Acid-fast: Retains the stain even when treated with acid

This information can be obtained rather quickly and helps determine the class of antibiotic to prescribe.

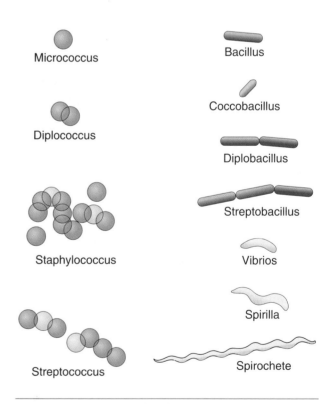

Figure 10–1 Bacterial cells vary in shape and arrangement.

It is estimated that each of us carries 10^{14} bacteria (100,000,000,000,000, or 100 trillion) in and on our bodies and that the total population of our planet excretes 10^{22} bacteria in feces every day (Thomas, 1989).

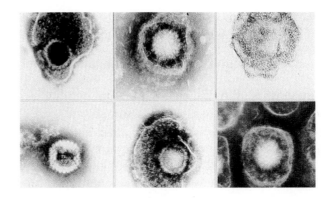

Figure 10–2 Herpes simplex viruses. (Electron Micrographs Courtesy of the Centers for Disease Control, Atlanta, GA).

Another laboratory method usually performed at the same time is to grow the microorganism in various culture media (material that promotes the growth of microorganisms). It can take 24 to 72 hours for colonies to form, but the information obtained can result in the identification of the exact bacteria. Based on this more specific diagnosis, the choice of antibiotics can be reevaluated to determine if a more specific medication should be prescribed.

Almost all bacteria can be destroyed with antibiotics. However, there are several types of bacteria that are resistant to antibiotics and are challenging to treat. They create a threat to the health of both patients and health care workers. Resistant strains of bacteria are discussed later in this chapter.

Some bacteria have the ability to form spores. A *spore* is a thick capsule that the bacteria creates for self-protection. Spores are created when life-supporting conditions are not favorable and are referred to as the "resting stage." Spores are extremely difficult to kill and can lay dormant for months or even years. In this stage, bacteria are still alive but inactive and very resistant to heat, drying, and the action of disinfectants. When supportive conditions return, the bacteria become active again. Extremely high temperatures, such as that reached by steam, must be used for sterilization to ensure that all spores are killed.

Viruses

Viruses are the smallest of the microbes and cannot be seen under the traditional light microscope. A special piece of equipment called an electron microscope is necessary to identify them. See Figure 10–2. Viruses are not whole cells but depend on other living cells to provide food, nutrients, and a means of reproduction. Since they can only live inside another living organism, they are referred to as *obligate intracellular parasites.*

Over 300 viruses have been identified by researchers. Some appear to be harmless, but others can cause infections that result in the common cold, influenza (flu), pneumonia, chicken pox, croup, hepatitis B, acquired immune deficiency syndrome (AIDS), measles, mumps, herpes, warts, and polio.

Viral infections can be extremely difficult to treat because viruses multiply rapidly and are easily transmitted by blood and other body secretions. They are resistant to many disinfectants and are not killed by the antibiotics, which kill bacteria.

Fungi

Fungi are a large group of simple plants. Two forms of fungi are potential pathogens: yeast and mold. Yeasts are one-celled and molds are multicelled plants. Both are present everywhere. Fungi cannot produce their own nutrients, so they rely on other *organic* (animal and vegetable forms of life) materials. Some use live and others use dead organic materials for nutrients. Fungi thrive in warm, moist, dark conditions.

Many yeasts and molds are nonpathogenic. In fact, penicillin, an important antibiotic, is produced from a mold. But as with other types of microorganisms, fungi can become pathogenic when the right conditions exist. When this happens they create an opportunistic infection. Fungal infections can range from merely annoying to life-threatening.

Some fungi cause chronic, recurrent infections. Superficial, or *cutaneous*, infections refer to infections of the skin or mucous membranes, and these include fungi that cause ringworm, athlete's foot, and infections of the skin, hair follicles and scalp. The most serious of the fungal infections are the systemic infections such as *histoplasmosis* (a systemic respiratory disease). Infections that go

Fungus is the organism that causes food spoilage. Who has not seen fuzzy or dark moldy spots on spoiled bread, fruits, and vegetables? And you are probably familiar with the characteristic "musty" smell of mold. But there are also the commercial uses of fungus, such as the use of yeast for making wine from grapes and beer from malt and the creation of carbon dioxide necessary for dough to rise. Molds are also responsible for the flavor of Roquefort and Camembert cheeses (Fong, 1994).

beyond the cutaneous level are always difficult, if not impossible, to treat or cure. Treatment of systemic infections requires medications that are toxic to humans. Patients, therefore, must be closely monitored.

Rickettsia

Rickettsia are much smaller than bacteria and have rod or spherical shapes. They do not move independently; they stain as gram negative. Rickettsia must live inside the cell of another living organism and so are, like the viruses, referred to as obligate intracellular parasites.

Rickettsia cause several types of typhus and Rocky Mountain spotted fever. The microorganism is passed through the bite of fleas, lice, ticks, and mites. Epidemic typhus is the only rickettsial infection transferred by humans. Once the killer of entire villages, typhus is rarely seen today.

Protozoa

Protozoa are the only microorganisms that are classified as animals. Consisting of one cell, they are very plentiful in the environment and reside in and on the body. Like other microorganisms, they seek locations that provide nutrients, warmth, and moisture. This is why some of the 45,000 identified types of protozoa are constantly present in the intestines and on the skin and mucous membranes of the nose and throat.

Protozoa are also found in decayed materials, water contaminated with sewage waste, food washed in contaminated water or handled by unwashed hands, bird and animal feces, and insect bites. See Figure 10–3.

Some of the most common diseases caused by the pathogenic protozoa include:

- Dysentery, an intestinal infection resulting in abdominal pain, cramping, and diarrhea. *Giardia lamblia*, commonly referred to as "traveler's diarrhea," is the most common intestinal parasite in the United States. It is acquired through contaminated water or food and is diagnosed by examination of the feces.

- *Trichomonas* is a sexually transmitted genital infection.

- *Toxiplasmosis* is of particular significance in pregnant women because it can pass to the unborn child and result in death, blindness, or mental retardation. It is found in the feces of birds and animals.

Here is a chilling fact that emphasizes the need to follow strict infection control procedures: Rickettsials get their name from the physician who first identified the causative agent of Rocky Mountain spotted fever, Dr. Howard T. Ricketts, an American pathologist. *He subsequently died from typhus, having been infected through his own research on the disease.* (Fong, 1994, p. 194)

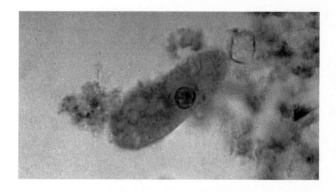

Figure 10–3 Intestinal protozoa, Entamoeba coli. (Electron Micrographs Courtesy of the Centers for Disease Control, Atlanta, GA).

- *Pneumocystis pneumonia* is caused by a protozoa that is normally not pathogenic. But, in patients with weakened immune systems, it is very serious and is a frequent cause of death among AIDS patients.

- *Malaria* is caused by a parasite that attacks the red blood cells and is characterized by periodic (every 48–72 hours) chills, fever, and sweats. The parasite is acquired through the bite of a specific kind of mosquito or through a blood transfusion.

Chain of Infection

The **chain of infection** is a useful model for explaining how infectious diseases occur and are transmitted. It consists of six elements that must be present for an infection to develop. (See Figure 10–4.)

1. Infectious agent: A pathogen must be present.

2. Reservoir host: The pathogen must have a place to live and grow. Examples of reservoir hosts are the human body, contaminated water or food, animals, insects, birds, and dead or decaying organic material. When humans or animals are capable of transmitting the pathogen, but have no outward signs of the disease, they are referred to as *carriers*. Individuals who are carriers may not even be aware that they are spreading an infectious disease.

3. Portal of exit: The pathogen must be able to escape from the reservoir host where it has been growing. Examples of portals of exit are blood, urine, feces, breaks in the skin, wound drainage, and body secretions such as saliva, mucus, and reproductive fluids.

4. Route of transmission: When the pathogen leaves the reservoir host through the portal of exit, it must have a way of being transmitted

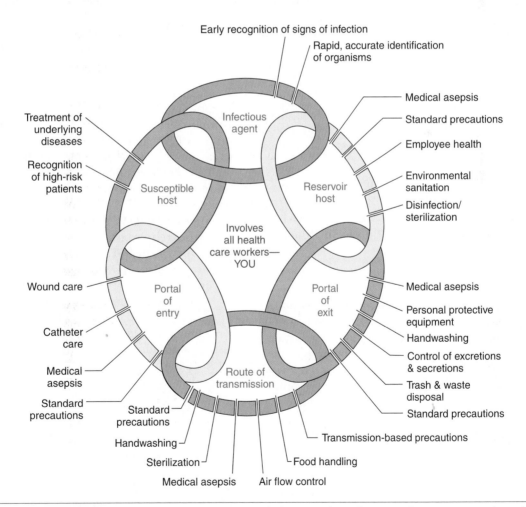

Figure 10–4 The chain of infection. Breaking at least one link stops the infectious disease. Examples of health care practices and procedures that will break the cycle are included.

to a new host. Examples are air, food, insects, and direct contact with an infected person.

5. Portal of entry: The pathogen must have a way of entering the new host. Common ports of entry are the mouth, nostrils, and breaks in the skin.

6. Susceptible host: An individual who has a large number of pathogens invading the body or does not have adequate resistance to the invading pathogen will get the infectious disease.

Defense Mechanisms

One of the marvels of the body is the number of defense mechanisms present to resist infections. If the defense mechanisms are intact, along with a strong immune system, the individual can frequently resist the microorganism and not become ill. Examples of the body's natural defense mechanisms include:

- Cilia in the respiratory tract that catch and move pathogens out of the body

- Coughing and sneezing to propel pathogens outward

- Tears, which contain chemicals to kill bacteria

- Hydrochloric acid in the stomach, which destroys pathogens

- Mucous membranes of the respiratory, reproductive, and digestive systems, which serve to trap pathogens

- Rise in body temperature (fever) to a temperature that will kill microorganisms

- Production of additional leukocytes (white blood cells), which have the specific function of destroying pathogens

Scope of the Problem

It is important to realize that a health care facility by the very nature of its business, assisting patients with infections, has a higher concentration of microorganisms than is found in other environments. Combine this with patients who have lowered levels of resistance due to illness and health care personnel who have frequent contact with body fluids, and there exists a potentially deadly situation.

The result is that infections are sometimes acquired through association with health care facilities. The term **nosocomial infection** refers to an infection that occurs while a patient is receiving health care. It is estimated that at least 5–10% of the patients admitted to a hospital contact a nosocomial infection and that these infections result in 80,000 deaths per year in the United States (Taylor, 1997).

When it is an employee who contracts an infectious disease while at work, it is called an industrial illness. Hepatitis B is one of the most serious risks for health care employees. As many as 300 U.S. health care workers die each year from this disease (Taylor, 1997). Hepatitis B, as well as the HIV virus, is transported by the blood of infected patients. Needle sticks are a common means of blood transport from patient to health care worker. It is estimated that 800,000 needle sticks occur each year in this country. It is essential that health care workers learn and apply the means to avoid all types of risks encountered in the workplace.

Regulatory Agencies

Two very important regulatory agencies have led the way in the battle against pathogens. They are responsible for developing the guidelines to safeguard health care workers, their patients, and the public. An essential part of health care training is understanding the purpose of these agencies and learning the guidelines that pertain to specific occupations.

The **Centers for Disease Control and Prevention (CDC)** is a government agency that is part of the United States Department of Health and Human Services. By studying the causes and distribution of diseases (*epidemiology*), the CDC is able to formulate safety guidelines to help prevent and control the spread of infectious diseases. Other major tasks include the licensing of clinical laboratories, maintenance of laboratory reference centers for microorganisms, and operation of extensive disease research programs.

Occupational Safety and Health Administration (OSHA), established in 1970, is a government agency that is under the Department of Labor. Its two main functions are to establish minimum health and safety standards for the workplace and to enforce those standards. OSHA is the "watchdog" of employee safety and has the authority to conduct onsite inspections to verify compliance with its standards. It is the agency that requires employers to have an exposure control plan and provide hepatitis B vaccines to employees with occupational exposure risk.

PREVENTION THROUGH ASEPSIS

The practice of **asepsis**, or **aseptic technique**, refers to the methods used to make the patient, the worker, and the environment as pathogen-free as possible. There are two types: medical and surgical.

1. **Medical asepsis**, or **clean technique**, includes procedures to decrease the number and spread of pathogens in the environment. Examples include handwashing, good personal hygiene, the cleaning of rooms between patient use, and disposal of gloves after contact with body fluids or contaminated objects.

2. **Surgical asepsis**, or **sterile technique**, includes procedures to completely eliminate the presence of pathogens from objects and areas. Examples of surgical asepsis are wearing sterile caps, gowns, masks, and gloves during surgery; sterilizing and using special techniques to handle instruments to be used with patients; maintaining sterile fields; changing dressings; and disposing of contaminated materials.

Breaking the Chain of Infection

The chain of infection demonstrates how infectious diseases occur and are spread. The most important concept to remember is *that breaking at least one link stops the infectious disease.* The practices and techniques that health care workers use daily are designed to break the chain.

Recall that the Chain of Infection consists of six elements. These six elements are frequently summarized into the following three components:

1. Source of infecting microorganisms (elements 1 and 2—infectious agent and reservoir host—both involve the source of infection)

2. Means of transmission for the microorganism (elements 3, 4, and 5—portal of exit, route of transmission, and portal of entry—all affect transmission)

3. Susceptible host (element 6—susceptible host—is unchanged in this summarized format)

The best defenses, then, are to decrease the sources of microorganisms, prevent the transmission, and maximize the resistance of the host. Here are examples of how the health care worker can have an impact in each of these areas (see Figure 10–4 for other examples):

1. How can I decrease the source of microorganisms?
   - Perform proper handwashing
   - Decontaminate surfaces and equipment (antiseptics, disinfectants, sterilization)
   - Avoid contact with patients and others when harboring infectious microorganisms. For example, the force of a sneeze can propel microorganisms for many feet (the spray travels in the shape of a cone so as the distance increases from the nose, the spray widens)

2. How can I prevent the transmission of microorganisms?
   - Wear PPE (person protective equipment) when indicated. PPE includes caps, gloves, gowns, masks, booties, and eye protection.
   - Follow isolation procedures when indicated. These are additional precautions used when working with patients who have highly contagious diseases.

3. How can I maximize the resistance of the host?
   - Provide good hygiene
   - Ensure proper nutrition and fluid intake
   - Decrease stressors that weaken the immune response

The first line of defense in medical asepsis and the most effective way to help prevent the spread of microorganisms is good handwashing technique. Many microorganisms are normal flora, always present on the body. For example, staphylococci occur naturally on the hands. But when transferred to a wound site, they can cause pus-producing infections.

Two types of normal flora are found on the hands. *Transient flora*, whether pathogenic or nonpathogenic, are picked up during our activities of daily living, and are easily removed from the hands with frequent and thorough handwashing. *Resident flora* are present at all times and considerable scrubbing is required to remove these deeply imbedded microbes. It is not possible to completely remove all the microorganisms from the hands, but the transient flora can be removed and the resident flora diminished with diligent handwashing. In individuals who do not maintain proper hygiene, it is possible that even the transient flora will become resident flora. This results in the person becoming a carrier of that particular organism (Taylor, 1997).

Standard Precautions

It is impossible to know which pathogens a patient may carry, so specific procedures have been developed by the CDC. Known as **Standard Precautions**, it is essential that they be followed at all times and applied to every patient in the health care environment.

Standard Precautions must be followed to prevent contact with potentially infectious body fluids. Specifically, these fluids include:

- Blood
- All body fluids, secretions, and excretions except sweat, regardless of whether or not they contain visible blood
- Nonintact skin
- Mucous membranes
- Any unidentified body fluids

The following sections summarize the specific standard precautions needed by health care workers.

Handwashing

Always perform proper handwashing technique as indicated to avoid transfer of microorganisms to patients, yourself, others, or the environment. Examples of appropriate times to do handwashing are:

- When coming on duty
- When taking a break or leaving work
- Between patient contacts
- Before applying and immediately upon removing gloves
- Before and after touching your face in any way (manipulating contact lenses, applying lip balm, blowing your nose, coughing, sneezing)
- After contact with anything considered contaminated (picking up items from floor, touching equipment or environmental surfaces that may be contaminated, handling soiled linens)
- Before touching any items considered clean such as a patient's food or drink; before and after eating, drinking, or using the restroom

It is necessary to wash the hands between tasks and procedures on the same patient if there is the possibility of cross-contaminating different body sites. The hands must also be washed and the gloves changed before touching nonintact skin or mucous membranes and after touching nonintact skin, mucous membranes, blood, or any moist body fluid, secretions, or excretions.

Check the Infection Control Program policy in your facility to determine which type of soap to use. It may state to use plain (nonantimicrobial) soap for routine handwashing and an antimicrobial agent for specific circumstances. See Figure 10–5a–d and Procedure 10–1.

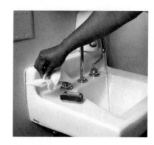

Figure 10–5a Use a clean, dry paper towel to turn the faucet on and off.

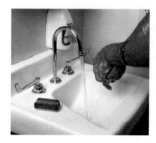

Figure 10–5b Keep the fingertips pointed downward. Scrub hands and wrists with a circular motion.

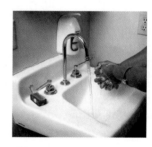

Figure 10–5c Scrub between fingers with back and forth motion by interlacing fingers.

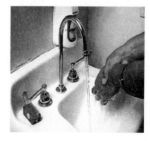

Figure 10–5d Rinse each hand thoroughly with running water from the wrists down to fingertips.

PROCEDURE 10-1

Handwashing

PROCEDURE	RATIONALE
1. Turn faucet on using a clean, dry paper towel (Figure 10–5a).	Faucets are always considered contaminated.
2. Run warm water over hands and wrists.	Warm water helps remove superficial dirt and microorganisms.
3. Do not lean against the sink and avoid splashing clothing with water.	The sink is always considered contaminated; water splashed from the sink is contaminated, and wet material easily conducts microorganisms.
4. Keep hands lower than arms during procedure and fingertips pointing downward.	Prevents contaminated water from running up the arms and dripping on clothes.
5. Apply liquid soap to hands.	Bar soap can carry microorganisms.
6. Scrub palms in a circular motion while clasping hands together.	Creates lather, and the friction helps to remove microorganisms.
7. Scrub wrists 1 to 2 inches above the hands by encircling one wrist with the other hand; then repeat for other wrist.	Same as above.
8. Scrub the back of each hand with a circular motion by cupping one hand over the other (Figure 10–5b).	Same as above.
9. Scrub between the fingers with a back and forth motion by interlacing fingers (Figure 10–5c).	Same as above.
10. Scrub each individual finger and clean under the nails with a cuticle stick, a brush, or a fingernail on the other hand, or by rubbing it against the palm of the other hand.	Microorganisms can easily hide under the nails.
11. Scrub hands for at least two minutes.	Provides thorough cleaning of all surfaces.
12. Rinse each hand thoroughly with running water from the wrists down to the fingertips (Figure 10–5d).	Soap residue can cause skin irritation.
13. Dry thoroughly with a disposable towel(s).	Moisture remaining on the skin can cause irritation; reusable towels can harbor microorganisms.
14. Use another dry towel to turn off the faucet handle (Figure 10–5a).	Prevents recontamination of hands from microorganisms on the faucet handles; a wet towel would allow microorganisms to travel from the faucet handle back to the hands.
15. Clean sink area using dry towels and being careful not to recontaminate hands by touching any surfaces.	Leaves the area ready for the next person; the faucets and sink are always considered contaminated; wet towels are considered contaminated.
16. Use lotion if desired.	Keeps hands soft and helps prevent chapping and cracking of hands, which are more susceptible to growth of microorganisms.

Personal Protective Equipment

Personal protective equipment, commonly referred to as PPE, includes gloves, masks, protective eyewear, gowns, and caps. To be effective, these must be properly used in all situations that have the potential to infect the health care worker.

Gloves

Wear clean, nonsterile gloves when you touch, or have the potential of coming in contact with blood, body fluids, secretions, excretions, or contaminated items. Put on clean gloves just before touching mucous membranes and nonintact skin. Gloves should be changed between tasks and procedures on the same patient if there is contact with material that may contain a high concentration of microorganisms. Remove gloves promptly after use, before touching noncontaminated items and environmental surfaces, and before going to another patient. After gloves are removed, wash your hands immediately to avoid transfering of microorganisms to other patients or environments. See Figure 10–6a–g and Procedure 10–2.

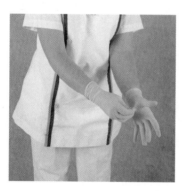

Figure 10–6a Grasp the outside of one glove at palm site with the other gloved hand.

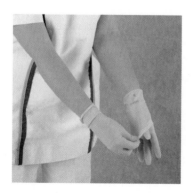

Figure 10–6b Pull the glove down.

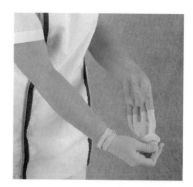

Figure 10–6c Turn the glove inside out while removing it.

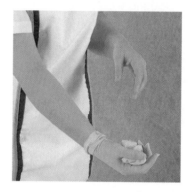

Figure 10–6d Hold the removed glove in the palm of the remaining gloved hand.

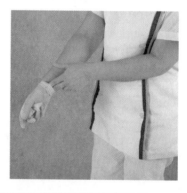

Figure 10–6e Take the ungloved hand and slide it under the cuff of the remaining glove.

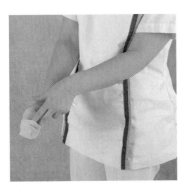

Figure 10–6f Push the glove off.

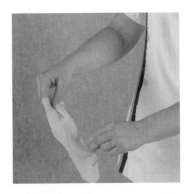

Figure 10–6g The first glove is now inside of the second glove that was removed. Dispose of gloves in appropriate container according to facility policy.

PROCEDURE 10-2

Nonsterile Gloves (applying clean gloves and removing contaminated gloves)

PROCEDURE	RATIONALE
1. Applying Nonsterile Gloves:	
2. Use proper handwashing technique before applying gloves.	To remove microorganisms from hands.
3. Remove appropriate-sized clean gloves from the box and apply. Once the hands are washed, no specific technique is necessary for applying gloves, but touch only the gloves you will be using when removing them from the dispenser.	Gloves that are too small can split and expose skin and gloves that are too large are difficult to work with and can expose skin by slipping down; do not contaminate the remaining gloves in the dispenser by touching them.
4. Removing Contaminated Gloves:	
5. Grasp the outside of one glove at the palm with the other gloved hand (Figure 10–6a); pull the glove down (Figure 10–6b) and turn it inside out while removing it (Figure 10–6c).	At no time should the hands touch the outside of the contaminated gloves.
6. Hold the removed glove in the palm of the remaining gloved hand (Figure 10–6d).	Same as above.
7. Take the ungloved hand and slide it under the cuff of the remaining glove (Figure 10–6e) and push the glove off (Figure 10–6f). The first glove is now inside of the second glove that was removed (Figure 10–6g).	Same as above.
8. Discard the gloves in an appropriate container according to facility policy.	Isolates the contaminated gloves from contact with other surfaces.
9. Wash hands immediately after removing gloves.	To remove microorganisms from hands.

Mask, Eye Protection, Face Shield

Wear a mask and eye protection or a face shield to protect the mucous membranes of the eyes, nose, and mouth during procedures and patient care activities that are likely to generate splashes or sprays of blood, body fluids, secretions, or excretions. See Figure 10–7.

Gown

Wear a clean, nonsterile gown to protect the skin and to prevent soiling clothing during procedures and patient care activities that are likely to generate splashes or sprays of blood, body fluids, secretions, or excretions. Select a gown that is appropriate for the activity and amount of fluid likely to be encountered. Remove a soiled gown as promptly as possible and wash your hands to avoid transfer of microorganisms to other patients or environments.

Application of PPE

When working in contaminated areas, there are guidelines for applying and removing PPE. The following guidelines include the most commonly used equipment:

1. Wash hands (Procedure 10–1).
2. Put on cap, mask, protective eyewear, and gown. No specific sequence of applying these items is required. Be sure that the cap covers all the hair, the mask fits snuggly to the face, eyewear extends to protect the side of the face, and the gown completely covers the clothing.
3. Apply gloves last and pull the cuffs over the sleeves of the gown to create a seal.

See Figure 10-8a–c.

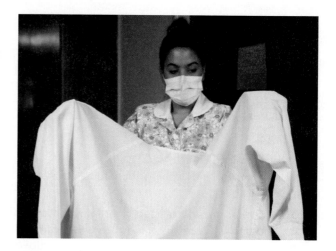

Figure 10–8a Put on the gown by placing your hands inside the shoulders.

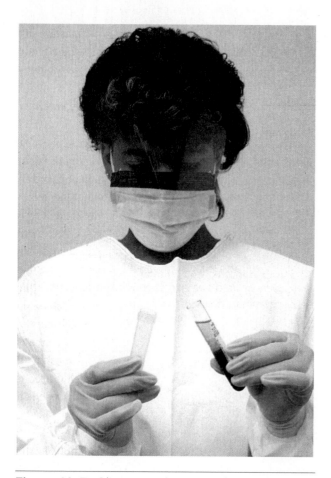

Figure 10–7 Gloves, mask, eye protection, and gown should be worn during procedures and patient-care activities that are likely to generate splashes or sprays of blood, body fluids, secretions, and excretions.

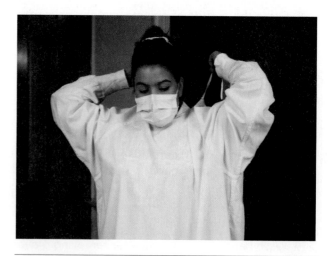

Figure 10–8b Slip your fingers inside the neckband to tie the gown at the neck.

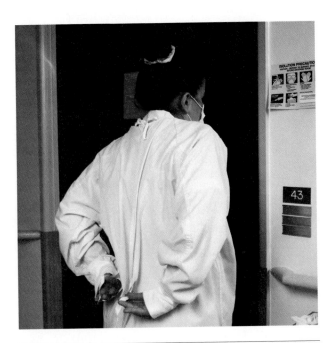

Figure 10–8c Overlap the back edges of the gown so your uniform is completely covered before tying the waist ties.

Remove PPE prior to leaving the contaminated area, as follows:

1. Untie the waist ties of the gown.
2. Remove gloves (Procedure 10–2).
3. Wash hands (Procedure 10–1).
4. Remove cap and protective eyewear.
5. Untie the neck tie of the gown and remove the gown, following the correct procedure (Figure 10–9 a–c).
6. Remove the mask. Hold the mask by the strings to discard it. The mask is always removed last if the contaminants are airborne.
7. Wash hands.

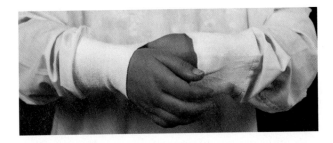

Figure 10–9a To remove the gown slip the fingers of one hand under the cuff of the opposite arm and pull gown down until it covers the hand.

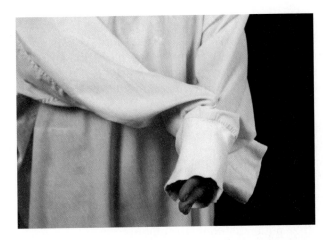

Figure 10–9b Using the gown-covered hand grasp the outside of the gown on the opposite arm and pull the gown down until it covers the hand.

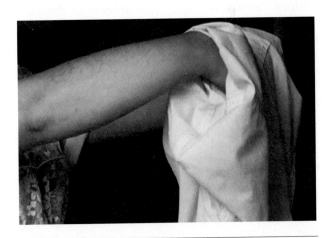

Figure 10–9c Both hands are now inside the gown and can be used to grasp the outside of the gown. Use your covered hands to grasp the gown at the shoulders and turn the gown inside out (contaminated side on the inside) as you remove it. Roll it up and place in appropriate container according to facility policy.

Patient-Care Equipment

Handle used patient care equipment that is soiled with blood, body fluids, secretions, and excretions in a manner that prevents skin and mucous membrane exposures, contamination of clothing, and transfer of microorganisms to other patients and environments. Ensure that reusable equipment is not used for the care of another patient until it has been cleaned and reprocessed appropriately. Be sure that single-use items are discarded properly.

Environmental Control

Procedures must be followed and consistently performed for the routine care, cleaning, and disinfection of environmental surfaces, beds, bed rails, bedside equipment, and other frequently touched surfaces.

Linen

Handle, transport, and process used linen that is soiled with blood, body fluids, secretions, and excretions in a manner that prevents skin and mucous membrane exposures, contamination of your clothing, and transfer of microorganisms to other patients and environments.

Occupational Health and Blood-borne Pathogens

Take care to prevent injuries when using needles, scalpels, and other sharp instruments or devices; when handling sharp instruments after procedures; when cleaning used instruments; and when disposing of used needles. Place used disposable syringes and needles, scalpel blades, and other sharp items in appropriate puncture-resistant containers. See Figure 10–10. These should be located as close as practical to the area in which the items are used. Place reusable syringes and needles in a puncture-resistant container for transport to the reprocessing area.

The following additional precautions must be followed when using needles:

- Never recap used needles. The health care worker needs to be familiar with the facility policies on how to handle contaminated needles because there may be an exception to this rule. Examples include using either a one-handed "scoop" technique or a mechanical device designed for holding the needle sheath.

- Do not remove used needles from disposable syringes by hand, and do not bend, break, or otherwise manipulate used needles by hand.

Use mouthpieces, resuscitation bags, or other ventilation devices as an alternative to mouth-to-mouth resuscitation methods. Keep these devices available in areas where the need for resuscitation is predictable.

Patient Placement

Patients with infections who contaminate the environment or who do not–or cannot be expected to–assist in maintaining appropriate hygiene or environmental control should be placed in a private room. If a private room is not available, consult with infection control professionals regarding patient placement or other alternatives.

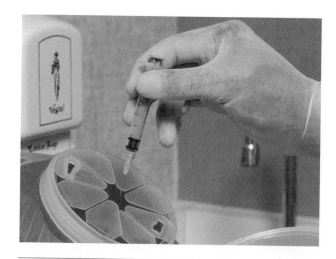

Figure 10–10 All needles and sharp objects should be discarded immediately in a puncture-resistant sharps container.

Transmission Precautions

Certain pathogens are especially dangerous because they are easily transmitted and have the potential of causing epidemics. The CDC recommends the use of **Transmission-Based Precautions** with patients who are documented or suspected to be infected with these pathogens. There are three types of Transmission-Based Precautions: Airborne Precautions, Droplet Precautions, and Contact Precautions. See Table 10–1. They may be combined for diseases that have multiple routes of transmission. *When used either singularly or in combination, they are to be used in addition to Standard Precautions* (Gardner, 1996, CDC Online).

Placing a patient on transmission precautions, however, often presents certain disadvantages to the hospital, patients, personnel, and visitors.

- Requires the patient to be in a private room unless it is shared with another patient with the same disease. The rationale for this is to confine the pathogen to the patient's unit.

- May require specialized equipment and environmental modifications that add to the cost of hospitalization

- Makes frequent visits by nurses, physicians, and other personnel inconvenient, and may make it more difficult for personnel to give prompt and frequent care that sometimes is required

- Using a multipatient room for one patient uses valuable space that otherwise might accommodate several patients.

Table 10–1 Transmission-Based Precautions (Isolation Precautions)

Type of Precaution	Description	Examples
Airborne (Figure 10–11)	• Airborne droplets or dust particles containing the infectious agent remain suspended in the air for long periods of time. • Can be dispersed widely by air currents within a room or over a long distance • Can be emitted during talking, sneezing, coughing and whispering	• Mycobacterium tuberculosis • Rubeola (measles) • Varicella (chicken pox)
Droplet (Figure 10–12)	• Propelled short distances through the air • Deposited on the host's conjuctiva, nasal mucosa, or mouth • Can be emitted during talking, sneezing, or coughing, and during the performance of certain procedures such as suctioning and bronchoscopy	• Some forms of pneumonia, meningitis, and sepsis • Streptococcal pharyngitis • Mumps • Influenza • Rubella
Contact (Figure 10–13)	• The most important and frequent mode of transmission of nosocomial infections • Divided into two subgroups: direct-contact transmission and indirect-contact transmission • Direct-contact transmission occurs when touching the infectious patient's dry skin—for example, when performing patient care activities, such as turning a patient or giving a bath. Direct-contact transmission also can occur betweentwo patients, with one serving as the source ofthe infectious microorganisms and the other as a susceptible host. • Indirect-contact transmission occurs when a contaminated object is touched. For example, coming in contact with instruments, needles, dressings, environmental surfaces, or patient care items.	• Some gastrointestinal, respiratory, skin, and wound infections • Herpes simplex virus • Impetigo • Scabies

■ Forced solitude deprives the patient of normal social relationships and may be psychologically harmful, especially to children and confused patients. As part of the health care team, you must do all you can to decrease these psychological stresses, not only for humanitarian reasons, but also because they compromise the immune system. So, even if it is inconvenient, check on the patient frequently. Remember you are isolating the pathogen, not the patient.

These disadvantages, however, must be weighed against the hospital's mission to prevent the spread of microorganisms that may cause an epidemic.

Another consideration is whether to post a precaution sign by the patient's door. Some hospitals prefer to protect the patient's privacy and post a simple note stating to report to the nurse's station prior to entry into the room.

The proper disposal of hazardous waste (contaminated materials) is also essential to maintaining a safe environment. When a patient is in isolation, there will be specially marked hazardous waste containers for trash and for linen located in the room. The only way to remove the

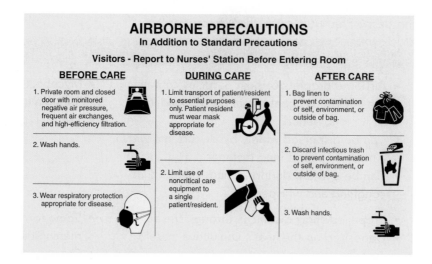

Figure 10–11 Airborne Precautions (Compliments of Briggs Corporation).

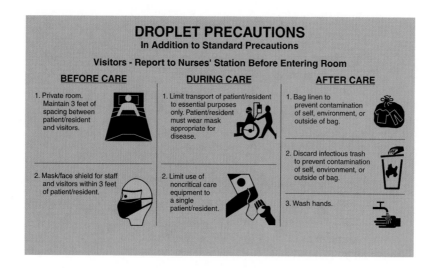

Figure 10–12 Droplet Precautions (Compliments of Briggs Corporation).

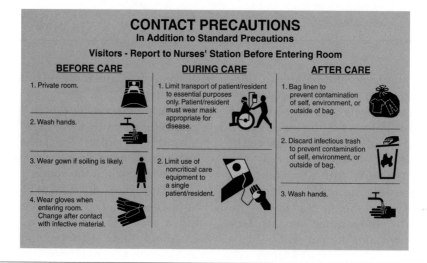

Figure 10–13 Contact Precautions (Compliments of Briggs Corporation).

contaminated items from the room is by using a *double-bagging* technique. Double-bagging is taking the contaminated bag from the isolation room (the health care worker has appropriate PPE on) and slipping it into another bag held by a coworker outside the isolation room. Care is taken so that the coworker does not touch the contaminated bag, and the health care worker in the room does not touch the clean bag. The bags are labeled according to the facility policy with hazardous waste or linen markers to alert other personnel to the need for special handling.

Antiseptics, Disinfectants, and Sterilization

There are a number of chemical agents and physical methods used to inhibit the growth of or destroy microorganisms. If the method used only inhibits the growth of the microorganism, the action is described as **bacteriostatic**. If the method results in the microorganisms being killed, the action is **bacteriocidal** or *germicidal.* The methods used can be broken into the following three categories:

- **Antiseptics**: Chemical agents that are antiseptics are only bacteriostatic. They are mild enough to be used on the skin. An example is cleaning with a 70% isopropyl alcohol wipe before giving an injection.

- **Disinfectants**: Agents or methods that destroy most bacteria and viruses. This method of cleaning is used for instruments that do not penetrate the skin and for cleaning the environment (floors, bathroom, equipment). *Chemical disinfectants* can be caustic or harmful to the skin. Using a solution comparable to a 10% dilution of common household bleach in water for cleaning the environment (including blood spills) meets OSHA recommendations because it kills hepatitis B, HIV, and tuberculosis organisms. Alcohol was mentioned earlier as an example of an antiseptic, but if instruments are soaked for 20–30 minutes, it acts as a disinfectant. See Figure 10–14. Glass thermometers cannot tolerate the high heat of other methods and are disinfected in this manner. Carefully read and follow the manufacturer's directions, when using chemical agents. *Physical disinfectant methods* include boiling instruments in water. This was once commonly used in home health settings, but with the availability of one-time use equipment, it is rarely used today.

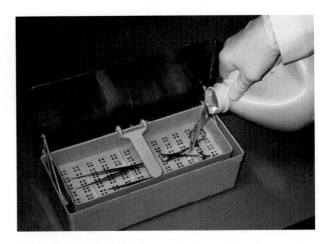

Figure 10–14 Chemical agent used as disinfectant. Pour in enough solution to completely cover all instruments.

- **Sterilization**: Agents or methods that totally destroy all microorganisms, including viruses and spores. Examples include chemical agents, gas, radiation, and dry or moist heat under pressure. The most common method used is the autoclave, which sterilizes by steam that is created by a pressurized heating system. The size can vary from a small unit for a medical office to a large unit for a hospital. See Figure 10–15.

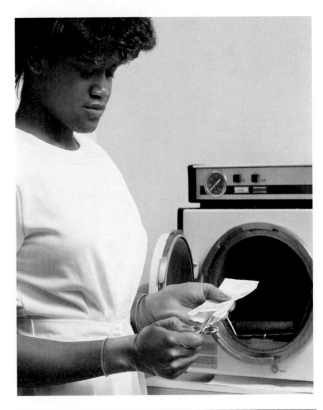

Figure 10–15 An autoclave is a pressurized heating system that sterilizes by steam.

Surgical Asepsis

Surgical asepsis (or sterile technique) refers to a group of principles and related procedures that eliminate the presence of pathogens from objects and areas. To correctly perform these procedures, it is necessary to understand the concept of a sterile field. A **sterile field** is an area that has been designated as free of microorganisms. An example is a sterile towel placed on a clean, dry surface. The towel now represents a sterile field. Many health care procedures, such as surgeries, require the use of sterile fields.

When working with a sterile field or sterile items, it is essential that contaminants not be brought into the field through actions such as touching it, allowing it to become wet, reaching across it, or talking directly over the surface. Sterilized items, such as instruments and surgical gloves, come in sealed packages that must be opened and handled properly to avoid contamination. It is also necessary for the health care worker to use sterile gloves, applying them in a way that prevents them from being contaminated. See Figure 10–16.

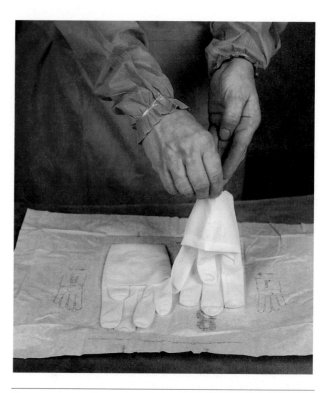

Figure 10–16b Pick up the first glove by grasping the glove on the top edge of the folded-down cuff.

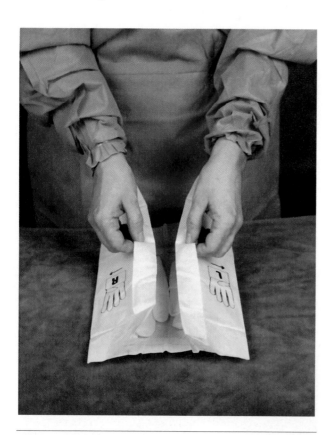

Figure 10–16a Open sterile gloves by pulling back on the tabs.

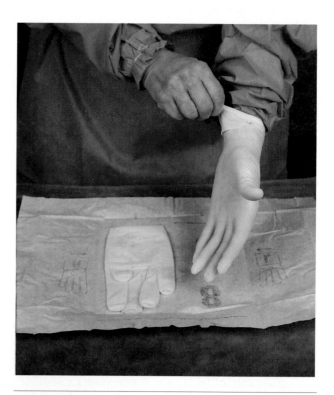

Figure 10–16c Maintain the grasp on the cuff, insert your other hand, and pull the glove on by the cuff.

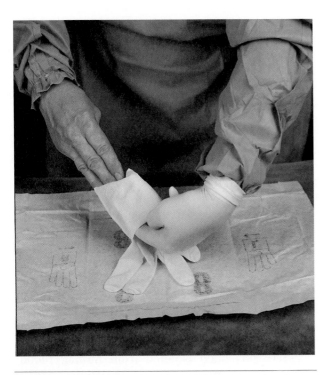

Figure 10–16d Slip the gloved fingers under the cuff of the second glove to lift it from the package and insert the other hand into the glove.

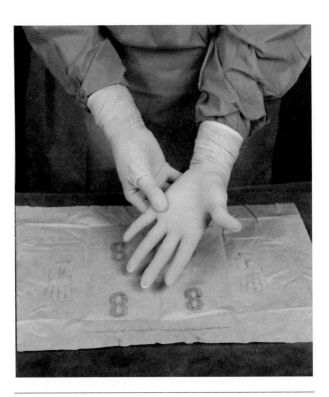

Figure 10–16f Check the gloves for tears, holes and imperfections.

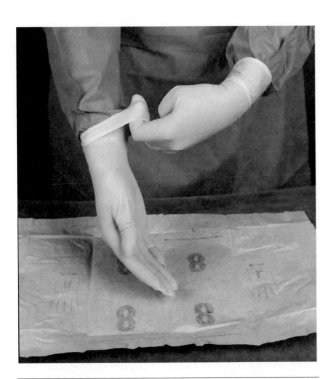

Figure 10–16e Pull glove on and adjust the glove into position being careful not to touch the skin with the gloved hands.

THE RISKS

Certain diseases pose special risks to the health care worker. These include two blood-borne pathogens, hepatitis B (HBV) and human immunodeficiency virus (HIV), and an airborne-transmitted disease, tuberculosis (TB). Also, of great concern are two drug-resistant infections that create unique challenges.

The term *blood-borne pathogens* is used to identify pathogenic microbes that are spread through contact with blood. Blood, however, is not the only route by which they can be transmitted. Infections can also be transmitted through contact with nonintact skin, mucous membranes, secretions, excretions, or any moist body fluid except sweat.

Hepatitis B

Hepatitis B virus (HBV) infection is the major infectious bloodborne occupational hazard for health care workers. The CDC estimates that each year in the United States there are approximately 8700 infections in health care workers who are exposed to blood and other infectious materials. HBV can be spread via several routes:

- Parenteral: Blood transfusion, needle sharing by IV drug users, needlestick, or other sharp instrument
- Mucous membranes: Blood contamination of the eye or mouth
- Sexual contact
- Perinatal: From infected mother to newborn infant
  (Source: OSHA Online)

When an individual becomes infected, the liver, in its attempt to destroy the hepatitis virus, causes an inflammation and subsequent destruction of liver cells. Symptoms range from very mild to severe jaundice (yellowing of the eyes and skin), dark urine, extreme fatigue, loss of appetite, nausea, abdominal pain, and sometimes joint pain, rash, and fever.

Efforts for prevention in health care are focused on the administration of hepatitis B vaccine, use of PPE, prevention of puncture injuries, and disinfection and sterilization of equipment and surfaces. OSHA mandates that employers provide hepatitis B vaccine for all employees who have an occupational exposure risk. The hepatitis B vaccines are given in three doses over a 6-month period. These vaccines, when given according to manufacturer's directions, induce protective antibody levels in 85–97% of healthy adults. If there is some doubt about a person's immunity, a blood test can be done to verify presence of the antibody (OSHA Online). An employee has the right to refuse the Hepatitis B vaccine, but if declined, the employee must sign a form stating their refusal. This releases the facility from responsibility should the health care worker become infected.

Human Immunodeficiency Virus

Human immunodeficiency virus (HIV) is the virus that causes acquired immune deficiency syndrome (AIDS). The virus destroys cells in the host that are vital to the proper functioning of the immune system. Individuals infected with the virus are said to be **HIV positive**. This is not the same as having **AIDS**, which means that the immune system has become weakened as a result of the action of the virus. Some individuals carry the virus without becoming ill; most, however, eventually develop AIDS and die as the result of severe opportunistic infections. These are infections that individuals with normal immune systems rarely experience. The most common opportunistic infection and cause of death of AIDS patients is *Pneumocystis carinii.*

Common signs and symptoms of AIDS include weakness, chronic fever, night sweats, swelling of the lymph nodes, weight loss, and diarrhea. There is no vaccine against AIDS and no known cure. It is primarily managed by treating the symptoms, but there are efforts to find more effective and safer antiviral drugs to prolong life.

Carriers of HIV may not have symptoms or even detectable amounts of the virus in the blood during the first 6 months of infection. It is essential, therefore, that health care workers understand how the virus is transmitted and follow Standard Precautions with *all* patients.

Infection with HIV may be identified through testing the blood for the presence of HIV antibodies. Most people infected with HIV have detectable antibodies within 6 months of infection, with the majority generating detectable antibodies between 6 and 12 weeks after exposure. Once individuals are HIV positive, they become lifelong carriers and can spread the virus to others.

HIV has been isolated from human blood, semen, breast milk, vaginal secretions, saliva, tears, urine, cerebrospinal fluid, and amniotic fluid; however, only blood, semen, vaginal secretions and breast milk have been proven to transmit the virus. Common modes of transmission are sexual intercourse, using contaminated needles, blood exposure via parenteral, mucous membrane or nonintact skin contact, transfusions, transplants, semen used for artificial insemination, and contact with perinatal fluids.

HIV is not transmitted by casual contact. No evidence exists that HIV is transmitted by shaking hands or talking; by sharing food, eating utensils, plates, drinking glasses, or towels; by sharing the same house or household facilities; or by "personal interactions expected of family members," including hugging and kissing on the cheek or lips. HIV is also not transmitted by mosquitoes or other animals (OSHA Online).

The rate of infection from exposure is in relationship to the amount of infected material introduced into the body. For example, a person receiving a contaminated blood transfusion has a much greater chance of infection than a health care worker injured with a contaminated needle. In fact, only 3–5 health care workers out of 1000 will became infected when injured with contaminated needles (OSHA Online). This is *not* to downplay the impact of acquiring such a devastating disease, but only to put the risk in perspective. Most health care workers fear being infected by AIDS more than HBV, and yet, the infection rate and death rate of HBV far exceeds that from AIDS.

Thinking it Through

Monica Stokes is a volunteer at a local extended care facility. Her duties include pushing a cart with books around to the patients' rooms to ask if they would like to borrow a library book. When she enters Mr. Haskin's room, the nurse asks her if she would please take the dirty linens and place them in the linen basket down the hall. She is new and unclear if this is one of her duties, but also desires to be helpful and surely the nurse would not ask her if it were not appropriate. So she picks the linens up from the floor, carries them close to her and places them in the linen basket. She notices some stains on her clothes, so she goes to the sink and rinses them off with cold water in the hope there will be no permanent stain. She then returns to her duties of distributing books to patients.

1. Was it appropriate for the nurse to ask the volunteer to assist with the linens?

2. Are all the links present in the chain of infection?

3. What breaks in Standard Precautions can you identify?

Tuberculosis

Tuberculosis (TB) is caused by *Mycobacterium tuberculosis,* an airborne pathogen. Working with tuberculosis patients requires the use of special PPE, such as special masks fitted to the individual health care worker, to avoid inhaling the tiny droplets that carry the virus through the air.

Once considered to be virtually eliminated from the United States, cases of TB have increased and some viruses have become resistant to drug therapy. This is because medications must be taken for at least 6 months. Failure by some patients to complete the full length of treatment has resulted in certain strains of the virus developing immunity to the drugs.

While renewed efforts to control TB have resulted in a steady decrease in cases since 1992, it remains one of the most common infections in the world and is the leading infectious killer of young adults. Globally, 8 million people develop TB every year (18,000 in the United States) and there are 3 million deaths annually from the infection (CDC Online).

The screening test for TB is a skin test. A positive test result does not necessarily indicate active disease, but does indicate that the person has had an exposure to the pathogen. A chest x-ray and other tests are done to determine if active disease is present. The signs and symptoms are lethargy, fever, night sweats, cough, weight loss, coughing up blood-tinged sputum, chest pain, and shortness of breath. TB primarily affects the lungs, but can affect other parts of the body as well. Patients hospitalized with suspected TB are placed in isolation for 2 to 3 weeks during which time antibiotic treatment is begun.

Drug-Resistant Organisms

The development of drug-resistant organisms is a fairly recent occurrence. It is a result of the way that antibiotics are used in the United States. They have routinely been overused by being prescribed for minor conditions. In addition, many patients fail to complete an entire course of antibiotic as prescribed. These two actions create conditions that encourage pathogens to become resistant to antibiotics. It is important to explain to patients why they must take all the medication prescribed for them, because they have a tendency stop taking the antibiotic when they feel better.

There are currently two drug-resistant organisms commonly encountered in health care. They are *methicillin-resistant Staphylococcus aureas (MRSA)* and *vancomycin-resistant Enterococcus (VRE)*. Both are difficult to control and treat and can cause very serious infections. If there is a treatment available, it is usually very

Fascinating Facts

Imagine ¼ teaspoon of HBV mixed into a 24,000-gallon swimming pool of water. Someone draws a ¼ teaspoon of that water into a syringe and injects you with it. Although the virus is diluted well, you will become HBV positive. Now imagine that 10 people are in a room. Someone takes a ¼ teaspoon of HIV and mixes it into a quart of water. A ¼ teaspoon of this solution is injected into each person. Only one person in the room will become HIV positive. Hepatitis B is thus a much greater threat to health care workers than HIV. (Acello, 1998).

[Fascinating Facts]

Persons exposed to TB may develop *latent* (inactive) TB infection. Almost 2 billion people (*one third of the world's population*) have latent TB infection, and about 10% of these infected individuals will develop active disease sometime during their lifetime. In an era marked by increased international travel and a global marketplace, no region of the world is immune from outside influences. International collaboration will be essential to eliminate TB. (Source: CDC Online).

expensive and can have very severe side effects, such as liver, kidney, and hearing damage. Because these infections occur most frequently in elderly patients who are more susceptible to the side effects and already have weakened resistance, they often result in death.

The seriousness of these infections emphasizes the importance of always following Standard Precautions and any additional procedures developed by the health care facility to prevent their spread. Actions on the part of the health care worker can determine whether infections are kept under control or are spread among patients and other workers.

REPORTING ACCIDENTAL EXPOSURE

Any injury or accident that involves exposure to blood or body fluids must be reported immediately to the supervisor. This must then be followed up by completion of a written incident or injury report per facility and/or agency requirements. Prompt reporting allows for evaluation, appropriate treatment, if indicated, and follow-up of any problems resulting from the exposure. Failure to report an incident can result in negative health consequences for the health care worker and others, as well as the need to take time off from work to recover.

OSHA regulations require every facility to have an Exposure Control Plan. This plan has many components, including the predetermination of employee exposure risk to blood-borne pathogens, description of how employees at risk

will be protected, and training and annual retraining and testing requirements for employees. Plans must also include policies and procedures to be followed if exposure does occur, such as those noted by Taylor (1997):

- Actions to take immediately upon exposure, such as washing the exposed area immediately with warm water and soap, or, if the eye or mucous membranes are involved, rinsing with normal saline
- Timeframes for reporting
- To whom the incident must be reported
- Form(s) to complete and information that must be included, such as how exposure occurred and the name of the patient
- Recommended procedure for evaluating the risk and outcome of the exposure. For example, a baseline blood test would be run on the health care worker and then repeated at specified intervals, the patient's blood would be drawn to determine HBV and HIV status, and post-exposure treatment would begin if indicated. Blood draws and treatments require the consent of the involved individual.
- Plan for counseling and information on safe practices to protect self and others

SUGGESTED LEARNING ACTIVITIES

1. If you have access to a microscope, take samples from various areas, such as your skin or mucous membranes, stagnant pond water, or decaying food, and look for microorganisms.
2. Watch a medical program on television and evaluate it for breaks in aseptic technique (medical and surgical).
3. Practice handwashing technique in your home environment.
4. Observe the handwashing techniques of others when out in the community.
5. Research additional sources and read about the lives and contributions made by Louis Pasteur, Oliver Wendell Holmes, and Lord Joseph Lister.
6. Practice using PPE by using a robe as a gown, any type of gloves you may have, and a mask made with paper and a plastic strap.

REVIEW QUESTIONS

1. Why is it critical for health care workers to apply infection control practices in the workplace?

2. What theories and discoveries led up to microbiology as we know it today?

3. Name and describe the characteristics of each of the five types of infectious microbes. Include examples of diseases caused by each type.

4. What are the elements in the chain of infection, and how can it be broken?

5. What are three examples of defenses used by the body against infection?

6. What are the roles of the CDC and OSHA in protecting the public against infectious diseases?

7. What are the requirements of Standard Precautions?

8. What are medical and surgical aseptic techniques?

9. What are the requirements outlined by the Standard Precautions?

10. What are the three types of transmission-based precautions?

11. Which three infectious diseases are major risks for health care workers?

12. Name two drug-resistant organisms. What has caused the development of this resistance? What are the specific risks caused by these organisms?

13. What is the purpose and contents of an Exposure Control Plan?

APPLICATION EXERCISES

1. What are the behaviors demonstrated by Mr. Romero in The Case of the Traveling Microorganisms that jeopardize both him and his patients?

2. Nurse Kristie Rudzinski oversleeps and has barely enough time to dress and get to work on time. She decides to wait until she gets to the hospital to change the Band-Aid on the finger she cut while fixing dinner last night. When she arrives at work she hears a patient calling for help. No one else is there, so she immediately goes to the patient's room. On entering, Kristie discovers that the patient's IV has become disconnected and blood is running from the patient's vein onto the linens. Without delay she is at the bedside and solves the problem by reconnecting the tubing. The patient is very grateful for her prompt assistance. Kristie leaves the room very pleased that she was able to help, especially since this is a patient she has cared for many times. He is an elderly gentlemen who is undergoing chemotherapy and has already had more than his share of problems.

   a. Evaluate the scenario to determine which elements in the chain of infection were present.

   b. What revisions to Kristie's actions would have to occur to follow the principles of medical and surgical asepsis?

   c. Which microorganisms would most likely be a threat to Kristie and to the patient?

SUGGESTED READINGS AND RESOURCES

Centers for Disease Control and Prevention: http://www.cdc/.gov

Fong, E., Grover-Lakomia, L., and Ferris, E. (1994). *Microbiology for health careers* (5th ed.). Albany, NY: Delmar.

Nielson, R. P. (1999). *OSHA guidelines for healthcare providers*. Albany, NY: Delmar.

OSHA: http://www.osha-slc.gov

CHAPTER

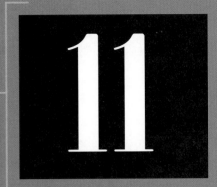

ENVIRONMENTAL SAFETY

OBJECTIVES

Studying and applying the material in this chapter will help you to:

■ Understand and explain the importance of environmental safety in maintaining the safety of the health care worker, the patients, and others.

■ Identify general safety guidelines that will help prevent injuries and accidents in health care facilities.

■ Describe and give examples of how changes in the physical and mental health of a patient can increase the risk of injuries and accidents.

■ Describe and explain the purpose of an incident report.

■ Identify the appropriate steps to take in the event of a fire.

■ Identify the different classes of fire extinguishers and type of fire on which to use each.

■ List ways to prevent electrical hazards.

■ Discuss chemical, radiation, and infectious hazards and the role of the health care worker in their prevention.

■ Describe the precautions necessary when oxygen is in use.

■ Explain when an emergency disaster plan would be implemented and define a triage system.

KEY TERMS

compatibility
emergency disaster plan
environmental safety
flammable
incident report
inflammable
PASS
RACE
toxic
triage system

The Case of

the Bomb Threat

Johanna Welks is a clinical assistant at the community hospital. As she sits at the nursing station, she reflects on how lucky she is to have a job she loves and one that is located only a few blocks from where she lives. When the phone rings, she answers the phone in a cheerful, professional manner, "Hello, this is 4West, Mrs. Welks speaking, how may I help you?" What she hears next, sends chills down her body. The caller states, "Your hospital killed my little girl, and now I will get my revenge. I have placed a bomb in the hospital." Mrs. Welks feels on the verge of hysteria. She thinks of hanging up and leaving immediately, calling home to make sure no one is at the hospital since it is close by, or perhaps starting to yell for everyone to evacuate the hospital immediately. But then her head clears, and she thinks about what would be the smartest thing to do in this situation. She tries to keep the caller on the telephone as long as possible in order to determine more specifically where the bomb is located and when it will explode. At the same time she is listening closely to the voice on the phone (i.e., to determine the sex, the age, and if the caller has an accent) and also for any background noise (e.g., car horns, trains, bells, music). This chapter will address the many environmental hazards found in health care facilities and how to keep patients and workers safe. Also discussed is the nature of an Emergency Disaster Plan, when it is initiated, and the role of the health care worker when the plan is in effect.

IMPORTANCE OF ENVIRONMENTAL SAFETY IN HEALTH CARE

Environmental safety means identifying and correcting potential hazards that can cause accidents and injuries. Examples include faulty wiring, slippery floors, and infectious waste left in open containers. The health care worker must understand and follow workplace safety policies and procedures that reduce hazards, prevent accidents, and know how to handle incidents correctly if they do occur.

OSHA, in addition to the infection-control measures presented in Chapter 10, has many regulatory requirements that apply to other workplace safety issues. The exact policies and procedures may vary among health care facilities,

but they must all meet the regulatory requirements of OSHA.

GENERAL SAFETY GUIDELINES

The best approach to safety is focus on *prevention*. There are many ways that health care workers can contribute to the prevention of common accidents and injuries that occur in the health care environment. Personal safety practices include ways to move safely within and dress for the workplace, work with patients, provide protection for oneself and others, and determine what, when, and how to report any accidents that do occur. The guidelines in this section present specific safety behaviors.

Moving Safely

Movement creates the potential for accidents such as falls. The following practices will limit such occurrences:

- Never run, even in an emergency. You can move swiftly without running if the situation warrants a fast pace.

- Stay to the right in hallways and be cautious when approaching intersections in order to prevent collisions. Pay attention to warning mirrors on corners.

- Remove any loose rugs from floors to prevent tripping or slipping.

- Open doors slowly to avoid injury to someone on the other side.

- Use handrails when climbing or descending stairs.

- Never run up or down stairs.

- Never carry uncapped syringes or sharp instruments in hallways or between rooms.

Dressing for Safety

Work in health care requires specific types of clothing and grooming to ensure the safety of both workers and patients:

- Wear long hair tied back or up to prevent contact with contaminated material or the contamination of clean materials.

- Do not wear earrings that extend beyond the earlobe so that they cannot be grabbed or caught.

- Wear enclosed shoes with no more than a 1–1½ inch heel to prevent injury to the feet.

- Limit jewelry to a smooth wedding band.

- Keep fingernails short.

Working Safely with Patients

Patient safety is always a primary concern. Focusing on the task at hand and thinking through patient care activities are essential ways to promote safety.

- Do not perform any procedure on patients until you have received adequate training and do not alter the correct procedure (avoid shortcuts).

- Observe and note conditions in patients that might increase their risk of accident and injury. See Table 11–1.

- Be absolutely positive you have the correct patient. Always identify your patient with their wristband against the patient's record. In some health care settings, patients will not have a wristband (e.g., a physician's office). These patients can be identified by asking them to tell you their full name. Do not ask, "Are you Mr. Jones?" because many confused patients will reply affirmatively.

- Always verify that the patient has given consent, because patients have the right to refuse any procedure or medication.

- Observe patients closely and report any changes immediately and/or assist them as needed. Do not leave patients unattended on treatment tables.

- Leave the bed in low position, side rails up (if needed), wheels locked, and call signal, telephone, and bed controls within the patient's reach.

- Keep the work area clean, dry, and organized for efficient use. Place all supplies and equipment in their proper storage location.

Protecting Yourself and Others

Health care environments contain many potential hazards. It is essential to apply safety practices that consider the well-being of others:

- Follow the Standard Precautions discussed in Chapter 10.

- Do not open more than one file cabinet drawer at a time to prevent tipping.

- Do not leave cabinet doors open because someone may hit his or her head or trip.

- Do not place food in a refrigerator that contains lab specimens or medications.

- Do not wear uniforms in nonwork settings.

- Keep floors clear by immediately picking up dropped objects. Use OSHA standards when cleaning up glass, spilled specimens, and liquids. Broken glass is best picked up with a brush or broom and dustpan (Figure 11–1) and placed in puncture-resistant wrap or container, prior to placing in a plastic bag. This will prevent cuts on the hands of anyone who handles the bag. When the spill involves bodily secretions or blood, follow Standard Precautions by using gloves and disposing of waste in special bags designated for biohazardous waste. See Figure 11–2.

Table 11–1 Physical and Mental Changes that Increase the Risk of Injuries and Accidents

Physical or Mental Change	The Risk	Health Care Considerations
Changes in vision	Unable to see unsafe conditions and/or unable to judge distances	Identify yourself when approaching or entering the room. Provide unobstructed walkways. Place items needed by patients within their visual field. Explain the location of items orally.
Changes in hearing	Unable to hear warnings or approaching carts and equipment	Face the patient when speaking. Speak clearly, but do not yell. Notice when patients do not react to warning sounds.
Altered neurological function	Shaking or tremors can affect balance and increase the risk of falls; decreased sensation can prevent normal warning signals (e.g., can step on sharp object and not be aware of injury).	Pay increased attention to physical signs of injury. Give extra assistance, as needed. Do not leave patient alone or on treatment table or under any conditions where falls might occur.
Changes in blood vessels	Dizziness when attempting to stand and increased risk of falls	Instruct patients to get up slowly. Assist patients as necessary.
Slowed reflexes (automatic reactions that cause us to pull away from danger)	Unable to move away quickly from danger (e.g., removing hand from hot surface or from under hot water, or unable to stop in time to avoid collision)	Provide patient and family with information about possible unsafe behaviors and ways to safeguard the home.
Changes in mental function	Confusion and forgetfulness can impair good judgment and decrease awareness of common dangers.	Provide family with information about medications, home health resources, and safeguarding the home.
Weakness from illness or injury	More prone to falls	Observe patients carefully. Provide extra assistance. Instruct the family about extra precautions needed.
Taking medications	Side effects of some medications cause dizziness, visual disturbances, and other problems that increase the risk of injury.	Instruct patient and family about reporting symptoms immediately. Monitor patients carefully when administering medications and do not leave them alone immediately afterwards; watch for possible reactions.

Adapted from *Patient care: Basic skills for the health care provider*, by B. Acello, 1998, Albany, NY: Delmar.

Reporting for Safety

Properly reporting unsafe conditions and accidents provides a means of making corrections and preventing future problems.

■ Report any unsafe conditions immediately, such as burned out exit sign lights, equipment or flooring in need of repair, frayed electrical cords, and siderails or signal lights that don't work.

■ Report any accidents or injuries immediately and complete an incident report. An **incident report** is a written document completed when any unexpected situation occurs that can cause harm to a patient, employee, or any other person. It contains only factual information, and most facilities have policies that specify not to include the report in the patient's chart or to refer to it in the documentation.

FIRE AND ELECTRICAL HAZARDS

Fires in health care facilities can result from a number of hazards, such as damaged equipment, overloaded circuits, defects in heating systems,

spontaneous combustion, improper trash disposal, and smoking. It is important to familiarize yourself with the recommended policies and procedures for the health care facility in which you work. Once a fire starts, there is no time to read the policy and procedure manual, and valuable minutes are lost if you hesitate in acting promptly and correctly.

It is critical to stay calm during an emergency. A number of decisions must be made, and clear thinking is needed to properly assess the problem. If your safety is at risk, leave the area and sound the alarm. If the fire is small and contained, and your safety and that of others are not at risk, determine which type of extinguisher is appropriate to use and proceed with the proper handling procedure. Remember that your safety and that of others come first.

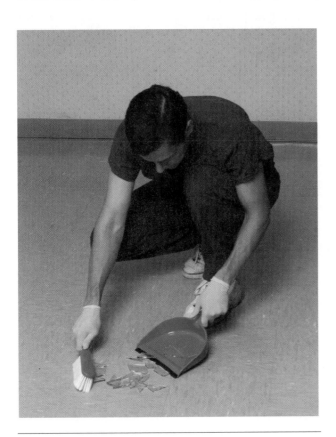

Figure 11–1 Sweep up broken glass. Wear gloves.

Thinking it Through

Peta Fry works as a respiratory therapist at a busy medical center. This particular day is busier than usual and it seems no matter how quickly Peta works, she cannot get her assignments done to keep on schedule. It is important to Peta to finish on time because she has a friend picking her up in front of the hospital right after work to go out for dinner. While working with Mrs. Homer, a bottle of water is accidentally tipped over because the patient did not see it due to her poor vision. Peta makes a mental note to call housekeeping when she finishes, so they can clean up the spill. When she finishes with Mrs. Homer, Peta realizes that she is going to be late and is afraid her friend will be upset. In an effort to save time, she decides not to change into the street clothes she brought with her to work and runs as quickly as she can to meet her friend.

1. Identify at least three behaviors of Peta that jeopardize environmental safety. What are the possible consequences of these unsafe behaviors?

2. What health care considerations could Peta have followed when working with the patient with impaired vision that may have prevented the bottle of water from spilling?

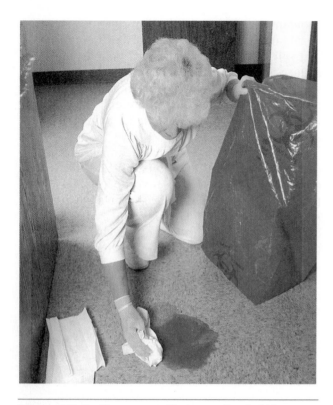

Figure 11–2 Clean up spills immediately. When bodily secretions or blood are involved, follow Standard Precautions.

Fires require three things to start: oxygen or air, an item that will burn to supply fuel (trash, linen, chemicals), and a source of heat (sparks, flames, matches). See Figure 11–3. To respond promptly and correctly to a fire, you must be knowledgeable in the following areas:

- The location of fire alarms and extinguishers
- How to use a fire extinguisher–carry the extinguisher upright. To help remember the proper sequence of operation, think **PASS**:
  1. **P**ull the pin
  2. **A**im the nozzle at the *base* of the fire
  3. **S**queeze the handle
  4. **S**weep back and forth along the *base* of the fire. See Figures 11–4a–c.
- How to respond to each type of fire. Fire extinguishers vary as to the type of fire. Using the wrong type of fire extinguisher can result in spreading a fire, rather than putting it out. See Table 11–2.

- The emergency evacuation routes. (See Figure 11–5.)
- What procedures to follow. Although procedures may vary at individual facilities, there are generally accepted guidelines to use when a fire occurs. These are outlined in Procedure 11–1. To help you remember the proper sequence, think **RACE**:
  1. **R**emove patients
  2. **A**ctivate Alarm
  3. **C**ontain the fire
  4. **E**xtinguish the fire or **E**vacuate the area (See Figure 11–6.)
- In case of a major fire, follow all instructions carefully. Your duties may include assisting patients into wheelchairs or onto stretchers. Advise ambulatory (able to walk) patients about evacuation routes.
- A policy that many facilities have is that no personal electrical equipment can be brought into the hospital because the possibility of it being defective is a fire risk. Larger facilities will have Environmental Safety personnel that verify the safety of facility equipment. Check the policy manual to determine if the Environmental Safety personnel will also check personal equipment. If so, they will attach a tag verifying the completion of the safety check.

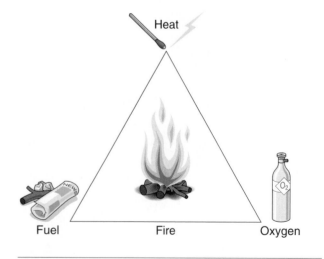

Figure 11–3 The fire triangle—elements needed for combustion (burning).

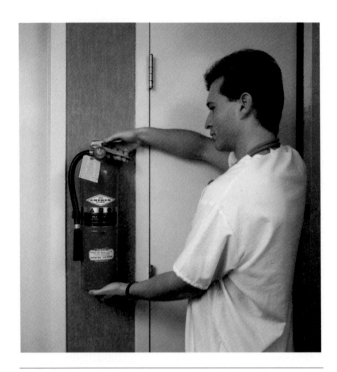

Figure 11–4a Verify that the fire extinguisher is the correct class to use.

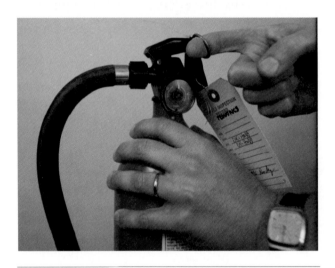

Figure 11–4b Pull the pin.

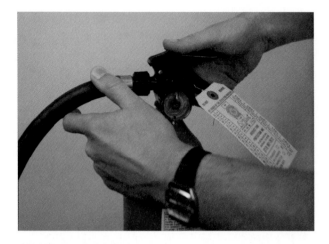

Figure 11–4c Aim the nozzle at base of the fire and squeeze the handle. Sweep back and forth along the base of the fire.

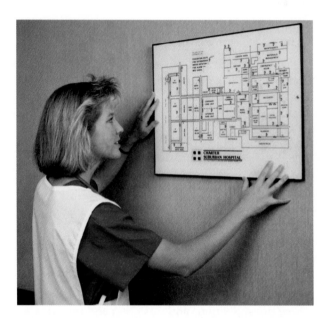

FIGURE 11–5 All personnel should be familiar with the emergency evacuation plan established by the facility in which they work.

TABLE 11–2 Types of Fires and How to Extinguish

Type of Fire	How to Extinguish	Cautions
Class A Most common type of fires (ordinary combustibles, such as paper, cloth, rubber, plastic, and wood fires e.g., trash or mattress fires)	Use either water, a Class A fire extinguisher, or a Class ABC fire extinguisher. Class A extinguishers are water-based and contain pressurized water or aqueous film-forming foam (AFFF). Class ABC extinguishers release a multipurpose dry chemical (monoammonium phosphate) that blankets the burning area and interrupts the chemical chain reaction.	Class A extinguishers—no special precautions; follow the proper sequence of operation (PASS) required with all extinguishers. Class ABC extinguishers—leave a white powdery residue irritating to skin and eyes. Do not stand too close to fire. Take care when using extinguisher. Wash skin as soon as possible after extinguishing fire. The chemical is corrosive and will damage computers and electrical equipment.
Class B **Flammable** (easily set on fire; same as **inflammable**) and combustible liquids (e.g., gas, oil, paint, solvents, and cooking fat fires)	Use Class B, BC, or Class ABC fire extinguishers. Class B extinguishers release carbon dioxide (CO_2) that forms a cloud of dry ice or snow. The cloud displaces air and cuts off the fire's oxygen supply, thereby providing a smothering action.	Do not use water or a Class A fire extinguisher on a Class B fire as most burning liquids will float on top of the water, which spreads the fire further. Class B extinguishers—no special precautions; they are noncorrosive and do not damage computers and other electrical equipment, but are heavy and have a shorter discharge range. Class ABC extinguishers—see above.
Class C Electrical fires (e.g., electrical equipment, fuse boxes, wiring, and appliances)	Use Class C, BC, or ABC extinguisher. Same as Class B because carbon dioxide is used, which is nonconducting and provides a smothering action.	Do not use water or Class A extinguisher on this type of fire unless the electricity has been disconnected. Electrical fires are particularly hazardous because the possibility of electrocution is present. Class ABC extinguishers—see above.
Class D Burning metals (not typically seen in the health care environment)	Use Class D extinguisher or smother with dry sand. Class D extinguishers release a sodium chloride powder, that when heated, forms a crust. The crust excludes air and fire is smothered.	Do not use any of the other types of fire extinguishers on this type of fire.

PROCEDURE 11-1

What to Do When You Discover a Fire

Procedure	Rationale
R Remove any patient who is in danger. Ambulatory patients can walk to safety; others may need wheelchairs or can be pushed in beds. Never use elevators during a fire; instead, carry nonambulatory patients in a linen sling, held at each end by a health care worker, while descending steps.	Places patient safety first. Fires can travel through elevator shafts, cables can be damaged, and elevators can get stalled between floors if power fails.
A Activate the fire alarm and notify the facility telephone operator/receptionist.	Pulling the fire alarm sends an alarm call to the fire station. The facility telephone operator(s) are often key to communication, and an exact location of the fire should be given to them.
C Contain the fire by closing all windows and doors. Follow facility procedure for turning off oxygen and electrical equipment.	Decreases the amount of air available to the fire. Drafts (air currents) cause fire to spread more rapidly. Prevents explosions and further fueling of the fire.
E Extinguish small fires with an extinguisher. Stand 6–10 feet from the nearest edge of the flame and aim at the base of the fire. For large fires, follow or start evacuation procedures.	Allows for immediate extinguishing of fire before it spreads further. If fire is too large, do not attempt to put out; instead, use that time to initiate further evacuation procedures.
Keep exits clear at all times.	Allows patients and workers to leave if necessary.
Maintain an exit at all times—never let the fire get between you and the exit.	Traps the health care worker and patients in a confined area.
If smoke is present, workers and patients should crawl or move close to the floor toward the exit.	Decreases inhalation of smoke because smoke rises. More oxygen is available closer to the floor. All fires give off toxic gases, which are in the smoke.
A damp towel or similar cloth may be used to cover the mouth and nose for breathing.	Decreases the temperature of inhaled air and filters soot particles from the air.
Always check the temperature of a door before opening it. If a door is hot to the touch, do not open it. If you are trapped in a room and the door is hot to the touch, stay in the room (lie on floor for more oxygen and less smoke) and place wet towels or blankets under door.	Prevents burns caused by a sudden burst of flames escaping room when door is opened. Wet towels decrease the smoke entering the room.

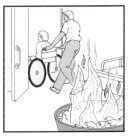
Remove

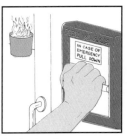
Activate alarm

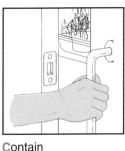
Contain

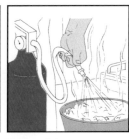
Extinguish or

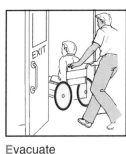
Evacuate

Figure 11-6 Remember the sequence of critical actions to follow in case of fire.

Most electrical hazards can be avoided by following a few general safety practices:

- Always be thoroughly familiar with any equipment before attempting to use it independently for the first time. Know and follow all safety precautions.

- Review and follow the manufacturer's operating instructions. The health care worker should not use shortcuts or experiment with unfamiliar equipment.

- If any damage to the equipment is noted, do not attempt to use it, but report it to the proper person for repair. If the health care worker is not trained in the repair of a particular piece of equipment, he or she should never attempt to repair it.

- Never use electrical cords that are not completely intact, use plugs that have been altered (i.e., have third prong removed), or use excessive force to insert plug into an outlet.

- Never handle any electrical equipment around water because electrocution can occur (water conducts electrical currents). Holding electrical equipment with wet hands, standing in water, or removing equipment that has been accidentally dropped in water can be life threatening. Always dry hands, clean up any spilled water, and remove the power source.

- If someone is being shocked (electrically), do not touch the person or pull the plug from the wall because this places you at risk. Instead, turn the main source of power off immediately and be prepared to administer emergency care and call for help.

CHEMICAL HAZARDS

Hundreds of chemicals are used in health care, such as cleaning solutions, anesthesia, and drugs used for chemotherapy. Chemicals can often cause harm if swallowed, inhaled, or absorbed through the skin or mucous membranes. Some also create a fire hazard. Great care must be taken when working with or near these agents. As discussed in Chapter 10, OSHA requires all health care facilities to have an exposure control plan. In addition, Material Safety Data Sheets (MSDS) must be available to all employees. The MSDS includes the precautions to take when handling the chemical, safety instructions for use, requirements for clean-up and disposal, and first aid measures to take if exposure occurs. See Figure 11-7. There are some general guidelines that apply whenever chemicals are handled:

- If the container is not properly labeled or if it cannot be read clearly, do not use it.

- Recheck labels at least three times. Read the label carefully when you first locate it, and then reread it after removing the solution, and again before returning it to its proper location.

- Never mix any two chemicals together without first verifying **compatibility** (can be combined without unfavorable results).

- Avoid contact with the eyes and skin and do not inhale.

- Take precautions not to slash or spill solutions.

- Wear PPE (personal protective equipment) as indicated.

- Make sure chemicals are used only for their intended purpose.

- Store chemicals as directed on the labels. For example, does the chemical require room temperature storage or refrigeration? Can it be stored on the counter or does it require a dark environment? Never place chemicals in direct sunlight or close to heat.

- Do not pour **toxic** (poisonous), flammable, foul-smelling, or irritating chemicals down the drain. Instead place them in the specified container as per the policy and procedure manual.

■ If you spill any solutions, clean up immediately according to established procedures and dispose of the debris properly.

■ If a chemical does come in contact with the skin, rinse immediately under cool water for at least 5 minutes. Splashes in the eye should be rinsed a minimum of 15 minutes, preferably with normal saline. Report any accidents immediately to the supervisor and seek medical assistance for evaluation and follow-up.

RADIATION HAZARDS

Health care workers in areas where x-rays or radiation therapy are used must practice safety precautions to prevent exposure to radiation waves and particles. Excessive radiation exposure can put the employee at risk for developing tissue damage, contracting cancer, or becoming sterile (unable to have children), or may lead to infants being born with birth defects. Employees at risk for radiation exposure must wear safety monitoring film badges that record the amount of exposure. Safety guidelines have been developed that determine the maximum level of radiation exposure allowed per employee.

There are strict guidelines for the proper disposal of radiological waste. Radioactive waste must be placed in a special container and labeled as "radioactive." It should never be placed in the trash, incinerated, placed in a bag with other waste products, or put down a drain. Only a licensed removal facility can remove these wastes from the health care facility.

INFECTIOUS WASTE

Infectious waste is any item or product that has the potential to transmit disease. Infectious waste must be handled using standard and transmission-based precautions, placed in containers or bags labeled as to type of waste (e.g., linen, sharps, trash), decontaminated onsite, or removed by a licensed removal facility for decontamination. It is the health care worker's responsibility to follow the facility's policies and procedures in the proper handling, containment, clean-up of spills, and disposal of infectious waste. Any direct contact with waste that puts the worker at risk for infection should be reported per facility policy.

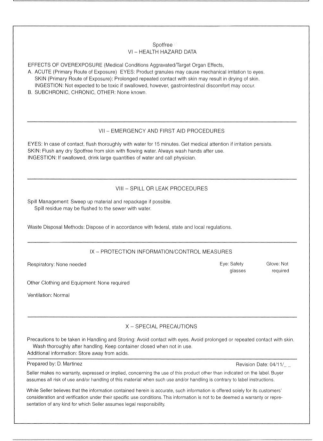

Figure 11–7 Example of a Material Safety Data Sheet (MSDS). (Courtesy of The Clorox Company, Pleasanton, CA.)

OXYGEN PRECAUTIONS

When a patient is unable to take in adequate oxygen on his or her own, the physician may order the administration of oxygen. The physician will order how much oxygen to give, what device to use for oxygen delivery (Figures 11–8a–b), and how long it is to be administered.

Special precautions are necessary when oxygen is in use:

- Most facilities have signs stating "Oxygen in Use" that are posted as specified in the facility policy.
- Sparks may come from some electrical appliances, equipment ,or toys. Before using any of these, always check with the supervisor. Examples include hair dryers, heating pads, space heaters, fans, radios, electric shavers, and hand-held computer games.
- Never use flammable liquids, such as alcohol, oils, adhesive tape remover, nail polish, or nail polish remover.
- An oxygen tank should be secured to prevent it from falling over. Do not place it in the sunlight or near heat.
- Smoking is not allowed when oxygen is in use, and smoking materials must be removed from the room. Fortunately, most facilities no longer allow smoking at any time, due to the health risk to the person and others. Always be alert for those who disregard the rules. No lighted matches or open flames should be permitted in the area.
- Use cotton blankets, gowns, or clothing. Wool and synthetics are more apt to create static electricity.

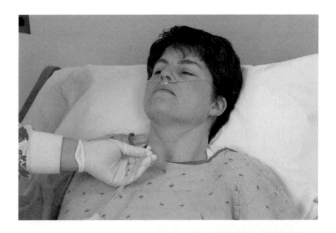

Figure 11–8a Oxygen being delivered by nasal cannula.

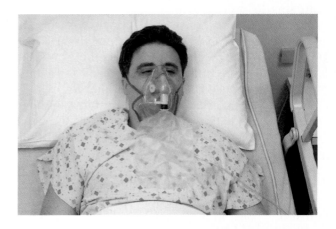

Figure 11–8b Oxygen being delivered by mask.

EMERGENCY DISASTER PLAN

OSHA requires health care facilities to have an **emergency disaster plan** for handling large numbers of patients in the event of a catastrophic event such as an earthquake, a flood, a tornado, a hurricane, or a bombing. It is the responsibility of health care workers to be familiar with the requirements and understand their roles. Procedures will vary based on type of facility, but some examples of what may be included are:

- Whether you should report to work
- How to protect yourself and your patients
- Your specific duties
- How to get communications and updates.

Whatever your role, always remain calm. This will help you think clearly, as well as provide needed stability to those who are confused, injured, and frightened. This is a critical time for the health care team to work efficiently and cooperatively.

The following general guidelines are to be followed when an emergency disaster plan is in effect:

- Stay calm. There will be a great deal of chaos and confusion in a severe disaster, but panic can escalate the fear and related difficulties. Everyone involved will benefit from an approach by the health care worker that communicates control of the situation, competence, and compassion.
- Know who is in charge and report your availability.
- Report to person in charge at regular intervals for further directions or changes in assignments.
- If unsure about what to do in a particular situation, ask someone in authority.
- Communicate clearly and be cooperative.
- Use telephones only for official business, not for personal calls.

Triage

An effectively managed disaster response rests on an established **triage system**. Triage is a French word that means "to select." Specially trained personnel follow established triage guidelines to assess patients' conditions and determine where they should be sent and what treatment they should receive.

Triage systems are not just for major natural disasters, but are also used in the emergency room when there are multiple patients needing medical care. For example, a bus accident with multiple passengers or a passenger train that derails, sending multiple victims to the emergency room. When there are multiple victims, the available services are overstrained, so the triage personnel must determine who to treat first, what lab or diagnostic tests receive priority, what procedures to perform immediately, and who to send to surgery. They continually reassess patients who are waiting for services to determine if their condition has changed and if their priority needs to be updated.

A less obvious triage system is in place at all times in the Emergency Department. For example, there may be a patient waiting to be seen for an earache or another who fell off a bike and may have a possible broken collar bone. Then a third patient arrives with complaints of chest pain and may be having a heart attack. The patient with the potential heart attack will be seen first, because his or her need is more urgent, and lack of immediate care could lead to death.

SUGGESTED LEARNING ACTIVITIES

1. Visit your local fire station and ask for information about common fire hazards, prevention, use of fire extinguishers, and availability of training sessions for the public.
2. When you enter a health care facility, look for the fire alarms and evacuation route plan (usually posted on a wall).
3. Look around your own home and when you are out in public. What potential hazards can you identify?
4. If someone in your family required oxygen to be administered at home, would anything need to be changed to make the situation safe?

REVIEW QUESTIONS

1. What are the general safety guidelines to prevent injuries and accidents in the health care workplace?
2. What are the different hazards commonly encountered in a health care environment?
3. What are the physical and mental impairments that make patients more prone to injuries and accidents?
4. What is an incident report, and when should it be completed?
5. What do RACE and PASS mean?
6. What types of portable fire extinguishers are available? How would you decide which one to use? What are the precautions for their use?
7. What are the guidelines for preventing electrical hazards?
8. What precautions must be taken when oxygen is being administered, and why?
9. What is an emergency disaster plan, and what is the health care worker's role?
10. What is the meaning of "triage"?

APPLICATION EXERCISES

1. Refer back to The Case of the Bomb Threat at the beginning of the chapter and answer these questions:

   a. What would have been the possible consequences if Mrs. Welks had acted on her initial response to flee, call home, or yell out for an evacuation?

   b. How could the outcome of this situation be affected by obtaining more information as to location of the bomb and what time it was set to explode?

   c. Why do you think she was trying to listen so carefully to the voice and background noise?

   d. What should Mrs. Welks do when the telephone call is terminated?

   e. Should an Emergency Disaster Plan be initiated?

2. While at work, Jack Thompson, a health care worker, smells smoke and goes to investigate. He discovers the trashcan in the restroom has smoke billowing from it, and he runs to get a fire extinguisher. The fire extinguisher is not where he thought it was, and by the time he returns to the restroom, there is smoke coming out from under the door. Jack opens the door, pulls the pin out of the extinguisher, moves as close as he can to the flames, and aims directly down into the trash can. He then hears someone coughing in one of the bathroom stalls and discovers a patient slumped on the floor. Jack pulls the patient out of the bathroom, but in the process, some of the white powdery residue from the fire extinguisher gets on the patient's skin. Jack is pleased with his actions and thinks to himself, "This patient might have died if I hadn't smelled the smoke and put the fire out."

   a. Evaluate the scenario to determine if Jack followed the recommended procedure. Did he follow RACE and PASS?

   b. What revisions to Jack's actions would have to occur to ensure safety for him, patients, and coworkers?

   c. Can you determine from the information given which class of fire extinguisher was used? Was it the correct extinguisher for a trash fire?

   d. Is it of concern that the patient has some of the white powdery residue on his skin?

SUGGESTED READINGS AND RESOURCES

American Association of Poison Control Centers: http://www.aapcc.org

Klinoff, R. (1997). *Introduction to fire protection.* Albany, NY: Delmar.

National Safety Council: http://www.nsc.org

UNIT

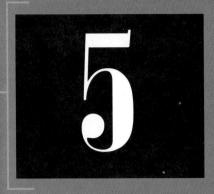

BEHAVIORS FOR SUCCESS

LIFESTYLE MANAGEMENT

OBJECTIVES

Studying and applying the material in this chapter will help you to:

■ Explain the importance of developing a healthy lifestyle.

■ State the principles of habit formation.

■ Describe the following components of healthy living: diet, exercise, sleep, and preventive measures.

■ Define stress and list several common causes.

■ Describe five ways of effectively dealing with stress.

■ Explain the major health risks encountered by the health care worker.

■ List the causes, symptoms, and preventive measures for burnout.

■ Explain how patients can be assisted in developing good health habits.

KEY TERMS

aerobic

anorexia nervosa

assertiveness

attitude

binge eating

bulimia

burnout

calories

carbohydrate

cholesterol

fat

fiber

meditation

food guide pyramid

prioritize

protein

relaxation

stress

stressor

The Case of
the Cardiac Unit Nurse

Gracie Chin is a registered nurse working in the cardiac care unit at a large metropolitan hospital. Many of the patients in the unit are recovering from open heart surgery and require continual monitoring and attention. Gracie works three 12-hour shifts each week, and her duties require that she be on her feet during much of that time. She checks each patient frequently and performs such tasks as turning and bathing patients, adjusting the levels of their beds, placing patients on and removing them from bedpans, repositioning and maintaining equipment, and reaching to change intravenous fluid bags or adjust monitoring devices that are located above bed level. In addition to the physical requirements of her job, Gracie must remain mentally alert throughout her shift. Her work requires keen observation skills and good judgement because in patient care, there is no room for error. She must also deal with the stress of working with patients who suffer from serious, often fatal conditions. In this chapter you will learn about personal habits that enable health care workers like Gracie to maintain the physical and mental fitness necessary to promote their own and their patients' welfare.

IMPORTANCE OF A HEALTHY LIFESTYLE

The human body consists of systems that are extremely complex and delicately balanced. Cared for properly, the average body is capable of repairing itself and giving many years of service.

One's state of wellness is largely under one's own control. While the causes of many conditions are still unknown, the top three causes of death–heart disease, cancer, and stroke–in the United States today are often influenced by personal habits. Unlike previous generations who did not understand the causes of and ways to prevent disease, we have the knowledge and power to make healthy choices. To a great extent, individuals today can choose what to eat, how to deal with stress, and how much to exercise each day. Opportunities to raise our level of wellness lie within us, but *each person must accept the responsibility to take advantage of these opportunities.*

Practicing good health habits is especially important for the health care worker. The health professions require adequate physical energy and the ability to handle stress, two important benefits of healthy living practices. Health care workers owe it to themselves and to their patients, employers, and families to take care of themselves. In this way their effectiveness and level of professional contributions are increased.

In addition, today's health care worker has an important responsibility to serve as a role model for patients. Patient education is a growing part of the health care worker's duties, because patients are assuming more responsibility for their own health. People tend to learn more from example than from words and advice. The behavior of the health care worker can have a positive effect on others.

Habits and Health

Maximizing health often requires a change in habits, and this is not always easy. As you read this chapter, you may find that there are areas you would like to improve. Perhaps it is to improve time management skills, develop an exercise program, or change eating habits. Being *willing* to change current behavior is the first step. Here are some additional ideas for changing old habits and developing new ones:

1. Recognize that it may not be easy at first. Accepting this fact will help prevent you from becoming discouraged in the beginning.

2. Be patient with yourself. Changes do not occur overnight.

3. Set reasonable goals. Do not try to make so many changes at once that you feel defeated from the start.

4. Focus on the positive. Think about the long-term benefits you will enjoy.

5. Track your progress. Make a chart, write a journal or diary, or create another personal recording system.

6. Plan rewards for your achievements.

Some habits, such as smoking, involve the use of addictive substances. These habits are particularly difficult to change. Many people have found that seeking professional assistance or participating in self-help groups is the most effective way of dealing with these addictive behaviors.

COMPONENTS OF HEALTHY LIVING

The purpose of attaining good health is more than hoping to prevent disease and extend the length of life. It includes improving the *quality* of life. It means waking up refreshed with the energy and well-being necessary to enjoy each day. The following sections of this chapter contain general guidelines and suggestions for achieving maximum wellness. What is appropriate for each individual will vary. Identify your strengths and weaknesses, and develop a plan that works for you.

Proper Diet

Diet has been proven repeatedly to contribute to the promotion of good health and prevention of disease. Excessive weight is a major health problem in the United States. It is estimated that at least 33% of adults in the United States are overweight (www.coloradohealthnet.org). The number may be actually closer to 50%, according to recent reports, because official statistical reports lag by several years and the trend is toward higher numbers of overweight individuals. Excess weight contributes to a number of uncomfortable conditions as well as serious diseases:

- Shortness of breath
- Back and joint pains
- Reduced ability to enjoy physical activities
- Diabetes mellitus
- High blood pressure
- Heart disease
  (National Institutes of Health, Federal Obesity Clinical Guidelines, 1998)

Recent studies also show that excess weight may contribute to breast and other forms of cancer. (National Institutes of Health, Federal Obesity Clinical Guidelines, 1998).

The percentage of overweight Americans continues to grow even as we learn more about the benefits of diet and exercise. There is disagreement among health professionals and researchers about why this is occurring. The majority view is that individuals who are overweight take in more **calories** (energy content of foods) than are needed for daily activities. The body stores unused energy in the form of fat. Losing weight and maintaining a healthy weight requires reducing the number of calories taken in and/or increasing the level of activity.

Another opinion currently gaining popularity among individuals who are trying to lose weight is based on the theory that excess weight is the result of eating too many carbohydrates. **Carbohydrates** are food substances which are composed of units of sugars and provide the body with immediate energy. Common sources of carbohydrates include fruits, breads, cereals, and pasta. Recommendations include drastically cutting down the number of carbohydrates in the diet, while increasing the intake of proteins and fats. **Proteins** are food substances that contain amino acids, necessary for both building and maintaining the structural components of the body. Common sourses of proteins are meat and eggs. **Fats** consist of fatty acids and provide the most concentrated form of energy for the body. In addition to oils and butter, fats are found in meats, fish, nuts, eggs, and certain plants such as olives and avocados.

Proponents of low-carbohydrate diets claim that they result in weight loss as well as other benefits, such as lowering **cholesterol** (fatty substance that can clog artery walls) levels. At the same time, opponents warn that drastically reducing carbohydrates while increasing the intake of proteins and fats is too extreme and dangerous to overall health. They also point out that many people find restrictive diets too difficult to maintain and eventually return to their previous eating habits with a corresponding weight gain.

In fact there are many reasons for the increasing number of overweight Americans. These include:

- Lack of active recreational exercise
- Number of hours spent watching television and using the computer
- Heavy use of the automobile
- Consumption of processed foods that contain high amounts of sugar, as well as fats
- Increase in technology and decrease in tasks that require manual labor

Decreased activity results in a loss of muscle mass, which in turn leads to a decreased number of calories needed to maintain the body's weight, because muscle tissue uses more energy to support itself than does fat tissue. Lack of exercise contributes to increased weight both by lowering the number of calories burned throughout the day and by reducing the body's caloric requirements.

Eating disorders, often the result of a fear of obesity and the desire to conform to an unrealistic body image, are a growing problem. The three most common conditions are:

1. **Anorexia nervosa**: The distorted belief that one is overweight, even when severely underweight, and the cutting of calories below the number necessary to maintain health. Exact causes are not known but may be related to social pressures to achieve the unrealistic slimness promoted by the entertainment industry and fashion models. Anorexia can be life-threatening, ending in death by starvation. Medical intervention is almost always necessary, and hospitalization may be required.

2. **Bulimia**: A condition characterized by the compulsive eating of huge quantities of food, followed by self-induced vomiting and/or the use of large amounts of laxatives. These actions may be accompanied by feelings of guilt and the fear of being "found out." Stomach acids in vomit may cause the erosion of tooth enamel, development of dental cavities, and eating away of the esophagus.

3. **Binge eating**: The compulsive consumption of large quantities of food, beyond that needed to satisfy hunger. This uncontrolled eating is sometimes used as an escape from boredom, as a means to handle anger, and for other reasons related to handling emotional issues.

Medical assistance, counseling, and support groups offer help with various eating disorders.

The best practice among otherwise healthy individuals who are not suffering from an eating disorder is to avoid extremes and eat a variety of healthy and appealing foods. Eating patterns begin early, so children should be encouraged to develop good eating habits. This is especially important today because there is a growing number of children today who are obese. They will suffer the consequences of poor eating habits throughout their lives.

It is important to choose foods that provide all the nutrients needed for maintaining body functions and good health. This includes an adequate supply of vitamins and minerals. Vitamins and minerals are both essential to life and perform various functions: building and repairing body tissue, regulating fluids and body processes, and enabling the body to use the energy supplied by foods.

Improving eating habits may require the individual to make significant adjustments, because the typical American diet contains many processed foods that are high in calories and low in nutritive value and fiber. Fiber contributes to a sense a fullness and signals the body to stop eating. In addition, many people eat on the run and depend on fast food suppliers—or worse, vending machines—for at least one of their daily meals. The United States Department of Agriculture has developed an eating plan, known as the **food guide pyramid**, for ensuring that the daily diet contains all the components necessary for good health. See Figure 12–1.

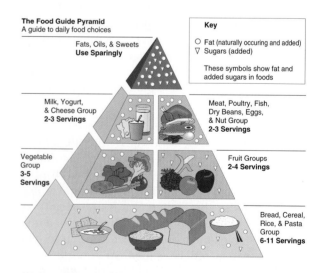

Figure 12–1 The Food Guide Pyramid contains recommended daily servings from the five major food groups (Courtesy of the U.S. Department of Agriculture).

Other important recommendations when planning a healthy diet include:

- Eat moderate amounts. Go for flavor, not quantity.
- Look for nutritional value. Find foods you enjoy eating that contain essential nutrients.
- Avoid excessive amounts of salt and sugar. Everyone enjoys a chocolate bar, popcorn, or bag of chips from time to time, but these should not be eaten every day or substituted for meals.
- Eat adequate amounts of **fiber**, food that cannot be fully digested. This helps maintain colon health by forcing the muscles to work to remove the fiber from the body. The main sources of fiber are vegetables, cereals, and fruits.
- Prepare your own sack lunches and dinners. Find foods that can be carried well such as fruits, raw vegetables, nuts, seeds, cheeses, and peanut butter. (Note: while the last four foods listed are high in calories, eaten *in moderation,* they are good sources of protein.
- Eat slowly and enjoy each bite. You may find that you are satisfied sooner and don't need to eat as much.
- Drink lots of water: six to eight glasses a day. This is one of the easiest, yet most overlooked, weight control methods available. It is also essential for good health. The body consists of 55–65% water and depends on it to bathe cells and tissues, remove waste, and dissolve substances necessary for normal body function (Fong, 1998).
- Take vitamins, as needed, to make up for nutrients not provided in your diet.

Stress, anxiety, and boredom are sometimes the cause of overeating. If you believe this to be true for you, try the stress-reducing techniques discussed later in this chapter. Eliminating the causes of overeating may not only resolve a weight problem, but can improve other areas of life as well.

Sufficient Exercise

Like diet, exercise has been found to have a significant influence on health. Its many benefits include the following:

- Promotes feelings of well-being through the body's production of endorphins, substances that naturally raise the pain threshold and produce sedative effects (Miller-Keane, 1997)
- Relieves stress and improves mental outlook

- Improves the quality of sleep
- Helps with weight control
- Increases energy level

Exercise is also believed to raise the body's resistance to various diseases, including heart disease and certain types of cancer. The heart is a muscle and needs regular exercise that forces it to work by increasing the heart beat beyond its normal resting rate. This type of exercise, known as **aerobic**, increases the heart's strength.

In addition to periods of planned exercise, activity should be incorporated into daily life. A few alterations can result in a built-in exercise program that does not take too much time in an already busy life. Here are a few ideas:

- Whenever possible, leave the car at home. Walk to the store, library, church, and so on. When using the car, park at the far end of the mall or grocery store parking lot.
- Use the stairs instead of elevators.
- Wash the car instead of going to the car wash.
- Do jobs yourself that require physical effort, such as mowing the lawn and washing windows.
- Find a sport or activity you enjoy, such as swimming or dancing. Or shoot baskets with the kids and walk around the neighborhood with a friend. Substitute activity for a few hours of television each week.

Adequate Sleep

An adequate amount of sleep is necessary because it is during sleep that the body recuperates from the day's activities. Body functions slow down and its temperature drops. It is believed that during that the last few hours of sleep before awakening, the time when most dreams occur, mental recuperation takes place. The brain is preparing itself for learning and taking in new information (Miller-Keane, 1997). This is why it is especially important that students and others who are engaged in learning activities make it a point to get enough sleep. "Enough" varies among individuals, but is generally believed to be 6 to 9 hours for adults.

Sleep provides the energy necessary to function efficiently throughout the day and deal with stress. Getting enough sleep is a good investment because it can increase productivity. Busy students may appreciate the benefits, but are wondering just how to get the recommended amount of sleep when trying to balance the responsibilities of school, work, family, and personal activities. This is a common problem. Here are some suggestions for increasing the length and quality of sleep:

- Avoid caffeine–found in coffee, tea, cola drinks, and chocolate–late in the day if it keeps you awake.

- Try to avoid stressful activities or communications just before going to bed.

- Keep a "worry log" to write down things to think about at a set "worry time." Keep the "appointment" and use the time to focus on finding solutions. Knowing that it is possible to get back to worries later can help clear the mind at bedtime.

- Use the time management techniques described later in this chapter to increase personal efficiency and increase the time available for sleep.

- Engage in some form of exercise each day, but avoid very vigorous exercise just before going to bed.

- Develop a routine for getting ready for bed and try to use it every day. This will signal the body to become sleepy.

- Keep the bed for sleeping. Don't do homework and other chores there or the body may program itself to become alert when getting into bed.

Preventive Measures

Many health problems can be avoided by practicing preventive measures. These include:

- Regular visits to physician or health care practitioner for routine checkups. See Figure 12-2.

- Periodic screening for risks associated with your gender and age group.

- Regular visits to the dentist and the practice of proper dental hygiene, including regular flossing. Most gum disease, which can cause the loss of teeth, can be avoided. Untreated tooth decay and abscesses can result in serious infections in other parts of the body.

- Treatment of illnesses in their early stages. Positive outcomes are more likely with early treatment.

- Immunizations. Many health care employers offer hepatitis B vaccinations for all employees whose work requires them to be exposed to body substances.

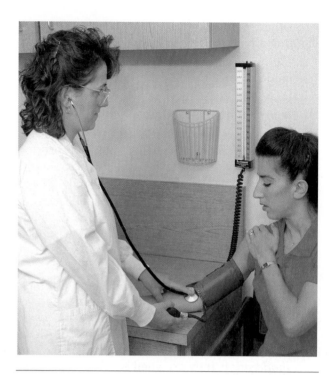

Figure 12–2 Regular checkups are important for maintaining good health.

STRESS IN MODERN LIFE

Stress refers to the body's reactions when it responds to danger, either real or imagined. In seeking a state of readiness for action, the body undergoes a series of physical changes that include:

- Increased heart rate

- Elevated blood pressure

- Raised level of blood sugar

- Dilated blood vessels in the muscles to give them the immediate use of sugar

- Dilated pupils of eyes (Miller-Keane, 1997)

These reactions, characteristic of the "fight or flight response" introduced in Chapter 7, serve individuals well when they must protect themselves or run from the scene. But the body cannot distinguish between physical danger and fears and worries experienced in the mind. For example, worries about losing a job or handling financial problems create the same reaction as being in danger of physical attack. When psychological pressures are continuous or occur frequently, the body can literally wear itself out making preparations to face danger. Responses originally meant to be helpful become sources of harm.

Thinking it Through

Mikel Korsov is a recent graduate of a licensed practical nurse program. He has been hired to work in the pediatric ward at Samuelson Hospital. Mikel loves working with children and has a real talent for calming their fears and helping them cope with necessary procedures and medications. He finds, however, that he is physically exhausted at the end of each day. He has little energy left to do much more than drag himself home, eat whatever is available or quick to prepare, and then watch television until bedtime. Mikel weighs about 60 pounds more than the weight suggested for his height and does not participate in much physical exercise beyond that required on the job.

1. What might be the long-term consequences of Mikel's current habits? Consider this from both personal and professional viewpoints.
2. Discuss the possible impact of his health habits on the attitudes of his patients regarding their health.
3. Suggest five things he can do that can help increase his energy level.

Research studies in recent years have focused on finding a correlation between stress and various illnesses. While the evidence is not conclusive, some researchers and physicians believe that the experience of chronic stress weakens the body's immune system. This reduces the body's ability to defend itself against disease. Stress is also believed by some to contribute to high blood pressure, heart disease, cancer, and other diseases. In addition to possibly increasing the risk of serious health problems, excessive stress interferes with personal effectiveness, productivity, relationships, and the enjoyment of life.

External and Internal Stressors

Modern life presents many **stressors** (causes of stress). External stressors are those outside one's immediate control. They include the fast pace of life, the high cost of living, crowded cities and freeways, demanding patients, and physical disabilities. We have limited control over external stressors, although changes can be made in how we perceive and deal with them. (See the section on attitude in this chapter.)

Internal stressors are self-generated and within the individual's control. Examples include a negative attitude, unrealistic goals, poor time management skills, and lack of problem-solving ability. Internal stressors can be controlled by acquiring additional skills, making changes in personal habits, and adjusting one's mental outlook.

Dealing with Stress

There will always be stressors in life. The future may bring achievements and satisfaction, but there is no perfect job or ideal set of conditions that is stress-free. And some degree of stress is healthy because it provides the motivation for action. Health care work, by its very nature, can be stressful because workers must be able to:

- Interact with people who are ill or injured
- Remain calm in difficult situations
- Remain constantly attentive
- Apply thinking skills
- Perform tasks accurately
- Work under time constraints
- Respond to changing needs of patients and the facility

Dealing effectively with stress starts with identifying the major stressors in life. Are they internal or external? Which are within your control? Are you adding to your own stress level with ineffective personal habits? Which stressors are outside your control and require adaptive and coping techniques?

Marcos, a respiratory therapy student, worries that his class assignments are never quite good enough. He goes over each one several times, reworking them until they are "perfect." As a result, Marcos frequently turns in assignments late and never feels caught up. The need for perfection is causing Marcos stress and may be a serious problem when he becomes employed. Workplace tasks, while needing to be performed correctly, must also be completed in a timely way. Knowing when work is satisfactory can alleviate unnecessary stress.

Setting Priorities

Stress can be created by the inability to prioritize. **Prioritizing** means ranking items that need to be done in order of importance. Adult students often experience conflicts between their many responsibilities. School and work are priorities and, at times, choices must be made in order to reduce stress. Ellen, a mother of three, agreed to serve on a parents' committee at her children's school. After enrolling in a dental hygiene program, she found that she did not have the time for both the committee meetings and responsibilities, and studying for her classes. She completed the tasks she had already committed to do, then met with the chairperson to explain her situation and resigned from the committee.

Examining your values and determining which current activities will result in long-term benefits can help you decide what is most important to you. Where can you make compromises now in exchange for future benefits? The time and effort you invest in your studies, for example, will determine your future employment success. And time spent with children is essential to their healthy development. See Figure 12–3. The ability to prioritize will continue to be an important skill both on the job and as you balance professional, family, and personal responsibilities.

Time Management

Poor time management is a major cause of stress. Fortunately, it is possible to have more control over time than we may realize. While it is impossible to increase the number of hours in a day, the ones that are available can be used more effectively. Improving the use of time can reduce stress, improve personal performance, and increase feelings of personal power.

Start by doing an honest review of your daily habits. It will help to keep a record for a week, listing the amount of time spent on each activity. Are there hours when time is simply "killed" instead of being used effectively or enjoyed? Television, the telephone, and the Internet can eat up hours. They may not provide enjoyment in proportion to the time spent. Are there others? Is

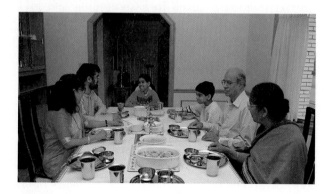

Figure 12–3 Time spent with family and friends is an important priority.

there adequate time built in for resting and thinking, or is everything too rushed? Are there actions you can take to prevent a future crisis that can be very time-consuming? Try prioritizing activities to identify those that bring the most benefits and/or enjoyment for the time invested.

Procrastination is a stress-producer for many people. This is illustrated by Mohammed, a health information management student. He has assignments that are due throughout the semester. Last semester he was in a continual state of panic and last minute rushes to complete them. Unexpected delays and interruptions created a sense of emergency. Feelings of desperation mounted and made it difficult to concentrate. Mohammed thought about why he procrastinates and realized that he was afraid to start projects because they seemed overwhelming. He developed the following plan:

1. Break large projects into smaller steps that are more manageable.

2. Set completion dates for each step, starting with the project deadline and moving backwards on the calendar.

3. Schedule time to work each day or every other day in order to feel a sense of accomplishment and keep the project moving. (It is important to work even when not in the mood for it.)

4. Seek appropriate help and gather information as needed.

5. Focus on the feelings of accomplishment and control being experienced.

There are many time management techniques that can be incorporated into a busy daily schedule:

- Keep a calendar of assignments, tests, field-trips, appointments, birthdays, and other "must-remember" activities.

- Write a daily to-do list in the order of most to least important tasks. At the end of each day, cross off completed tasks and carry over undone tasks for the next day.

- When possible, do the hardest things first.

- Keep other lists to help stay organized: shopping, freezer contents, children's chores.

- Organize errands so that several can be accomplished in one trip.

- Keep things in their place so that time is not wasted looking for them.

- At work, know the priorities of your supervisor and/or department.

Time management is a critical work skill. With emphasis on cost containment and efficiency, health care workers are expected to use time well

Thinking it Through

Janice Nelson, dental assistant for Dr. Grady, is worried about the conversation she had with Dr. Grady this afternoon. He spoke with her privately and expressed concern about her time management practices. He pointed out that Janice had arrived late for work three times in the last two weeks, had left early one day due to child-care problems, and had several times failed to complete assigned work tasks in the designated time. Dr. Grady explained that in a small practice with only a few employees, Janice was having a significant impact on work flow in the office. He warned her that she must improve if she was to continue working there.

1. Discuss the possible impact of Janice's actions on patients, coworkers, and Dr. Grady.
2. Suggest ways that Janice can improve her personal organization and time management.

Box 12–1   Muscle Relaxation Technique

1. Choose a time and place where you can arrange not to be interrupted.

2. Sit in a comfortable position with the spine straight and feet flat on the floor.

3. Starting at the toes, tighten the muscles of each section of the body, experience the feeling of tension, and then relax. Move up as follows:

   A. Toes (flex)
   B. Legs
   C. Hips and abdomen
   D. Chest and upper back
   E. Hands (make a fist) and arms
   F. Shoulders (lift toward ears)
   G. Face, head, and neck (be sure to relax the jaw afterwards)
   H. Raise and lower eyebrows, pull together and release

4. Tighten the entire body at once, hold as long as possible, then relax as much as possible. (Important note: this is not recommended for people with hypertension—high blood pressure.)

5. Repeat to yourself: "I am relaxed."

6. Sit for several minutes and experience the lack of tension. If you become aware of any areas of tension, tighten and then release the muscles in that area.

(Adapted from Understanding human behavior *(6th ed.), by M. E. Milliken, 1998, Albany, NY: Delmar.)*

and accomplish required duties within prescribed time periods. Learning to manage time now will contribute to workplace success. See Chapter 26 for more ideas about time management on the job.

Relaxation Techniques

Relaxation, as used here, refers to releasing tension in the muscles. This reduces stress by improving blood circulation and allowing the release of blood lactate, a substance that is associated with anxiety (Milliken, 1998). Using relaxation techniques also produces the sensation of being rested. With practice, it is possible to quickly identify and release muscle tension when it begins to occur.

There are several methods for doing muscle relaxation. While it is outside the scope of this book to provide extensive information, instructions for one popular method can be found in Box 12–1.

Meditation

When individuals are awake, the mind is continually engaged in thinking. **Meditation** is a process for quieting the mind by clearing it of thoughts. It slows the rate of brain waves experienced during normal activity. The regular practice of meditation has been shown to bring about physiological changes that result in both psychological and physiological well-being (Milliken, 1998). An increasing number of health care professionals are recommending meditation as a therapeutic technique, even for serious illnesses such as cancer.

The positive, long-term effects that can be achieved through daily meditation, when it is practiced over an extended period of time, include:

- Release from negative emotions
- Better self-awareness
- Increased capacity to love oneself and others
- Sense of peace
- Improved coping abilities (Milliken, 1998)

[Fascinating Facts]

It has been found that 20 minutes of meditation is equivalent to a 2-hour nap. (Milliken, 1998.)

You may have had the experience of finding the solution to a problem when you stopped focusing on it and just "let the mind go." Meditators report similar experiences occurring after completing a meditation session.

There are a number of meditation methods. See Box 12–2 for an example.

The meditation procedure may sound incredibly simple, but it has been proven over the centuries to be effective. Like many practices that result in improved health and stress relief, it is free and fairly easy to learn. It does take practice, however, and must be done regularly over time. This requires the willingness to set aside 20 minutes each day.

Attitude

The close relationship between the mind and body is increasingly becoming recognized. One's quality of life is dependent to a great degree on whether one's thoughts are generally positive or negative. Every situation in life can be viewed in many different ways. **Attitude** refers to how a situation is viewed mentally. For example, problems can be viewed as dreaded difficulties or as challenges that keep life interesting.

Health care workers find themselves faced with many situations that can be approached as problems or challenges. Let's look at an example:

Mr. Chang is an 86-year-old resident in an extended care facility. He spent most of his life in Hong Kong, moving to the United States when he was in his 60s. His wife died two years ago, and his children live in other parts of the country. He rarely has visitors. Mr. Chang is difficult to understand because of his accent, complains a lot about being in the care facility, and is considered generally unpleasant to be around. Two staff members have contrasting experiences with Mr. Chang:

1. Anne dreads having to enter Mr. Chang's room each morning. He complains and grumbles as she gets him up and dressed. Anne hurries through her tasks and limits her conversation to necessary instructions.

2. Charles works the evening shift and looks forward to working with Mr. Chang. Charles has learned something about Chinese culture and understands that for Mr. Chang, living in a care facility away from family, is different from how life would have been in Hong Kong, where senior family members are highly respected and cared for at home. Charles asks Mr. Chang questions and listens carefully. As a result, he has learned a lot about life in another culture and has learned to appreciate the importance of family ties. He has shared stories about his family with Mr. Chang and offered the elderly resident friendship and relief from loneliness.

When faced with difficult situations, try to turn them into learning experiences or deal with them in ways that create the least amount of stress. Ask yourself:

1. Do I fully understand the situation?

2. Is my behavior contributing to the problem?

3. If so, what can I do differently?

4. Are there any positive possibilities, such as those that Charles found, that I have overlooked?

Box 12–2 A Meditation Method

1. Choose a time and place where you can arrange not to be interrupted.

2. Set a timer. Twenty minutes is best; ten is the minimum.

3. Sit in a comfortable position in a chair or on the floor. Straighten the spine and place the hands on the thighs.

4. Take a few deep breaths and let your body relax.

5. While breathing naturally, start counting each time you exhale. When you reach four (four breaths), start over.

6. Focus on the counting, not on the breaths.

7. If thoughts enter your mind, let them go by, refocusing on the counting.

(*Adapted from* Understanding human behavior *(6th ed.), by M. E. Milliken, 1998, Albany, NY: Delmar.*)

Thinking it Through

Mary Payongayong is stressed out from her job as a radiologic technician in a mid-city orthopedic clinic. Her work load has increased as the result of staff reductions, and her current supervisor is demanding. Mary finds it difficult to communicate with him and feels that he is unresponsive to the needs of the staff.

1. How might Mary's attitude be contributing to her stress level?
2. What might she do to better handle the conditions at work?

Some situations, in spite of the health care worker's best efforts, do not turn out to be as positive as the example with Charles and Mr. Chang. The best approach in these cases is to perform work in a professional manner, keep emotions under control, and avoid mentally dwelling on the negative aspects of the situation.

MINIMIZING HEALTH RISKS

Being aware of the health risks commonly encountered by health care workers enables them to take preventive measures. This provides benefits for workers themselves as well as for the patients they serve. Armed with knowledge about health risks, workers are better equipped to educate patients about ways to achieve maximum wellness.

Smoking

Most people are familiar with the risks associated with cigarette smoking. It has been linked to many serious health conditions and is estimated to contribute to approximately 400,000 deaths in the United States each year (www.oncolink.upenn.edu).

Unfortunately, understanding the dangers does not necessarily make it easy to stop smoking. Nicotine is a physically addictive substance. While the long-term benefits of quitting are many, the discomfort of withdrawing from the use of tobacco discourages many people who would like to quit.

Several methods have been found to be successful:

- Groups that meet regularly and offer a structured program that involves quitting gradually. Leaders are usually ex-smokers who offer

encouragement. Buddy systems are often organized to provide support between meetings.
- Classes and support groups offered by health care facilities
- Hypnosis
- Methods that allow the gradual withdrawal from nicotine through the use of skin patches and/or gum

Withdrawal symptoms vary among individuals. They may include anxiety, inability to concentrate, headaches, irritability, and strong cravings for a cigarette. (These are an indication of just how strong the effect of nicotine is on the body!) Knowing what to expect and keeping in mind that the symptoms *will disappear* may offer encouragement to stay with the quitting process. Most ex-smokers agree that the discomfort is worth the long-term benefits.

Substance Abuse

Substance abuse is a growing problem that increases the risk of stress, disease, and injury. In an effort to escape from stress, some individuals engage in behaviors that create new problems that become *additional* sources of stress. Drinking excessive amounts of alcohol in an effort to "relax" after work is an example. At best, alcohol offers only temporary relief. At worst, it can result in poor job performance and dismissal, in addition to health problems such as liver damage and increased risk of accidents.

Drug abuse has become a problem for an increasing number of health care workers. Studies have indicated two factors common to those nurses who experience the highest levels of substance abuse:

1. They had jobs with high-level stress, such as assignments in emergency departments.
2. They had the greatest or most frequent access to controlled substances. (Storr, Trinkoff, and Anthony in Danis, 2000.)

The dangers of drug abuse, whether with illegal substances or prescription drugs, cannot be overemphasized. Patient care is compromised when health care workers perform under the influence of either drugs or alcohol because this can cause:

- Faulty judgment
- Blackouts
- Memory loss (Bugle in Danis, 2000)
- Inability to adequately perform tasks requiring physical coordination
- Temptation to take drugs that are prescribed for patient use
- Illegible written documentation

There are negative physical effects on the health care worker, along with the problems caused by the need to use larger amounts of the substance as the degree of physical tolerance rises. Stealing prescription drugs from a facility is a crime. Even in cases not involving theft, the use of any type of drug or alcohol on the job can result in severe consequences. The fortunate employee may be required to enter a rehabilitation program. The less fortunate one faces imprisonment and a lifetime ban from working in certain areas of health care. Health care students should be aware that a conviction for using illegal drugs may permanently disqualify them from licensure in certain occupations.

There are many effective programs for treating substance abuse. The counseling office at most schools is a good source of community services. Anyone who believes that he or she has a problem with drugs or alcohol should seek help immediately.

Occupational Hazards

Health care workers encounter various risks on the job: exposure to infectious disease, to chemicals, and to potentially dangerous equipment. Most risks can be minimized by using proper safety precautions and following facility rules. Occupational safety is discussed throughout this text:

- Avoiding injury through the use of proper body mechanics: Chapter 9
- Protecting oneself against infection and bloodborne pathogens: Chapter 10
- Practicing environmental safety: Chapter 11
- Using the computer safely: Chapter 9

At each facility where you are employed, carefully read all the safety manuals and instruction books that apply to your work. Never hesitate to ask questions about anything you do not understand.

Your safety, and that of patients and coworkers, depends on your knowledge and use of safe practices.

Safe Sex

Sexual practices have become a necessary topic of discussion due to the global spread of the HIV virus. And while not fatal, genital herpes has reached epidemic proportions in the United States. According to the Centers for Disease Control and Prevention, one person in five is infected with the virus that causes genital herpes. The number may actually be much higher because many people do not experience symptoms.

The only 100% effective means of preventing sexually transmitted diseases (STDs) is abstinence from sexual activity. For individuals who choose to be sexually active, there are basic precautions that minimize the risk of contracting sexually transmitted diseases (STDs):

- Discuss risk factors with your potential partner before beginning a sexual relationship. Ask if he or she is aware of having a STD. Herpes is problematic because many people do not know they have it, since the symptoms can be very mild.
- With any new partner, mutually agree to be tested for HIV. (Note: this is only effective if it has been at least 6 months since the last sexual contact. It can take that long for the virus to become detectable.)
- Use condoms.
- See a physician immediately if symptoms of any STD are experienced. These include sores in the genital area, unusual odors, discharges, and itching.

Burnout

Burnout is a form of physical and emotional exhaustion that is caused by a variety of personal and environmental stressors that are experienced over an extended period of time. Burnout occurs in all professions, but health care workers can be particularly susceptible, due to the nature of their work. Examples of stressors that can lead to burnout include:

- Long hours working under difficult conditions
- Lack of adequate rest
- Inability to deal effectively with frustrating situations
- Inadequate emotional support

- No time for recreational activities
- Emotional involvement with patients who are suffering from terminal diseases
- Poor diet and insufficient exercise

The symptoms of burnout vary among individuals. Commonly noted changes in behavior include:

- Negative feelings about work
- Feelings of not being appreciated
- Increased absences due to minor illnesses
- Irritability
- Making errors and taking longer than previously required to complete tasks
  (Adapted from *Understanding human behavior* (6th ed.), by M. E. Milliken, 1998, Albany, NY: Delmar.)

Health care workers should be on the alert for signs of burnout. The habitual practice of good health habits and regular use of stress-prevention techniques are the best ways to prevent its occurrence. Developing good **assertiveness** (expressing feelings freely in a nonthreatening manner) and communication skills (see Chapters 15 and 16) will help resolve workplace issues that might otherwise result in burnout.

Working cooperatively in high-risk situations can help everyone deal with a difficult workload. The nurses in a neonatal unit at a northern California hospital found the stress of caring for heroin-addicted newborns who cried constantly for days at a time to be overwhelming. They agreed to share their assignments so that no one had more than two consecutive shifts working with these babies. (Source: personal communication.)

HELPING PATIENTS DEVELOP HEALTHY LIFESTYLES

In addition to your serving as a role model, your job may require you to provide patient education. All the health-promoting techniques described in this chapter can be applied to patients. You may also be expected to give specialized instructions, like the dental hygienist who teaches proper flossing and brushing techniques. Including information about healthy lifestyles is an excellent form of preventive care. Some dental patients, for example, will also benefit from learning the nutritional guidelines that improve dental and general health.

Physical therapy assistants teach exercises as part of their daily work. But other health care workers, such as medical assistants, may also have opportunities to explain the benefits of exercise.

(Note: Be sure that your supervisor is aware of and has approved the information and materials that you share with patients.)

SUGGESTED LEARNING ACTIVITIES

1. Read articles about the benefits of proper nutrition and exercise. What does current research report about best practices?
2. Start a scrapbook of articles and information from journals and the Internet about healthy habits.
3. Read packaged food labels. What are the major components of your favorites? Are you surprised by what you discover?
4. Try eating new foods that are high in nutritional value.
5. Start a collection of recipes for healthy dishes.
6. Create a food chart using pictures from magazines or your own drawings.
7. Develop a personal exercise program. Set a reasonable goal such as three times a week for 20 minutes. Record your progress.
8. Look for examples of stressors in your environment. Which are internal and which are external?
9. Try the relaxation and/or meditation exercises for 2 weeks. Do you notice any benefits?
10. Explore the following Web sites to see the type of information that is available for health professionals and their patients:
    a. National Clearinghouse for Alcohol and Drug Information: http://www.health.org
    b. Tobacco Fact Sheets: http://www.nswcc.org.au/pages/health/schpubs/smokefact/facts1.htm
    c. Eating Disorders and Excess Weight: http://health.yahoo.com/health/Diseases_and_Conditions/Disease_Feed_Data/Bulimia/
       http://health.yahoo.com/health/Diseases_and_Conditions/Disease_Feed_Data/Anorexia_nervosa/

See how many other sites you can locate by using key terms such as "obesity" and "stress."

REVIEW QUESTIONS

1. Why is it important for the health care worker to practice good health habits?
2. How can old habits be changed or new habits be formed?
3. What are five health problems caused by obesity?
4. Why is it important that the diet contain a variety of items from all the food groups?
5. What are five benefits of physical exercise?
6. What are the consequences of an inadequate amount of sleep?
7. What preventive measures help ensure good health?
8. How can the health care worker deal effectively with stress?
9. What are the major health risks faced by health care workers today?
10. Explain the symptoms of burnout and preventive measures.

APPLICATION EXERCISES

1. Refer to The Case of the Cardiac Nurse in the beginning of this chapter. Describe the lifestyle habits, based on what you learned in this chapter, that enable Gracie Chin to stay fit for her job as a cardiac nurse.
2. Jorge Chavez is a surgical technician at a busy ambulatory surgical center. His full-time job requires that he spend many hours on his feet, that he stay mentally alert, and that he quickly and correctly respond to surgeons' requests. Jorge must balance his job with a busy family life. He and his wife have two small children whom he cares for while his wife attends college two evenings a week. Using the information in this chapter, develop a plan that will help Jorge stay healthy, avoid burnout, and remain a positive member of the health care team.

SUGGESTED READINGS AND RESOURCES

Alcoholics Anonymous:
http://www.recovery.org/aa
American Dietetic Association. "Role of Nutrition in Health Promotion and Disease Prevention Programs." Available:
http://www.eatright.org/adap0298b.html
American Heart Association:
www.americanheart.org
Department of Agriculture, Center for Nutrition Policy Promotion:
http://www.usda.gov/cnpp
Drug Abuse Information and Treatment Referral Line:
1-800-662-HELP
Health Care Costs of Smoking:
http://www.urel.berkeley.edu/berkeleyan/1998/0916/smoking.html
McGraw, P. C. (1999). *Life strategies: Doing what works, doing what matters.* New York: Hyperion.
National Clearinghouse for Alcohol and Drug Information:
http://www.health.org
National Council on Alcoholism and Drug Dependence:
http://www.ncadd.org
National Eating Disorders Organization:
http://www.kidsource.com/popup.html
National Institute on Drug Abuse Hotline:
1-800-662-HELP
Public Health Service AIDS Hotline:
1-800-342-AIDS
Sexually Transmitted Diseases:
American Social Health Association:
http://www.ashastd.org
Tobacco Fact Sheets:
http://www.nswcc.org.au/pages/health/schpubs/smokefact/facts1.htm

CHAPTER

PROFESSIONALISM

OBJECTIVES

Studying and applying the material in this chapter will help you to:

- Explain the meaning of professionalism for health care workers.

- Identify the four major components of professionalism.

- Describe the characteristics and behaviors of workers who display professionalism.

- Explain how health care workers can effectively handle difficult situations.

- Explain the meaning of "professional distance."

- Describe how to use criticism constructively.

- Explain how professional organizations help health care workers increase their level of professionalism.

- Identify the characteristics of a leader.

KEY TERMS

continuing education
leadership
objective
professional distance
professionalism

The Case of

the Lost Opportunity

Gerald Lenz has worked as an ultrasound technician for just over 3 years. He performs a variety of duties at a large imaging center. Gerald does what is necessary to complete his work, but believes that his job consists of using his technical skills. He performs them adequately but makes no effort to "go out of his way" for either his coworkers or patients. While he isn't actually rude, it is clear to patients that, for Gerald, working with them is simply a job he performs in exchange for a salary. Gerald never volunteers to work on extra projects, to contribute new ideas at staff meetings, or to participate in special activities offered outside working hours. Ultrasound technicians are in short supply in Gerald's city, so he remains employed. He was recently passed over for a promotion because his supervisor believes he lacks professionalism. Gerald was disappointed and couldn't understand why someone who had worked there for just a year and a half got the position. In this chapter you will learn about behaviors that make the difference between just getting by on the job and making a positive, professional contribution.

THE MEANING OF PROFESSIONALISM

Professionalism is an essential quality of the health care worker. We often hear someone described as being "very professional" or "acting professionally." Professionalism is difficult to define because it consists of many characteristics and behaviors. Health care workers display professionalism by dedicating themselves to doing their best on the job and providing and maintaining high-quality service. "Caring competence" is one way to express the meaning of **professionalism** in health care.

The confidence patients have in the care they receive is influenced by each individual they have contact with in the health care system. Health care workers represent the facilities in which they work. Their actions are a reflection of all the services and people who work there.

Professional Attitude

Attitude, discussed in Chapter 12, refers to the way a person thinks and feels. Health care workers with professional attitudes approach work positively and enthusiastically. They think in terms of what they can give rather than what they can get. Patient welfare is the primary focus of the worker

with a professional attitude. This is true whether the task is to prepare accurate billing statements or provide direct patient care.

A professional attitude in health care work can be expressed in many ways:

- Be committed to your work. Believe in the value of what you are doing and your ability to do it.

- Keep in mind your impact on patient care and services. Aim to contribute positively to the well-being of patients and their perception of the facility.

- Use an **objective** approach to situations. This means considering the facts rather than responding emotionally. For example, if a patient you have assisted is rude, think about possible causes. The rudeness may be a reaction to fear or pain, and have nothing to do with you personally.

- View problems as opportunities for positive action. Problems are part of everyday life, and learning to deal with them effectively is essential for achieving work success and satisfaction.

- Develop and practice self-discipline. Knowing you can depend on yourself to accomplish what needs to be done results in both competence and self-confidence.

The National Study of the Changing Workforce reports that "personal satisfaction for doing a good job" is the most frequently mentioned measure of success in worklife—cited nearly two to three times more often than "getting ahead" or "making a good living."
(Galinsky, Bond, and Friedman quoted in Kouzes and Posner, 1995, p. 131.)

According to Stephen Covey, author of best-selling books on personal effectiveness, the average person spends 80% of his or her time interacting with others. For most people, then, the majority of their waking hours are spent interacting or communicating with other people—or dealing with the poor results of that interaction.

Professional Behaviors

A professional attitude provides a foundation for developing professional behaviors, and these behaviors are what demonstrate "caring competence." The actions of health care workers directly influence the level of patient satisfaction. Poor outcomes as well as malpractice lawsuits increase when patients are dissatisfied with the service they receive. Patients are health care consumers, and good service increases consumer loyalty. See Chapter 23.

The following behaviors are important expressions of professional conduct:

- Be dependable. Follow through on assignments, meet deadlines, and be on the job and on time as scheduled.

- Perform all duties as assigned and needed. "It's not my job" is rarely heard in today's facilities because employees who say it are not employed for long. Willingness to always do one's best is the sign of a true professional.

- Be flexible. Health care work is continually changing. Willingness to adapt to these changes is essential.

- Accept differences. Today's patient population is increasingly diverse. See Chapter 15 for information on cultural diversity.

- Treat everyone with courtesy and consideration. Be aware of how your actions affect others.

- Practice good communication skills. See Chapters 15 and 16.

- Put personal problems aside during work time. Do not discuss them with coworkers or patients. And *never* complain about your work, supervisor, or the facility. Patients who hear such complaints may lose confidence in the care they are receiving. Complaining can

also negatively affect the morale of coworkers. See Figure 13–1.

- Be well organized and plan your work. For example, gather all equipment and supplies before beginning a procedure so that the patient does not have to wait.

- Behave ethically at all times and set high personal standards. See Chapter 3.

- Conduct yourself calmly. This is especially important in emergencies and upsetting situations, when it is necessary to think clearly. Remaining calm also helps patients, who look to health care workers for reassurance.

- Serve as a role model for good health. As a health care worker, you have an opportunity to encourage good health habits in others. See Chapter 12.

- Set professional goals and aim for continual improvement.

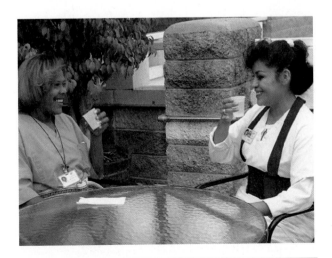

Figure 13–1 Keep conversation positive. Avoid complaining about the workplace with coworkers.

Professional Appearance

The appearance of health care workers is an outward sign of their professionalism. It strongly influences the way they are perceived by patients and coworkers. A professional appearance communicates the message, "I take my job and myself seriously. I have self-respect and want patients to have confidence in my abilities."

Professional appearance in health care is generally conservative. Some popular fashion trends, such as tattoos and body piercing, are usually unacceptable at work because many patients may find them offensive and frightening. Extremes in appearance can undermine patient confidence. Maintaining a fairly conservative appearance, whether or not this includes wearing a uniform, helps project an image of competence. It is a sign of respect for patients to

consider their feelings when planning your appearance. See Figures 13–2 and 13–3. Maintaining a professional appearance includes the following:

- Practice personal cleanliness. This includes the hair, hands and fingernails, clothing, and shoes.
- Use a deodorant or antiperspirant daily.
- Pay attention to dental hygiene. Flossing and regular dental care help prevent bad breath.
- Avoid the use of perfumes and strong-smelling hair sprays and other personal products. Some people are allergic to fragrances. Many others find them offensive, especially when they are ill.
- Avoid extreme styles in dress and grooming, such as unnaturally colored hair and green nail polish. When possible, wear clothing that covers tattoos.
- Consider personal safety and that of others. Avoid wearing anything that can be grabbed or caught, such as dangling earrings and untied long hair. Wear closed-toed shoes to protect your feet from injury.

Professional Health Care Skills

Achieving and maintaining a high level of skill is a critical component of professionalism. Tasks must be performed correctly and carefully. Pay attention

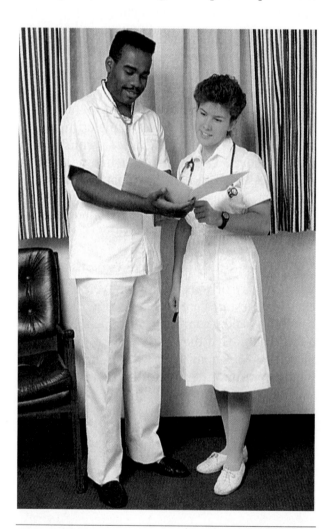

Figure 13–2 What messages are communicated by the appearance of these health care workers?

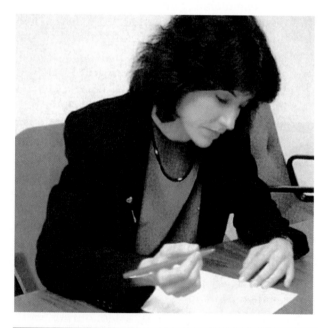

Figure 13–3 Regular clothing worn to work should be neat and conservative.

and think about what you are doing at all times. Nothing can be taken for granted or become routine. Approach each patient as an individual who deserves your best efforts.

- Develop an in-depth understanding of your work. Learn as much as possible about the theories that support your skills. This will increase the level of your performance and improve your decision-making and problem-solving skills.

- Observe and listen carefully. Question situations that do not seem right given the circumstances.

- Consult the employee manual and/or ask questions if you are unsure about a policy or procedure.

- Perform all work as neatly and accurately as possible.

- Dedicate time to acquiring new knowledge and skills. See Chapter 14.

Professional Distance

Professional distance refers to a healthy balance in the worker-patient relationship. It means demonstrating a caring attitude toward patients without the goal of becoming their friend. While it is appropriate to seek personal satisfaction from work, it is inappropriate to personally depend on the friendship and approval of patients. Working to please, rather than serve appropriately, can be counterproductive. Keep the focus on the patients' health goals and what must be done to achieve them. (See Figure 13–4.)

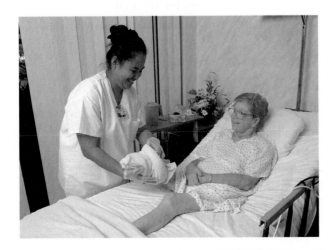

Figure 13–4 Professional distance requires focusing on the health care needs of the patient while expressing caring concern.

Thinking it Through

An important part of Torst Borgen's work as a physical therapy assistant is working with postoperative patients in their homes. His job is to help them regain strength and range of motion. Exercises prescribed by the supervising physical therapist, are often uncomfortable and Torst must encourage, as well as instruct, patients to perform them. Torst lives alone and enjoys the social aspects of working with patients. He wants them to like him. This sometimes makes it difficult for him to insist that they engage in necessary exercises that are extremely painful.

1. How might Torst's need to be friends with patients interfere with their full recovery?

2. What changes are needed in his view of his role as a physical therapy assistant?

3. What actions can he take to achieve the professional distance necessary to best assist patients in their recovery?

Professional Handling of Difficult Situations

Health care workers sometimes deal with challenging and stressful situations. It is natural to react emotionally when faced with an emergency, the death of a child, or an angry patient. Such a response, however, can interfere with the worker's effectiveness. An objective, although not unfeeling, response is necessary for the health care worker to perform professionally and constructively.

Being professional requires that you know yourself well and attempt to understand the basis of your reactions to workplace problems. Learning to recognize the causes of a behavior can help you change it, if necessary. For example, Keith has always had a quick temper. He finds it difficult to be patient and becomes easily irritated by incidents involving disorder, delays, and disorganization. His work as a pharmacy technician in a busy hospital does not always go smoothly, and Keith's impatience is negatively affecting his relationships with coworkers. When he takes time to analyze his behavior and sees that it follows a lifelong pattern, he realizes that he must learn to make adjustments and adapt to workplace conditions.

The problem-solving model described in Chapter 1 provides a constructive way to deal with difficult situations. Reviewing and gathering information, as described in the model, helps to separate fact from emotion. Facts help form a basis on which to make sound decisions and identify effective resolutions.

Professional Acceptance of Criticism

Criticism and correction can be valuable learning resources. These opportunities to learn are often lost because it is hard for people to admit that they might be wrong. It is common to react defensively in these situations and miss the message. Responding gracefully to criticism is a sign of professionalism and self-confidence. Health care workers who feel secure about themselves are comfortable with suggestions about their work and conduct. They are able to evaluate the information received and decide if it applies to them. Being willing to recognize and work on imperfections is a sign of emotional maturity and professionalism. See Figure 13–5. Chapter 23 contains more information about giving and receiving criticism.

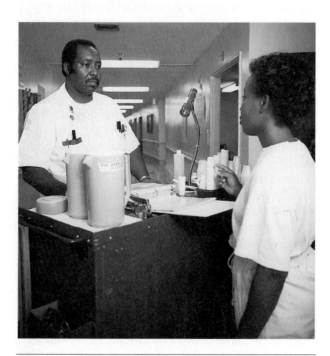

Figure 13–5 Accepting criticism gracefully is the sign of a professional who is willing to see it as a learning opportunity.

Thinking it Through

Certified nursing assistant Barbara Sterndorf has difficulty working independently in her job at Pinehurst Care Home, an extended care facility. Barbara was raised by parents who were quite critical, and she lacks self-confidence. She is afraid of making mistakes and only does exactly what she is directed to do by her supervisor, Carla Thomas. In spite of her self-doubts, Barbara always performs high-quality work and is well liked by the residents. Carla believes her to be well trained and among the most competent CNAs on the staff and tells her this during Barbara's performance evaluation.

1. Discuss how Barbara's attitude may be affecting her actions at work.

2. What might she do to increase her self-confidence at work?

PROFESSIONAL ORGANIZATIONS

Participating actively in a professional organization can contribute positively to professional development. Most health care occupations have an organization whose purposes include:

- Promoting the profession
- Sponsoring **continuing education** (learning experiences beyond those needed to earn the initial certificate or degree to work in an occupation)
- Encouraging networking among members
- Supporting legislation on behalf of the profession and health care in general

Serving on committees, volunteering to help with projects, and running for office are excellent ways to become involved. There are many advantages for health care workers who participate at any level:

- Learning to work in a group toward common goals
- Meeting established professionals who can offer career advice, as well as serving as a positive role model for others

- Keeping current in the field
- Developing management skills
- Receiving the support and encouragement of colleagues

See Appendix 1 for a list of health care organizations.

PROFESSIONAL LEADERSHIP

Leadership means encouraging people to work together and do their best to achieve common goals. Leaders combine visions of excellence with the ability to inspire others. They promote positive changes that benefit their professions and the people they serve. A leader may or may not be a supervisor. It is possible to set an example of excellence and encourage others without having a position of authority.

Characteristics of effective leaders in health care include:

- A high level of competence in their profession
- Commitment to providing high-quality service
- Willingness to recognize and support the work of others
- Dedication to meeting high standards
- Belief that necessary changes and improvements can be accomplished
- Willingness to serve as an example and complete whatever tasks are necessary for achieving the goals
- Ability to communicate effectively

SUGGESTED LEARNING ACTIVITIES

1. Find examples of people you consider to be "professional." Explain why you chose them.
2. Rate yourself in each of the following professional categories:
   - Attitude
   - Conduct
   - Appearance
   - Health Care Skills
3. Interview a health care supervisor about his or her definition of professionalism.

4. Using the material in this chapter as a guide, create your own description of "professionalism" in your occupational area.
5. Send for information about the professional organization in your area of interest or explore its Web site. How does it define "professionalism" for its members? What opportunities does it provide for members to develop professionally?

REVIEW QUESTIONS

1. What is meant by "professionalism" in health care?
2. What are five examples of professionalism in each of the following areas?

   Attitude

   Conduct

   Appearance

   Skills
3. Explain the meaning of "professional distance."
4. How can criticism be received constructively and professionally?
5. What are the advantages of participating in the activities of a professional organization?
6. What are the characteristics of a leader?

APPLICATION EXERCISES

1. What changes does Gerald Lenz, described in the Case of the Lost Opportunity at the beginning of the chapter, need to make in order to increase his level of professionalism as an ultrasound technician?
2. Shelley is a dental receptionist for Dr. Sims. She arrives at the office on Monday morning to face the beginning of "one of those days." A long-time patient who has suffered all weekend with a toothache is waiting at the door. The dental hygienist is ill and will not be in, leaving seven patients without appointments. When notified that they will have to reschedule, two patients are very unhappy and express their irritation to Shelley. Later in the morning, the office computer freezes up, and

the scheduling and billing programs cannot be accessed. In the afternoon, an elderly patient returns to the office after his appointment to say that his car won't start. He asks for help to get it started or to find other transportation home.

a. Discuss how Shelley can handle each situation professionally. Include professional attitude as well as actions.

SUGGESTED READINGS AND RESOURCES

Adams, P. (1998). *House calls: How we can all heal the world one visit at a time.* San Francisco: Robert D. Reed Publishers.

Chapman, E. N. (1995). *Attitude: Your most priceless possession.* Menlo Park, CA: Crisp Learning.

Kouzes, J. M. and Posner, B. Z. (1995). *The leadership challenge: How to keep getting extraordinary things done in organizations.* San Francisco: Jossey-Bass Publishers.

Purtilo, R. and Haddad, A. (1996). *Health professional and patient interaction* (5th ed.). Philadelphia: W. B. Saunders Company.

CHAPTER

LIFELONG LEARNING

OBJECTIVES

Studying and applying the material in this chapter will help you to:

- Understand and explain the importance of lifelong learning for the health care worker.

- List the reasons for participating in continuing education opportunities.

- Describe ways you can earn continuing education credits.

- Create a personal plan for self-directed learning.

KEY TERMS

continuing education unit (CEU)

continuing professional education (CPE)

lifelong learning

self-directed learning

The Case of Lifetime Success

Mabel Bennett has worked in medical records for many years. So many that she likes to joke and tell people that records were handwritten with feather pens when she started. Mabel enjoys tasks that involve detail and order. She has always received satisfaction from the challenge of maintaining complete and accurate records and has risen to the position of medical records manager at a large suburban rehabilitation hospital. Over the years, Mabel has seen many changes in her field. Her first position was keeping paper records for a country doctor at a time when no one had even thought about desktop computers. Through the years, Mabel pursued every available opportunity to learn more about her field and enjoyed her learning experiences, both alone and with others in her field. She was one of the first in her profession to realize the potential of computer applications in medical records and became an expert user of computer technology. Mabel credits her long-term career success to her interest in learning all she can and working with the future in mind. In this chapter you will learn ways that successful health care workers like Mabel acquire the knowledge they need to stay current and advance in their fields.

IMPORTANCE OF LIFELONG LEARNING

The world is changing today faster than at any other time in history. It is hard to imagine that until recently people could expect to live much the same way as their parents and grandparents. Current advancements in technology now produce changes not only between generations, but within a single lifetime. For example, people who are only in their sixties today grew up without television. They began their professional lives without personal computers, hand-held calculators, cellular phones, and many other products that are now considered necessities in the workplace.

Most people take change for granted and incorporate it into their lifestyles. They are no longer surprised by the constant stream of new products available or the speed of the changes in these products that require them to be updated before they are even worn out by use. What health care workers may find surprising is *how much learning will be required after graduation* in order to keep up with the many changes that affect the way jobs are performed. For example, the majority of people in the workforce today learned to use a personal computer *after* they completed their formal education and were already employed. They had to take time to read manuals, attend workshops, watch videos, or use tutorials to learn to use what has now become an essential tool in most workplaces. And the need to learn in the area of computers alone will continue as new applications and updated versions are developed.

Lifelong learning refers to all purposeful learning activities, both formal and informal, that take place throughout our lives. The need for these activities was formally recognized by the federal government in 1976 when it passed the Lifelong Learning Act:

> American society should have as a goal the availability of appropriate opportunities for lifelong learning for all its citizens without regard to restriction of previous education or training, sex, age, handicapping condition, social or ethnic background, or economic circumstance (Section 131; Cross, 1981, p. 27).

Keeping up with Changes in Health Care

Changes in the delivery of health care are taking place continually. Knowledge quickly becomes outdated and within a few years of entering the health care field, a worker who fails to keep up with current information will become incompetent. Your graduation, then, marks the end of formal training and the beginning of lifelong learning.

In addition to technology, the social and demographic changes and trends discussed in Chapter 2 require that health care workers acquire new knowledge and skills. See Table 14–1 for examples of changes and the corresponding learning requirements for health care workers. Standard Precautions, explained in Chapter 10, are now "common knowledge" in the workplace. And yet they are actually a recent development, created in 1987 in response to the spread of the HIV and hepatitis B viruses. All health care workers must be trained and tested on the Standards, including undergoing annual reviews. The increasing number of HMOs is another recent change that has

Table 14–1 Changes that Affect Healthcare

Changes	Corresponding Learning Needs of Health Care Workers
People living longer	Developmental stages and needs of older adults Patient care skills for long-term care
Hospital stays are much shorter than in the past	Home health patient practices and techniques Patient education delivery techniques
Recognition of increased ethnic and cultural diversity of United States population	Diverse customs and health habits Languages other than English
Growing patient interest in complementary health care practices such as acupuncture and holistic medicine	Knowledge of complementary health practices and practitioners Understanding of how the use of complementary health care practices may affect Western medical practices
Increase in third-party payers	Coding and billing practices Contract administration, obtaining preauthorizations for treatment, and permission for referral to specialists
Emphasis on wellness and patients' responsibility for their own health	Prevention practices to ward off diseases and disorders Patient education on wellness and prevention techniques
Increased computerization	Computer applications in health care: administration, diagnostics, treatment, and education Computer operation skills and knowledge of software programs
Spread of HIV and hepatitis viruses and the return of tuberculosis	Standard Precautions Symptoms, treatment, and prevention of specific diseases
Expansion of roles for health care workers	Increased skill base Flexibility and willingness to perform a variety of tasks
Increased specialization and use of teams to provide patient care	Teamwork skills Intraprofessional and interprofessional communication skills
Development of increasingly sophisticated equipment	Operation of equipment and interpretation of results

resulted in the need for further education of all health care workers. Administrative workers in particular must continue to update their knowledge of contract management, patient eligibility, and billing procedures. And the shift in patient demographics has meant that a large percentage of health care workers will spend much of their time working with older adults. See Figure 14–1.

Many health care occupations have expanded their scope of practice in an effort to increase the efficiency of patient care delivery. Workers who previously performed a limited set of tasks are now being cross-trained and becoming multi-skilled. This section from the 2000–2001 *Occupational Outlook Handbook* explains what is happening in the field of respiratory therapy:

> Therapists are increasingly asked to perform tasks that fall outside their traditional role. Tasks are expanding into cardiopulmonary procedures like electrocardiograms and stress testing, as well as other tasks like drawing blood samples from patients. Therapists also keep records of materials used and charges to patients. Additionally, some teach or supervise other respiratory therapy personnel. (*Occupational Outlook Handbook*, 2000, pg. 205)

CONTINUING EDUCATION UNITS

Continuing education units (CEUs) refer to the credits granted for certain types of learning that take place after the completion of formal education. This type of education is also referred to as **continuing "professional education" (CPE)**. Most forms of professional approval, such as licensure, certification, and registration, require that a specific

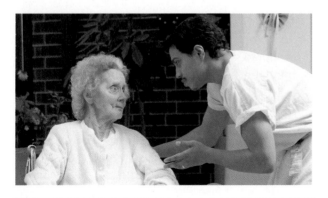

Figure 14–1 Health care workers must continue to learn about the needs of older patients.

[Fascinating Facts]

In an effort to keep health care workers provided with information on advances in health care, it is estimated that 20,000 biomedical journals are available and more than 2,000,000 medically-related journal articles are published each year. (DeLaune and Ladner, 1998)

number of CEUs be earned in order to be renewed. Health care workers should find out the requirements for their occupations well in advance of licensure and certification renewal dates in order to allow adequate time to meet them. Many professional organizations have sites on the Internet that explain their continuing education requirements.

A CEU commonly represents 50 to 60 minutes of instruction or other learning activity, although this amount varies. Some CEUs are granted for assignments completed or tests passed, rather than for hours of class or workshop attendance. Many schools and organizations offer classes and various activities that award CEUs. However, the organizations that grant licenses, certifications, and registrations decide which CEUs they will accept. Not all courses and activities are accepted by all organizations. Before engaging in any activity for the purpose of earning CEUs, be sure that it has been approved by the necessary professional or regulatory organization.

If you participate in workshops or other activities, be *sure* to sign in. Also, ask for a certificate verifying attendance or completion of work. These will be needed as proof that units were earned. Keep certificates in a safe place. Some approval agencies require that they be kept for at least 4 years. Inquire whether your professional organization maintains a tracking system for CEUs earned by members. Some make a practice of sending out regular "statements" of units earned. This is a good way for health care workers to avoid getting caught short at renewal time.

Ways to Earn CEUs

There are many ways to earn CEUs. Health care professional organizations offer a variety of convenient ways to help their members stay current in their field. They can provide you with information about how many CEUs are needed, which subject areas they must be in, and how they can be earned. In addition to traditional classes and workshops, there are a variety of other ways to obtain CEUs:

- Special sessions and workshops offered at annual meetings, conferences, and conventions sponsored by professional health care organizations. These may require taking a quiz, completing an assignment, or demonstrating in some other way that you have met the objectives.

  Example: pharmacy technicians can earn up to 16 units by participating in learning activities at the American Association of Pharmacy Technicians annual convention (Harteker, 1998).

- Home study materials published in professional journals

  Examples: members can read designated articles published in *The Professional Medical Assistant* (American Association of Medical Assistants) and the *Journal of Practical Nursing* (the National Association for Practice Nurse Education and Service) and earn units by submitting written answers to questions about the articles' content. The American Association for Respiratory Care allows members to earn CEUs once a year by taking a test on the material covered in specific articles that appeared in its professional journal, *Respiratory Care*, during the previous 12 months (AARC Guide for Members, 1999).

- Home study courses offered by approved educational providers

  Example: Tech Lectures is a company that offers a series of printed lectures and exams that enable pharmacy technicians to earn CEUs, which are accepted by the American Pharmaceutical Association. Their Web address is http://www.geocities.com/Athens/Forum/3098

- Study packets

  Example: The American Association for Respiratory Care offers Individual Independent Study Packages (IISPs), a series of 30 self-study modules that cover clinical topics.

- Distance education courses offered by colleges and universities

  Many courses are now available over the Internet. A growing number of institutions provide for-credit classes that include interaction with the instructor and other students.

Thinking it Through

Jan Summers loves her work as an occupational therapy assistant. One of the reasons that Jan wanted to be an occupational therapy assistant was because she likes to interact with other people. Her outgoing personality helps her develop good relationships with patients, and her cheerful disposition makes her a popular assistant. Jan looks forward to the annual occupational therapy conferences, held in different cities around the country. They provide opportunities to see friends she has made in the profession and catch up on all the news. What Jan does not enjoy is attending the informational meetings and workshops. She finds them "boring." She has talked some of her friends into signing her name on the attendance rosters and, so far, has not been caught. In this way she manages to accumulate the credits needed to renew her certification to practice.

1. Even if Jan is not caught, what are the possible future consequences of her failure to attend the meetings and workshops?
2. Is Jan maintaining professional ethical standards with this practice? Why or why not?
3. What is the possible impact on her patients?
4. On her future career?

Example: University of Phoenix, based in Phoenix, Arizona, is one of the leaders in developing and offering distance education courses for credit. Their Web address is http://www.phoenix.edu.

- Internet courses designed for continuing education

  Many companies and organizations are developing courses specifically designed for health care providers.

  Examples: Institute for Continuing Education at http://ceu.org, CE4U at http://ceu4u.com, and CE Connection at www.springnet.com/ce.htm

Not all providers of learning opportunities are high quality. And not all courses are beneficial simply because they grant CEUs. Consider the following criteria for choosing courses and materials that offer maximum value for the time and money invested:

- Skill and knowledge requirements of your current job
- Future career goals
- Credibility and reputation of the educational provider
- Areas of personal and/or professional weakness that need improvement
- Personal and/or professional interests

SELF-DIRECTED LEARNING

Knowing how to learn is essential to updating your knowledge and acquiring new skills throughout your career. Learning is not limited to formal classroom settings or experiences for the purpose of earning CEUs. **Self-directed learning** refers to all activities that you plan and participate in to increase your knowledge and skills. There are many ways to incorporate learning into your daily life:

- Observe others: Watch how successful, experienced workers perform their duties. See Figure 14–2.

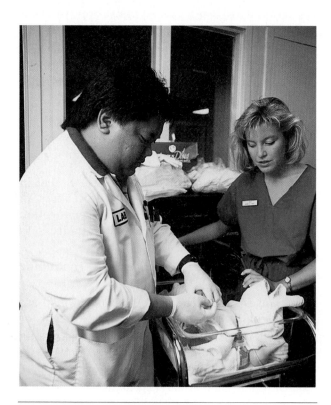

Figure 14–2 Health care workers can learn a lot by observing others at work.

- Ask questions: Learn from the expertise of others. Most people are happy to share what they know. Be sure to choose an appropriate time to ask questions. For example, do not ask questions about patients in their presence or when the other person is very busy and cannot stop to answer questions.
- Read books and journal articles: Plan a regular time to keep up on publications related to your area. Most professional organizations publish a newsletter or journal. Many large health care facilities have libraries available to employees. Many universities and colleges allow the public to use their libraries. Some offer check-out privileges for an annual fee. Libraries have become highly computerized, so don't hesitate to ask the librarian for assistance if you have trouble locating materials.
- Study in a small group: Organize a study group with other employees at work. Or, if you belonged to a study group at school, consider encouraging the members to meet regularly. You can learn by sharing workplace experiences and working on selected topics to keep current in your field. See Figure 14–3.
- Study with a partner or mentor: You may prefer to work with just one other person who can support your learning efforts.
- Attend professional conferences and meetings: These often include lectures, workshops, and discussions of current topics.

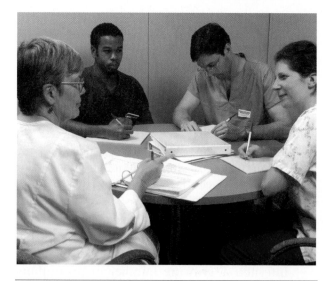

Figure 14–3 Studying in a small group can allow for an exchange of ideas and can be a productive way to learn.

- Watch videos and educational television programs: Videos are available for check-out at public libraries. Learning channels, along with those managed by local universities, often feature programs of interest to the health care worker. There are also cable channels devoted exclusively to medical issues.

- Explore the Internet: There is information available on all kinds of topics. To get started, see the *Directory of Internet Sources for Health Professionals* listed at the end of the chapter.

Planning your own study activities allows you to take advantage of your preferred styles of learning, discussed in Chapter 1. Look for ways to make learning enjoyable and incorporate them into your daily life. Think of the world as a giant classroom that offers endless opportunities for learning. Keeping up with changes and adding to your knowledge and skill base should be part of your work routine. You will have the satisfaction of knowing that you are staying current and competent.

In addition to developing health care skills, you can advance your career by improving nontechnical skills. Oral and written communication, interpersonal relations, computer applications, and time management are examples of important skills that will help you get ahead.

SUGGESTED LEARNING ACTIVITIES

1. Develop the habit of scanning popular magazines, such as *Newsweek*, and your local newspaper for health-related articles.

2. Visit your local library. Review periodicals and books on health care. Are there helpful resources in your subject area?

3. Request a continuing education catalog from a local college or university. What types of courses are offered? Do you see any that might help you develop your personal or professional skills?

4. Choose a health topic you find interesting and conduct an Internet search. Record your findings and develop a Webliography (a list of sites with name, Web address, and brief description of contents) of useful sites.

5. Contact the professional organization for your occupational area and request information about continuing education requirements and ways to earn CEUs.

6. Explore the Internet sites mentioned in this chapter.

REVIEW QUESTIONS

1. Why it is essential for health care workers to participate in lifelong learning activities?

2. What are five recent technological and demographic changes that required experienced health care workers to acquire new knowledge and skills?

3. What is a continuing education unit (CEU)?

4. Who determines which CEUs are accepted by professional and regulatory organizations?

5. What are five methods of earning CEUs?

6. What are eight ways to continue learning after graduation?

APPLICATION EXERCISES

1. Describe the methods for keeping up to date that Mabel Bennett, described in the Case of Lifetime Success, may have used throughout her career.

2. Debbie Yano is a licensed vocational nurse working for Dr. Cerutti in a single-physician office in a small town. Dr. Cerutti is a general practitioner and, because of the limited number of health care facilities in the area, many long-time patients rely on this caring physician for the majority of their health care needs. Debbie enjoys the variety of experiences encountered in her work with Dr. Cerutti: patients of all ages with all types of health issues. An important professional goal is to keep her skills up to date and to continue to acquire new ones. Learning opportunities are limited by her busy work schedule, family responsibilities, and living in a small town.

Develop a comprehensive, long-term plan for Debbie to achieve her goal.

SUGGESTED READINGS AND RESOURCES

American Pharmaceutical Association
   http://www.geocities.com/Athens/Forum/3098
CE4U: http://ce4u.com
Griffen, A.D. (1998). *Directory of internet sources for health professionals.* Albany, NY: Delmar.
Institute for Continuing Education: http://ceu.org

UNIT

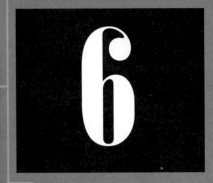

COMMUNICATION IN THE HEALTH CARE SETTING

6

CHAPTER

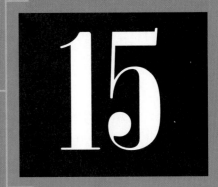

THE PATIENT AS AN INDIVIDUAL

OBJECTIVES

Studying and applying the material in this chapter will help you to:

- Explain the meaning of the Philosophy of Individual Worth and how it applies to work in health care.

- Define culture and describe how it influences all aspects of human beliefs and behavior.

- Give examples of how different cultural groups approach issues of health.

- Describe ways that the health care worker can determine the individual needs of patients that take into account cultural influences.

- List the five levels of needs described by Maslow and give an example of each.

- Recognize common defense mechanisms encountered in health care situations.

- Explain how the health care worker can help patients deal with the experience of loss.

KEY TERMS

culture

defense mechanism

dominant culture

Maslow's Hierarchy of Needs

personal space

Philosophy of
    Individual Worth

physiological needs

prejudice

self-actualization

self-esteem

The Case of

the Polite Patient

Shortly after graduation from a medical assistant program, Carley Ford moves from her small town to a large city 50 miles away. She has always wanted to experience city life and is excited when she is hired to work in a large downtown clinic. During her first week at the clinic, she meets with Mr. Alvarez, who has been recently diagnosed with diabetes. His physician, Dr. Washington, believes that if Mr. Alvarez follows a diabetic diet and regular plan of exercise, he may avoid having to take insulin injections. Carley spends about 10 minutes carefully explaining the eating plan recommended by Dr. Washington. She speaks slowly and clearly because she has noted that Mr. Alvarez does not speak English fluently. From time to time Carley asks Mr. Alvarez if he understands, and he nods vigorously to indicate that he does. She gives him a set of written instructions, including an eating plan, which she advises him to follow carefully. When Mr. Alvarez arrives for his follow-up appointment 6 months later, Dr. Washington is surprised that his condition has worsened. When he questions Mr. Alvarez—in Spanish—he learns that the elderly widower did not understand much of what Carley had explained to him. The written instructions were not helpful because Mr. Alvarez reads very little Spanish and no English at all. He hasn't cooked for himself since his wife died. Mr. Alvarez didn't say anything to Carley about not understanding because "she was so nice and took her time" so he "didn't want to hurt her feelings." He also didn't want to inconvenience the neighbors and family members who supply his meals by asking them to cook in a different way than they do for their families. This chapter discusses how to learn about individual patients in order to best help them meet their health care needs.

PATIENTS AS INDIVIDUALS

The well-being of patients depends on more than the technical competence of health care workers. It is also very much affected by the attitude and concern expressed by everyone who works with them in the health care setting. Each patient is a complex individual who represents a combination of cultural influences, personal experiences, and basic human needs. Working effectively with patients, as well as with coworkers, requires understanding and appreciating the differences that make each person unique. The wide variety of people that characterizes the population of the United States today has been compared to a garden filled with flowers of every color and shape. While each one is different, they all contribute to the overall beauty of the garden. The lesson for the health care worker is that having a variety of patients will enrich the worker's experience of giving service to fellow human beings.

Philosophy of Individual Worth

The **Philosophy of Individual Worth** is based on the belief that every human being, "regardless of personal circumstances or personal qualities, has worth and is entitled to respect as a human being" (Milliken, 1998, p. 23). Health care workers have the obligation to strive to give the same level of care to every patient, regardless of race, cultural background, economic status, behavior, physical condition, and/or sexual orientation. This is not always easy because patients can be rude, demanding, and uncooperative. Health care workers have many tasks to accomplish in a limited amount of time. It is natural to resent people who are unpleasant and make life more difficult. But it is at precisely these times that the Philosophy of Individual Worth should serve as a reminder and motivator for health care workers to do their best for every patient. Providing equal care to all, even under demanding circumstances, demonstrates the highest level of professionalism. Florence Nightingale, the founder of modern nursing, stated that "Souls deserve to be cared for." (Portillo in Steefel, 2000). Caring for them effectively requires that sincere efforts be made to understand and accept them as they are (Figure 15-1).

Dealing with Prejudice

Prejudice means having negative feelings about a person because he or she belongs to a specific cultural or racial group. It means assigning certain characteristics to an individual, often negative, based on assumptions about a group. Prejudice prevents people from being considered as the unique individuals that they are. Prejudice also refers to making unfavorable judgments about individuals because of characteristics such as obesity and poverty.

Almost everyone has prejudices of some type. They are not always easy to recognize because they become incorporated into belief systems. They are taken for granted and become part of one's reality. It is difficult to see that there are other possibilities that are acceptable ways of viewing the world. Health care workers should make an

[**Fascinating Facts**]

Perhaps the greatest example of the application of the Philosophy of Individual Worth was demonstrated by the life of Mother Teresa who dedicated her life to working with, in her words, "the poorest of the poor." From 1948 until her death in 1997, Mother Teresa worked in Calcutta, India, caring for desperately poor people who were ill, abandoned, and dying. She founded the House for the Dying in 1952 to provide a place for people to die in peace and dignity. Over the years she created other sites that offered medical care and shelter to the needy all over the world. Mother Teresa put into action her belief that *every* human being is worthy of respect and loving care.

effort to recognize their own prejudices by examining honestly how they judge others.

It is not necessary to agree with all the beliefs and actions of others. In fact, some behaviors may be harmful to the health of the individual, and it is the duty of health care workers to encourage positive changes. In order to do this, they must understand patients' beliefs and motivations. And this understanding is the result of careful listening and resisting the temptation to judge what is heard. When hearing information believed to be "incorrect," a common reaction is to stop listening. This prevents the gathering of the very information needed to begin to understand other people's points of view and the reasons for their beliefs.

THE MEANING OF CULTURE

Every individual is influenced, to a great extent, by his or her cultural background. The term **culture** refers to a wide range of factors that include values, shared beliefs and attitudes, social organization, family and personal relationships, language, everyday activities, religious practices, and concepts of time and space. Belief systems and customs are developed over time to help people make sense of their world. Accepted customs provide guidelines for behavior and action so that daily life can proceed without constant decision making.

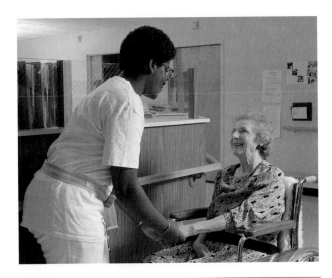

Figure 15-1 Every patient is worthy of your full attention and respect.

They give life predictability and stability and provide the means for people to live together in relative harmony.

Culture gives direction to all aspects of life and provides a set of lenses through which the world is seen and interpreted. It is natural to take one's own beliefs and way of life for granted. This is a frequent source of miscommunication because behaviors that are considered positive in one culture may be a sign of disrespect in another. For example, in the United States direct eye contact is considered a sign of honesty and sincerity. In other cultures, it is a sign of boldness and disrespect. It is important for the health care worker to recognize that everyone sees the world through a set of cultural lenses.

Individuals and Culture

The United States is home to an increasingly diverse number of people from a variety of cultural backgrounds. Significant portions of the population are made up of people once considered to be members of "minority groups." Table 15-1 contains demographic information for a city and a county on the West Coast. Note how Hispanic and Asian populations are expected to grow during the 10-year period between 2000 and 2010, while the percentage of white people in the population decreases, i.e., the white population may also continue to increase, but at a slower rate than the Hispanic and Asian populations.

Immigrants come to the United States for a variety of reasons. Many who have arrived over the last thirty years fled wars and unstable political conditions in their own countries. These immigrants are the most likely to live in close communities. Older members tend to retain their native language and many customs.

There also exist other sub-cultures whose members, although born in the United States, have not fully integrated. The Chinese community in San Francisco is an example of a group that has retained the language and customs of the original culture over many generations. This does not mean that most members of ethnic groups, including recent immigrants and those who choose to retain traditional beliefs and customs, fail to learn the customs necessary to be successful in the United States. Many customs are quickly learned and integrated into daily life. Some behaviors, however, are based on deeply held beliefs about what is important in life. Making the required changes may involve adapting new behaviors that are considered inappropriate in the original culture. Attitudes are much more difficult to recognize and change when they are based on important values.

Health care workers must recognize that differences exist among people and that sometimes these differences are based on cultural background. At the same time, they must take care to identify which cultural characteristics each individual

Table 15–1 Sample Population Trends in California

Group	July 2000 % of Population	Projected July 2010 % of Population	Projected Increase or Decrease
City of San Francisco			
Asian	33%	35%	+ 2%
Hispanic	16%	18%	+ 2%
White, non-Hispanic	40%	37%	- 3%
County of San Diego			
Asian	9%	11%	+2%
Hispanic	25%	29%	+4%
White, non-Hispanic	59%	54%	-5%

(Source: California State Department of Finance, Demographic Research Unit)

patient or coworker has chosen to identify and integrate into their lifestyle. Making assumptions about individuals based on the group to which they are believed to "belong" is disrespectful because it *takes away from their worth as individuals*. It is essential that health care workers learn to observe, ask meaningful questions, and listen carefully to the responses. Using these skills, described later in this chapter, they can best meet the needs of all patients.

There is value to be gained from learning about the general beliefs and practices of the various cultural groups that might be encountered by health care workers in their geographic areas. Gathering this information enables them to:

- Realize and appreciate that there are many valid approaches to life. There is never an "only way" or even a "best way".

- Enrich and improve their own lives by increasing their knowledge of other cultures and discovering differences they might want to incorporate.

- Avoid making the assumption that everything health care workers do and say will be understood and appreciated.

- Understand that certain beliefs *might* be held and certain customs *might* be practiced because of an individual's background.

- Be sensitive to the possible needs of individuals who *appear* to be from specific cultural backgrounds and avoid taking actions that might be offensive until more information can be obtained.

- Ask appropriate and useful questions.

When learning about different cultural groups, it is important to recognize that many common cultural groupings are actually composed of many subgroups that differ in customs and beliefs. For example, Asian Americans come from a wide variety of countries, including China, Japan, the Philippines, Korea, Laos, Cambodia, and Vietnam. Each of these countries has its own history, language, and customs. Spanish-speaking peoples, collectively called "Hispanics," come from dozens of different countries and represent a variety of races and cultures.

Dominant Culture

The term **dominant culture**, as used here, refers to what are generally considered to be the foundational beliefs and ideal behavior of a society or country. These beliefs and behaviors are taught in public schools. They are considered to be necessary in order to be successful. This text, for example,

contains examples of attitudes that belong to the dominant culture of the United States:

- The importance of "being on time" and "using one's time effectively": Not all cultures believe that time is something to be controlled—or even that it *can* be controlled. Nor is punctuality an important concern. The belief is that everything will happen in its "own time" with or without the intervention of humans.

- The need to work efficiently: Interactions with people, even if a medical appointment or work assignment takes longer as a result, are given high priority by some cultures. If a health care worker moves quickly, even though competently, through a procedure and fails to inquire about the patients' family and engage in personal conversation, this indicates a lack of interest in and respect for the patient.

- The need to shake hands firmly when meeting new people: Recommended and even rehearsed for important occasions such as job interviews, this behavior is not universally practiced. In some cultures, only men are expected to shake hands. In others, handshakes are not common among persons of either sex. Other forms of greeting, such as a bow, may be used.

Personal Space and Personal Contact

Customs regarding personal space and personal contact should be understood by health care workers because they have close daily interactions with patients and coworkers. **Personal space** refers to the distance at which people feel most comfortable when carrying on a conversation. In the dominant culture of the United States, a distance of about 18 inches is considered appropriate for people who do not know each other very well. In other cultures, such as some Middle Eastern societies, people stand very close together when talking. It is appropriate that each speaker feels the breath of the other. People from some of the Asian cultures, on the other hand, tend to maintain more distance when engaged in conversation.

The issue of touch is relevant in health care. Many medical procedures involve areas of the body considered private by all cultural groups. It is important to be aware that the degree to which any type of physical contact is tolerated varies among cultures. For example, some cultures consider the examination of a female by a male physician to be inappropriate.

Thinking it Through

In a study of the culturally diverse workplace, European-American nurses saw the quiet, observant, tactful, patient, and slow-to-respond behaviors of Filipino nurses as unassertive. The Filipino nurses saw the outspoken, bold, and fast-moving behaviors of European-American nurses as crass and insensitive. (Source: Spangler, Z. "Culture care of Philippine and Anglo-American nurses in a hospital context." In: Leininger, M. L. ed. (1991). *Culture Care Diversity and Universality: A Theory of Nursing*. New York, NY: National League for Nursing Press.)

1. Why do you think each group of nurses saw the behavior of the other group in negative terms?

2. Do you believe the characteristics listed for each group are necessarily positive or negative? Explain your answer.

3. What might the nurses in the hospital in this study learn from each other?

4. How would you suggest they accomplish this?

Harmless touching in one culture may be improper in another. For example, patting a child on the head can cause extreme distress for some Vietnamese because they believe that the spirits of their ancestors reside there. People who believe in reincarnation (rebirth of the soul in another body) may consider the issue of touch to be important even after death. The Hmongs, a group from Asia who immigrated to the United States as a result of the Vietnam War, fear that autopsies will cause the deceased to be born mutilated in the next life (Wilner, 1995).

The most important point to understand is that there are no "correct" customs. The most important consideration for health care workers is to establish an environment that is comfortable and reassuring for patients and that promotes their welfare.

HEALTH CARE BELIEFS

Health care beliefs and practices vary widely among cultural groups. Traditional Western medicine, defined here as that which is practiced by most physicians in the United States, focuses on the physical aspects of the body and employs scientific methods of diagnosis and treatment. The effect of the mind on the body is not generally considered to be of great importance. An exception is stress, which is becoming recognized as having an impact on health. Illness is generally attributed to factors that can be measured and explained such as infection, environmental conditions, and physical changes in the body's structure. Treatment methods, such as medications, must be proven to be both effective and safe through carefully controlled clinical trials. There is emphasis on formal training and official verification of the competence of health care practitioners through licensing and certification.

Traditional Western medicine is only beginning to acknowledge the possible effects of the mind on the functions and health of the body. Some cultures have always believed that there is a strong connection. Traditional beliefs of many Native Americans, for example, emphasize the relationship between the mind, body, and spirit. Illness, they believe, results when the harmony between these three human components is disrupted.

Religious Beliefs and Health

Religious and spiritual beliefs influence the health practices of many cultural groups and individuals. For example, the traditional healers in some Native American communities have religious status. Known as *shamans* or medicine men, they receive a calling similar to that experienced by spiritual leaders in other cultures. Shamans serve as the mouthpiece of the spirits, which are believed to exist throughout the universe. They employ diagnostic and healing methods that have been used for centuries. These include the widespread use of herbs and special healing ceremonies.

Faith healing is practiced by some Christians. They believe they can be cured from illness and disabilities through prayer and strong religious faith. Some Christians believe that certain members of the clergy have the power to assist with healing. Christian Scientists believe that illness and health are controlled by God and that the patient's mind, not medical treatment, is the means to recovery.

The Moslem religion is predominant in many parts of the world, including North Africa, the Middle East, and Indonesia. Many Moslems believe that what happens in life, including illness, is due to the "Will of Allah" (God's will). Illness, then, can be avoided by religious means. These include the use of prayers, reciting verses from the Koran (the Moslem equivalent of the Bible), and wearing charms.

Some cultures believe in the effects of evil spirits and the evil eye, a stare from someone believed to have the power to cause harm. Some Caribbean peoples, for example, wear charms and carry special objects, such as engraved stones, to ward off evil spirits. This is not unlike athletes who have lucky objects, such as a special pair of shoes, that they believe they need to perform well. Some Latin American peoples have special customs to avoid encountering the evil eye. They are especially protective of young children.

The Catholic religion plays a major role in the life of many people and is the predominant religion in Spanish-speaking countries. Illness is considered by many Catholics to be a form of punishment for sins. Prayers are believed to be helpful, especially when they call upon specific saints for help and are accompanied by the purchasing and lighting of votive candles.

Harmony and Health

The concept of harmony as necessary for good health is common to many cultures. The balance of mind, body, and spirit, mentioned earlier in relation to Native American beliefs, is part of the belief system of some African Americans. The phrase "mind-body" connection is being heard more often in the United States as people are discovering the benefits of a more holistic approach to medicine. See the section in Chapter 2 on complementary therapies.

The Chinese civilization is thousands of years old and has developed many time-honored health care practices. Chinese medicine is based in part on the belief that the body has two energy forces, known as *yin* and *yang.* Illness occurs when these forces are out of balance. Diseases and treatments are classified by their relationship to these forces. Activities and treatments that are believed to promote the integration of the mind and body and enhance the flow of the life force (*chi*) are widely practiced. An example is *t'ai chi,* an ancient form of martial arts, in which slow, relaxed movements are carried out while focusing the mind. T'ai chi is now becoming a popular method in the United States for promoting relaxation, balance, flexibility, and healthy joints.

Traditional beliefs among some Hispanic groups include the theory that the body is controlled by four basic body fluids, known as *humors.* These humors are classified as follows: hot and wet, hot and dry, cold and wet, and cold and dry. Illness results when the humors are out of balance. Disorders and corresponding treatments are organized according to the hot-cold principle. It is recommended that cold illnesses be treated with hot remedies, and hot illnesses with cold ones. For example, a headache is classified as a cold condition. Appropriate hot foods include cereals, eggs, beef, and spicy foods; appropriate medical remedies include aspirin, cinnamon, and garlic.

Herbs and Plant Medicines

Plants and herbs have been used for thousands of years to treat various ailments. Asian cultures have developed thousands of herbal remedies that are widely used today. There has been growing interest in the use of medicinal herbs in the United States by many people who believe that, because they are natural, they have fewer dangerous side effects than pharmaceutical drugs. (Note: It is important that health care workers are aware that "natural" treatments are not necessarily safe. Many plants and herbs *can* have harmful side effects. Herbal remedies and food supplements are not under government regulation as are pharmaceutical products.) The Chinese also prescribe specific foods as treatments for various conditions.

Some older members of African American communities are recognized for their ability to provide effective home remedies, including the preparation of medications from herbs and roots. As with other cultural groups, popular remedies may be handed down from one generation to the next.

See Boxes 15–1 through 15–4 for examples of culturally influenced approaches to health.

Box 15–1 Definitions of Health

Absence of disease

Balance of body energy (yin and yang)

Balance of hot/cold and wet/dry forces in the body

Harmony with nature

Integration of body, mind, and spirit

Box 15–2   Sources of Good Health

Nutritious food, rest, and practice of good hygiene

Gift from ancestors

Good self-care practices such as exercise and not smoking

Reward from God

Will of God

Good luck

Box 15–3   Causes of Illness

Blockage or imbalance of body energy

Disharmony between self and environment

Disharmony caused by demons or spirits

Punishment for sins

Receiving the evil eye or a bad fright

Scientifically explained phenomena such as microbes

Supernatural forces

Violation of taboo (prohibited activity)

Will of God

Box 15–4   Methods of Treatment

Acupressure

Acupuncture

Consultation with traditional healers

Exercise and changes in eating habits

Fasting (giving up eating all or certain foods for a specific period of time)

Herbs

Meditation

Pharmaceutical drugs

Prayer

Roots from plants

Restoration of balance of energy or other bodily forces

Restoration of mind-body-spirit harmony

Rituals and ceremonies

Surgery

DETERMINING INDIVIDUAL NEEDS

The effectiveness of the health care worker's interactions and communication with patients depends largely on understanding and respecting individual differences. While it is not suggested that the practice of modern health care be compromised to accommodate all the traditional beliefs of patients, knowing something about the content and basis of these beliefs can help provide a foundation on which to build effective helping relationships. Being sensitive to the variety of perceptions that patients bring to the health care setting enables health care workers to better meet patient needs. There are several methods to learn about patients as individuals:

1. Observe the patient's behavior and ways of interacting with others.
   - Eye contact
   - Degree of formality in conversation and body movements
   - Outward signs of possible emotions such as nervousness, fear, or suspicion
   - Presence of family members
   - Interactions with family members
   - Reaction to touch and close personal contact
2. Determine whether language barriers are present.
   - Ask patient in what language he or she is most comfortable communicating.
   - Ask about language preferences for written information and instructions.
   - Ask if patient needs an interpreter when discussing health care information and treatments.
3. Ask questions to determine individual preferences.
   - Health beliefs and practices
     - What do you do to help you stay healthy?
     - What do you usually do when you are sick or not feeling well?

- Who do you go to first when seeking help with health problems?
- Who in your family is primarily responsible for making health care decisions for members of the family?
- Who will help you at home if you need assistance with health problems?
- In coping with this illness/injury, what are your expectations of the health care team and of yourself?
- What do you think will be the most important factor in your recovery?
- Are you aware of any medical procedures or practices that contradict your spiritual beliefs?
  - Communication styles
    - What are the ways you show respect and disrespect?
    - Do you have preferences or restrictions related to touching, personal space, making eye contact, or social behaviors that you would like to tell me?
  - General
    - Is there anything you would like to tell me that might help us understand your needs? (Adapted from *Health assessment and physical examination*, by M. E. Z. Estes, 1998, Albany, NY: Delmar.)

4. Listen carefully to the patient's responses.
5. Explain what you are doing and why when performing procedures or asking questions that may be difficult for the individual based on what you have learned.

MASLOW'S HIERARCHY OF HUMAN NEEDS ✓

Cultural backgrounds form the frameworks for the physical, psychological, and spiritual development of human beings. Within these frameworks, however, each individual develops a unique combination of characteristics and behaviors.

There are many approaches to describing and explaining the complexities of human behavior. One useful approach for the health care worker is based on understanding basic human needs. A model that has helped health care professionals to better understand their patients was developed by American psychologist Abraham Maslow. According to Maslow, human behavior is motivated by each individual's efforts to fulfill certain requirements for complete physical and mental well-being (Miller-Keane, 1997). He developed five categories of human needs which

Thinking it Through

Kelly O'Connor handles the billing for Dr. Sinclair's busy orthopedic practice. Patients are sent to Kelly to give her information about their insurance coverage, make payment or payment arrangements, and pay their portion of office calls. One day she is collecting a payment from an elderly patient who came to Dr. Sinclair for treatment of arthritis. He had moved to the United States from a small island in the South Pacific a few years ago. The patient is visibly upset. Kelly asks if Mr. Juarez is all right. He says, "Well, everything here is so rush-rush. The doctor has no time."

1. How can Kelly appropriately respond to the patient?
2. Are there questions she might ask him to learn more about his feelings?
3. How should she follow up?
4. Should she share this encounter with anyone else in the office? Why?

he then ranked in order of importance for human fulfillment. Figure 15–2 contains a triangle that shows the relationship of these five groups. This is known as **Maslow's Hierarchy of Needs**, a hierarchy being an arrangement in order of rank or grade.

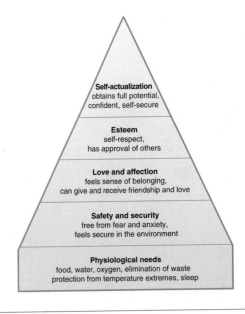

Figure 15–2 Maslow's hierarchy of needs.

- Level 1: **Physiological needs**, which must be satisfied in order to maintain life. These include necessities such as oxygen, water, and food.

- Level 2: Need for physical and psychological security such as living free from the fear of physical harm.

- Level 3: Need for maintaining satisfying relationships with other people, in the form of love and affection. This need is met by enjoying friendships and attaining intimacy with another. See Figure 15-3.

- Level 4: Need for **self-esteem**, the opinion that an individual has of himself or herself. People with high self-esteem are comfortable with themselves and usually able to cope satisfactorily with stress. Being accepted into peer groups is an important influence on self-esteem.

- Level 5: **Self-actualization**, which Maslow defined as the achievement of one's greatest potential. The individual who reaches this level experiences a sense of personal control and accepts responsibility for creating a satisfying life. Another characteristic of individuals at this level is their willingness to help others.

Individuals change and develop over time. They do not remain at one level until every need at that level is met. Life is a dynamic process that involves movement up and down the hierarchy in response to events and experiences and in an ongoing effort to satisfy various needs.

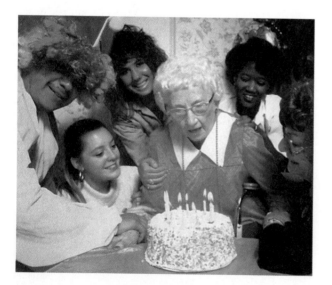

Figure 15–3 Celebrating with friends helps fulfill the need for love and affection.

The behaviors used at any given time to meet the needs described by Maslow are determined by the characteristics of the individual, the current situation, and the opportunities available. For example, securing food for survival can be achieved in several ways: earning money, farming, trading, begging, or stealing. The method selected will be influenced by such factors as parental training, educational level, economic status, job availability, physical condition, level of self-esteem, and moral beliefs.

Patient Needs

Illness and injury alter the nature of human needs and the means that are available to satisfy them. When patients enter the health care world as a result of illness or injury, they must develop new strategies for adjusting and coping. Health care workers must be aware of how the need to meet basic needs affects patient behavior and recovery. They should also recognize that they can play a significant role in helping patients meet these challenges.

We will use the example of a patient named Carlos to illustrate the application of the hierarchy of needs throughout the recovery process. Carlos is a 29-year-old welder. His wife cares for their two children and maintains their home. Carlos is involved in a motorcycle accident in which he suffers a spinal cord injury that results in paraplegia, paralysis from the waist down. His injuries will make it impossible for him to ever walk again.

Carlos's needs are significantly changed as a result of the accident. His progress through the long recovery process begins with the most basic physiological need, which is to survive the physical trauma of the accident. If Carlos is able to meet his needs at each level, his chances of moving up the hierarchy and achieving self-actualization are increased. His progress will not necessarily be smooth and steady and may not take place in an orderly way. Maslow's hierarchy, like other models developed to explain human behavior, can only serve as a guide to assist understanding.

Physiological Needs

Carlos's survival depends on whether his physiological needs can be met to deal with his injuries. This is carried out by emergency room staff who provide immediate medical care. He is now dependent on others to meet his physical needs. The emphasis at this time is providing the medical care necessary to save his life. His needs at this time, like those of other patients in similar situations, include:

- Reassurance
- Knowledge that they are receiving competent care
- Information about where they are and what has happened

After receiving the basic care necessary to save his life, Carlos will remain dependent on the health facility for some time to attend to his physical needs. These include the food and shelter that he used to provide for himself and others.

Safety and Security Needs

Being confined to a health care facility can threaten the patient's feelings of safety and security. Carlos feels uncomfortable in this strange environment, separated from the familiar surroundings of his home and the presence of family members. Feelings of security are increased for patients when they know:

- The names of the staff providing their care
- How to contact staff when they need assistance
- The routine for their care, including when to expect meals, personal care, and treatments
- Pain or discomfort they are likely to experience
- Availability of pain medication

Carlos faces a future full of unknowns, and this is causing him considerable anxiety. He often expresses concern about how he will be able to pay for his medical expenses and continue to support his family. Trying to minimize his worries, even if well-intentioned ("Now, you shouldn't worry about that. Just concentrate on getting well.") does not show respect for Carlos nor does it help him find solutions for his problems.

As Carlos learns to trust the members of the health care team, his feelings of security will increase. Team members can encourage the development of trust by demonstrating acceptance of and respect for the patient. This can be accomplished by listening attentively, withholding judgment, and providing answers to questions. Questions from patients that the health care worker is not qualified to answer should be referred promptly to his or her supervisor.

Love and Affection Needs

Paraplegia brings a set of serious challenges, and one of the most difficult areas is how it affects the need for friendship, love, and affection. Before the accident, Carlos's social life centered on active pursuits with his friends. He knows that he will no longer join in on Saturday soccer games and that his days of riding motorcycles are over. Many of the guys have visited him in the hospital, but he wonders how long they will go on hanging around someone who is confined to a wheelchair. Worse yet are his fears about how his wife is adjusting to having a disabled husband. Does she still love him? Will they be able to have sex?

All aspects of Carlos's previous social life seem altered, and the future looks very lonely. He is experiencing intense frustration and fear, and these emotions lead to occasional angry verbal attacks on the health care workers who provide his care. Understanding the motivation for this behavior, a reaction to threats against the fulfillment of his basic needs, helps the health care team realize that Carlos's outbursts are not meant to be personal attacks, but are the result of his frustration. While it is a natural response to avoid prolonged contact and communication with an angry patient, it is often at this time that human contact is most needed. If Carlos fears rejection and loneliness, avoidance will only reinforce his belief that he is unlikable and unlovable.

Ways to help patients meet their need for love and affection include:

- Expressing sincere interest in them and their well-being
- Behaving in a compassionate way when patients are difficult
- Listening attentively
- Touching patients on the hand or shoulder as a form of greeting or reassurance
- Allowing them to express themselves even if the topic is difficult or unpleasant
- Helping family and friends feel welcome and comfortable during visits
- Encouraging family and friends to come and celebrate holidays or special events with patients

The health care worker can also alert the supervisor or other appropriate members of the health care team about Carlos's current behavior and possible needs. For example, occupational therapists help patients like Carlos rebuild their lives and achieve the highest level of activity possible, including sexual function. (Remember, however, that legal considerations of confidentiality restrict any discussions about patients to ONLY those health care practitioners who work with them.)

Self-Esteem Needs

The feelings that individuals have about themselves at a given time and their opinions of their value as people are known as self-esteem. Self-esteem can fluctuate, and whether it is high or low depends on the person's experiences and perceptions at the moment. Injuries and illnesses that disfigure and cause loss of function often result in a decrease in self-esteem that can last for extended periods of time. Most people place importance on what others think of them and base their self-esteem, to a great extent, on the opinions of others. Before the accident, Carlos defined himself in terms of his roles as husband, father, son, friend, and worker. In other words, his personal value was based on *what* rather than *who* he was. His relationships with others and his role in the community were sources of self-esteem. He took pride in his ability as a welder and was confident of his ability to provide for his family.

In the weeks following the accident, Carlos's self-esteem has plummeted. Maslow's hierarchy can help explain why. Carlos has lost control over his ability to meet the needs that make up the first three groups of the hierarchy. Let's look at each one. In caring for his physical needs, he will learn to perform many tasks for himself when he enters rehabilitation. For now, however, he must depend on others to take care of these requirements. Regarding security, he has not yet determined how he will provide for the future financial security of himself or his family. Finally, he still has doubts about how he will be treated by friends and family during his long rehabilitation and subsequent life as a paraplegic.

Health care workers can help reinforce Carlos's self-esteem by sending the message that "You are worth my time. Your disability does not detract from your value as a person." Ways to express this idea to patients include:

- Taking the time to listen
- Showing interest by referring back to something the patient said in the past or remembering an occasion or event that is important to the patient
- Allowing patients the opportunity to express their needs
- Asking for and respecting their preferences
- Protecting their privacy
- Treating them with respect and dignity
- Asking for their approval before giving care
- Asking for patients' opinions of what works best for them *if* there are options

Self-Actualization Needs

While the means available for Carlos to reach his highest potential have been altered by his accident, it is still possible for him to achieve self-actualization. Some people who have suffered serious health problems see their circumstances as an opportunity to make positive life changes. They even find that their quality of life improves, because they realize the value of each day and more fully appreciate what they have. Common life changes include:

- Finding work that is more meaningful
- Making time for things they have always wanted to do, such as painting or working with children
- Sharing their recovery experiences with others who are suffering from similar injuries or illnesses
- Becoming involved in health care fund-raising activities to pay for research into and treatment of their condition

Actor Christopher Reeves, star of the Superman movies, was paralyzed from the neck down when he was thrown from his horse in 1995. He has returned to films as a director and is working vigorously to promote research that is focused on developing new treatments for spinal cord injuries. He is an example of responding in a self-actualized manner to a catastrophic event. Another example is popular television and movie actor Michael J. Fox, who left acting as a result of Parkinson's Disease. He is now working to raise public awareness of the disease and funds for research to find a cure.

Many factors will influence to what extent Carlos attempts to achieve self-actualization. The treatment he receives in the various health facilities during his recovery are important. Health care workers must realize how their interactions with patients can affect their ability to move up the hierarchy and meet their needs at the highest level possible.

Maslow's Hierarchy of Needs serves as a useful model for understanding the behavior of all patients, not just those like Carlos who are suffering from very serious conditions. For example, one's sense of security can be threatened by visits to the dentist and physician for annual exams. And the self-esteem of an overweight patient can be undermined during a procedure that requires disrobing. It is important that health care workers keep in mind that what is routine to them can be threatening to their patients. Being sensitive to the needs of patients is a prerequisite for establishing good communication.

DEFENSE MECHANISMS

The need to maintain one's self-esteem at an acceptable level is a driving force in shaping human behavior. **Defense mechanisms** are a special category of responses to perceived threats to self-esteem. They help provide relief from the mental discomfort and anxiety caused by internal conflict and are usually performed unconsciously (Miller-Keane, 1997). For example, a student may believe that his inability to arrive on time to class is due to sleep patterns inherited from his father, when in reality, it is due to his habit of partying late at night. Although they provide temporary relief, defense mechanisms do not resolve the underlying, anxiety-producing problems that need to be addressed. For example, Mrs. Azordegan discovers a small lump in her left breast. She is afraid that it might be cancer and refuses to take any action. She puts off calling her physician or telling anyone in the family about the lump. Her *denial* is a defense mechanism whose purpose is to avoid facing a potential unpleasant truth. By the time she seeks medical attention, she learns that she does have cancer and that delaying treatment has allowed it to metastasize (spread to other parts of the body). The use of a defense mechanism has worsened the very problem that Mrs. Azordegan feared most and hoped to avoid. Even if the lump had not been cancerous, Mrs. Azordegan would have experienced prolonged and unnecessary stress caused by the delayed diagnosis. In either case, ignoring the situation only caused additional problems.

Defense mechanisms are commonly used at times of stress and anxiety, such as those experienced during illness or injury. Table 15–2 describes some of the defense mechanisms that health care

workers may encounter when working with patients. Milliken (1998) states that it is not the role of health care workers to point out that patients may be using defense mechanisms. Rather, it is their role to reduce the amount of threat experienced by patients. Examples of ways the health care worker can do this include:

- Demonstrating acceptance
- Showing sincere interest in their well-being
- Providing education and instructions to increase patients' control over their own health issues (Figure 15-4)
- Allowing them to discuss what is really bothering them, if they wish to do so
- Respecting their need to use defense mechanisms, which may be needed to get through a very difficult situation

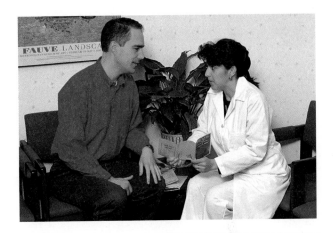

Figure 15-4 Educating patients about self-care techniques can reduce their anxiety by increasing their control over personal health issues.

Table 15–2 Common Defense Mechanisms

Defense Mechanism	Definition	Example
Compensation	Attempting to meet a need by substituting something that does not actually satisfy the need	Recently divorced woman overeating to deal with loneliness
Control	Trying to exert excessive control over others to make up for a loss of control elsewhere	Hospitalized patient insisting on being given an exact time schedule for care
Denial	Pretending that something is not true, especially something unpleasant	Business executive refusing to acknowledge testing positive for HIV

(continues)

Table 15–2 (continued)

Defense Mechanism	Definition	Example
Displacement	Transferring feelings that one has about one person to a different person	Nurse becoming angry with her children after working with a demanding patient
Malingering	Pretending to be ill when one is not	Student faking symptoms to avoid taking a test at school
Projection	Failing to see one's own weaknesses and/or problems while seeing them in others	Overweight mother criticizing her overweight daughter's "poor eating habits"
Rationalization	Explaining behavior by using a socially acceptable reason	Graduate nurse delaying taking a licensing exam because she is "too busy" when in reality she is afraid she will fail
Regression	Behaving in ways that are more appropriate for a younger aged person	A 10-year-old boy returning to thumb-sucking after being hospitalized
Repression	Keeping unpleasant thoughts or memories in the unconscious and out of awareness	A young woman lacking conscious memory of having been sexually assaulted as a child
Withdrawal	Refusing to communicate with others or participate in social activities	A teenage boy refusing to take calls from friends or attending social activities after being diagnosed with leukemia

DEALING WITH LOSS

Having to deal with loss can significantly influence patient behavior. Suffering an illness or injury or even undergoing the normal aging process can result in many types of loss. These include loss of independence, a body part or function, control over one's life, appearance and self-image, privacy, financial security, familiar surroundings, and significant other. The patient who must remain in a health care facility for a long period of time is likely to suffer multiple losses. However, even the removal of a tooth in the dentist's office represents a loss. It can be traumatic for the middle-aged patient who experiences this as the beginning of the dreaded aging process and only the first of future physical problems and losses. Any health care encounter can represent loss of control for patients.

Just as the methods used to fulfill basic needs vary among individuals, so will their reactions to loss. Some common examples of ways of dealing with loss include:

- Seeking support from family and friends
- Finding comfort in religion
- Drawing on self-esteem
- Employing problem-solving techniques
- Using the defense mechanisms
- Becoming angry
- Experiencing depression

Health care workers can help patients deal with loss by realizing its significance to patients, understanding their reactions to loss and their need to grieve, and by being willing to talk with patients who wish to discuss their loss. This gives patients the opportunity to share their feelings, if they wish to do so, and to explore ways to grieve and deal with their loss (Figure 15–5).

THE PATIENT AS AN INDIVIDUAL

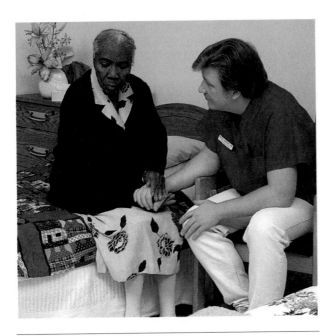

Figure 15–5 Listening and expressing concern can help patients deal with loss.

SUGGESTED LEARNING ACTIVITIES

1. Brainstorm ideas on how you can apply the Philosophy of Individual Worth, described in this chapter, in your personal and future work life.

2. Learn more about the various cultural groups in your area. Attend local cultural events such as diversity fairs and informational workshops.

3. Research two cultural groups that are different from your own. Choose five aspects to compare and contrast between the two groups and with your own.

4. Use illustrations from magazines to create a poster that represents the cultural groups represented in the United States today.

5. Observe the behavior of people around you. Identify attempts to meet the needs described by Maslow.

6. Explore the Web site at: http://members.tripod.com/~HmongAmerican/HmongAmerican to see how and why one group of recent immigrants are attempting to retain their language and customs.

7. Start a journal of your own behavior in which you observe and note your attempts to meet the needs described by Maslow.

8. Watch for examples of possible defense mechanisms used by people around you: friends, family members, and classmates. Why do you think these mechanisms were employed?

REVIEW QUESTIONS

1. Explain the Philosophy of Individual Worth and how it relates to work in health care.

2. What is the definition of "culture"?

3. Give three examples of different cultural approaches to health care for each of the following categories:
   - definition of health
   - sources of good health
   - causes of illness
   - methods of treatment

4. What are four ways that the health care worker can determine the individual needs of a patient?

5. Give five examples of questions to ask to discover a patient's needs.

6. What are the five levels of needs described by Maslow?

7. Give an example to demonstrate the meaning of each level of need.

8. What are the common defense mechanisms encountered in health care situations?

9. What are three ways the health care worker can help patients deal with the experience of loss?

APPLICATION EXERCISES

1. Refer back to the case involving Carley and Mr. Alvarez. What assumptions did Carley make? How could she have learned more about Mr. Alvarez? Once she learned about his situation, what could she have done to better help him understand and carry out the diet and exercise program prescribed by Dr. Washington?

2. You are working as a medical assistant in the private medical office of an oncologist (cancer specialist). Mrs. Ramirez, an elderly woman who lived in Guatemala until she was 56, comes to the office accompanied by her granddaughter. Mrs. Ramirez speaks very little English, but her granddaughter is bilingual. This visit was at the granddaughter's insistence after her grandmother admitted finding a small lump in her breast. Mrs. Ramirez is very anxious about the visit. Describe how you would work with this patient, including a review of cultural factors and individual needs.

SUGGESTED READINGS AND RESOURCES

Dienemann, J. (Ed.). (1997). *Cultural diversity in nursing: issues, strategies, and outcomes.* Washington, DC: American Academy of Nursing.

Luckmann, J. (2000). *Transcultural communication in health care.* Albany, NY: Delmar.

Purtilo, R. and Haddad, A. (1996). *Health professional and patient interaction* (5th ed.). Philadelphia: W. B. Saunders Company.

Van Servellen, G. (1997). *Communication skills for the health care professional: Concepts and techniques.* Gaithersburg, MD: Aspen Publishers, Inc.

Wieland, D., Benton, D., Kramer, B., and Dawson, J. (Eds.). (1994). *Cultural diversity and geriatric care: Challenges to the health professions.* New York: Haworth Press, Inc.

CHAPTER

THE COMMUNICATION PROCESS

OBJECTIVES

Studying and applying the material in this chapter will help you to:

- Explain the importance of effective communication in health care delivery.

- Describe the relationship between effective communication and patient well-being.

- Identify and describe the six steps of the communication process.

- Define and explain the use of the four types of questions.

- Apply communication techniques successfully.

- Explain the meaning of nonverbal communication and give examples of three types.

- Explain the meaning of active listening.

- Define "empathy" and explain its application in health care.

- Explain the meaning of feedback and how it is used in communication.

- Recognize common barriers that can prevent effective communication.

- List the techniques to use when communicating with patients who have special needs.

- Demonstrate professional telephone techniques and explain why it is important to apply them in the health care facility.

- Describe the elements that make up effective patient education.

- List strategies for preparing and giving presentations to groups.

- List three ways to handle situations involving gossip.

KEY TERMS

barriers

closed-ended questions

communication

empathy

feedback

leading questions

learning objectives

nonverbal communication

open-ended questions

pantomime

paraphrasing

probing questions

receiver

reflecting

sender

The Case of

the Coder Who Lacked Confidence

Jenny McAbee has worked as a medical insurance coder and biller for Appleton Medical Clinic for three years. She enjoys working with detailed information and performing tasks on the computer. Her coding is accurate and very few claims to insurance companies are denied. One of Jenny's reasons for choosing this career is her shyness and desire to work by herself. Dr. Morton, the director of the clinic, has noted that many patients are confused about their insurance coverage, which payments are their responsibility, how to fill out and submit the proper paperwork, and other insurance details. He decides to provide Jenny with an assistant so that she can make herself available to answer patients' questions and explain their insurance plans. Jenny wants to help the clinic's patients but does not feel confident about her communication skills. She realizes that many patients have hearing impairments or don't speak very much English. She wonders how she can best help them.

This chapter covers the communication process and techniques for becoming an effective communicator.

IMPORTANCE OF COMMUNICATION IN HEALTH CARE

Communication is a process in which messages are exchanged between a sender and a receiver. The **sender**, also referred to as the speaker, is the person who creates and delivers a message. The **receiver**, also known as the listener, is the person to whom the sender directs the message. Communication is successful when the receiver interprets the sender's message as it was sent. Throughout a communication encounter, the sender and receiver will exchange roles. Messages can be exchanged in at least four ways:

1. Orally
2. Nonverbally (examples: facial expressions, gestures)
3. In written form (see Chapter 17)
4. Electronically (see Chapter 18)

In order to function effectively, modern health care systems rely on the efficient and accurate delivery of large amounts of information. Diagnoses and treatments are often based on a variety of data that must be shared among many health care providers. There are vast networks of primary care providers, specialists, therapists, testing centers, medical facilities, and insurance companies that work together to provide and coordinate patient care. It is critical that all information be both accurate and delivered in a timely way.

Several of the health care trends discussed in Chapter 2 have increased the need for communication excellence:

1. Growth of managed care systems: Effective delivery of patient care depends on the coordination of information among various facilities and staff members. Chances for miscommunication increase as systems become larger and more complex.

2. Significant decrease in the length of time patients spend in hospitals and other health care facilities: They are now more responsible for their own follow-up care and need clear instructions to correctly carry out necessary self-care procedures.

3. Shift in major causes of death from infectious diseases to cancer, heart disease, and stroke: There has been an increase in chronic illness

because people are living longer. An increasingly important part of health care workers' responsibilities is providing patient education about factors that promote wellness. Good education is achieved through effective communication.

The ability to communicate well is as important to the professional success of the health care worker as the phlebotomist's ability to safely draw blood and the respiratory therapist's command of ventilation therapy. The well-being of patients depends on more than technical competence. For example, if a nurse is instructing a patient about how to change the dressing on a wound, the patient's understanding of these instructions is critical for successfully carrying out self-care practices at home.

Communication and Patient Well-Being

The ability of health care workers to communicate effectively is influenced by their attitude. The first step in achieving communication excellence is to develop respect for and an understanding of individual patients and their needs, as discussed in Chapter 15. Effective communication skills involve more than applying a set of techniques. They must be based on sincere compassion and concern for patients and their welfare (Figure 16–1).

The health-care world can be intimidating for patients. They may be anxious about receiving negative test results and learning that they have serious medical conditions. Or they may be fearful about experiencing pain and discomfort during necessary treatments. Still others are worried about losing control over portions of their lives as a result of their physical conditions. These concerns, combined with the physical stress caused by illness or injury, can negatively affect patient recovery. Health care workers can help relieve patient stress by giving reassurance, providing appropriate information, and answering questions. *Good communication can increase the speed of patient recovery.*

Loneliness and depression are commonly experienced by patients during their stay in health care facilities. Health care workers may be their principal contact with the outside world. Being willing to talk and, even more important, to *listen* to patients, can lift their spirits. One of the most important goals in health care communication is to help others to feel good about themselves (Collins, 1983).

Situations do not have to involve a direct threat to one's health to be stressful experiences for patients. As discussed in Chapter 15, any health care encounter can represent a loss for the patient and be a source of anxiety. Well-chosen words and a willingness to listen can help relieve anxiety. Patient satisfaction is determined, to a great extent, by the quality of their communication with health care staff (Lindh, et al., 1998).

Patient care delivery is dependent on communication among members of the health care team, as well as on health care worker-patient interactions. The quality of care can be negatively affected when poor interpersonal and interprofessional relations exist among members of the team (Kreps and Kunimoto, 1994). As a future member of this team, it is your responsibility to make every effort to ensure that patient care is never compromised by a lack of attention to communication skills. Poor communication can lead to fatal consequences.

THE COMMUNICATION PROCESS

It is commonly believed that communication consists of simply talking and listening, activities that most people have been doing all their lives. Dozens of conversations are carried on daily with family members, friends, classmates, and coworkers. Effective communication in health care, however, is specifically aimed at meeting the needs of patients. It involves the application of a highly developed set of skills, and acquiring these skills takes effort, concentration, and practice.

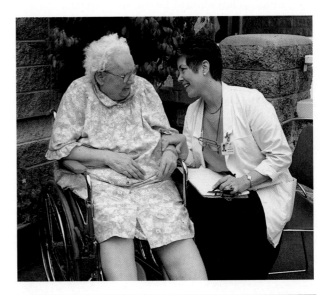

Figure 16–1 Communication skills are essential for effective patient care.

These skills have been organized into a six-step process. This process provides a structured approach for studying and learning the variety of skills that make up effective communication. Like other healthcare skills, communication cannot be taken for granted or performed in a routine manner. Each communication encounter presents its own set of circumstances and demands the health care worker's full attention. It requires the application of the thinking skills presented in Chapter 1.

The Six Steps of the Communication Process

1. Set communication goals: Determine what is to be accomplished. This involves considering patient needs, current circumstances, and the duties assigned to the health care worker.

2. Create the message: Select and organize appropriate content based on the communication goals.

3. Deliver the message: Choose the delivery method best suited for ensuring that the receiver will understand the intent of the message.

4. Listen to the response: Employ listening and observational techniques to determine whether the message was received as intended.

5. Offer feedback and seek clarification: Rephrase what is heard or ask questions to check your understanding of the response.

6. Evaluate the encounter and revise the message: Determine whether the goal was met. If not, why not? What other options are available? What should be the next step?

Step One: Set Communication Goals

The first step in the communication process is to determine the goal. What is to be accomplished? Much of everyday communication is spontaneous and superficial and requires little or no planning. This includes everyday greetings ("Hi, how are you?"), which are said automatically and from which little real information is usually expected. Interactions in health care settings are more purposeful and contribute to providing appropriate patient care. They require skill. For example, instead of asking a patient, "How are you?" which usually results in a programmed response of "fine," health care workers need to ask more specific questions. These will be based on communication goals. Examples of specific questions include:

- What is your pain level?

- Do you have any questions about your care?

- Are you feeling nervous about the procedure?

Health care communication often takes place at a deeper level than everyday conversation and must be clear and accurate. It may involve the sharing of very personal information, such as a patient's fears. Health care workers must learn to carefully observe and listen for clues.

Communication goals come in many forms. The following examples are typical goals in health care situations:

- Gather as much objective and subjective information as possible from a patient.

- Instruct individuals on postsurgical home care procedures so family members will understand and follow them correctly.

- Inform a patient about the benefits of the treatment procedure you are administering.

- Report patient care information to a coworker who is taking over the care of the patient.

In addition to goals that are specific to the situation, there are three that should be included in every patient interaction:

1. Demonstrate sincere concern for the patient's welfare
   - Have a warm smile.
   - Use a gentle manner.
   - Do not act hurried.
   - Listen carefully.

2. Establish trust.
   - Establish eye contact.
   - Explain why a procedure, treatment, or test is necessary.
   - Explain in advance everything you are going to do.
   - Follow through with anything you say you will do (return in 5 minutes, call patient at home to check on progress, and so on).

3. Enhance the patient's self-esteem.
   - Involve the patient in decision-making whenever possible.
   - Clarify the patient's communication if you're unsure of meaning.
   - Address the patient properly and respectfully.
   - Provide for privacy.
   - Ask the patient for input on how he or she wants things done, when appropriate.

These goals are based on the Philosophy of Individual Worth discussed in Chapter 15. It may seem unrealistic to try to achieve these goals in the brief time the health care worker spends with patients. There are other tasks to accomplish, such as taking a blood sample or performing a breathing treatment. Good communication, however, depends more on quality than quantity. A warm smile and informative reassurance are not time-consuming and can be included in any encounter. Patients today receive much of their care from strangers who are in a hurry. It is for this very reason that an effort should be made to personalize interactions and treat patients as individuals.

Collect Information

An important part of goal-setting is to collect and review information that might affect communication. This includes the cultural and behavioral factors discussed in Chapter 15 as well as circumstances specific to the situation, such as the amount of pain the patient is experiencing or the effects of medication. The following factors should be considered:

- Patient's level of understanding
  - Is patient very young?
  - Does patient speak English?
  - If so, is English the second language?
  - Does patient have a learning disability that affects his or her ability to understand?
  - Does patient appear to be confused or disoriented?
  - What is the patient's ability to retain information? Is there short-term memory loss?
  - What is the appropriate terminology to use?
- Emotional factors
  - Does patient's behavior indicate fear and/or anxiety?
  - Are there signs that patient is using a defense mechanism? See Chapter 15.
  - Is patient ready to accept the information that is to be offered?
- Physical factors
  - Is patient in pain?
  - Is patient on medication that causes drowsiness or affects the ability to concentrate?
  - Does patient have a hearing, visual, or speech impairment that affects the communication process?
- Urgency of the communication
  - Must the communication take place now?
  - Is this the appropriate setting for the communication?
  - What are the consequences if it does not take place? Or if it is unsuccessful?

Learning to make these determinations quickly is an important health care skill that is developed over time. New health care workers should strive to develop mental checklists to help them prepare for communication encounters.

Step Two: Create the Message

Creating an appropriate message requires the selection of content and language that are based on the answers to the questions listed above. Information must be presented in a manner that the receiver understands. For example, while the use of medical terminology helps ensure accuracy in communications with other health care workers, it can confuse and intimidate patients. Even everyday language may have to be simplified into common terms for some patients, depending on their age and language skills. For example, "number two" might be substituted for "bowel movement." Take care, however, not to talk down to patients.

It is best to use language that is not limited to specific age or cultural groups. For example, the current use of the verb form "goes" to mean "says" can be confusing for many people. Similar to clothing, the language appropriate for professional settings may differ from that used in social situations. The overuse of filler words such as "you know" and "like" should also be avoided. They can be irritating to the receiver and distract from the message. Television news announcers are good models for standard American speech.

Long messages should be organized so that they are easy for the receiver to follow. Here are some examples of organizational strategies:

- Explain what you plan to do and what the patient should expect to hear, feel, and so on.
- Rank information in order of importance.
- List a sequence of steps for the patient to follow.
- State facts and follow each with an explanation.
- Present an overview of a procedure before detailing the individual steps.
- Give instructions along with a description of possible consequences if they are not followed.
- Break information into smaller sessions, if possible, so the patient can grasp each step before moving on to the next.
- Ask clarifying questions or have the patient demonstrate understanding by explaining the information or performing the task or exercise being taught before going on to the next level.

Asking Questions

Some messages may be phrased as questions. There are several types of questions as well as a variety of ways to maximize their effectiveness.

1. **Closed-ended questions** can be answered with a single word or a response of "yes" or "no." This type of question is used to gather factual information. For example, the health care worker may ask closed-ended questions when obtaining background information about a patient. Closed-ended questions are not recommended when checking for understanding. Many patients will answer "Yes" to the question, "Do you understand?" even if they do not. They are afraid of appearing stupid or do not want to "bother you" by having the information repeated.

2. **Open-ended questions** cannot be answered with a simple "yes" or "no." They require a more complete response and are used to encourage patients to provide more detailed information or explanations. These questions can be used to learn about the patient's symptoms, to encourage the sharing of feelings and opinions, or to check understanding of the message.

3. **Probing questions** are requests for additional information or clarification. For example, they can be used to lead a patient to more fully discuss the symptoms being experienced. If a patient states, "My stomach hurts," appropriate probing questions would inquire about the exact location and type of pain, when it first appeared, and at what time it occurs. It is important not to confuse the purposeful use of probing questions with digging for unnecessary personal details, which patients may find offensive.

4. **Leading questions** are those in which all or part of the answer is included in the wording of the question. Leading questions should be avoided when they encourage the receiver to give the answer believed to be correct or what the sender wants to hear. This is most likely to happen when a patient is concerned about appearing to be stupid or does not understand the question. Leading questions can be useful when used with patients who have difficulty speaking or who do not understand English well enough to phrase a complete answer. In these situations, take extra care to check for understanding to ensure that the patient is not simply agreeing with you. See Table 16–1 for examples of each type of question.

After a question is asked, it is important to pause and give the receiver sufficient time to respond. Some people need more time than others to formulate answers. Do not interrupt or finish sentences for the receiver. If it is obvious that a question is not understood or that the receiver is unable to reply, reword it and provide another opportunity for a response. The state of each patient and his or her ability to answer questions must be considered. For example, Mrs. Feinstein is an elderly patient who has difficulty remembering. Hospitalized for severe back pain, she cannot accurately respond to questions about how she is feeling today compared to yesterday. A more effective way to get the needed information is to ask her to rate her pain level on a scale of zero to ten, with zero being no pain and ten being the highest level tolerable. See Chapter 20 for more information about assessing pain.

Table 16–1 Common Types of Questions

Question Type	Examples
Closed-ended	What is your date of birth? Are you taking any medications?
Open-ended	How did you fall? Why do you think you are feeling sad?
Probing	You said that you've been experiencing pain in your chest. Where, exactly, in your chest do you feel the pain? When is it the most severe? Can you tell me more about when you get these headaches?
Leading	Would you describe the pain as sharp, dull, throbbing, or aching? Do you feel more nauseated in the morning, afternoon, evening, or during the night?

Thinking it Through

Robin Winters is starting her career as a dental hygienist for Dr. Castro at an urban dental clinic. Robin has noted that many of the patients appear to have poor dental care habits: their teeth have accumulations of plaque and a high number of caries (cavities), and the patients suffer from gingivitis (inflammation of the gums). When she asks patients if they take care of their teeth at home, most respond, "yes."

1. How can Robin use questions more effectively to learn about her patient's dental care habits?

2. Give examples of questions that she might ask.

Using Humor

Messages need not always be serious. The careful use of humor can offer temporary escape from the difficult situations faced by patients and their families. It can help relieve tension and promote the open discussion of sensitive issues. Humor, however, should *never* be at the expense of anyone, even in their absence.

Patients will sometimes joke about their condition as a cover-up for fear or embarrassment, but the health care worker should never initiate this type of humor. Listen carefully in these situations, because these jokes may indicate the patient's need for help in dealing with a difficult condition. It is appropriate to let patients know that if they wish, they can discuss fears they have or request information they need.

Step Three: Deliver the Message

It is important to determine to whom the message should be delivered. This is not always obvious. For example, if the patient is a child or elderly person, should communication be directed to the patient or to a family member? Patients who are able to understand any or all of the message should be addressed directly. Detailed information or instructions can also be given to a family member later. For example, a medical assistant who greets 87-year-old Mrs. Hernandez by asking her daughter, "How is your mother doing today?" is failing to show respect for the patient. This can undermine the self-esteem of the elderly, who are frequently faced with the biases of a youth-oriented society. Using titles, such as Mrs., Ms., and Mr., demonstrates respect for patients. A common guideline for health care workers is to address patients older than themselves more formally than those who are the same age or younger. If in doubt, it is best to ask patients how they wish to be addressed.

Some cultural groups designate a family member, often the oldest or a male, to make decisions on behalf of the patient. While it is important for the health care worker to understand the dynamics of the patient's family, this does not suggest that the laws governing confidentiality can be broken in order to accommodate cultural preferences. Well-meaning family members and friends, the patient's insurance company, and others who may appear to have a valid right to know *cannot* be given information unless the patient has signed a release. It is essential to recognize which messages have a restricted audience and exactly who that audience is.

Advance directives and a health care power of attorney, discussed in Chapter 3, serve as the links between health care workers and patients who have lost their ability to communicate. It is essential to know what medical treatments patients desire to be performed and who may receive information and speak on their behalf.

It is believed that many patients who cannot speak or respond can hear and experience touch. Health care workers can provide comfort by maintaining communication. They should speak reassuringly and make physical contact, such as touching the patient's hand or shoulder when speaking.

Nonverbal Communication

The manner in which a message is delivered can either reinforce or change the intended meaning. It can communicate more than the words that make up the content. For example, an otherwise friendly remark, stated in a sarcastic voice, distorts the intended message. The words "that's a nice thing to say" can be delivered in a way that indicates the sender's pleasure. The same words, delivered in a mocking tone with stress on the word "that's," convey the opposite meaning. It sends the message that what was said was hurtful.

Nonverbal communication includes tone of voice, body language, gestures, facial expressions, touch, and physical appearance. Up to 70% of the meaning of messages is expressed nonverbally.

Nonverbal communication is usually the best expression of what the sender truly feels and believes. This is because it comes from within, outside the awareness of the sender. It takes place unconsciously.

Health care workers must be aware of the nonverbal communication of both themselves and others. The nonverbal communication of patients should always be observed. For example, if a patient reports feeling "fine," but appears very tense and nervous, the verbal and nonverbal messages do not match. In such cases, the health care worker needs to ask questions and provide opportunities for the patient to share what is really being experienced.

The appearance of the health professional is a form of nonverbal communication. It can influence the confidence of the patient in the worker's competence and, therefore, can affect how messages are perceived. See Chapter 13 for a complete discussion of professional appearance.

Body Language

Body posture and movements convey messages. Some body language can have a negative impact on the receiver. Examples include crossing the arms, shrugging the shoulders, tapping the fingers or feet, clenching the fists, and rolling the eyes. These communicate disagreement, lack of interest, disbelief, and impatience.

Positive body language conveys interest, caring, and the willingness to listen to the sender's message, even if there is disagreement. It encourages the sharing of information and promotes the exchange of honest messages. Positive body language includes the following:

- Looking at the other person
- Directing the body toward the other person
- Leaning slightly toward the person being addressed
- Holding the body in a relaxed position
- Nodding or verbalizing (uh huh, yes, tell me more) occasionally to indicate acknowledgement
- Having open and warm facial expressions
- Approaching the patient, if standing at a distance
- Stopping the performance of tasks to give your full attention

Positive body posture communicates "I am focused on and paying attention to you and what you are saying." See Figure 16–2. Actions must match words. For example, if a patient wants to discuss a sensitive matter and the health care worker listens while facing toward the door, the message to the patient may be "I'm really in a hurry to leave." In another example, a health care worker wants to reassure a patient but looks away nervously while speaking. The message will seem false and the patient will sense that important information, probably negative, is being left unsaid. The establishment of trust, an essential ingredient in effective communication, requires that spoken and nonverbal communication match.

Facial Expressions

Facial expressions are an important form of nonverbal communication. The health care worker's expressions can be a source of reassurance or anxiety for patients, so it is important to learn to be aware of and control them. This can be difficult when dealing with situations that are challenging, unpleasant, or offensive. For example, you may feel very frustrated with the behavior of an angry patient. Efforts at calming will be less effective if your face reflects signs of impatience and annoyance.

Patients look to the health professional for reassurance while receiving care, and facial expressions such as surprise or disgust can alarm them and undermine their faith in the services they are receiving. It is important not to react negatively to the sight of wounds or deformities, and the smell of unpleasant odors. Patients are very sensitive to the reactions of health care workers to these potentially embarrassing conditions. The health care worker's face should reflect warmth, confidence, and interest in the welfare of the patient.

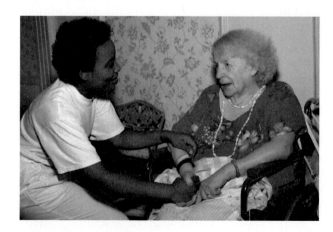

Figure 16–2 What positive body language is being demonstrated by this health care worker?

Gestures can help emphasize and enrich spoken messages. The use of **pantomime**, using body movements to convey ideas or actions, can increase patient understanding. For example, acting out the movements a patient must make when performing an exercise can demonstrate exactly what needs to be done. Pantomime can also be effective when patients cannot hear or understand the spoken word.

Gestures and facial expressions are effective when patients cannot be attended to immediately. Acknowledging their presence conveys respect and creates good will. For example, if the medical receptionist is speaking on the telephone when a patient arrives for an appointment, the patient should be greeted with a smile, nod of the head, and quick hand gesture to indicate that he or she will be attended to shortly.

Use of Touch

The use of touch has become a difficult issue in health care today. While a friendly pat or squeeze of the hand has been a traditional way of communicating care and interest, any touching that a patient considers to be inappropriate can lead to legal problems. It is essential that health care workers always practice good judgment and use common sense. Many health care activities require entering personal space that is normally reserved for only the closest and most trusted people in the patient's life. It is important that patients be told what is to take place and why. Explain what they should expect to see, hear, and feel. For example, when administering an injection, the patient should be informed of its purpose, where is will be given, and what sensations might be experienced.

The health care worker should avoid touching areas that are considered sexual (buttocks, breasts, genital area), unless it is necessary in the performance of a procedure. Any unnecessary roughness, even done in a playful manner, can be interpreted as abusive and should be avoided.

Gestures and body movements that are either positive or neutral to one person may be unacceptable to others. As discussed in Chapter 15, health care workers should be sensitive to the existence of such differences, willing to learn about various cultural practices, and observant of patient reactions. If a patient seems uncomfortable with any contact that was intended to be a sign of caring or reassurance, seek clarification by stating your intention and asking if the gesture was unacceptable.

Physical Environment

The physical environment and how the health care worker is positioned in relation to the patient can affect the delivery of the message. Sitting behind a desk or standing over the other person projects a sign of authority or dominance. Other factors to consider include the following:

- Light sources: Can the patient see you clearly? Is there a glare on anything the patient is expected to see? Is light shining in the patient's eyes?
- Sounds: Can the patient hear you clearly? Are there unnecessary noises that are distracting? Should the television or radio be turned off?
- Privacy: Are there other people in the area who can hear the communication? If privacy is necessary, how can it be arranged? Are you speaking directly to the patient and only as loudly as necessary?
- Activity: Are you more focused on taking notes or entering data into a computer than on the patient?
- Comfort: Is the patient exposed or in an awkward position? Can communication wait?

Being aware of the effects of the environment and positioning on communication can assist in the delivery of appropriate messages that achieve communication goals.

Step Four: Listen to the Response

Listening is not passive, but an active process that requires:

- Concentration
- Attention
- Observation

Hearing and taking in words takes place at a rate that is several times faster than the rate of speech. This is helpful when taking notes, but it allows time for the mind to wander. Hearing too quickly can actually detract from hearing well.

Effective listening can also be hindered by the receiver's reactions to what the sender is saying. For example, if the receiver strongly disagrees with the message, his or her thoughts may stray from listening to what the sender is actually saying to forming mental arguments against what is being said. Or the receiver may think about how to respond. The mind becomes engaged in self-talk and listening stops.

Good listening also requires that receivers do not interrupt senders or complete messages for them. Allow enough time for messages to be given. Encouraging remarks and gestures may be used as prompts: "I see," "Go on," or a nod of the head. Interrupting can convey a lack of respect and impatience. It can also distort the sender's intended message.

Box 16–1 Summary of Good Listening Skills

Clear your mind of distractions.

Face the sender.

Focus your full attention on the sender.

Maintain eye contact as appropriate for the culture.

Turn off "self-talk."

Do not make value judgements about what you hear.

Mentally note anything that needs clarification.

Do not interrupt.

Effective listening skills can be developed. Concentrate on being aware of lapses in attention. When a loss of focus is noted, bring your mind back to the speaker. With practice, internal interference and poor attention can be eliminated. See Box 16–1 for a summary of good listening habits.

Periods of silence can be a meaningful component of communication. The purpose of health care encounters is not to maintain a steady stream of conversation, but to help patients solve their health problems. Silence allows time for thought and reflection. Some cultures have a high respect for the value of silence. Allowing periods of silence may feel awkward at first, but they can be a valuable tool in promoting good communication.

Empathy

Good listening skills are necessary to achieve **empathy**, which means understanding another person's thoughts, feelings, and behavior (Miller-Keane, 1997). To experience empathy is to look at the world from the other person's viewpoint. The old expression "Walk a mile in my shoes" is a good description of the concept. Empathy is a critical component of health care communication, because it enables the health care worker to understand and address the needs of each patient. It allows each person to be considered as an individual.

Assumptions cannot be made about other people. This is especially true today when patients come from a variety of age groups and cultural backgrounds. Older adults, who make up a significant portion of today's patients, have a whole set of life experiences very different from

their children and grandchildren. What seems common sense to one person may in fact make no sense to another. Health care workers must understand before they can help, and understanding only comes when close attention is paid to what patients say and do.

Empathy includes communicating that you are aware of the other person's feelings. Sharing in this way demonstrates care and respect. It can help relieve the loneliness and anxiety often experienced by patients and encourage them to feel safe about sharing feelings and discussing concerns. Empathy should not be confused with "sympathy," which means feeling sorry for or taking pity on the other person.

Step Five: Offer Feedback and Seek Clarification

Feedback is a way for the sender to check the understanding of the receiver. Was the message received as intended? Everyone has had the experience of sending what was thought to be a very clear message, only to discover that it was completely misinterpreted. Obtaining feedback is a way to avoid misunderstandings.

Here are four ways to obtain feedback:

1. **Paraphrasing**: The receiver restates the sender's message in his or her own words and then asks the sender for confirmation.

   Example: I understood you to say that you have experienced these headaches every day for the past 2 weeks. Is that correct?

2. **Reflecting**: This is similar to paraphrasing, but prompts the receiver to either complete or add more detail to the original message.

   Example: You say that it's difficult for you to do the exercises the therapist has recommended because _____. (Pause and allow time for response.)

3. Asking questions: Request clarification and additional information. Many words, such as "difficult," "painful," and "a lot," have different meanings for people. In health care, the skillful use of questions can help patients describe their conditions more clearly. Accurate diagnoses and appropriate treatments depend, in part, on the clarity and completeness of information supplied by the patient.

   Example: What symptoms are you experiencing when you say you are feeling terrible?

   Questions can be used to check the receiver's understanding of important information.

Instead of asking if the receiver understands, ask a question whose answer will demonstrate understanding.

Example: Can you list for me the three steps you'll take when giving your son his medication?

Open-ended questions can be used to encourage patients to talk about their values and beliefs. While it is not the role of the health care worker to make value judgements about patients, what is learned can help you better understand the behavior and motivations of patients and find ways to meet their needs.

Example: Why do you say that you deserved to have the accident?

This question may help in understanding why a patient is making no effort to perform the exercises that will assist in recovering from injuries.

4. Requesting Examples: Examples can help more clearly explain and fill in meaning.

Example: Tell me about the kind of situations in which you feel lightheaded.

Establishing clear channels of communication through the use of feedback also helps maintain good relationships with coworkers and supervisors. Developing as a health care worker requires the monitoring of personal progress and learning from mistakes. Feedback can be an important tool in this development. For example, Rosie's supervisor informs her that a report she has prepared is "unacceptable." Rosie can request more specific feedback by asking questions such as "What did I do or not do that made my performance on this task unacceptable?" and "Can you tell me exactly what it is that makes the report unacceptable?" These questions encourage the supervisor to be specific and provide details from which Rosie can learn. If Rosie were to say "I don't know what you mean" or "I don't understand," the supervisor might not provide her with the needed information (Figure 16–3).

Step Six: Evaluate the Encounter

The purpose of evaluation is to determine whether the communication goals were met. This can be demonstrated by either the response or behavior of the receiver. If the goal was not met, the following questions can serve as guidelines for identifying the difficulty:

- Were the messages clearly stated?

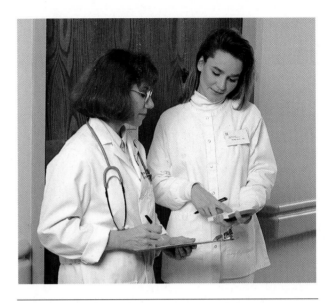

Figure 16–3 Good communication between members of the health care team improves the quality of patient care.

- Were they presented at a level appropriate for the receiver?
- Did you listen actively?
- Which part of the message was misunderstood?

The evaluation process actually continues throughout every communication encounter. A good communicator constantly checks for understanding by listening, observing, and asking for feedback. Adjustments can then be made as needed.

Some communication goals are achieved over a period of time, and the evaluation is delayed. For example, if cardiac patient Heinrich Mueller is instructed about improving his eating habits, it may be weeks before the dietician finds out if he understood and was motivated to follow the low-fat eating plan. Another example of a long-term communication goal is working over time to improve a relationship with a coworker.

Communication Barriers

Obstacles known as **barriers** sometimes block communication. Barriers include:

- language differences
- cultural influences
- defense mechanisms (see Chapter 15)
- physical distractions
- sensory impairments
- medication effects
- pain

Craig Segal is a recently graduated LVN who has been hired at an oncology clinic in his home town. Craig works with patients who are dealing with a potentially fatal disease. This is difficult because he has known many of them and their families for many years. He finds himself wondering how he can best communicate with patients and their families. Craig wants them to know that he cares and wants to be of assistance, but he is not sure how to approach what he believes to be emotional topics and finds himself keeping conversation to a minimum.

1. How can Craig use the steps of the communication process to help him feel more confident about communicating with patients?

2. Which techniques do you think he might find most effective?

Identifying and overcoming barriers require the use of empathy, observation, questions, and feedback. Serious barriers may require the help of a supervisor such as in the case of a patient who refuses to follow directions during a treatment procedure. If a language barrier cannot be overcome, it may be necessary to secure the assistance of a family member or translator.

PATIENTS WITH SPECIAL NEEDS

Health care workers assist patients who have a variety of special needs. Meeting these needs calls for extra consideration and attention. Special techniques can be employed and extra time allowed in order to promote effective communication.

Patients Who Are Terminally Ill

Patients who are dying have reported that the loneliness they encounter is worse than the prospect of death itself (Purtilo and Haddad, 1996). As the dying process advances, they may receive fewer visits and feel abandoned and cut off from the outside world. At the same time, many believe that they are given less attention than patients for whom there "is hope." See Figure 16–4. Some health care workers view death as a failure of the system to help the patient. Others find it difficult to deal with because it brings up issues about their own mortality. It is important to come to terms with these difficult subjects in order to be truly effective and helpful when caring for terminally ill patients.

Terminally ill patients may have strong needs to share their fears and concerns, and health care workers may serve as their major remaining links with life. Some patients want to talk about death and their desire to complete unfinished life tasks. The health care worker can improve the quality of this final phase by seeking, rather than avoiding, opportunities for communication. Be willing to listen and show that you care. See Chapter 8 for a discussion of death and dying.

Patients Who Are In Pain, Medicated, Confused, or Disoriented

Under these conditions, patients often have difficulty communicating. Health care workers can assist them by taking extra time and following these guidelines:

- Identify yourself and say the patient's name.
- Maintain eye contact.
- Speak slowly and clearly in a moderate pitch of voice.
- Use simple language. Avoid slang and expressions that do not mean exactly what they say.
- Keep each message short and to the point. For example, do not give a series of instructions or ask more than one question at a time.

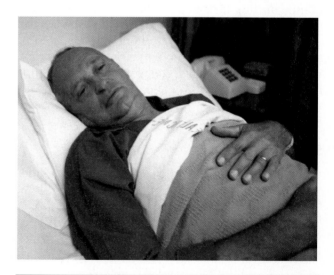

Figure 16–4 Dying patients often suffer from loneliness and feelings of isolation.

- Give the patient time to respond.
- Use touch if the patient is comfortable with it.
- Try to schedule interactions when patients are in the least amount of pain.
- Repeat the message as needed, without changing the content or words.
- Review the content with the patient to assess retention of the message.
- When appropriate, give the patient written information that can be referred to later.
  (Adapted from *Nursing assistant: A nursing process approach* (8th ed.), by B. Hegner, E. Caldwell, and J. Needham, 1999, Albany, NY: Delmar.)

Patients Who Have Hearing, Visual, or Speech Impairments

According to the Alexander Graham Bell Association for the Deaf, 10% of the American population has a significant hearing loss (1996). Half of these people are older adults. When initiating conversation, especially with the elderly, carefully observe the receiver and use appropriate feedback to check for understanding. It is important not to assume that people can hear just because they are not wearing a hearing aid or do not ask you to speak up. Many people who experience hearing loss are unaware of it or too embarrassed to admit it. Signs that a person may have difficulty include:

- Leaning forward and turning the head
- Asking you to repeat information
- Failing to hear when not facing the sender

American Sign Language (ASL) provides a means of communication for people with serious hearing losses. It consists of hand movements and shapes, facial expressions, and corresponding body postures to convey meaning (Figure 16–5). It is now the fourth most used language in the United States (Jondreau, 1998). Partly due to the difficulty experienced in trying to communicate with people who have normal hearing, many hearing-impaired individuals consider themselves to be members of a unique cultural group that has its own history, background, and identity (Jondreau, 1998).

The following suggestions can help improve communication with the hearing impaired:

- Position yourself close to the receiver and speak face to face.
- Remove or turn off sources of noise.
- Have the light source directed to your face.
- Make sure your mouth is visible to the listener.
- Speak distinctly and do not mumble.
- Speak slowly.
- Do not shout or exaggerate words.
- Maintain a low to moderate pitch of voice.
- Use short sentences.
- Watch for signs of comprehension.
- Do not change the subject without warning.
  (Alexander Graham Bell Association, 1996.)

Patients who have visual limitations need special consideration, too. They do not have visual clues with which to orient themselves physically. With 70% of the meaning of communication being conveyed nonverbally, it is understandable that the visually impaired person experiences special communication challenges. Here are some ways to assist visually-impaired patients:

- Start all communication by announcing your presence and identifying yourself.
- Before starting a procedure, describe any equipment to be used and its position in relation to the patient.
- As you proceed, explain what will be done and where you will be touching the patient.
- Explain what noises will be heard.
- Give clear and complete directions. For example, say, "Raise your left arm directly in front of you to a 45-degree angle" not "Raise your arm like this," or "Lift your arm."

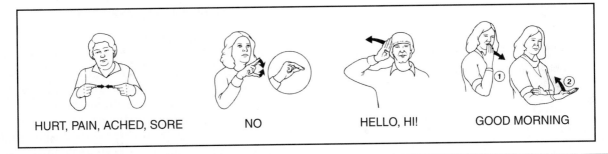

HURT, PAIN, ACHED, SORE NO HELLO, HI! GOOD MORNING

Figure 16–5 Sign language is a means of communication for many people who are hearing impaired.

- Let the patient know when you are leaving the area.
- If the patient is to leave, give specific instructions about doorways and other landmarks and obstacles, such as uneven surfaces, that will be encountered.
- Give extra verbal information to describe anything that would usually be expressed through facial expressions, gestures, head nods, and other movements.
(Adapted from *Nursing assistant: A nursing process approach* (8th ed.), by B. Hegner, E. Caldwell, and J. Needham, 1999, Albany, NY: Delmar.)

Patients may be unable to speak because of injury or a stroke. Communication can be aided by the use of pantomime, pictures and drawings, writing, and specially designed communication boards that have the most frequent patient requests, to which they can point. It is a good idea to have a calendar and clock available for patients to orient themselves. While it is important to clarify mutual understanding with all patients, it is especially critical to spend the time necessary with those who have special communication difficulties.

Patients Who Are Angry

Anger is the emotional response to a perceived threat to one's self, possessions, rights, or values (Miller-Keane, 1997). The loss of personal control experienced due to illness or injury, worries about the expense of health care, and the inconvenience of having to wait for service can all result in patient anger. Anger can also be caused by problems unrelated to health care such as family difficulties or the loss of a job.

When dealing with an angry patient, try to determine the cause. In most cases, the anger is not the fault of the health care worker. Recall the defense mechanisms discussed in Chapter 15. Anger may be a form of displacement in which the patient is unable to direct anger at the real cause. If, however, you discover that you have done something to upset the patient, apologize sincerely and try to establish good communication aimed at meeting the patient's needs. The following guidelines are helpful when dealing with angry patients:

- Never respond in anger or argue with the patient.
- Remain calm and courteous.
- Listen attentively to the patient's concerns.
- Offer a sincere apology, if necessary.
- Do not raise your voice.

- Be aware of your body language. Look at the patient.
- Express concern and interest, not annoyance.
- Answer the patient's questions.
- If you cannot resolve the problem, discuss it with your supervisor or other appropriate person.
- If the patient is cursing or being verbally abusive, state politely that you are willing to listen but will not tolerate cursing or threatening language.
- Ask for help from a coworker or security, if necessary.

Patients Who Do Not Speak English

Imagine yourself as a tourist in a country whose language you do not speak and where the health care practices are different from those of the United States. You are involved in an accident and taken to a hospital where no one speaks English. You cannot explain your needs, the location of your pain, or ask questions about your condition. The treatments are different from anything you have ever experienced.

The fear and confusion experienced in this scenario are similar to those of some immigrants and non-English speaking patients in the United States. Health care workers can demonstrate care for these patients by learning at least a few common phrases of the major languages spoken in their area. In addition, the following ideas are helpful when working with non-English speaking patients:

- A smile is a universal sign of good will.
- Determine if the patient speaks or understands any English.
- Find out if an English-speaking family member or friend is available to help. (Be sure that the patient agrees to having the other person involved so that confidentiality is not violated.)
- Do not raise your voice. It will not help the other person understand.
- Use gestures and pantomime to demonstrate what you need the patient to do.
- Use pictures, if available.
- Request the services of a translator, if necessary.

Hispanics make up the largest population in the United States who speak a language other than English. As of 1997 they constituted 11% of the total United States' population (Hispanic Association on Corporate Responsibility, 1998). While many Hispanics speak English as well as Spanish, there is a significant number who do not. If a patient speaks a little English, take care not to assume that health care communication will be understood. Health care workers who are likely to work with Spanish-speaking patients can better help patients by learning a few words and phrases. See Appendix 2 for a list of conversational and health-related phrases.

SPECIAL APPLICATIONS OF COMMUNICATION SKILLS

There are a variety of special applications of communication skills in health care work. Each application requires the use of specific techniques.

Telephone Communication

The telephone often provides the first means of contact between patients and health care facilities. The impression that patients, other professionals, and the general public receive at this time influences their perception of the facility and helps set the tone for all future communication. It is essential that interest, competence, and professionalism be projected.

Employers report that the inability to properly handle telephone calls is a major weakness among new hires. The health care worker who develops excellent telephone skills is a valuable asset. It is a mistake to take these skills for granted or consider them to be unimportant.

The quality of the voice is an important factor in all types of oral communication, but it is especially significant when speaking on the telephone. The receiver has no visual clues and must depend on words and voice to understand the message. The following guidelines can help create a telephone manner that is both welcoming and professional:

- Speak clearly and pronounce words correctly and distinctly.
- Speak at a moderate rate of speed. When giving instructions or directions, speak more slowly.
- Strive for a pleasant tone, not too high-pitched.
- Project warmth, friendliness, and caring.
- Smile as you speak unless it is inappropriate in the situation, as in a call for emergency help.
- Put expression in your voice. Avoid speaking in a monotone.

- Allow appropriate periods of silence to give the other person an opportunity to speak.
- Never chew gum or eat when speaking on the telephone.

Patient Education

Patients today are taking more responsibility for their own health. They want to know about preventive measures, such as diet and exercise, to avoid disease and injury. More hands-on care is being performed by patients themselves as a result of the decreasing length of hospital stays. As a result, a significant portion of your time as a health care worker may be spent on patient education. See Table 16–2 for major categories of patient education topics.

Providing effective patient education can be one of the most satisfying responsibilities of health care work. Education requires the application of many general communication concepts. Its purpose is to provide knowledge and/or skills that result in a change in patient behavior. The steps in the communication process described in this

Table 16–2 Patient Education Subject Categories

Category	Examples
Promote Wellness	Hygiene Nutrition Exercise
Prevent Illness	First aid Safety Immunizations Management of risk factors
Restore Health	Orientation to treatment Introduction to staff Information about the illness Self-care practices
Improve Coping Skills	Stress management Grief counseling Community resources

(Adapted from *Fundamentals of Nursing: The art and science of nursing care* (3rd ed.), by C. Taylor, C. Lillis, and P. LeMone, 1997, Philadelphia, PA: Lippincott-Raven Publishers.)

chapter can be adapted to provide a process for delivering patient education:

1. Set educational goals.

   Educators call these **learning objectives** and create them to describe what students will be able to do as a result of the instruction. Examples of goals for patients include:

   - Self-administer insulin injection following correct procedure
   - Follow a daily physical exercise program
   - Explain medication side effects that require calling the physician

2. Create the instructional message.

   This means deciding how the instruction will be provided. As with any other communication, it is based on the patient's needs and current condition. When creating effective instruction, additional facts about the patient should be determined:

   - Level of knowledge: What does the patient already know about the topic? It is frustrating to be given information that either repeats what is already known or is too advanced for comprehension.
   - Preferred learning style: Ask patients whether they learn best by listening, seeing, or doing. See Chapter 1 for more information.
   - Motivation: How important the patient believes the information to be
   - Ability to learn: The patient's ability to acquire and retain new information

   Use nontechnical language that patients are likely to understand. Break information into sections and relate it to something the patient already knows. Finally, try not to give too much information at one time so that the patient is not overwhelmed.

3. Deliver the instruction.

   Instruction can be delivered in a variety of ways. In order to address the various learning styles of patients and to reinforce the material presented, as many methods as possible should be used:

   - Oral explanations, presented either to an individual or a group
   - Audio visual materials such as videos, diagrams, and charts
   - Written materials such as instructional sheets, lists, informational reports, pamphlets, reprints of journal articles (see Chapter 17 for information about creating written documents)
   - Discussion groups
   - Demonstrations of procedures, exercises, self-care techniques
   - Computerized instruction such as interactive software programs and information available on the Internet (see Chapter 18 about computer uses in education)

4. Listen.

   Encourage patients to ask questions as material is presented and then listen carefully to find out what they do not understand and what they want to know.

5. Check for understanding (obtain feedback and seek clarification).

   Ask patients to summarize what they have learned or to explain how they will apply the new information. If appropriate, have patients demonstrate what was learned. They must be able to perform the task without prompting. Allow them to repeat the task, as necessary to demonstrate mastery.

6. Evaluate.

   - Were the instructional goals met?
   - Does the patient appear to understand the instruction? Is the patient able to repeat information and/or satisfactorily demonstrate the skills?
   - Does the patient achieve the results intended by the instruction?

Group Presentations

You may not expect to give formal speeches as a health care worker, but there are occasions when it is necessary to talk to a group. Examples include explaining home-care procedures to a patient's family members, giving a report at a professional meeting, and demonstrating a new procedure to coworkers. Developing the ability to organize and present information orally can increase your effectiveness in helping others.

It is important to plan in advance what is to be said, even when the audience is a small, informal group. Patient health may depend on the clarity of the presentation. The following strategies can help improve its effectiveness:

- Be clear about the purpose and most important points.
- Determine the needs and level of understanding of the audience.

Thinking it Through

Robin Winters, the dental hygienist with Dr. Castro, wants to create a patient education program to teach effective dental home care and nutritional practices. Her patients range from toddlers to the elderly. They come from a variety of cultural backgrounds. Some speak English as a second language.

1. What should Robin take into consideration when planning a patient education program?
2. What types of methods would you suggest she use?
3. How can she check for patient understanding?
4. How can she evaluate the effectiveness of her program?

- Organize material so that it is easy for the audience to follow.
- Avoid jumping from topic to topic or adding unnecessary information that can be confusing.
- Speak at a moderate rate.
- Prepare notes or prepare a checklist to prevent forgetting important points.
- Look at the audience while you are speaking.

Handling Gossip

Gossip is unnecessary conversation, often negative, about people who are not present. It serves no constructive purpose and should always be avoided. Gossip about one's coworkers can disrupt the harmony of the health care team and compromise the quality of the patient care delivered. If it involves the inappropriate sharing of patient information, it can result in a lawsuit. See section on patient confidentiality in Chapter 3. Any type of gossip is a time-waster and cannot be justified in the busy schedules maintained by health care facilities. If a coworker tries to engage you in gossip, the following techniques may be helpful:

- Explain that you believe such conversation is unfair to the subject of the gossip. ("I don't think we know enough about the situation to discuss it." or "I don't think it's fair to talk about people behind their back.")

- State that you believe it is inappropriate for discussion. ("You know, I really don't feel comfortable talking about that.")
- Change the subject. ("What I really need to talk to you about is ....")

Take care that private patient information is not included in social conversations with coworkers. Avoid making comments in public areas that might be overheard by the patient's friends or family members. Even sympathetic remarks such as, "I feel so bad. My favorite patient, Mr. Phillips, was just diagnosed with lung cancer," can be damaging if overheard. Patient names, along with personal information, should not be used during telephone conversations that can be heard by others. For example, when transferring a telephone call from the front desk, say "A patient is calling to follow up as you requested," *not* "Mr. Sanders is calling to get the results of his HIV test." If patient information is shared with another health professional in the patient's presence, it is best to include the patient in the conversation. Being "talked about," even by health care workers discussing the patient's condition, can cause anxiety. Patients want to be acknowledged as individuals and not made to feel like "cases."

SUGGESTED LEARNING ACTIVITIES

1. Make a poster to illustrate the six steps in the communication process.
2. Observe people as they communicate. What communication techniques are they using? Do they appear to be effective? Why or why not?
3. Apply what you have learned in this chapter to your everyday life. Use the listening techniques when communicating with your instructors, friends, and family members.
4. Practice asking different types of questions and requesting feedback in your everyday encounters.
5. Look for examples of nonverbal communication. List the instances when the nonverbal message does not seem to match the verbal message.
6. Create a list or chart of various forms of nonverbal communication.
7. Mentally monitor your telephone conversations over the next week. Note the conversations you

find most pleasant; those that are most unpleasant. Explain why in each case.

8. Create a teaching situation with a friend or family member. Apply the education process presented in the chapter and describe the results.

REVIEW QUESTIONS

1. Why is effective communication an important factor in health care delivery?

2. How does communication affect patient well-being?

3. What are the six steps of the communication process?

4. What are the four types of questions? Give an example of each.

5. What is nonverbal communication? Give three examples.

6. What is the meaning of "active listening"?

7. What is the meaning of "empathy"? Why is it important in health care?

8. What is "feedback"? How can its use improve communication?

9. What are five common barriers that can interfere with communication?

10. Describe two specific considerations when communicating with patients who are:
    a. Terminally ill
    b. Hearing impaired
    c. Visually impaired
    d. Speech impaired
    e. Angry
    f. Unable to understand English well

11. What are eight ways to project a professional impression when speaking on the telephone?

12. What are the six steps for developing and delivering effective patient education?

13. What are five ways to improve presentations given to groups?

APPLICATION EXERCISES

1. Refer to The Case of the Coder Who Lacked Confidence at the beginning of the chapter. What would you recommend that Jenny do in order to increase her communication skills?

2. Compare and contrast how you would initiate communication with each of the following patients. Include your communication goal, what information you would need to gather about the patient, and important factors to consider in preparing your message.
   a. You are a medical assistant. The patient has a severe hearing impairment. She is seeing the physician for a routine physical examination.
   b. You are a dental hygienist. The patient is 5-years-old and terrified of the dentist's office.
   c. You are a physical therapist assistant. The patient is a well-to-do man in his fifties. He is furious about having had to wait for 20 minutes while you finished working with your previous patient.

SUGGESTED READINGS AND RESOURCES

Alexander Graham Bell Association for the Deaf: http://www.agbell.org

Colbert, B. (2000). *Workplace readiness for health occupations.* Albany, NY: Delmar.

Jondreau, F. American Sign Language Institute. (Online). Available: http://www.asli.com

National Federation for the Blind: http://www.nfb.org

Tamparo, C. and Lindh, W. (2000). *Therapeutic communications for health professionals* (2nd ed.). Albany, NY: Delmar.

Wilber, C. and Lister, S. (1990). *Medical Spanish: The instant survival guide* (2nd ed.). Boston: Butterworth-Heinemann.

CHAPTER

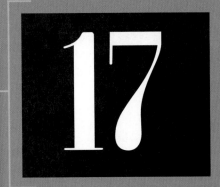

WRITTEN COMMUNICATION

OBJECTIVES

Studying and applying the material in this chapter will help you to:

- Explain why the ability to write clearly and correctly is an important skill for the health care worker.

- Describe effective techniques for planning and organizing written documents.

- Use correct spelling and grammar in all written communication.

- Explain how to write, format, and send effective business letters.

- Identify what should be included in meeting agendas and minutes.

- Describe techniques for creating effective written patient education materials.

- Discuss the proper handling of written documents to protect patient confidentiality.

- List ways to improve proofreading skills.

KEY TERMS

agenda
block letter
contraction
cross-training
etiquette
full block letter
grammar
independent clause
justified
modified block letter
quotation
salutation
suffix
syllable
vowel
word processing

The Case of

the Surprised Therapist

Al Trent was recently hired by Cathy Barnes, a physical therapist in private practice. When Al started work, he imagined that his tasks would consist mainly of working with patients. He was surprised when Cathy asked him to help her with several special projects that required good writing skills. She is active at both the local and state level of two professional organizations. Believing that professional organizations are important for the promotion of physical therapy, she has encouraged Al to become active and has requested his help in preparing agendas and reports for the meetings. Cathy has also asked him to prepare written instruction sheets for patients to use when doing exercises at home. While there is an administrative assistant who does the billing, bookkeeping, and other clerical tasks, Cathy believes that Al's physical therapy education better qualifies him for writing materials that are directly related to physical therapy.

This chapter covers the basics of effective written communication that may be required of today's health care worker.

WRITTEN COMMUNICATION: A VITAL LINK IN HEALTH CARE

The quality of modern health care delivery depends heavily on the completeness and accuracy of written communications prepared by health care workers. Many kinds of documents are created daily. They range from notes made in a patient's medical record to technical reports to formal business letters. The type of writing done by each health care worker depends on his or her specific occupation and employment circumstances. However, even workers who spend most of their time providing hands-on patient care may prepare written documentation and may be required to write an occasional letter or patient instruction sheet. The ability to write clearly and correctly is a mark of professionalism and increases the health care worker's value and promotional opportunities.

Written documents provide important links among the many workers and facilities that make up the web of care for today's patients. While the growth in specialty services raises the level of care, it also increases the chances for miscommunication and lost information. Consider the paper trail created during the routine annual exam of Mrs. Kardinski, a 55-year-old patient of Dr. Landau:

1. Dr. Landau's administrative medical assistant, Denise Carter, sends Mrs. Kardinski a *reminder letter* to encourage her to make an appointment for her annual physical exam.

2. On the day of the appointment, Denise locates the patient's *file* for the clinical medical assistant, Lachelle Hayes.

3. Lachelle updates the *medical record* with Mrs. Kardinski's weight, blood pressure, and other vitals signs.

4. Lachelle adds further notes to the *medical record* at the direction of Dr. Landau during the exam.

5. Dr. Landau signs *request forms* for routine tests to be performed at other faciites.

6. Mrs. Kardinski visits an offsite lab to have blood drawn for routine tests, and the lab sends the results in a *report* to Dr. Landau's office.

7. Mrs. Kardinski then visits an imaging center for a mammogram, and the center sends a *report* to Dr. Landau's office.

8. The cytology lab that examines the pap specimen sends a *report* to Dr. Landau's office.

9. All reports are normal, so Denise sends a *letter* to Mrs. Kardinski, notifying her of the results.

10. Denise sends a *statement* to Mrs. Kardinski's insurance company.

Mrs. Kardinski's routine visit involves at least ten paper documents that contain essential information for ensuring that she receives consistent and appropriate care. This care depends on the smooth flow of clearly and accurately prepared paperwork among health care providers and between them and their patients.

The Components of Good Writing

Good writing is characterized by logical organization and attention to detail, including spelling, grammar, and format. In addition to aiding in the provision of good patient care, complete and accurate written documents are viewed by many as the sign of a competent professional. Writing that contains errors and is poorly presented reflects negatively on the quality of the facility. Patients may question the competence of the facility to deliver quality health care if written documents are sloppily prepared, contain spelling errors, and are difficult to understand.

Organizing Content

All types of written communication, whether they consist of one paragraph or several pages, must be organized in a way that is easy for the reader to follow and understand. Unlike oral communication, during which the speaker can

Thinking it Through

For each of the documents involved in Mrs. Kardinski's routine visit, discuss the possible consequences for the patient and health care providers if it were:

1. Written inaccurately
2. Sent to the wrong facility or person

request feedback and make necessary adjustments, writers rely strictly on words as they are printed. Writers also lack the ability to use non-verbal language to enhance and emphasize their messages.

The steps for organizing written content described in this section are designed as a guide for creating all types of written communication. The specific techniques used and the time spent on each are determined by the type of document being prepared. For example, a short memo might take 10 minutes to plan and write, while a research report could take more than a month and require attention to each step in the process. Whatever the length of a document, good writing requires that consideration be given to planning and organizing.

Preparing to Write

1. Determine the purpose for writing.
   - Inform
   - Persuade
   - Gather information
   - Encourage action

   It is possible to have more than one purpose. A patient information sheet about physical exercise, for example, may be designed to provide information about the health benefits of exercise *and* encourage patients to participate in regular physical activity.

2. Generate ideas for content based on the purpose of the document.
   - List as many ideas as come to mind. Write down everything without rejecting anything that seems silly or unusable. "Dumb ideas" often stimulate "smart ones."
   - Gather facts. Sources include professional journals, books, publications from professional organizations, and credible sites on the Internet (see Chapter 18 for evaluating the quality of sites).
   - Talk with others. Get content information from experts. Ask potential readers what they want to know.

3. Consider the reader's:
   - Knowledge of the subject matter
   - Reading level (age, native language, level of education)
   - Interest in the subject
   - Importance of the subject to their well-being

It is appropriate to use medical terminology and abbreviations in writing that is directed to health care professionals. The same language, however, might confuse patients who lack a background in health care.

The tone must be appropriate for the situation. For example, collection letters for late payment should be adapted to the circumstances. A patient who always pays medical bills promptly but is currently experiencing financial difficulties might receive a different letter than the one directed to a patient with a history of late payments.

4. Organize the content.

The material should flow in a way that makes sense to the reader. The traditional structure of a written document includes three parts:

- Introduction

  State the topic and purpose. Interesting facts and questions can be used to attract the reader's attention.

- Body

  Fully develop the topic or message. Focus on supporting facts and information.

  Ways to present information

  - Examples and illustrations
  - Description, using specific details
  - List of steps in a process
  - List of reasons
  - Grouping of items into categories

- Conclusion

  Summarize the body. Effective endings include restating the purpose or pointing out how the facts given support the purpose.

Starting to Write

The task of writing can be simplified by using one of the following organizing techniques. Even short documents can be improved by making a few notes before preparing the "real thing."

- Create a formal outline. Use letters and numbers and to create a detailed outline, which is fleshed out when you begin to write. See Figure 17–1 for an example.
- Create an informal outline. Omit letters and numbers. Simply list major ideas and indent supporting ideas.

- Draw a diagram, also known as a mind map, using circles and lines to connect major and supporting ideas. This is especially helpful for visual learners, who may also include the use of colors to clarify the relationships of ideas. See Figure 17–2 to see how the information organized in the formal outline looks in mind map form.

(Adapted from *A writer's reference*, by D. Hacker, 1999, Boston: Bedford/St. Martins.)

Using an Outline to Organize Content
Subject: Hepatitis B

I. Introduction
    A. Threat to health
    B. Vaccine available
II. Symptoms
    A. Loss of appetite
    B. Fatigue
    C. Nausea
    D. Headache
    E. Fever
    F. Jaundice
III. Transmission
    A. Contact with virus
        1. Sexual contact
        2. Blood
        3. Body fluids
            a. Vaginal secretions
            b. Semen
            c. Fluids from body cavities
            d. Sputum
IV. Treatment
    A. Dietary measures
        1. Decrease dietary fat
        2. Low protein
        3. Small, frequent high-calorie meals (if nausea present)
        4. Decrease fluids (if retaining)
    B. Bed rest
V. Prevention
    A. Hepatitis B vaccine for employees at risk for exposure
    B. Standard Precautions
        1. Handwashing
        2. Gloves
        3. Personal protective equipment
        4. Proper handling of needles
        5. Proper disposal of hazardous waste

Figure 17–1 Sample formal outline to organize content for writing.

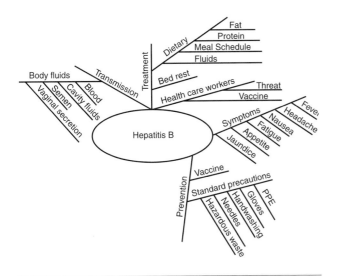

Figure 17–2 Mind maps can help the writer organize content.

When starting to write a long document, many professional writers suggest writing as quickly as possible. Content, rather than grammar and spelling, should be emphasized at this time. Creativity can be lost when the focus is on detail. Trying for perfection on the first draft can be so intimidating that the writer becomes overwhelmed. The final draft, however, should contain perfect spelling and grammar.

Spell Your Way to Success

Spelling errors in medical documents can have serious consequences. Apart from giving the impression of carelessness, misspelled words can cause confusion that negatively affects patient care. As discussed in Chapter 4, many medical terms can present difficulties because they were borrowed from Latin and Greek, are long, have silent letters, or have spelling that is similar to other words with different meanings.

If in doubt about the spelling of any word, take the time to check it. Not doing so is negligent. There are many tools available to assist with proper spelling:

- General English dictionary. If English is your second language, you may also need a bilingual dictionary.
- Medical dictionaries
- Word books for health care specialties

- Spell-checkers for **word processing** software (program for creating written documents on a computer). These are available for general English and medical vocabulary. Do not depend on spell-checkers to catch all errors, because the computer cannot identify words that are spelled correctly but used incorrectly. For example, "to" is spelled correctly, but is incorrect if you meant to write "toe."
- Pharmaceutical reference guides such as the Physician's Desk Reference (PDR) and American Hospital Formulary Service (AHFS)

Spelling Tips

Everyday English, as well as medical spelling, can be challenging, but it is well worth the time and effort necessary to achieve mastery. Here are a few suggestions for improving spelling:

1. Learn the major spelling rules listed in Table 17–1. Each rule governs the spelling of many words and prevents having to learn to spell each word individually.

2. Memorize words that are look-alikes, exceptions to the rules, or ones you usually misspell. Try a method that complements your learning style (Chapter 1).
   - Write each word several times.
   - Spell each word out loud several times.
   - Make flashcards for practice and self-quizzes.
   - List words on a wall chart and place it where it will be seen frequently.
   - Create rhymes or associations. For example, the sentence "he was v<u>ai</u>n about owning a big v<u>a</u>n" might help distinguish between "vain" and "vein."
   - Create a personal dictionary of words with which you have trouble. This can be handwritten or stored on the computer. Review the list regularly.

3. Review troublesome words regularly for mastery. See Table 17–2 for a list of frequently misspelled words that are commonly used in health care.

4. Set weekly goals. Challenge yourself to learn a certain number of new words. Create self-quizzes and give yourself small rewards for perfect scores.

Table 17–1 Major spelling rules

Rule	Examples
Place i before e except after c or in words in which the ei sounds like ay. EXCEPTIONS: seize either weird height foreign leisure	relieve receive weight
Drop the final silent *e* before adding a **suffix** (word ending) that begins with a **vowel** (the letters a, e, i, o, u). Keep the *e* if the suffix begins with a consonant (all letters except a, e, i, o, u).	care → caring → careful achieve → achievable → achievement
Change the final *y* to *ie* when adding *s* or *d* when the *y* is preceded by a consonant.	laboratory → laboratories dry → dried
Double the final consonant when adding a suffix if all the following conditions are met: 1. The final consonant is preceded by a vowel. 2. The suffix begins with a vowel. 3. The word is only one **syllable** (part of a word that has a single spoken sound) OR the final syllable is stressed.	sit → sitting commit → committed
Add **k** to words ending in *c* before adding suffixes that begin with *e, i, y*.	panic → panicking, panicked
Add **s** to make most words plural.	patient → patients x-ray → x-rays
Add **es** to make the plural form of words that end in *s, sh, ch, x*.	abscess → abscesses dish → dishes crutch → crutches suffix → suffixes
Add **s** to make the plural form of words that end in *o* if it is preceded by a vowel. Add **es** if *o* is preceded by a consonant.	ratio → ratios tomato → tomatoes
Some words that were borrowed from other languages keep their original plural forms, which do not use the letter *s*.	diverticulum (singular) → diverticula (plural) (pouch in mucous membrane lining) curriculum (singular) → curricula (plural)

Table 17–2 Frequently misspelled words

abscess	eligible	maneuver	resuscitate
absence	eliminate	miscellaneous	rhyΩthm
accidentally	embarrass	necessary	schedule
accommodate	emphasize	negligible	scissors
accumulate	encourage	negligence	secretary
address	enthusiastic	neighbor	seize
aggravate	environment	noticeable	seizure
analyze	equipped	occasionally	separate
appropriate	equivalent	occur	severely
assistant	especially	occurrence	significance
association	exaggerate	often	similar
behavior	exercise	pamphlet	strategy
belief	exhausted	parallel	strictly
beneficial	experience	particular	substantial
business	extremely	patience	succeed
cafeteria	fatigue	persistent	success
caffeine	February	physically	surprise
calendar	fluctuation	physician	sympathy
cancel, canceled	foreign	pneumonia	technique
column	forty	possession	temperature
commitment	fourth	practical	though
communicate	fragile	precede	thorough
comparative	friend	prejudice	tongue
cooperate	government	privilege	transferred
correspond	harass, harassment	proceed	typical
criticism	height	prominent	urgent
criticize	intelligence	psychology	vacuum
decision	judgment	psychiatry	vague
deficiency	knowledge	qualified	vegetable
definitely	knowledgeable	quantity	Wednesday
describe	label	questionnaire	weight
disease	laboratory	recommend	writing
efficiency	license	reference	
eighth	maintenance		

(Adapted from *Delmar's comprehensive medical assisting: Administrative and clinical competencies*, by W. Lindh, M. Pooler, C. Tamparo, and J. Cerrato, 1998, Albany, NY: Delmar.)

Grammar At a Glance

Every language has a set of rules that determines proper word order, sentence construction, punctuation, and capitalization. Collectively these are referred to as **grammar**. The use of correct grammar is a sign of a good education, competence, and professionalism. As representatives of the facilities in which they work, it is important for health care workers to achieve a level of grammar that gives a favorable impression of both them and their employers.

The following sections are designed to provide a quick review of English grammar. If you are unsure about your knowledge of grammar, plan to take an English class, purchase educational software, or locate a workbook with review exercises. Time spent now can make a significant difference in your professional life. A good grammar reference book will be useful now and on the job. Most word processing software programs have grammar-checkers.

Capitalization Rules

Capitalizing correctly is an important mark of good written English. The following conditions require capitalization:

- First word in a sentence
- Names of people, countries, organizations, companies, products, holidays, and so on
- Names of months and days of the week
- Medical acronyms: AIDS, ECG
- Titles used with a person's name: Dr. Castanedo, Mrs. Cranston
- First word of a **quotation** (words written exactly as spoken): The patient stated, "The medicine didn't seem to help me."

Punctuation Rules

Punctuation marks help the reader understand written messages. Incorrect or missing punctuation can lead to confusion and distorted meanings. Here are guidelines for the most common uses of punctuation marks:

1. The *period* is used at the end of a sentence and after abbreviations, except for names of states and organizations.

   Example: Respiratory therapists must have good technical skills.

2. The *comma* is used:

   a. to join two **independent clauses** (parts of a sentence that can stand on their own as complete sentences) joined by *and, but, or, nor, for, so, yet*

   Example: Brushing the teeth after each meal is important, but flossing is also necessary.

   b. to separate three or more words or phrases that appear in a series

   Example: The three energy nutrients are carbohydrates, fats, and proteins.

   c. At the end of an introductory group of words

   Examples: When the patient arrived at the office, he was having trouble breathing.

   Efficient and well-organized, Dr. Bancini's office staff rarely got behind schedule.

   Buried under piles of papers, Mrs. North's medical chart was nowhere to be seen.

   d. Around inessential phrases that describe or add information

   Example: The patient, who lives in my neighborhood, came to the clinic on Monday. (*Phrase only adds interesting but unnecessary information.*)

   The physician who specializes in pulmonary disorders agreed to see the patient this afternoon. (*Phrase adds important information about the physician.*)

   e. to set off transitional expressions: *however, therefore, for example, in other words, as a matter of fact*

   Example: Taking blood pressure, for example, is an important medical assisting skill.

   Giving medical advice, however, can only be done by the physician.

   f. With dates and addresses

   Examples: The clinic first opened on June 2, 1985, in Omaha, Nebraska.

   The nearest hospital is located at 417 Kearny Road, San Diego, California.

3. The *semicolon* is used:

   a. between independent clauses that are NOT joined with connecting words such as *and, but, or, nor, for, so, yet*

   Example: The physician referred Mr. Denton to a physical therapist; his leg requires special exercises to regain strength and range of motion.

   b. between independent clauses joined by transitional expressions such as *also, besides, finally, furthermore, for example, in conclusion, on the contrary*

   Example: Good health is influenced by proper nutrition; also, exercise plays an important role.

4. The *colon* is used:

    a. at the end of an independent clause that introduces a list or a quotation

    Example: The major functions of the integumentary system include the following: provide protection from the external environment, control body temperature, and maintain homeostasis.

    b. after the **salutation** (greeting) in a business letter

    Example: Dear Dr. Phillips:

5. The *apostrophe* is used:

    a. to create the possessive form of a noun

    Example: The nurse's stethoscope lay on the counter.

    b. to indicate the **contraction** (combining) of two words

    Example: It's a busy day at the clinic. (It's = It is)

6. *Quotation marks* are used:

    a. to enclose direct quotes (exact words of a speaker)

    Example: "I need you to help me turn Mrs. Sands," said Nurse Ames to the CNA.

    b. around titles of magazine and newspaper articles, chapters in books, stories, songs, and poems. (Note: titles of books, plays and movies and names of magazines and newspapers are put in italics–*like this*–or underlined.)

Using More Than One Punctuation Mark

- Always place periods and commas inside quotation marks.

  Example: This month's journal had an interesting article entitled "Postoperative Pain in Knee-Replacement Patients."

- Place exclamation and question marks inside unless they apply to the entire sentence.

  Examples: When Dr. Pedersen told Mr. Watson that his cholesterol was lower as a result of the new medication, the patient exclaimed, "That's great news!"

  Have you read Chapter 20, "Physical Assessment" ?

Writing Numbers Correctly

The general rule when using numbers in sentences is to write them out as words when:

1. They are made up of two words or less.

2. They are the first word in a sentence.

[Fascinating Facts]

Computer grammar-checkers are helpful for catching common grammatical errors. But they don't replace proofreading by the writer. According to a study by Diana Hacker, author of *A Writer's Reference*, grammar-checkers flagged only 20 to 50% of the run-on sentences in a sample. (A run-on sentence consists of two independent clauses that are not joined with a connecting word. Example: I saw Dr. Anderson, he was in a hurry and couldn't answer my question.)

Otherwise, they are written as figures. See the following examples:

1. There were five patients waiting to see the doctor.

2. There were 25,000 cases reported last year in the United States.

3. Twenty-five thousand new cases were reported last year in the United States.

In technical writing, such as that used in health care, using figures rather than writing out words for numbers is sometimes preferred. Check the preferences for your specific profession and facility. Figures are also used in the following situations:

- When expressing time with A.M. or P.M. (a.m. and p.m. are also correct) Your next appointment is scheduled for 3:15 P.M. on Wednesday, January 10, 2001.

  Otherwise, write the numbers out in words.

  Mr. Hashimoto's surgery is scheduled to begin at eight o'clock in the morning.

- Percentages

  The range of normal hematocrit (volume percentage of red blood cells in whole blood) values for newborns is 45–60%.

- Temperature

  His temperature was below normal at 97.6 degrees.

- Fractions and decimals

  A quart is equal to ¼ gallon.

  The specific gravity (weight compared to equal volume of water) of normal urine ranges from 1.003 to 1.035.

Writing Titles Correctly

Use standard abbreviations if the title appears immediately before or after names (never in both places). Note that not all abbreviations require the use of a period.

Dr. Joanna Carter	OR	Joanna Carter, M.D. (Doctor of Medicine)
Dr. Esteban Alvarez	OR	Esteban Alvarez, Ph.D. (Doctor of Philosophy)
Dr. Mary O'Leary	OR	Mary O'Leary, D.D.S. (Doctor of Dental Surgery)

Thomas Kirk, MA

Sally Hines, OTR

BUSINESS LETTERS

A trend in health care employment today is **cross-training** employees. This means that they learn to perform tasks in addition to those traditionally performed by individuals with their job titles. For example, more administrative tasks are being required of health care workers. The ability to write business letters correctly is a necessary skill for an increasing number of occupations.

Business letters create an important link between health care providers and their patients and colleagues. The following types of letters are commonly used in health care:

- Appointment: Reminds a patient of the date and time of the next appointment
- Recall: Requests a patient to call and make an appointment
- Collection: Requests a patient to pay a bill
- Follow-up: Summarizes reports regarding test results, outlines further treatment needs
- Consultation: Requests another professional to examine a patient
- Explanation: Provides an excuse from work or school, explains special needs for patient accommodation
- Inquiry: Requests information about products or processes
- Special occasion: Accepts an invitation or sends regrets, offers congratulations
- Announcement: States new office hours or other policies, announces new associate or retirement of staff member

Thinking it Through

Karin McFarland is the office manager for Drs. Kern, Wilkes, and Ruiz. She recently hired a new medical receptionist, Wanda Belini, whom patients like for her warm, friendly personality. Wanda has excellent telephone skills and good judgment about handling calls appropriately. Karin is concerned, however, about Wanda's writing skills. The short documents such as memos and meeting announcements that she has prepared have contained spelling and punctuation errors. Karin believes that Wanda is a valuable asset to the office and wants to help her improve.

1. Why is it important for memos and meeting announcements to be written properly if they are only seen by people who work in the office?

2. What might Wanda do to improve her writing skills?

3. What impact might Wanda's poor writing skills have on her future career if she does not improve them?

Using Form Letters

Many letters are sent out repeatedly with the same information. Creating form letters can save time. Some patients are offended by obvious form letters and believe that they reflect an uncaring attitude. With today's word processing software, it is possible to personalize form letters and print them without the telltale signs of repeated passes through the copy machine. The patient's name and address can be entered, and personal notes included within the text. Form letters should be personally signed whenever possible.

Creating Effective Letters

Effective business letters are courteous, clear, and direct. Getting to the point, without being abrupt, is a sign of respect for the reader's time. While being businesslike, letters to patients should never be so formal as to seem uncaring. The message of a letter is organized in the same way as for other types of writing:

1. State the purpose in the introduction.
2. Develop ideas in the body. Provide necessary information and explanations. Use an appropriate tone. For example, a collection letter should be written in a firm manner.
3. Summarize, and state what you want the reader to do.

Carefully proofread all letters for content, grammar, and spelling. A letter that contains even a single error is not considered mailable.

Business Letter Formats

There are certain traditions that govern the appearance of business letters. Like dressing appropriately for a business occasion, the correct use of a prescribed letter format is a sign of proper business **etiquette** (manners). Remember that the quality and appearance of correspondence represent the level of professionalism of the sender.

Thinking it Through

Kendra Washington is the administrative assistant for Dr. Benson, the director of an inner-city community clinic. The clinic depends on charitable contributions for a significant portion of its operating funds. Dr. Benson has asked Kendra to draft a letter to past and potential contributors in anticipation of the clinic's annual fund-raising drive. The purpose of the letter is to explain the progress of the clinic over the last year and how it contributes to the community. The most important part is to ask the recipient to make a donation. Kendra knows that the organization and wording of the letter are important in order for it to be effective.

1. What must Kendra consider when deciding how to write this letter?
2. What steps should she take to plan its content?
3. Which style of letter do you think would be most appropriate?
4. If she decides to use a form letter, how could it be personalized for the recipients?

The three most commonly used letter formats are **full block**, **block**, and **modified block**. The main difference between the formats is how the lines of text are **justified** (lined up with the margins).

- Full block: All lines are flush (lined up evenly) with the left margin. This is the most efficient format to use because it eliminates the need for extra keystrokes to indent the lines. See Figure 17–3.
- Block: All lines are flush with the left margin except the date, closing, and signature. These begin just to the right of the center of the page. See Figure 17–4.
- Semi- or modified block (also called "semi-block"): The same as block except that paragraphs are indented five spaces and the subject line begins just to the right of the center of the page. This format is considered the least formal of the three. See Figure 17–5.

Preparing Letters for Mailing

When a letter requires more than one sheet, use a piece of plain matching paper (without the information about the sender and receiver) for the second page. The correct way to fold a completed letter depends on the size and type of envelope used. See Figure 17–6. Proper delivery is ensured if the envelope is addressed according to the following guidelines:

- Write the address in all uppercase (capital) letters
- Do not use punctuation in the address
- Use the ZIP code. Add the additional 4-number code when possible.
- Do not write in the lower-right corner.
- Include a complete return address in the upper-left corner.

MEMOS

Memos are written to share information within an organization. Examples of typical memo topics include policy changes, staff schedules, explanations of procedures, announcements about new staff or equipment, and safety reminders.

Memos should be written clearly, concisely, and to the point. It is important that they can be read and understood quickly and easily. The message should be useful to the recipient. Employees who receive too many memos begin to ignore them.

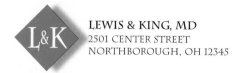

LEWIS & KING, MD
2501 CENTER STREET
NORTHBOROUGH, OH 12345

NORTHBOROUGH
FAMILY MEDICAL GROUP

Date Line

January 12, 20___ (approximately 15th line)

Inside Address

Jeremy Brown, MD (approximately 20th line)
111 S Main
Blossom, UT 10283-1120
            (double-space)

Salutation

Dear Dr. Brown:
            (double-space)

Subject Line

Blossom Medical Society Meeting
            (double-space)
Thank you for inviting me to speak at the Blossom Medical Society
Meeting June 15, 20___. As requested, my topic will describe the
use of the MRI in assisting physicians to make a more accurate
diagnosis without resorting to invasive procedures. The exact
title of my speech will be sent by next Friday.
            (double-space)
Please have your office manager send information regarding the
number of participants expected, time of meeting, location, and
any other details that will assist me in preparing my speech.

I will write or call if I have any additional questions.
            (double-space)

Complimentary
Closing

Yours truly,

Winston Lewis, MD (4-5 line spaces)

Keyed Signature

Winston Lewis, MD
            (double-space)

Reference Initials

WL:jg
            (double-space)

Enclosure Notation

Enclosure: Handout on MRI

Figure 17–3 Full block style letter. The contents of a standard business letter are labeled.

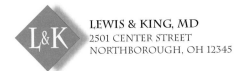

LEWIS & KING, MD
2501 CENTER STREET
NORTHBOROUGH, OH 12345

NORTHBOROUGH
FAMILY MEDICAL GROUP

January 12, 20___ (approximately 15th line)

Jeremy Brown, MD (approximately 20th line)
111 S Main
Blossom, UT 10283-1120

Dear Dr. Brown:

Blossom Medical Society Meeting

Thank you for inviting me to speak at the Blossom Medical Society
Meeting June 15, 20___. As requested, my topic will describe the use of
the MRI in assisting physicians to make a more accurate diagnosis without resorting to invasive procedures. The exact title of my speech will
be sent by next Friday.

Please have your office manager send information regarding the number of
participants expected, time of meeting, location, and any other details
that will assist me in preparing my speech.

I will write or call if I have any additional questions.

Yours truly,

Winston Lewis, MD

Winston Lewis, MD

WL:jg

Enclosure: Handout on MRI

Figure 17–4 Block style letter.

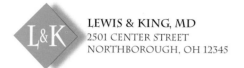

LEWIS & KING, MD
2501 CENTER STREET
NORTHBOROUGH, OH 12345

NORTHBOROUGH
FAMILY MEDICAL GROUP

January 12, 20____ (approximately 15th line)

Jeremy Brown, MD (approximately 20th line)
111 S Main
Blossom, UT 10283-1120

Dear Dr. Brown:

Blossom Medical Society Meeting

Thank you for inviting me to speak at the Blossom Medical Society Meeting June 15, 20____. As requested, my topic will describe the use of the MRI in assisting physicians to make a more accurate diagnosis without resorting to invasive procedures. The exact title of my speech will be sent by next Friday.

Please have your office manager send information regarding the number of participants expected, time of meeting, location, and any other details that will assist me in preparing my speech.

I will write or call if I have any additional questions.

Yours truly,

Winston Lewis, MD

Winston Lewis, MD

WL:jg

Enclosure: Handout on MRI

Figure 17–5 Semi- or modified block style format.

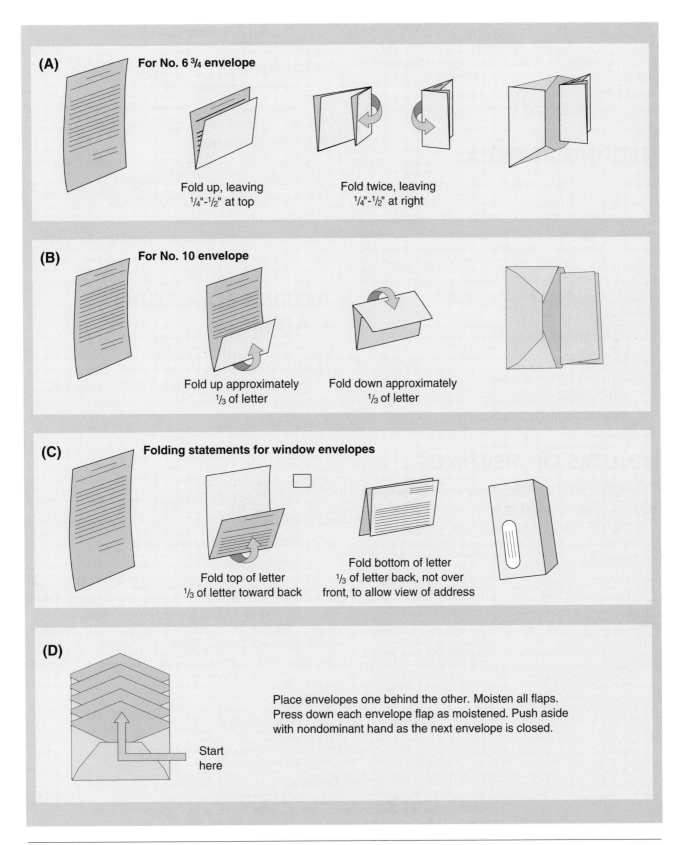

Figure 17–6 Proper methods for folding business letters for mailing.

Prepare memos with the same care given to outgoing letters. The quality of memos can set the tone for work standards at a facility. Poorly prepared memos and other internal documents can send the message that quality paperwork and attention to detail are not valued. See Figure 17–7 for a sample memo format.

MEETING AGENDAS

Whether for a meeting at work or for a professional organization, the health care worker may be called upon to prepare a meeting agenda. An **agenda** lists what is to take place at a meeting. Agendas promote efficiency by helping attendees prepare in advance and by keeping meetings focused on what needs to be discussed and accomplished. A good agenda should include:

1. Date of the meeting
2. Start and end times
3. Exact location
4. Topics to be discussed
5. What attendees should bring, if applicable
6. Guest speaker(s), if applicable

MINUTES OF MEETINGS

Minutes provide written documentation of what happens at meetings. They serve several purposes:

- Inform those who did not attend about important decisions and announcements that took place.
- Create a record of facility transactions. Document, for regulatory and accrediting purposes, that specific items were discussed.
- Serve as a guide for the next meeting's agenda.
- Provide a resource for future reference and a reminder of decisions made.

The following items are commonly included in minutes:

1. Date and time the meeting is called to order
2. Members present and absent
3. Acceptance of previous minutes, including any corrections or additions
4. Announcements
5. Short write-up of discussions, decisions made, and conclusions agreed on
6. Date and time of next meeting
7. Time of adjournment
8. Signature of person preparing the minutes and chairperson

PATIENT EDUCATION MATERIALS

High-quality written materials are an important part of effective patient education, introduced in Chapter 16. Written materials are appropriate for providing information on many topics:

- Diets
- Exercises
- Medications
- Postoperative instructions
- Preparing for a diagnostic test
- Self-exams
- Tips for quitting smoking
- Wound care

If original information or instruction sheets are created or if material is borrowed from other sources, it is important to verify the content for accuracy. Organize the material in an easy-to-follow format. Bulleted or numbered lists may be easier for patients to follow than solid text. Create a logical

---

Wilsonville Orthopedic Clinic

MEMO

To: Person(s) to whom the memo is being sent
From: Person sending the memo
CC: Names of other individuals to whom a copy of the memo is being sent
Date: Date memo is written and/or sent
Re: Subject of the memo. Helps recipient prioritize and organize
             memos if they are saved

Figure 17–7 Sample memo heading format.

order. For example, when listing possible postoperative complications, start with the most serious. Clearly indicate which ones require notifying the physician. When explaining the steps of a procedure, list them in the order in which they are performed.

Write at a reading level that is appropriate for patients. Avoid technical language that may be confusing or misunderstood. Use diagrams to illustrate important points or procedures. Use a larger-than-standard font size for patients with poor eyesight. Keep clear master copies so that repeated copying does not result in poor-quality print. Be sure that materials are kept up to date with medical advances and changing policies.

CONFIDENTIALITY OF WRITTEN MATERIALS

All written materials containing patient information must be secure from the sight or possession of any unauthorized person. As discussed in Chapter 3, patient confidentiality must be respected at all times. Seemingly innocent documents, such as appointment reminder letters, are considered confidential if patients' names are visible. These, along with similar written materials, should never be left out where they can be seen by other patients, vendors, or other office visitors.

PROOFREADING WRITTEN WORK

All written work should be proofread for content, grammar, punctuation, spelling, and appearance. It is easy to overlook errors, because most people read more than one word at a time. The mind, reading for content, fills in missing letters and even whole words. Here are some tips for proofreading effectively:

- Reread the document to verify content. Check all facts for accuracy.
- Check the organization of the material. Does it make sense? Does it flow well?
- Read aloud. Listen for odd-sounding phrases and words.
- Check spelling by reading backwards, word by word. This way, you concentrate on the appearance and spelling of words rather than on the meaning.

Box 17–1 Written Communicaton Checklist

____ Appearance: margins, formatting, print quality

____ Completeness: all information filled in

____ Accuracy: numbers, dates, facts verified

____ Grammar

____ Punctuation

____ Capitalization

____ Confidentiality protected

____ Corrections done properly

- Use the spell-checker and grammar-checker features on the computer.
- Print out documents created on the computer rather than proofreading from the screen. Most people find printed material easier to read.
- If you are unsure about any aspect of a document, ask a qualified person for help.
- Have your written work checked as required by your facility.

See Box 17–1 for a list of items to check when reviewing written work.

SUGGESTED LEARNING ACTIVITIES

1. Quiz yourself on the spelling of the words in the list of frequently misspelled words.
2. Start your own personal dictionary for words you misspell. Dedicate time each week to studying and mastering these words.
3. Collect samples of nonconfidential written documents such as instruction sheets, form letters, and office policies, from health care facilities. Compare the quality and look for examples that illustrate good written communication.
4. Pay attention to writing styles as you read your textbooks, magazine and newspaper articles, novels, etc. Identify characteristics you believe make writing effective. Start a scrapbook of good examples.

REVIEW QUESTIONS

1. What are three reasons why every health care worker should develop good writing skills?

2. What are the four steps that should be taken when planning a written document?

3. Why is it important that the health care worker use correct spelling and grammar?

4. Compare and contrast the three major formats used when writing business letters.

5. How should the content of an effective business letter be organized?

6. What should be done to ensure that business letters are delivered properly to the addressee?

7. What items should be included when preparing meeting agendas?

8. What are five strategies for preparing effective written materials for patient education?

9. What items should be included when writing the minutes of a meeting?

10. How can patient confidentiality be protected when handling written documents?

11. What are five good proofreading techniques?

APPLICATION EXERCISES

1. Refer to The Case of the Surprised Therapist at the beginning of the chapter. Explain what Al can do to ensure that the agendas, reports, and instruction sheets are written effectively and correctly.

2. Dental assistant Tanya Lucas is the chair of the program planning committee for her local professional organization. She has written the following letter to Dr. Samantha

```
                                        Tanya Lucas, RDA
                                        943 Castro Lane
                                        Oakland, CA 94662

November 15, 2001

Dr. Samantha Speares, D.D. S.
Speares Pediatric Dentistry
7920 Glenwood Circle
Oakland, Ca  94662

Dear Dr. Speares,
On behalf of the Oakland Dental Assistants Society, I would like to invite you speak
to our group about pediatric dentistry. Many of our members are interested in work-
ing with children, they are thinking about working in pediatric dentistry and would
like to know more about it. It would definitely be a priviledge to have you as our
speaker.
The meeting will be held on January 10 2002, at seven o'clock P.M. at the Town and
Country hotel located at 2275 Scenic Road Oakland. I sincerely hope you can attend.
Please call me or our secritary, Diana LaMer at (510) 123-4567.


Sincerely;



Tanya Lucas
Program Committee Chair
```

Speares, a local dentist, inviting her to speak to the group.

a. Should Tanya send her letter as written to Dr. Speares?

b. If not, explain what she should do to make it "mailable." Apply what you learned in this chapter about spelling, capitalization, punctuation, and letter formats.

SUGGESTED READINGS AND RESOURCES

Hacker, D. (1999). *A writer's reference.* Boston: Bedford/St. Martin's.
www.bedfordstmartins.com/hacker/writersref

CHAPTER

COMPUTERS IN HEALTH CARE

18

OBJECTIVES

Studying and applying the material in this chapter will help you to:

- Explain why computer literacy is important for today's health care worker.

- Describe ways that computers are used in the following applications in health care:
  - Information management
  - Creation of documents
  - Numerical calculations
  - Integration of operations
  - Diagnostics
  - Treatment
  - Patient monitoring
  - Research
  - Education
  - Communication

- Explain the difference between computer hardware and software.

- Describe how to properly handle and maintain hardware components.

- Identify and describe the two major storage devices.

- Explain the proper care of diskettes.

- List six important guidelines for using computers effectively.

- Explain precautions that the health care worker can take to ensure computer security.

- List ways that the health care worker can acquire computer skills.

KEY TERMS

application program
bioinformatics
browser
central processing unit
compact discs
computer literacy
database
diskette
download
electronic mail
electronic spreadsheet
expert systems
fiber optics
field
file
hard drive
hardware
Internet
modem
network
peripheral
point of care charting
RAM
record
site license
software
telemedicine
virus
virtual communities

The Case of

the Therapist Who Wants to Add to Her Computer System

Carol Lindstrom has maintained a physical therapy practice in a small community for over 30 years. Her interpersonal communication skills are excellent, and she is known for her ability to motivate her patients to reach their highest physical potential following accidents and surgeries. Carol is computer literate and has a computer system capable of word processing, bookkeeping, and accessing the Internet. Her assistant, Graciela, uses the computer mainly for correspondence and billing. Carol is aware that she and Graciela could be using computer technology in additional ways to make the practice more efficient and to help patients in more ways. Carol discusses this with Graciela and assigns her the task of investigating additional computer applications. This chapter includes a discussion of the many ways that computers are being used to provide expanded services to patients.

COMPUTERS IN HEALTH CARE

Computers and their applications have influenced every aspect of modern health care. From patient check-in procedures to diagnostics and research, computerization is changing the way that health care is delivered. All health care workers now function as information managers, and the ability to use computers has become an essential part of health care competency.

Computers perform three major types of operations:

1. Store huge amounts of information
2. Calculate and manipulate data quickly and accurately
3. Enable high-speed communication

Harnessing the capabilities of the modern computer relieves workers from having to perform repetitive jobs. Mathematical calculations and organizational tasks involving enormous amounts of data can be completed quickly and accurately. Additions, revisions, and corrections to, and deletions from documents can be made quickly and easily. Changes and updates are immediately available to those who need them. Information can be accessed simultaneously by many people.

We can see more clearly the impact of computers on health care by following one patient, Mr. Johnson. Mr. Johnson was mowing his lawn on a Saturday afternoon when he experienced chest pains and nausea. His wife took him to the emergency room at nearby Ames General Hospital. The following list includes some of the many ways that computer technology was used during his stay at Ames:

1. Mr. Johnson was taken to see a physician immediately, because of the possibility that he was suffering a myocardial infarction (heart attack). Mrs. Johnson gave information about Mr. Johnson and their health insurance coverage to the admitting clerk who entered it on the hospital's *computerized patient record system*.

2. An ECG (electrocardiogram, a diagnostic method used to measure the heart's electrical activity) was performed on Mr. Johnson. The results were interpreted by a *computer* and produced on a paper printout for qualified personnel to read and review.

3. Dr. Sanchez, the cardiologist on duty, examined Mr. Johnson and decided to admit him to the hospital for observation. He dictated his observations, which were then *word processed* by a hospital transcriptionist for entry into the medical record.

4. A room was scheduled for Mr. Johnson using the hospital's *computerized scheduling program.*

5. Orders for medications prescribed by Dr. Sanchez were sent via a *computer network* to the hospital pharmacy.

6. A hospital pharmacy technician used a *pharmaceutical software program* to compare the new medications with those that Mr. Johnson was already taking to check for possible drug interactions.

7. All supplies used for Mr. Johnson's hospitalization were tracked on a *computerized inventory system.* This information was used for reordering supplies and preparing billing statements.

8. Mr. Johnson's blood pressure and pulse were intermittently monitored at preset intervals by *computerized equipment* at his bedside.

9. Mr. Johnson is diabetic and the nursing assistant took his blood sugar level before meals and at bedtime. She used a hand-held piece of equipment called a glucometer that has *computer components* for testing blood and storing the readings.

10. Mr. Johnson had blood and urine samples sent to the laboratory for processing. As soon as the tests are completed, the results are available on *computer* for the staff to review.

11. Mr. Johnson's charge nurse entered nursing notes about his care and condition directly into the *computerized medical record system* to enable ready access to his health care team.

12. When Mr. Johnson was discharged, he was given instructions about diet and exercise that had been created with *word processing software.*

The health care workers who provided direct care for Mr. Johnson or provided support services needed to be computer literate. Sandra Anderson (1992), who writes about the use of computers in health care, lists the following competencies as the components of **computer literacy**:

1. Understand what a computer is and what functions it performs.

2. Perform basic operations to complete professional tasks.

3. Become aware of the impact of technology on the quality of human life, including social and ethical issues.

The type and number of computer-related tasks performed by health care workers depend on their specific occupations and factors such as the size of the facility in which they work. Duties range from simple data entry to interpreting diagnostic test results. Employees in small facilities sometimes need to have a wider variety of computer skills than those in larger facilities, which have computer specialists on staff. For example, a dental receptionist in a single-dentist office may be asked to research and purchase a computer system to upgrade the administrative functions of the office. Very large facilities, such as hospitals or groups of associated clinics, have computer departments consisting of specialized staff members who assist other departments with their computer purchasing and maintenance.

Information Management

Keeping track of huge amounts of data is a challenge in the health care world. Having quick access to information is necessary for tasks such as selecting appropriate courses of treatment, preparing reports for regulatory agencies, and justifying insurance bills. A major role of the computer is storing and making this information easily accessible in useful formats. See Box 18–1 for other examples of health care databases.

A **database** is a collection of information organized in a structured way. Databases can be set up by the user with application software that can be purchased at a relatively low cost. For example, a small medical office might use a software program to develop a database of all active patients served by a specific insurance company. Complex databases for large facilities are created by computer programmers to meet the specific needs of the facility.

Box 18–1　Examples of Health Care Databases

Disease profiles

Insurance company records

Inventory management

Mailing lists

Patient records

Personnel records

Pharmaceutical records

Production reports

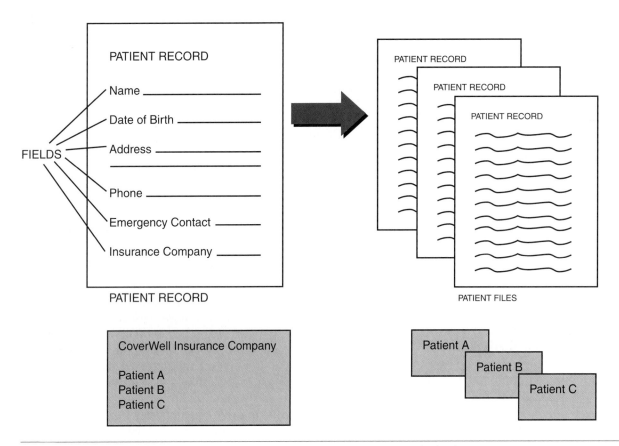

Figure 18–1 Databases are structured to provide easy access to needed information.

The basic structure of a database is the key to its usefulness. Each collection of related data is called a **record**. For example, the data about each individual is grouped together in a separate record. This data is entered into **fields**. Suppose that a computerized patient record contains 15 pieces of demographic information, such as name, address, telephone number, occupation, and insurance company name. Each of these items has its own field. A group of related records is called a **file**. See Figure 18–1 to see the relationship between fields, records, and files.

Computerized databases have many advantages over paper filing systems. The following features make them especially useful in health care information management:

- Records can be retrieved quickly and easily.

- Records can be sorted, accessed, and reported in many ways. For example, patient records can be organized alphabetically by last name, grouped by ZIP code, grouped by insurance company, or listed chronologically by date of last visit.

- Information can be accessed by more than one person at the same time.

- Additions and changes can be entered easily.

- Reports can be generated as needed.

- Quality improvement studies can be conducted (see Chapter 23).

Many health care workers are responsible for entering data on forms that are displayed on the monitor. Some forms use abbreviations or numerical codes to identify the various fields. The data is converted into a readable form such as the computerized medical history and physical examination in Figure 18–2.

Accuracy is critical when entering data. Patient diagnoses, treatment plans, and billing are negatively affected by incorrect data. Carefully review and verify all input. When an error is made when inputting data, be sure that only the intended sections are erased. Reconstructing records can be difficult and time-consuming, as well as being the cause of inconsistent patient care and legal problems.

Health care workers who function as information managers may be required to design and create databases. In these cases, it is important to carefully study the information needs of the facility. A computerized database is valuable only if it serves the needs of the users.

Patient: Leo McKay
Date of Birth: 01/22/44
Visit Date: 04/01/__

Chief Complaint: Abdominal pain
History: Has been ill over the last 2 weeks with progressively worsening abdominal pain.
Review of Symptoms: Patient denies the following:
- Chest pain, Chest pressure, Chest heaviness, Circulation problems, Palpitations, Rapid heartbeat, Irregular heartbeat, Ankle swelling
- Cough, Phlegm, Coughing up blood, Shortness of breath, Wheeze, Change in exercise tolerance
- Burning or pain on urination, Difficulty starting or stopping urination, Dribbling after urination, Incontinence of urine, Blood in urine, Cloudiness of urine
- Change in appetite, Unexpected weight loss, Nausea, Vomiting, Difficulty Swallowing, Belly pains, Gas pains, Change in bowel habit: change in frequency, shape, color, consistency, size of stool; Blood, Mucus, or Slime, Rectal pain or discomfort, Hemorrhoids
- Skin rash, New or changing moles, Excess bruising or bleeding
- Mouth sores, Denture problems, Sinus drainage or stuffiness, Facial pain
- Panic attacks, Anxiety, Depression, Sadness, Seizures, Problems with concentration or memory, Disturbance of sleep, Insomnia, Early wakefulness
- Dizziness, Fainting, Lightheadedness on standing, Headaches, Vision problems, Hearing problems, Numbness or tingling in arms or legs, Weakness in arms or legs

Medications:

Drug	Dose	Freq.	Started
none			

Medical Problem List

Problem	When Dx'd	Active?
Peptic Ulcer	1985	no

List of Surgeries.

Surgical Procedure	When
none	

Family History: Parents deceased, father died of heart attack, mother of breast cancer.
Social History: Divorced, no children
Habits: Smokes 2 ppd, Several beers daily
Allergies: Penicillin _____
                            Physical Examination
GENERAL: Well developed and well nourished gentleman in no distress. No jaundice, cyanosis, clubbing, or edema.
VITALS: Weight = 192, Temp = 97.6, Pulse = 78, BP = 152/88
HEENT: Normocephalic and without evidence of trauma, tympanic membranes and external auditory canals are normal. Pharynx and mouth are normal.
NECK: supple, no masses or thyromegaly.
NODES: No cervical nodes palpable. No axillary or inguinal adenopathy.
CARDIOVASCULAR SYSTEM: Heart sounds: no murmurs, rubs or gallops, carotids with good upstrokes, no bruits heard. Peripheral pulses including radials, brachials, and femorals intact. Posterior tibial, and dorsalis pedis pulses intact.
RESPIRATORY SYSTEM: resps 16/min, trachea central, expansion, fremitus, resonance, and breath sounds normal.
ABDOMEN: soft, no masses, organomegaly, or tenderness. No loin or costo-vertebral angle tenderness. Inguinal canals are intact without herniae. Bowel sounds active.
GENITOURINARY: Penis without lesions or discharge, scrotum, testicles, epididymis and cords all normal
RECTAL: no masses, tenderness, or hemorrhoids. Soft brown stool in vault. Prostate normal in size, and shape without nodules or tenderness.
MUSCULOSKELETAL SYSTEM: Joints with full ROM, no joint tenderness or swelling. Muscle bulk symmetric and normal.
SKIN: without masses, skin tags, rash, blisters or ulcerations. Nails are normal without splinter hemorrhages.
NEUROLOGICAL SYSTEM: Alert and oriented to place, person, and time. Communicates with good word recognition and appropriate word usage. Cranial nerves and spinal nerves grossly intact.

Assessment and Plan

Problem	Plan/Status
Abdominal pain	Reports about two weeks of epigastric and retrosternal chest pain radiating up and to the left. Episodes of pain occur usually during the day and last for 3-4 hours. No associated dyspnea, palpitations, sweats, dizziness. No nausea, vomiting or diarrhea. No blood in the stool. To get barium swallow, CBC, Chem 7 and UA.

follow-up appointment: 3 days
Mark Woo MD

Figure 18–2 Sample of computer-generated medical history and physical examination.

Thinking it Through

Tyler is an occupational therapy assistant who works for Kelly Graziano, an OTR with a private practice that specializes in hand therapy. In addition to assisting patients with their therapy and making splints, Tyler is helping Kelly computerize the administrative activities of the office. He wants to create a system to track the vendors used by the practice to supply equipment and materials. Use the following questions to help him design a useful database.

1. How can the database be organized?

2. What data would be useful in each record?

3. How will the database make it easier to order supplies?

4. What reports might be useful for the practice? How often should they be generated?

5. How would such a system help Kelly with the financial management of her practice?

Creation of Documents

The importance of accurate and professional-looking documents was discussed in Chapter 17. Computers are excellent tools to help create high-quality written material. Word processing software converts the computer into a "supertypewriter" that gives the user the capability to create customized documents that are error-free. Written materials of all types–letters, reports, forms, newsletters–can be produced with word processing software. See Box 18–2 for examples of word processed documents found in health care. There are a number of software programs available that enable the user to perform the following functions:

- Design the appearance of text and documents.
- Edit, correct errors, and check spelling and grammar.
- Store documents for later use.
- Print and/or send documents by e-mail, fax, or direct connection to other computers.

Spreadsheets

Electronic spreadsheet software permits the user to apply the computer's ability to perform high-speed calculations of numerical data. Spreadsheet software provides a worksheet that consists of intersecting rows and columns that form squares called cells. Numbers and formulas (instructions for performing calculations) are entered into the cells. To create a simple budget using spreadsheet software, the user enters the amounts of income and expenses and the formulas for the desired calculations. A formula may have several steps. The budgeting example would allow the user to calculate monthly income by adding all income and subtracting all expenses.

Accounting and financial management were two of the first computer applications in both business and health care. Electronic spreadsheets provide the basis for billing and accounting programs. In addition to speed and accuracy, these programs allow changes to be reflected throughout the spreadsheet. For example, if the cost of a clinic's rent increases, the effect on income can easily be calculated. All totals affected by the change in rent will automatically be adjusted. Changes or corrections that would take a person many hours to recalculate can be accomplished in seconds.

The methods used for patient billing have been significantly affected by computers. Amounts to be billed are not only calculated electronically, but they are now also sent electronically to payers instead of being mailed. Starting in the year 2000, all Medicare and Medicaid claims had to be submitted electronically. Standardized codes have been developed that correspond to various diagnoses and treatment procedures. See Chapter 22 for more information about medical codes. The computer matches the codes for various procedures to a fee schedule and prepares bills. Computerized billing is

Box 18–2   Using Word Processing in Health Care

Announcements

Business letters

Homecare instructions

Information sheets for patient education

Medical reports

Memos

Newsletters

Payment collection notices

Research reports

easier and more accurate. Additional numerical codes that identify specific insurance companies can be entered that result in automatic preparation of the proper bill format.

The high speed of computer calculations also enables the user to employ "if...then" scenarios to explore a variety of options. Questions such as the following can be posed:

- "If the number of patients visiting the clinic continues to grow at the current rate, how many full-time medical assistants will be needed next December?"

- "If we finance the purchase of new medical equipment at 6.5%, how much will the total cost be if the repayment period is 3 years? Five years?"

This type of information assists in the delivery of quality patient care and the making of sound business decisions. Electronic spreadsheet programs are also able to create graphs and charts that illustrate numerical concepts and statistics. See Figure 18–3.

As with databases, it is critical that data entered into the spreadsheet be accurate. One incorrect entry can affect hundreds of numbers. Carefully check all electronic spreadsheet entries.

Integration of Operations

The capacity to integrate various types of operations contributes to the power and value of computers. There are a growing number of commercially prepared integrated systems designed for the health care facility. Medical Manager and Medisoft are only two examples of the many that have been developed for medical offices. They include patient record maintenance, appointment scheduling, insurance coding, billing, and report creation. Using an integrated program helps coordinate administrative tasks and eliminates the need to enter data more than once. For example, a patient recordkeeping database that is tied to billing software allows information entered in one place to appear in the medical record and on a bill to be sent to the insurance company.

Diagnostics

Many types of diagnostic aids are available as a result of the computer's capacity to manipulate data and perform high-speed calculations. For example, the analysis of blood and other body fluids can be conducted quickly and accurately. Diagnostics is an area in which technology has advanced rapidly.

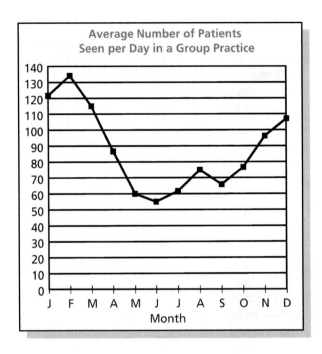

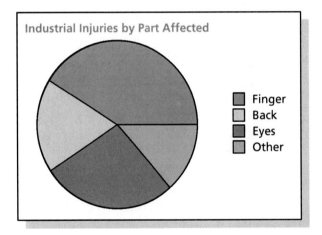

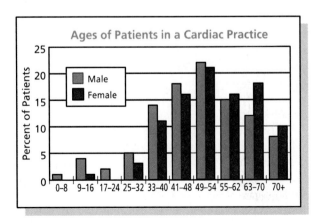

Figure 18–3 Graphs and charts can be easily created using computer software. (Courtesy of GE Medical Systems)

Thinking it Through

Sandra Carruthers has been entering patient billing data into the computer as part of her work as the administrative assistant and book-keeper at Chandler Sports Medicine Clinic. The last week has been difficult for Sandra, because she has out-of-town relatives staying at her house and she is dealing with a variety of family problems. She is usually able to concentrate on her work but has been so tired the last few days that it's been difficult for her to fully focus on the details of data entry.

1. What might be the consequences if Sandra makes the following types of errors:

   a. Enters the wrong medical procedure codes on a bill to an insurance company.

   b. Sends an appointment letter to the wrong patient.

   c. Directs laboratory test requests to the wrong lab.

   d. Enters the wrong numbers for expenses in the computerized accounting program.

2. What would you recommend that Sandra do to protect against making mistakes of this kind?

Diagnostic Imaging

The computer's ability to mathematically convert thousands of measurements into images has encouraged the growth of technology that permits the viewing of soft tissues not possible with traditional x-rays. Safer and more efficient ways of seeing the inner workings of the body continue to be developed and implemented in modern medical facilities. See Table 18–1 and Figures 18–4, 18–5, and 18–6.

The practice of dentistry has been improved by the introduction of safer methods of x-ray. For example, digital x-rays can now be taken, in which a small electronic chip is placed in the patient's mouth and an image sent to a computer. Viewed on the monitor, it can be enlarged, studied, and then stored in the patient's electronic record. The patient is exposed to a smaller amount of radiation than with traditional x-rays.

Fiber Optics

Fiber optics involve the use of hair-thin cables to transmit data. This technology has applications in both diagnostics and treatment. In dentistry, tiny fiber-optic cameras moved within the mouth create images that are projected onto a screen. Both the dentist and patient can see areas that are otherwise very difficult to access. Patient understanding of necessary dental procedures is greatly enhanced.

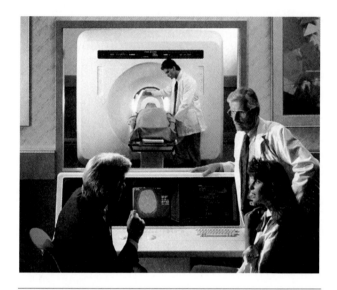

Figures 18–4 For magnetic resonance imaging (MRI), the patient is placed in the center of a large magnet.

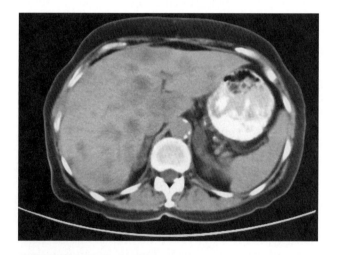

Figures 18–5 This CT scan shows a cross-section of an abdomen. The trained observer can see the presence of liver disease. (Courtesy of Harbor-UCLA Diagnostic Imaging Center)

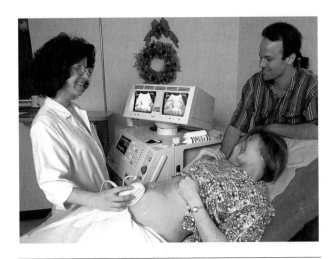

Figures 18–6 Ultrasonography is a safe procedure to use during pregnancy to determine the size, position, sex, and possible abnormalities of the fetus.

The use of fiber optics for both viewing and working inside the body has increased the safety of surgery. A tiny camera, inserted through a narrow tube, projects images along the cable onto a screen, allowing the physician to see the inside of the body without having to make a large incision. If surgery is required, tiny instruments are introduced though other tubes and the procedure is guided by images on the screen.

Patient Questionnaires

Health assessment software assists with identifying patient problems. Some facilities now use computer terminals (monitors) at which patients sit and use the keyboard to enter data on computerized forms that appear on the screen. Patients answer questions, which are designed to perform health screening and identify risk factors. It is believed that patients answer computerized questionnaires more accurately than those asked in person by health care personnel. (Anderson, 1992.)

Table 18–1 Diagnostic Imaging Techniques

Procedure	How it Works	Examples of Use
Computerized Topography (CT)	X-rays are taken from many angles. Measurements of the density of tissues are converted to cross-sectional views.	Evaluation of soft tissues for presence of disease and conditions such as blood clots, fractures, and tumors
Magnetic Resonance Imaging (MRI)	Patient is placed in a magnetic field. The activity of hydrogen atoms in tissues is measured and converted into cross-sectional images.	View tumors clearly View brain structure and abnormalities See movement in the body, such as blood flow
Positron Emission Topography (PET)	A radioactive substance is injected into the patient and detected by a scanner, resulting in three-dimensional images.	Determine how brain is functioning; used with Parkinson's and Alzheimer's disease, epilepsy, cancer Can study effects of drugs on brain and some forms of mental illness
Ultrasonography	High-frequency sound waves hit tissues and organs and bounce back as echoes. The signals obtained are used to create images.	View movement Use when x-rays might cause harm, as with a fetus Examine organs Detect tumors, aneurysms, and blood vessel abnormalities

Expert Systems

Computerized databases, known as **expert systems**, have been designed to assist health care professionals in diagnosing and treating specific conditions. One of the first successful systems, MYCIN, was developed at Stanford University to help identify and treat bacterial infections of the blood and cerebrospinal fluid. The system is used by answering a series of questions that narrow down the choices by matching symptoms with information that is stored in the database. (Anderson, 1992; Burke & Weill, 2000).

Other specialized databases used to assist with diagnosis include the following:

- INTERNIST: Developed at the University of Pittsburgh, contains 2900 symptoms that relate to 500 diseases
- POEMS (Post Operative Expert Medical System): Assists with diagnosis of illnesses that occur during recovery from surgery
- Databank for Cardiovascular Disease: Developed at Drake University, contains a large collection of information dedicated to this specialized area
  (Burke & Weill, 2000).

These expert systems are intended to *assist* health care professionals, *not* take the place of trained individuals. Their reliability varies, and they are never to be substituted for human input and decision making.

Treatment

Many new methods of treatment are based on computer technology. Patients have benefited from new applications that range from robotics to the computer's ability to quickly sort and match data.

Robots have been developed to assist with surgical techniques that are tiring for humans to perform and that require a steady hand. For example, robots hold endoscopic tubes in position as long as necessary. Advanced techniques, such as precise incisions, are performed by sophisticated robots that are programmed to carry out precise movements. Research is even being carried out to develop robots that can be matched to the surgeon's voice and follow oral commands. This may someday enable surgeons to perform procedures at a distance by watching a monitor to guide the movements of a robot (Burke & Weill, 2000).

Lasers, focused light rays that can cut and remove tissue, are guided by computerized measurements to make precise incisions. A common use is for corrective eye surgery.

The preplanning of complex and appearance-altering procedures can be aided by computer capabilities. The COMPASS system provides three-dimensional models of brain tumors created from CT scans and MRIs (Burke & Weill, 2000). Surgeons can use the models to create a detailed strategy for the tumors removal, increasing the speed and accuracy of the procedure. Plastic surgeons use computer-modeling capabilities to assist in reconstructive and cosmetic surgery. Many dentists employ computerized images to make perfectly fitting crowns.

Rehabilitation

The disabled have benefited from computer technology, which has made it possible for them to live more independently. Commands that can be activated with the touch of a button or pad, the voice, or simply by eye contact with the monitor allow the control of household functions. These include turning lights and appliances on and off, answering the telephone, and controlling room temperature.

Computer-aided design has contributed to improvements in prosthetic devices. For example, artificial legs can be designed that more exactly fit the physical characteristics of the individual. Tiny microprocessors can be inserted in prosthetics to improve their movement and to allow them to be better controlled by the user. In another application, computer technology enables the electrical stimulation of muscles that no longer receive stimulation from the brain through the nervous system (Burke & Weill, 2000).

Pharmaceuticals

Computers have improved many aspects of the dispensing of pharmaceutical products. Drugs, including anesthetics, are accurately measured and dispensed through computer-controlled devices. The chance for error is decreased as well as the potential for abuse by health care workers.

MEDI-SPAN is a database that assists in the prescribing of safe, effective medications. It contains information about drug-drug and drug-food interactions. It also has updates on the latest drug releases and those that are pending approval. Computerized patient medication records enable even more specific monitoring of potentially harmful drug interactions. Prescriptions currently taken and allergies, are entered for access by health care professionals at many locations. Approximately 7% of all hospitalized patients suffer adverse drug events (ADE), so having a system to help prevent these occurrences represents a significant positive contribution to patient care (Burke & Weill, 2000).

Patient Monitoring

Physiological monitoring systems employ computer technology to oversee critical body functions, such as heart and respiratory rates. Alarm systems may be connected to various types of monitoring systems to advise health care personnel when patients need intervention. See Figure 18–7. Obstetrical monitoring of the fetus has become a standard procedure.

In addition to performing actual physical measurements, computer systems enable health care workers to enter and track data for charting and recordkeeping. For example, bedside terminals allow keyboard entry of information such as vital signs, dispensing of medications, fluid intake and output, and other information about care. Many systems, known as **point of care charting**, allow information to be entered from the patient's home or hospital bedside. (See Figure 18–8.)

Laptop computers are used by home health workers, such as nurses and physical therapists, to record patient notes and progress. This information is then transmitted electronically into the patient's permanent record. Making sure that data is entered accurately when working in the field is extremely important.

Many specialized devices assist the health care worker to track patient recovery. For example, a camera connected to a computer allows hand therapists to store and compare photographs of the patient's hand taken over time. This aids in evaluating the effectiveness of the treatment plan.

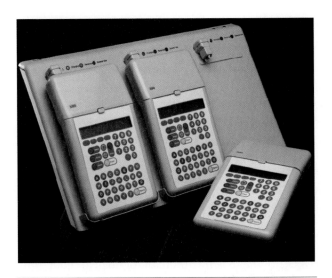

Figure 18–8 Hand-held portable computers can be used to record information at the patient's bedside. (Courtesy of NCR Corporation, Dayton, Ohio)

Research

Literature databases are like giant indexes, containing references to specific journal articles, books, and research reports. Each entry is accessible in various ways, such as the following:

- Preassigned key words that describe the content
- Words in the title
- Name of author(s)
- Name of journal
- Publication date

The National Library of Medicine has created 40 different databases, which are organized in a huge collection of resources called MEDLARS (Medical Literature Analysis and Retrieval System). The entire system contains over 18 million references. A major MEDLARS' database is MEDLINE, which contains bibliographic information on medical research from 3,700 journals.

Other specialized databases are available in addition to MEDLARS. One of potential interest to health care students is the Cumulative Index to Nursing and Allied Health Literature (CINAHL). The index includes references to articles in 1,000 journals, as well as books, pamphlets, software, and standards of practice. Three other large, specialized indexes of interest to health care workers include:

1. Educational Resources (ERIC)
2. Psychological Abstracts (PsychINFO)
3. BIOETHICSLINE

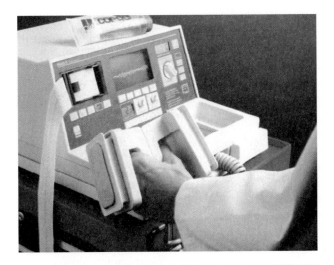

Figure 18–7 Computers are used to monitor the heart and correct abnormal heart rhythms. (Courtesy of Siemens Burdick, Inc.)

[Fascinating Facts]

The Food and Drug Administration Center for Drug Evaluation uses giant electronic spreadsheets of up to 300 million cells for the review of each drug. (Burke and Weill, 2000.)

In addition to providing published information, databases can serve researchers by their capacity to sort and match data. The term **bioinformatics** refers to the organization of biological data into databases. Such databases make information easily available to scientists all over the world. The sharing of information in this way is a significant factor in enabling scientific progress.

The Human Genome Project is an example of bioinformatics. Begun in the late 1980s, it is an international effort to collect the results of investigations relating to human genes (one of the biologic units of heredity). The goal is to enable the mapping of genes for the purpose of identifying the causes of genetic-based diseases.

Pharmaceutical research has benefited from the computer's ability to sort and match the results of thousands of tests carried out to explore the effectiveness and safety of new drugs. Results can be obtained more rapidly and sent to the Food and Drug Administration. This is decreasing the time needed to obtain approvals for new products.

Education

Computers offer new ways to learn for students, health care workers, and patients. Distance education is becoming more widely available. This is a method of accessing courses over the Internet and enables students to take a wide variety of courses in their own homes at times convenient for them. As discussed in Chapter 14, this is a way for health care workers to earn continuing education units.

Many subjects are also available on software. Sound, voice, and interactive components make these an effective way for students to learn at their own pace. CD-ROMs allow storage of vast amounts of reference information. Entire sets of encyclopedias are now available on a single disk. Medical reference books, including specialized dictionaries, have also been placed on disks. It is now possible to own an extensive reference library even if space is limited.

The Visible Human Project has harnessed the power of computers for the instruction of anatomy. Thousands of photographs of cross-sections of the human body have been input into a program, known as ADAM, that allows students to perform mock dissections using a computerized scalpel moved around the screen.

Computerized simulations provide scenarios that enable student interaction. A realistic situation is presented, followed by questions and opportunities for students to suggest appropriate action. The computer responds to the student's input, either indicating its correctness or requesting more information. Virtual reality technology, in which reality is simulated as closely as possible, is enabling individuals to practice procedures before working on patients. These include the insertion of needles or the performance of surgical tasks. Virtual reality provides opportunities for surgeons to practice before working on actual patients. This is especially helpful with very complex and delicate procedures.

Many professional licensing exams are now administered by computer. In the past, exams were offered only once or twice a year, and graduates had to wait until they were scheduled. Some testing programs now individualize the exams by selecting each question based on the response given for the previous question. Test-takers who answer all questions correctly may pass the exam with fewer total questions. An example of this type of test is the NCLEX (National Council Licensure Exam), which is administered to registered nurse candidates.

Communication

The sharing of data over cables and the telephone enables computers to be linked into systems, called **networks**, that allow all types of communication. A simple networked system may consist of four or five personal computers in a small medical office. Patient records are shared, and all staff use the same printer. A large facility may have hundreds of computers linked together that carry out many of the functions described in this chapter. The Internet is the ultimate networked system, consisting of millions of computers located all over the world.

The Internet

The **Internet** began as a method for government authorities to communicate in case of nuclear attack. It has rapidly grown to become a principal means of communicating, conducting business, shopping, learning, and securing needed information. Only four things are needed to access the Internet:

1. Computer
2. **Modem**: A device that converts outgoing messages from a computer into a form that can be sent over telephone lines
3. Access to a service that provides a link to the Internet
4. Special software, known as a **browser**, that allows the user to view Web pages and conduct searches for information

Using the Internet for Research

Health care workers can benefit from the Internet in many ways. Consider the case of Mark, a recently graduated nurse, who is hired by an orthopedic surgeon who specializes in joint replacements. Mark wants to learn more about these procedures and decides to see what he can find on the Internet. In one afternoon, he locates the following resources:

- Articles in medical journals
- Information produced by and about companies that manufacture artificial joints
- A newsgroup in which patients who have had joint replacement surgery share their experiences
- Articles in popular magazines, such as *Newsweek*
- A list of medical facilities and surgeons in the United States who specialize in joint replacement
- Government reports about the effectiveness of artificial joints
- E-mail addresses of university researchers who are experimenting with new types of artificial joints
- A medical bookstore that takes orders over the Internet

During his search, Mark discovers that many sites are linked to others that contain related information. Searches can be conducted by instructing the computer to search for all sites that contain key words. For example, Mark used "artificial joint" to begin his search. By pointing to indicated areas on the screen and clicking on a mouse, he moves quickly from one site (computer connection) to another. This linking capability dramatically increases the searching power of the Internet. In addition to linking, each site of the Internet has an address, much like a building. These can also be entered for instant access to that site.

Evaluating Internet Sources

At this time, material placed on the Internet is not regulated. Anyone can say anything and make any claims. Not all information is reliable. Much of it consists of personal opinions or is motivated by the desire to sell products. Health care workers must take care to determine the reliability of any information taken from the Internet. The following guidelines, suggested by Leshin (1998), are designed to help evaluate sites:

- Identify the source: Universities and government agencies tend to be reliable sources of information. Research and professional organizations, if not organized for the purpose of selling specific products, may also be reliable. For example, the American Heart Association and the American Association of Medical Assistants.
- Determine the author: Is the person an expert in the field? Does he or she have appropriate education and credentials? Is the purpose of the material to share information and/or report research findings? Or to persuade readers and sell ideas or products?
- Check for accuracy: Is a reference given for the information? Is the reference from a reliable source?
- Verify important data: Cross-check statistics and other numerical data.
- Look for signs of quality: Are the ideas well-supported? Is the spelling accurate and vocabulary used correctly?
- Check for currency: Is the information recent and up to date?

In 1998, there were over 10,000 health-related Web sites, visited by 27.1 million people. In 1997, a random selection of sites found that only 47% were created and administered by organizations considered to be reliable, such as universities, hospitals, and government agencies. (Burke & Weill, 2000.)

Electronic Mail

Electronic mail, also known as "e-mail," is a means of creating and sending messages from one computer to another, using the Internet system of networks. E-mail is becoming a standard professional communication tool. It provides a means to quickly send documents such as memos, announcements, and reports to one or more persons. Some physicians and other health care providers are using e-mail as an efficient means of communicating with patients.

It is important that e-mail messages be clear and accurate, just as with any written material.

The growing popularity of e-mail means that some people receive dozens of transmissions daily. Keeping messages brief and to the point is considered a professional courtesy.

Files created in other programs can be sent with an e-mail message. For example, a report created in WordPerfect can be sent as an "attachment" to an e-mail message without rekeying the document. This provides a convenient and economical way to send, review, revise, and return documents and share useful information. For example, two respiratory therapists in different states who are working together to write a journal article can send updated drafts of their work to each other for review. The sharing of research findings is another example of collaboration made easier through the ability to exchange documents electronically.

It is important for health care workers to understand that it is not appropriate to conduct personal e-mail correspondence or explorations on the Internet during work hours. Be aware that e-mail messages may be stored in the form of backup files that belong to the employer. Employers have the right to read and monitor any messages sent through their computers by any employee. Many organizations have increased their monitoring of employee activity on the Internet. Using work hours to write unflattering messages about the boss and to order personal care products are invitations for trouble on the job. They may be cause for disciplinary action and can lead to dismissal.

Telemedicine

Telemedicine is a growing technology in which medicine is practiced over telephone lines. Images, such as x-rays, can be transmitted. Telemedicine is especially helpful for the following functions:

- Allowing patient access to specialists who are located at a distance
- Communicating vital signs from home to allow monitoring at a health care facility
- Checking pacemaker function and performing EKGs over telephone lines
- Performing physical exams from a distance
- Providing more comprehensive emergency care by linking emergency medical workers in the field and during transport with physicians

An interesting barrier to the growth of telemedicine is state licensing laws that control the practice of medicine. Physicians are not allowed to practice medicine across state lines. A physician licensed in one state cannot legally give medical advice, via telephone, to patients in other states (Burke & Weill, 2000). This provides an example of technology advancing more quickly than society's ability to adapt and fully take advantage of it.

Telepharmacies

Telepharmacies allow the dispensing of drugs at sites other than pharmacies. Instructions for prescriptions are sent to a computerized dispensing unit over telephone lines. The unit prepares and releases the exact dosage. Safety features are built into the system to prevent incorrect types and amounts of drugs from being dispensed. This technology is especially useful in medical facilities that are located far from commercial pharmacies.

Virtual Communities

Virtual communities consist of individuals who use the Internet to communicate and share information. Discussion groups and methods for exchanging information have valuable health care applications. Both health care workers and patients can share information and experiences about specific health conditions. Chronically ill, bedridden, and disabled patients have used the communication capabilities of the computer to break from the isolation that often results from these conditions. There are at least three ways that this can be accomplished:

1. Chat rooms allow participants to correspond in real time, using typed messages. Many groups are organized to create communities of individuals who share similar interests.

2. Listserve mailing lists are automated systems that distribute e-mail on specific topics. It is like receiving a newsletter or magazine. There are mailing lists for thousands of topics.

3. Newsgroups provide opportunities for participants to contribute information and comment on items submitted by others. They are organized by subject, and range from general topics to specific local issues. Newsgroups can be accessed using Netscape Navigator or Microsoft Internet Explorer.

[Fascinating Facts]

As of 1998, there were more than 20,000 newsgroups, with 20 to 30 more being added weekly. (Leshin, 1998.)

Thinking it Through

Robin Winter, a dental hygienist, is working on creating a patient education program to teach effective dental home care and nutritional practices. Her patients range from toddlers to the elderly.

1. Describe how Robin can use computers and a variety of applications in her patient education program.

COMPUTER BASICS

While it is not within the scope of this text to teach computer operations, certain fundamental concepts are introduced to guide students who are not familiar with the basic terms and components of computer systems.

Computer Hardware

All computers, whether small laptops that fit into a briefcase or large mainframes that run the operations of a hospital, have physical components in common. These are known as **hardware** and consist of the following:

- **Central processing unit (CPU)**: Located inside the computer, the CPU has three major functions:
  1. Manage all operations
  2. Perform calculations and manipulate data (facts)
  3. Store program instructions and data
- **Peripherals**: Equipment that allows the user to interact with the CPU. Common devices that allow the input of data include:
  1. Keyboard
  2. Mouse, trackball (built into keyboard), and trackpoint (small eraser-like protrusion on keyboard)
  3. Scanner
  4. Microphone

  The three most common output devices are:
  1. Monitor
  2. Printer
  3. Speakers

Caring for Hardware

The physical components of a computer system require regular care. Health care workers should exercise the same care for them as for other medical equipment used on the job. All components of the system contain delicate parts and must be handled gently. A mouse, for example, should never be brought down sharply onto a hard surface. Wires and cables should not be jerked or pulled. Spilled liquids can permanently damage the inner workings of electronic equipment. Dust and food crumbs can also cause problems. For example, salt crystals attract moisture, so salty snacks should not be eaten over the keyboard.

Regular maintenance will help ensure the continued operation of computer equipment:

- Clean monitor screen with an antistatic cloth. Do not use a commercial glass cleaner.
- Vacuum keyboards periodically with a hand-held vacuum cleaner or attachment.
- Wipe the plastic cases with a soft, damp (not wet!) cloth.
- Clean printers according to manufacturer's instructions. Dust that collects on the moving parts can cause smears and fuzzy print.
- Use dust covers when equipment is not in use.
- It is important to read all directions carefully when using and caring for computer components. Follow the manufacturer's recommendations.

Storage of Information

The **hard drive** is a storage device located inside the computer out of the user's view. All types of work can be saved on the hard drive: letters to patients, medical records, accounting reports, and research articles. Today's computers can store very large amounts of data.

Occasionally hard drives cease functioning properly and become inaccessible to the user. This is known as a "crash" and can be caused by a number of factors, including problems with electrical power supplies. To protect against the loss of important data, all work should be saved in at least one other place. The most commonly used methods are diskettes and tape drives. This is called "backing up files" and is an essential habit to develop.

Diskettes consist of magnetic material enclosed in a flat hard plastic case. They are sometimes referred to as "floppy disks" or simply "floppies" because the original diskettes were flexible.

Diskettes are inserted into a slot on the computer called a drive.

Diskettes should be labeled clearly and stored upright in dustproof containers away from high temperatures. Protect against loss of data by following these guidelines for handling diskettes:

■ Do not place diskettes near magnetic fields, such as on top of a monitor or television set or near a cellular phone. An easily overlooked source of magnetism is paper clips and their magnetic holders.

■ Keep diskettes away from cigarette smoke.

■ Avoid touching the exposed surface of the magnetic material.

■ Never force the diskette into the slot on the computer.

■ Avoid spilling drinks, glue, correction fluid, and other liquids on their surface.

Computer Software

Software programs contain instructions that enable computers to function. Hardware components cannot perform a single operation without the direction of software. An **application program** is a type of software that performs a specialized task such as patient billing, performing diagnostics, or word processing. Some software provides information, such as entire medical dictionaries that can be loaded onto the computer. Software may be purchased in off-the-shelf formats, useful for health care applications, such as the following:

■ Microsoft Word and WordPerfect: Word processing programs

■ Excel: Spreadsheet program

■ Medi-Soft and Medical Manager: Integrated medical office management programs

■ Tabers Cyclopedic Medical Dictionary

Compact discs (CDs), the same type used for recording music, store computer data. They can hold much more content than diskettes. For this reason, they are becoming the standard method for selling application software. For example, a word processing program that previously required fourteen diskettes to install, is now available on one compact disc that also includes five other complete programs! Entire medical dictionaries and encyclopedias are available on a single CD.

USING COMPUTERS EFFECTIVELY

Developing good work habits when using computers will help increase their effectiveness as useful work tools.

■ Verify the accuracy of all data entered: When working on a large system, incorrect entries may affect the work of others. Health care work demands accuracy to ensure high-quality patient care as well as compliance with regulatory agencies.

■ Always back up work: Save work to the hard drive periodically. The computer workspace, called **RAM**, stores data only while the computer is on. If power is interrupted, any work not saved will be lost. Many software programs allow you to save work automatically at regular intervals. When a task or work session is completed, save all files on a diskette or other storage medium. Computers can break down, and emergencies can occur.

■ Stay legal: It is against copyright law to install software that has been installed on another computer. Purchase and register needed programs. **Site licenses**, giving permission to install software on more than one computer, can be purchased for programs that will be loaded on more than one computer at a facility. Never bring personal software to load onto the workplace computer.

■ Keep up with advancements: Software is continually updated with new versions that offer additional features. Many updates are available at reduced prices for owners of previous editions. New Internet sites, offering an increasing number of products and services, appear daily.

■ Don't panic: Computers are a relatively new technology, and the complexity of today's software results in occasional glitches. It is almost impossible to damage computer equipment through normal use. If the computer does not understand a command, an error message will appear on the screen. The message "Fatal Error" may sound rather serious, but the worst thing that can usually happen is that work performed since it was last saved, either by the user or automatically by the program, is lost and must be redone. As discussed above, this can be avoided by regularly saving work.

- Avoid injury: Prolonged use and improper positioning can result in physical injuries. See Chapter 9 for information about reducing the risk of workplace injuries related to computer use.

COMPUTER SECURITY

The very characteristics that make computers useful in health care can also be a cause for concern. For example, the increased accessibility to patient records also increases the risk of breaching patient confidentiality. The need for the protection of privacy has been addressed by both the government and private organizations.

- Federal government: Several major laws, such as the Electronic Communication Privacy Act of 1986, provide protection against unauthorized access or interception of data communications.

- American Medical Association: Guidelines to protect patient privacy were established by the Council on Ethical and Judicial Affairs and included in the 1996–97 Code of Ethics. They include the following recommendations:

  - Only authorized personnel may enter confidential patient information.

  - Any person or organization with access to data must be disclosed to patient and physician.

  - Patients must approve any distribution of reports in which they might be identified from the data.

- American Health Information Management Association: Guidelines have been created to protect the security of medical records.

There are simple precautions the health care worker can take to help ensure computer security. If assigned a password to gain access to a computer system, never give it to anyone else, even a coworker. Unauthorized users can destroy or falsify data, add hours to their payroll records, or illegally transfer funds. Entries can often be tracked to the password used. The following simple practices will increase computer security:

- If passwords are chosen rather than assigned, do not use something obvious, such as a nickname.

- Clear monitor screens containing private information before leaving the work area.

- Do not allow patients or other unauthorized persons to wander into the area where data entry is taking place.

- Shred discarded printouts before throwing them in the trash.

Viruses are a threat to computers. Viruses are programs that contain instructions to perform destructive operations, such as scrambling and erasing files and preventing the computer from operating normally. Viruses can get into the hard drive from "infected" diskettes and files that are **downloaded** (transferred onto the computer) from the Internet. It is not always obvious that a virus is present because the instructions may have been programmed to perform at a future date. Business, as well as home-based computers are susceptible to viruses. Entire organizations have been literally shut down by viruses coming through the Internet when employees opened e-mail messages.

The following practices will help prevent viruses from infecting workplace computers:

- Do not open e-mail messages or download files from unknown parties.

- Do not use your work e-mail address for personal correspondence.

- Never bring diskettes from home.

- Do not use diskettes from any outside source, such as friends or acquaintances.

- Use purchased software to load application programs, not copies secured from friends or other outside sources.

- Use antivirus software and keep it updated to protect against new viruses that are continually being created.

MAINTAINING THE HUMAN TOUCH

Computers are one of the factors that have led many patients to feel that health care is becoming depersonalized. They complain that they feel like a number in a vast system over which they have little control. This may result in feelings of intimidation and annoyance.

The health care worker should strive to provide a personal interface between patients and machines. Prevent the computer from becoming a barrier. Those responsible for inputting patient data should extend a friendly greeting before beginning the data entry process. Look up and make eye contact periodically.

If it is not obvious to the patient, explain what information you are entering and why. Make appropriate comments to convey a sense of caring to the patient. Communicate verbally and nonverbally that the patient is more important than the machine.

LEARNING MORE ABOUT COMPUTERS

Learning more about the capabilities and operation of computers can increase the efficiency and job satisfaction of the health care worker. Opportunities for promotion may be increased. The many ways to increase computer knowledge and skills include the following:

- Take classes.
- Read the manuals that come with hardware and software.
- Work through tutorials and help menus included with software programs.
- Explore the various functions of software programs.
- Read some of the many books that are available for all levels of users.

Thinking it Through

Stacey Petersen is the admitting clerk at a large urban hospital. The patients served come from a wide variety of cultural and economic backgrounds. Much of Stacey's work involves collecting and entering patient data into the hospital's computer system. While many patients are comfortable with this procedure, some find it intimidating or are uneasy about "just what is being put into the computer." Of particular concern to Stacey are elderly patients from cultures in which health care is very personalized and where practitioners are well known to the patient.

1. What can Stacey do to help these patients feel more at ease?
2. How can a lack of understanding on the part of patients about the health care system affect the way they deal with health problems?

Identifying effective ways to learn about computers will help you keep up with a rapidly advancing technology that will continue to change the nature of health care.

SUGGESTED LEARNING ACTIVITIES

1. Find out what types of computer classes are available at your school and in the community that are appropriate for your needs.
2. Explore the health-related Web sites in the Health category at www.yahoo.com. List the address and a brief description of each. (Add these to the Webliography started for Suggested Learning Activity # 4 in Chapter 14.)
3. Look for health-related mailing lists on the following Web sites:

   http://www.liszt.com

   http://www.tile.net/tile/listserv/index.html
4. Arrange a visit to a health care facility to learn about how computers are used for diagnosis, treatment, and administration.
5. Interview someone who is working in a field of interest to you. How are computers used in this field? How much work does this person perform using computers or computerized technology? What skills are considered essential to be successful in this occupation? Which will increase promotional opportunities? Write up a short report of your findings.

REVIEW QUESTIONS

1. Why is it essential for today's health care worker to be computer literate?
2. List at least three computer applications for health care in each of the following areas:
   a. Information management
   b. Creation of documents
   c. Numerical calculations
   d. Integration of operations
   e. Diagnostics
   f. Treatment

g. Patient monitoring

h. Research

i. Education

j. Communication

3. What is the difference between computer hardware and software?

4. What are five ways to properly handle and care for computer hardware?

5. What are the two primary means of storing computerized information?

6. What are five guidelines for caring for diskettes?

7. What are six guidelines for using computers effectively?

8. How can the health care worker help ensure the security of computerized records?

9. What are three ways the health care worker can learn more about using computers?

APPLICATION EXERCISES

1. Refer to The Case of the Therapist Who Wants to Use More Technology at the beginning of the chapter. Based on what you learned in the chapter, list ways that Carol can use computer technology in her practice.

2. The students in an Introduction to Health Care class have just completed their study of the application of computers in health care. The course was an overview and the students have been thinking about how they will use computer technology in their work. For each of the following students, suggest potential applications and skills they should acquire for on-the-job success.

a. Craig Kingman, paramedic

b. Otis Brownwell, radiologic technician

c. Christine Abbott, surgical technologist

d. Marta Singh, registered nurse

e. Jaime Bustamante, medical assistant

SUGGESTED READINGS AND RESOURCES

Burke, L. and Weill, B. (2000). *Information technology for the health professions.* Upper Saddle River, NJ: Brady/Prentice Hall Heath.

Griffen, A. D. (1998). *Directory of internet sources for health professionals.* Albany, NY: Delmar.

Leshin, C. (1998). *Student resource guide to the Internet: Student success online.* Upper Saddle River, NJ: Prentice Hall.

CHAPTER

DOCUMENTATION AND MEDICAL RECORDS

OBJECTIVES

Studying and applying the material in this chapter will help you to:

■ List and explain the purposes of medical documentation.

■ List the characteristics of good medical documentation.

■ Explain the proper method for correcting errors on medical records.

■ List the various sources of information that may be found in a medical record.

■ Describe three different formats used for progress notes.

■ Discuss the advantages and disadvantages of each progress note format.

KEY TERMS

assessment

charting

chief complaint

medical documentation

medical history

medical record

plan

progress notes

SOAP

The Case of

the Therapist Who Hates to Write

Joseph Lane, a respiratory therapist, enjoys working with patients and the technical aspects of his profession. But he has never enjoyed paperwork and dislikes writing documentation following the treatment he administers. His notes are hurriedly scribbled, and other health care workers find them difficult, if not impossible, to read. In this chapter the importance of accurate, complete, and legible documentation will be stressed. Inaccurate, incomplete, and illegible charting has consequences for patient care, jeopardizes regulatory compliance, and presents legal risks.

MEDICAL DOCUMENTATION

Medical documentation refers to notes and documents that health care workers add to the medical record. For example, patient statistics and information about care, results of tests performed, the patient's diagnosis written by a physician, treatments received, and medications given are the types of information that are commonly included in medical documentation.

A **medical record** refers to the collection of all documents that are filed together and form a complete chronological health history of a particular patient. A medical record is also frequently referred to as a medical chart, patient chart, or patient record. Recording observations and information about patients is known as **charting**.

Many health care workers are responsible for some aspect of charting. Tasks may include the following:

- Recording demographic information about new patients
- Interviewing patients and filling in the medical history form
- Recording vital signs (e.g., temperature, blood pressure)
- Noting comments made by the patient
- Making notes on the patient's record as dictated by the physician, dentist, or other professional
- Recording any procedures performed
- Transcribing notes or dictation from other professionals into the medical records

Purposes of Medical Documentation

Complete and accurate medical documentation is critical in providing consistent patient care. It is the lifeline of communication that supports the coordination of care. Information included in the medical record is a significant source of data on which other health care workers can base their approach to the patient.

In addition to ensuring good patient care, medical documentation serves other important purposes:

- Provides legal protection: Medical records are legal documents that are admissible as evidence in court. In the case of a malpractice lawsuit, for example, documentation provides proof of what has taken place with the patient. Only through written documentation can tests, procedures, and treatment be proven to have occurred. In the world of health care, "If it isn't documented, it isn't done."

- Helps ensure compliance with regulatory agencies: These include governmental bodies and accreditation organizations such as the Joint Commission on Accreditation of Healthcare Organizations (JCAHO). Participation in certain programs, such as Medicare, requires that specific documentation guidelines be strictly followed.

- Improves cost control: Proper documentation prevents repetition and the performance of unnecessary procedures. It also helps ensure that appropriate preventive measures, early intervention, and correct procedures are performed.

- Decreases denials from insurance companies: The need for care and proof that it is provided by appropriate personnel are supported by documentation.

Characteristics of Good Medical Documentation

- Complete: All requested information must be included. Each entry must include the date and signature of the appropriate health care personnel. Charting should be completed as soon as possible to prevent the omission of important information.

- Concise and factual: A lot of words are not better than a clear concise statement. Never use the chart to record guesses or opinions. State only what has been observed, done, or heard. If you are quoting a patient's statements, use quotation marks. For example, "I feel a sharp pain in my left leg every time I try to walk."

- Properly identified: The patient's name and identifying numbers should be visible on every page. It is critical that the record matches the patient so that correct entries are made.

- Legible: Notes that cannot be read are useless. They do not serve their purpose of providing continuity of care. Furthermore, they present a liability and cause for negative legal and regulatory outcomes.

- Use correct spelling, terminology, punctuation, and grammar: Poorly written documentation can be easily misinterpreted and gives the appearance of carelessness when the record is reviewed by others.

- Clearly and objectively expressed: Important details are correctly noted: temperature, size, amounts (fluids, drainage, medication, etc.) The words used are not subject to misinterpretation, such as "small," "a lot," and so on. Notes should be limited to what is observed. For example, write "ate 25% of the meal" rather than "ate poorly."

- Do not duplicate findings: Some facilities use graphic sheets on which the blood pressure, temperature, pulse, and respiratory rate are recorded. If so, it is not necessary to also repeat this information in the written record. With abnormal readings, it may be repeated in the written record along with the associated action taken or treatment given to correct the problem. The record would then also include a follow-up assessment of how the patient responded to the action or treatment.

- Use abbreviations only if they are approved and listed in the facility's policy: This will prevent confusion when the same abbreviation is used with different meanings. For example, does "pt" stand for patient, protime, physical therapy, or part-time?

[Thinking it Through]

Juanita is an RN who works for a home health agency. She enjoys the work, because she really cares about each of her patients and likes getting to know them as individuals. She tries to spend a little extra time on each home visit, chatting with them about their families, interests, pets, and so on. With more patients being released to their homes rather than being hospitalized, she has a heavy case load. Juanita finds that sometimes she doesn't have time to complete all her charting until late in the evening. Sometimes she doesn't get to it until the following morning. She tries to complete it while eating breakfast before leaving for another day of rounds.

1. Discuss the possible consequences of Juanita's current work habits in terms of legal compliance and reimbursement.

2. Discuss any changes you would recommend.

current date & times		Date & time of out of sequence note
10/10/01	1530	*Late entry (10/10/01 - 1230)*
		Skin appears slightly
		reddened and moist
		to the touch. Z. Hera RN

Figure 19–1 Sample of a late entry in charting.

■ Time and date of all entries: Accurate and chronological charting presents a picture of how the patient appears over time. If charting is not done in a timely manner, another health care worker may record an event with a time that occurred after what you were to chart. The only option then is to write "late entry" and then chart, but this out-of-sequence information can still create confusion for others. See Figure 19–1.

■ Signed by the proper person: Never sign for someone else or have anyone sign charting you have done. Recording false information is a serious offense and should not be done under any circumstances.

■ Completed without leaving empty lines: All charting that begins after the previous signature and runs to the next signature belongs to the latter entry. If an empty space or line is left above the entry and signature of the health care worker, it is possible for someone else to chart information that now becomes part of the other health care worker's entry. See Figure 19–2.

■ Never chart in advance of giving the medication or performing a procedure: Chart only after the event has occurred, never before, in anticipation of doing it. For example, if a nurse charts that medications were given and

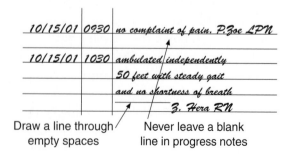

10/15/01	0930	*no complaint of pain. P.Zoe LPN*
10/15/01	1030	*ambulated independently*
		50 feet with steady gait
		and no shortness of breath
		Z. Hera RN

Draw a line through / empty spaces   Never leave a blank line in progress notes

Figure 19–2 Never leave empty lines in charting.

then is suddenly called away, the other health care workers will assume that the medications were given, and the patient will not receive the proper medications they need for treatment.

■ Written with black or blue ink (or as specified by the facility): Pencil is *never* acceptable.

Making Corrections on Medical Documentation

Medical records cannot be corrected in a way that covers up what was originally written. To do so can give the appearance that the records have been illegally altered and negates their value as legal records. Never use white out, erase, or use correction tape over errors. Observe the following practices:

1. Draw a single line through the error. The original entry must still be legible.

2. Write in the correct information where there is the most space: above, below, or following the original entry.

3. Note the error as required by your facility. For example, "M.E." may be used for "mistaken entry;" "correction" or "corr" may be acceptable. Be sure to learn the specific requirements for notations, and never create your own or assume that the facility will use the ones presented in textbooks. Regulatory agencies differ in the terms accepted, and it is important to carefully follow their guidelines.

4. Date and initial the correction.

5. If an error is made while typing or word processing a document, you may correct it as you work. If it is discovered later, correct it by hand following steps 1–4 above.

See Figure 19–3.

Contents of the Medical Record

The medical record will be organized according to facility policy, and the health care worker is expected to maintain the integrity of the record by following all policies and procedures. Many physician offices

11/1/01	1400	*Darvocette N*~~*Percocette*~~ *† given for complaints*
		error 11/1/01 zh
		of RU2 pain rated as 6 on
		a scale of 0 - 10. Z. Hera RN

Figure 19–3 Sample of how to make a correction in charting.

will have a continuous chronological record format, but in large health care facilities there may be a *source-oriented* approach. This approach divides the record into different sections separated by tabs for each health care specialty. This has the advantage of making it easy to find specific information related to a specialty, but has the disadvantage of increasing the difficulty of seeing the overall view of the patient because many sections need to be referred to for the complete picture. In a source-oriented charting format, the chart may be separated into the following sections:

- History and Physicals (H&P) and Consultations: Typed or handwritten reports on the initial finding of all physicians seeing the patient. The primary physician will do a complete **medical history**, which includes a personal, familial (medical problems of relatives that may show a family tendency for problems), and social history (if and how much patient smokes, drinks alcohol, or takes illegal drugs) of the patient. The personal history will include the patient's past medical problems and surgeries, allergies, current problems, assessment of each body system (see Chapter 20), and medications. The suspected diagnosis and plan for further assessment and treatments are also included. Consultations occur when the primary physician asks another physician to see the patient for further evaluation of a specific problem. Some facilities have transcription services in which the physician dictates the detailed findings and then the transcriptionist types from the taped message. This is then placed in the chart for the physician to review and sign.

- Physician's Orders: Written record of all orders for medications and treatments prescribed for the patient

- Diagnostic Tests: Any report that includes findings obtained in an attempt to diagnose or monitor the progress of patient. For example, the results of laboratory tests, x-rays, and EKGs

- Admissions: Completed forms and consents that deal with the admission process

- Surgical Procedures: Consents for and reports related to any surgical procedures performed

- Graphics: A graphed format for blood pressure, temperature, pulse, and respiratory rate. May also have spaces for height and weight.

- Flow Sheets: Forms for specialty needs such as monitoring blood sugar levels or measurements of a wound as it heals. Many specialty

fields create forms specific to their needs (Figure 19–4).

- Medication Record: Includes all medications administered by health care workers at the facility

- **Progress Notes**: Written chronological statements about a patient's care. For example, each time a physician sees a patient he or she will make an additional note to update findings and plan for the care of the patient. Therapists (e.g., physical, occupational, and speech therapists) and other services (i.e., social workers, chaplain services) will note what was done and their assessment of results. Nurses will record what treatments they perform, the patient's response, and any abnormal assessments, and plans for intervention. In large facilities, the physician, therapists, and nurses may have different sections of the chart in which to record their documentation.

When filing forms, reviewing charts, or charting, always verify that the correct form is in the chart by checking that the patient's name is on each document. An incorrectly filed form can lead to misunderstandings and errors. When filing or adding additional blank forms to the chart, always place them in the correct section in chronological order. The forms within each section will be chronological. The most current is usually on top, depending on facility policy.

Thinking it Through

Sally Jones is an administrative medical assistant for Dr. Yin, an orthopedist in a single-physician office. Sally takes great pride in the appearance of all her work, particularly patient records. She neatly corrects any mistakes made with white correction fluid and is pleased at how tidy the files are. Sally is shocked when Dr. Yin is sued by a patient and loses the case. Dr. Yin's attorney reports that the patient's medical records were largely at fault for the loss of the case.

1. What do you think happened?

2. How might Sally's handling of patient records have contributed to the loss?

3. What recommendations would you make to avoid this type of problem in the future?

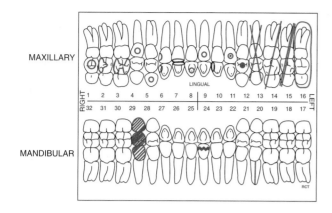

MAXILLARY

LINGUAL

RIGHT 1 2 3 4 5 6 7 8 | 9 10 11 12 13 14 15 16 LEFT
32 31 30 29 28 27 26 25 | 24 23 22 21 20 19 18 17

MANDIBULAR

RCT

Figure 19–4 A sample dental form that uses symbols to record conditions as they occur over time with an individual patient.

Sometimes a patient's chart becomes too thick, and another file on the patient is started. This is referred to as "thinning a chart." A note is then made in the new chart that an older file exists for this patient. When requesting charts, always make sure that you have all the charts on the patient for review.

The security of records is the responsibility of each health care worker. Never leave charts or the content of charts lying around for unauthorized individuals to see. There are specific rules and regulations on who can be given copies of the chart and what procedure must be followed to request copies. Ask your supervisor for these guidelines and follow them without exception.

Progress Notes

The progress notes make up the written record of every aspect of a patient's relationship with the health care providers. They are the primary tool used to record, communicate, and coordinate the care given to the patient. Keeping careful documentation is a critical skill for the health care worker. Before charting, it is important for the health care worker to take a moment and organize his or her thoughts. For example, health care workers can ask themselves what they observed while working with a patient, what has been done for the patient, and what the patient's response was to any interventions. It is important to always address the primary problem that required the assistance of health care services.

There are a number of ways to organize progress notes. It is the responsibility of health care workers to learn the formats used at the facilities in which they work. Several examples of common approaches are presented below.

Problem-Oriented Charting

Problem-oriented medical records are organized around the patient's health problems. After the initial assessment is completed, a list of problems and related plan of care are identified, and then all subsequent charting refers back to this problem list. If new problems develop, they are added to the list and dated. If a problem is treated and no longer exists, it is marked as resolved and dated. The advantage of this approach is that all health care workers focus their charting on the same problems. The disadvantages in this approach are keeping the problem list up to date and that the patient may be seen more as problems to be resolved, than as an individual human being.

The format for charting on each problem is known as **SOAP**. These letters stand for the following components of the documentation:

1. Subjective: Subjective information is that which is sensed and reported by the patient. Known collectively as symptoms, they describe how the patient feels as a result of a disease or injury. It is best to record the patient's own words as closely as possible. Use quotation marks when noting exact words. The **chief complaint** is the reason the patient is seeking medical care and is included in the subjective section of the record. Significant patient behavior, such as missed appointments, failure to follow directions, and statements about discontent with treatments, should also be included in this section.

2. Objective: Objective information includes the observations of health care personnel. These include measurements, such as temperature and blood pressure; lab test results; description of a wound; color, temperature, and moisture of skin; and how a patient walks (gait). These observations are known as signs.

3. Assessment: The **assessment** is the health care professional's impression of what is wrong with the patient, based on the signs and symptoms.

4. Plan: The **plan** documents the procedures, treatments, and patient instructions that make up the patient care. See Figure 19–5.

A variation of the SOAP is SOAPIE. The S, O, and A have the same meanings as described above. The P and the additional letters stand for the following:

1. Plan: What is planned for tests and treatment

2. Interventions: What interventions are actually carried out

3. Evaluation: Evaluation of the interventions. What were the results? Was the treatment effective?

Problem list

Date Opened	No.	Problem	Identified By	Date Resolved
1/15/01	#1	Angina related to coronary artery disease	B. Meed M.D.	
1/17/01	#2	Impaired mobility due to weakness of right lower extremity secondary to old stroke (1998)	Z. Hera RN	

Plan of Care

Date	Problem
1/15/01	#1 Angina related to coronary artery disease
	GOAL: Prior to discharge patient will be able to ambulate 300 feet with no angina
	PLAN: gradually increase walking distance & pace after starting on new medication regime

Progress Note

2/5/01	1700	Problem #1
		S: states "I had no pain in my chest when I walked. Twice around the floor."
		O: skin cool & dry. B/P 120/76 p. 84
		A: increasing walking distance with no angina
		P: continue to increase walking distance as long as stays angina free.
		Z. Hera RN

Figure 19–5 Sample of problem-oriented charting.

11/15/01	1800	Alert and oriented x3. No complaints of pain. Vital signs normal. Ate 100% of dinner. ———— Z. Hera RN

Figure 19–6 Sample of a narrative progress note.

clear lung sounds are normal and would not be charted. Rales is the exception to normal

12/5/01	2200	Rales noted in both lung bases. Will call Dr. Johnson to notify of change in condition ———— Z. Hera RN

Figure 19–7 Sample of a charting by exception progress note.

Narrative Charting

Narrative charting includes detailed written notes on all aspects of care. It includes routine care, normal and abnormal findings, and any other information related to the patient's plan of care. The advantage to this approach is that the health care worker can use his or her own approach to describing the patient and the care given. The disadvantage is that it is often time-consuming and results in an extensive written record that is difficult to read through to find specific information. See Figure 19–6.

Charting by Exception (CBE)

Charting by exception is an abbreviated format. Only abnormal findings are noted. This requires a well-defined understanding of the normal findings that are used for a comparison. If no abnormal findings are found then no written notes are required. The advantage in this approach is that it saves time and that the problems are easily identified by reviewing the notes. The disadvantage is that it is problem-oriented, so the preventative or wellness aspects of care are not included. See Figure 19–7.

SUGGESTED LEARNING ACTIVITIES

1. If you are currently working in a health care facility, review the written documents and evaluate the documentation. Why are the examples good or poor? Can you get a real picture of that patient by reading the chart?

2. Write samples using the three formats of progress notes presented and then check them against the characteristics of good documentation. If you make an error, remember to make the corrections according to accepted guidelines.

3. Work with another student to identify a specific situation that may occur in your health care specialty area. Then both write documentation, and compare the results.

REVIEW QUESTIONS

1. What are five major purposes of medical documentation?

2. What are five characteristics of good medical documentation?

3. How should errors be corrected on medical records?

4. What information is typically found in a medical record?

5. What are three different formats used for progress notes?

6. What are the advantages and disadvantages of each progress note format?

APPLICATION EXERCISES

1. Refer back to The Case of the Therapist Who Hates to Write.

   a. What are the possible consequences of the therapist's approach to charting?

   b. What characteristics of good charting is he not following?

2. Ms. Henrietta Jenkins, a nursing assistant at an ambulatory clinic is helping Mr. Wilkins off of the examining table. Mr. Wilkins suddenly feels faint, and his legs give out from under him and he falls to the floor. Ms. Jenkins notes that the patient never lost consciousness, but he is confused and asks where he is. She notes a 2 cm by 3 cm red mark on his forehead. His vital signs are B/P 100/60 T 98.6 P 92 R 20 (B/P-Blood pressure, T-Temperature, P-Pulse, R-Respirations). The physician examines the patient, finds no other injuries, and the patient is no longer confused. Another set of vital signs are taken B/P 124/80 P 78 R 18. Mr. Wilkins states he is feeling fine and leaves without further incident.

   a. What would be documented using problem-oriented charting?

   b. What would be documented using narrative charting?

   c. What would be documented using charting by exception?

   d. What additional information, if any, would be needed to complete the progress notes using each of the three charting formats.

UNIT

HEALTH CARE SKILLS

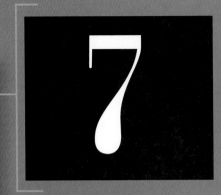

CHAPTER

PHYSICAL ASSESSMENT

OBJECTIVES

Studying and applying the material in this chapter will help you to:

■ State the purpose of a History and Physical and indicate what data the physician will obtain.

■ Discuss variances from the norm for each of the body systems.

■ Explain how to do a pain scale assessment.

■ Define what is included in assessment of the Activities of Daily Living (ADLs).

■ Correctly take the vital signs (temperature, pulse, respirations, and blood pressure).

■ Describe how the presence of an apical-radial deficit is determined and what it means.

■ Measure the height and weight of a patient.

KEY TERMS

afebrile

apnea

bradycardia

bradypnea

Cheyne-Stokes

dyspnea

eupnea

exhalation

hypertension

hypotension

inhalation

febrile

orthopnea

orthostatic (postural) hypotension

pulse deficit

pulse points

respiration

stethoscope

sphygmomanometer

tachycardia

tachypnea

vital signs

The Case of

the Missed Assessment

Mrs. Becker, age 83, arrives on time as usual for her appointment with Dr. Myers. Carrie Winsor, medical assistant, notes that Mrs. Becker seems unsteady as she walks across the room. When asked if she is all right, Mrs. Becker's answer is slightly garbled, but she states, "I must just be getting old." When Mrs. Becker speaks, Carrie notes a sweet, fruity smell that she thinks must be mouthwash. Carrie thinks Mrs. Becker seems depressed, but then thinks that she would be too if she had all the physical problems the patient has had with her diabetes, especially now that she has recently been diagnosed with renal failure and has started on dialysis. Dr. Myers is running behind with his appointments, and Carrie knows that it will be at least another 30 minutes and informs Mrs. Becker. Carrie continues with her other tasks, until she hears a sudden sound and finds Mrs. Becker on the floor and unconscious. This chapter will discuss how to assess patients and how important it is for the health care worker to observe and promptly report abnormal findings to his or her supervisor so early detection and treatment can be initiated.

GENERAL ASSESSMENT

The physician (or other primary care provider) takes a history and performs a physical on patients when they are seen for the first time or when they are admitted to the hospital. This is called the History and Physical, commonly referred to as the H&P. As discussed in the previous chapter, the physician then either writes the findings in the patient's chart or dictates them for someone else to type up and place in the chart. When the typed information is placed in the chart, the physician must review it for accuracy, and then sign the document.

An accurate and thorough H&P is very important, because it is the data on which the physician bases the initial diagnosis and treatment. The H&P consists of the following information:

- Date: This documents the day on which the H&P is actually done.
- Demographic data: Age, sex, race, place of birth, marital status, occupation, and religion
- Source of referral: Frequently one physician will refer a patient to another because of that individual's expertise in a specific area; if so, it will be stated as such.

- Chief complaint(s): This is the primary problem from the patient's view; why they are seeking medical care.
- History of present illness: This includes when the problem first started; how frequently it occurs; how long it lasts; description, location, and severity of symptoms; if they are aggravated by any specific activities; if anything relieves the problem; and if any treatments have been tried and their effect on the symptoms.
- Past history: This includes the general state of the patient's health and any previous physical or psychological illnesses, accidents, injuries, or surgeries, and hospitalizations.
- Current health status: List of allergies and immunizations; normal activity level and diet; current medications (prescription and over the counter); if tobacco, alcohol, or illegal drugs are used; if any environmental or safety hazards are present; and if there are any sleep pattern disturbances.
- Family history of illness: The age and health or cause of death of parents, siblings, spouse, and children. The physician will also ask if

any other family members have or are experiencing similar symptoms. The family history of specific diseases or conditions will be included (e.g., diabetes, heart disease, high blood pressure, cancer).

- Psychosocial history: Includes the home situation and support structure (family and friends) and any significant information that may affect the care of the patient.

- Review of all systems: Includes the height, weight, vital signs, and a review of each body system. When a complete physical assessment is done, it is frequently referred to as a head-to-toe assessment, which indicates all systems are being evaluated. It can also indicate a method that some health care workers use to organize their assessment. After assessing orientation, the process would include an examination in the following order:

  1. Head
  2. Neck
  3. Upper extremities
  4. Chest: respiratory and cardiac systems
  5. Abdomen: digestive, urinary, and reproductive systems
  6. Lower extremities

The musculoskeletal, integumentary, nervous, endocrine, vascular, and lymphatic systems are relevant to the entire body and are assessed as one moves along the body.

The information obtained during the H&P is considered the *baseline*. The baseline information is important to determine how the patient is progressing in relationship to how they were at a particular point in time. It is important for the health care worker to review the H&P because this information will increase the understanding of the patient's condition.

Noting Variances from Normal

A critical function of the health care worker is to be able to discriminate between normal and abnormal conditions and situations. Learning to observe patients, their symptoms, and their actions, and asking appropriate questions provide vital information that can be used by other health care workers and the physician in the care of the patient.

The observational skills needed are based on a thorough understanding of what is normal anatomy and physiology. Once the meaning of "normal" is understood, it is an easy step to identify abnormal

situations. A health care worker who observes an abnormal condition should immediately report the finding to his or her supervisor. Remember though that some patients begin with problems noted in the H&P. In this case, it is more valuable to compare a change in condition to this baseline.

Any change in a patient's condition may indicate a worsening of the condition, an improvement, a new problem developing, or a need for a change in treatment. The health care workers who interact with and observe a patient over a period of time may provide valuable information that the physician may not detect during relatively brief visits with the patient. It is for this reason that strong assessment skills are needed by all health care workers whose responsibilities include interaction with patients.

General Survey

A problem with dividing the body into systems for the purpose of study is that health care workers sometimes forget to look at the patient as a whole. To prevent this from happening, the health care worker should develop the habit of first performing a general survey of the patient. This means looking at and listening to the patient to secure an overall impression of presentation. How do they appear? What is the general impression you get from the patient? Another advantage of this approach is that it provides information on what area to focus on if time is limited. When doing a general survey on patients, the health care worker should look for answers to the following questions:

- Does the patient look strong or weak? Acutely or chronically ill?

- What is the posture (e.g., stooped, limping, any paralysis, walking normally)?

- Are there any signs of distress (e.g., difficulty breathing, face wincing in pain, sweating or trembling, holding part of body [hand over area or rubbing area on body may indicate pain])?

- Is body in proportion and normal size (e.g., very thin or obese, tall or short)?

- What is the color of the skin (e.g., pale, flushed [reddish], jaundice [yellow], or cyanotic [gray, dusty, or blue]? In noncaucasian patients, the nailbeds, whites of eye, and mucous membranes should be examined for color changes.

- Any odors noted from body or breath? For example, is there a sweet or fruity smell to the breath (may be untreated diabetic or severe restriction of food intake)? Alcohol?

- What is the character of speech (e.g., hesitant, slurred, fast, slow, or normal)?

- What are the vital signs (temperature, pulse, respirations, and blood pressure, to be discussed later in chapter)? During these procedures, you will be touching the patient's skin. This provides the opportunity to assess the skin for temperature changes and moisture (warm, cold, dry, moist); shaking the patient's hand upon greeting also provides an opportunity to assess the skin temperature and moisture.

- What is the height and weight? Has there been a recent gain or loss?

- What is the level of consciousness? When patients have a diminished level of consciousness, it is necessary to assess the extent of the problem, so comparisons can be made that indicate whether the patient is getting better or worse. Areas to assess are:

  - What is their best verbal response: are they oriented to time (can they tell you what day it is and what time), place (can they tell you where they are), and person (can they state their name)? Are they confused, inappropriate, or incomprehensible, or do they make no response?

  - If there is no verbal response, note whether the eyes open spontaneously, or perhaps only to speech or to pain, or if there is no response.

  - What is their best motor response–do they obey commands, move only in response to pain, or is there is no response?

Using appropriate communication skills is necessary when performing an assessment. How we communicate verbally and nonverbally often determines the quality of the response we get when interviewing patients. Refer back to Chapter 16 to review these special communication skills.

Psychosocial Assessment

When performing a general survey, both the physical and psychological aspects of the patient need to be considered. When incorporating a psychosocial assessment of patients, along with a general survey, the following questions can guide the health care worker:

- Emotional status: What are the emotional responses? For example, is the patient anxious, angry, depressed, indifferent? Are the facial expressions appropriate to what is being discussed?

- Mental status: Is the patient's behavior appropriate for his or her age? What is the attention span? Does the patient ask appropriate questions? Can the patient recall information and incorporate new information?

- Appearance: Is the patient dressed appropriately for the weather? Well groomed? Does the patient have good personal hygiene? (This may give clues on emotional status or ability to care for self.)

Physical Assessment

Skills frequently used during physical assessment are inspection, palpation, percussion, and auscultation.

- Inspection: Using the senses of vision, hearing, and smell for observation of patient condition

- Auscultation: Listening to sounds inside the body with the aid of a stethoscope (e.g., lungs, heart, and bowel sounds)

- Palpation: Using the hands and fingers on the exterior of the body to detect evidence of abnormalities in the various internal body organs

- Percussion: Using the fingertips to lightly tap on the exterior of the body to determine position, size, and consistency of underlying structures

These assessment skills will be briefly introduced in the following sections, as they relate to each of the systems presented in Chapter 7. Palpation and percussion of the body will not be covered, as these are more advanced skills. As health care students progress through their educational programs, additional and/or more advanced skills will be introduced that are specific to their specialties. Examples of advanced skills will be listed, but not expanded on, because they are beyond the scope of this text.

Musculoskeletal

- Is there any discomfort with movement (pain, muscle spasms, stiffness)?

- Is the gait (manner of walking) normal or altered? Observe the posture.

- Assess muscle strength–can the patient turn in bed without assistance; does the patient complain of weakness; is walking done with or without assistance?

- Examples of advanced skills are inspection of joints for any swelling or deformity, assessment of the range of motion (ROM) of joints in which discomfort is experienced, and assessment of the amount of counterresistance (pulling against an examiner's pull) to a force that a patient can maintain.

Integumentary

- Status of skin: color and temperature (warm or cold), hair distribution, dry or moist
- Any cuts, scrapes, swelling, rashes, incisions, or bruises on the skin

Circulatory

- What are the vital signs?
- What is the weight? Has there been a recent unexplained gain or loss of weight?
- Is there any pain in the extremities? Where does pain occur; how is pain relieved (resting, elevation, or placing extremity in dependent position); does it occur at night; how far can patient walk before pain occurs (claudication distance)?
- Palpate peripheral pulses for quality and strength (pulse points presented later in this chapter).
- Inspect extremities for swelling.
- Assess capillary refill–pinch the patient's fingertip and let go, then watch how long it takes for the nail bed to become pink again. The nailbeds of patients with poor circulation to the extremities will take longer to return to a pink color. Use fingers/toes if nailbeds are discolored or too thick to detect color changes.
- Inspect for neck vein distention–with the patient in erect or sitting position, inspect the neck for distention of jugular veins; normally there is no distention of neck veins when in erect position.
- Assess for activity intolerance–fatigue, palpitations (pounding felt in heart), or syncope (fainting) when engaging in any activities of daily living.

Examples of advanced skills include: palpating the calf area for tenderness, using dorsiflexion (movement of the foot backward at the ankle) to check for pain in the calf, an indication of possible clots in the leg; auscultating breath and heart sounds, using a Doppler probe if pulses are nonpalpable.

Respiratory

- What are the respiratory rate and rhythm?
- What color is the skin and mucous membranes?
- Is there obvious difficulty with breathing? Is there any chest pain when breathing?
- Is there a cough? Productive (coughing up mucus) or nonproductive? If productive, what is the color (clear, white, yellow, green, red) and consistency (thin, thick, frothy) of the mucus?
- If the patient is experiencing difficulty breathing, when does this occur? Is there **dyspnea** (difficulty breathing) on exertion? Does the patient use accessory muscles to assist breathing (lifting shoulders on inspiration, retraction of abdominal muscles with respiration, flaring of nostrils)?
- Assess for cyanosis: Do the skin or nailbeds appear cyanotic? The skin of a Caucasian patient who is receiving adequate oxygen is pink; in dark-skinned patients, a problem with oxygenation is noted by looking at the nailbeds, lips, and mucous membranes of the mouth.
- Does the patient have **orthopnea** (does the patient breath easier in a sitting or standing position)?

Examples of advanced skills are auscultation and percussion of lungs, determining if the chest expansion is symmetrical or asymmetrical, and determining which accessory muscles are used for breathing.

Digestive

- What is size and contour of abdomen? Is the abdomen round, flat, or distended? Soft or hard?
- Has there been a change in bowel pattern, color, or consistency of stools?
- When was the last bowel movement?
- Is there any abdominal discomfort? How is it relieved? What aggravates it?
- Have there been any sudden changes in weight and appetite?

Examples of advanced skills are auscultation of bowel sounds in all four quadrants and palpating for tenderness and masses.

Urinary

- What is the appearance of the urine (clear or cloudy, yellow or some other color)?
- Is there any burning when the patient urinates? Any urgency (sudden, strong desire to urinate), hesitancy (feel the urge to urinate, but have difficulty getting started), or frequency (urinate more often than normal)?
- Does the patient have nocturia (get up during the night to urinate)? If so, how often?

- Is the patient ever incontinent (inability to retain urine)? If so, does it occur all the time or only when coughing, laughing, or sneezing?
- Examples of advanced skills are palpation and percussion of the bladder.

Eyes and Ears

Eye:

- Are there any complaints of discomfort in the eye (pain, foreign body sensation, itching or irritation, fatigue)?
- Are there any complaints of visual disturbances–floaters or spots, loss of vision, tunnel vision (loss of peripheral vision), flashes of light, halos around lights, blurred vision, diplopia (double vision), curtain or veil over visual field, difficulty with color discrimination, photophobia (hypersensitivity to light)?
- Is there redness, swelling, drainage, tearing, squinting when attempting to read printed material, crusting of eyelashes?

Examples of advanced skills include using an ophthalmoscope to examine the internal structures of the eye and assessing the movement of eyeballs and eyelids and the reaction of pupils to light.

Ear:

- Is there any drainage from the ear?
- What is patient experiencing (e.g., feeling of fullness; unusual sounds, such as popping or cracking sounds when yawning or swallowing; heart beating in ear; tinnitus [ringing in the ears])? If a child is having discomfort in the ear, they are most likely to demonstrate it by rubbing the ear and crying.
- Does the patient use a hearing aid?
- Hearing acuity: Is there difficulty hearing in one ear or both? Does patient show behaviors consistent with diminished hearing, such as turning head and leaning closer when spoken to or frequently asking for statement to be repeated? Many patients compensate for a hearing loss by reading the lips of the speaker. To prevent this from disguising hearing loss, the health care worker can speak while standing behind the patient or when the patient's back is turned.

Examples of advanced skills include using an otoscope to look inside the ear canal to examine the internal structures, and conducting various hearing tests.

Nervous

- Is there any numbness or tingling?
- Many types of abnormal assessment data already discussed may indicate a neurological problem, such as changes in skin temperature or color, impairment of mobility, and problems with emotional or mental status.

Examples of advanced skills are testing the reflexes and conducting a neurological exam to determine the strength and movement of extremities, and cranial nerve testing. Another frequently used assessment technique is to test the response of the pupil to light. Normally, the pupils are equal in size and shape, and constrict symmetrically when exposed to a light source. Variances from this normal response may indicate neurological damage.

Endocrine

The endocrine system has such wide-ranging effects on the body that no additional questions will be listed here. The most common problems with the endocrine system (i.e., diabetes and thyroid disorders) are usually identified in the assessment of the other systems.

Female Reproductive

- Does patient menstruate? If so, how often, how long, and are there any problems related to this? When did menses begin?
- Any pain, discharge, itching, or discomfort with the vagina or genitalia? Any lumps in the breasts or discharge from the nipples?
- Any surgeries? For example, hysterectomy (removal of uterus), oophorectomy (removal of ovary), or mastectomy (removal of breast).

Male Reproductive

- Any discharge from or sores noted on the penis?

Pain Assessment

Pain is subjective information, and there is no test to confirm it in an objective manner. The best approach is to use a pain assessment scale. Most facilities use this approach and it helps to make the patient's assessment easier to compare. The patient is asked to rate his or her pain on a scale of 0–10. Zero is no pain, and 10 is the worst pain they can imagine. Each time a pain assessment is done, the same scale is used. For example, if a patient reports pain to be seven and then, after pain medication, they report it dropped to two, this is a good indication of the effectiveness of the medication.

But if it only dropped to a five or six, this would indicate that the pain medication regime needs to be reevaluated. It is also important to note any nonverbal cues that may indicate pain, such as limping, favoring an area, moaning, restlessness, and wincing.

ADL Assessment

Activities of daily living (ADLs) are the actions done on a regular basis to meet physical needs. These include bathing, eating, toileting, shopping, doing laundry, cleaning the house, paying bills, dressing, turning in bed, getting out of bed, and ambulating (walking). Conditions that effect the ability to perform ADLs may be temporary or permanent. For example, patients recovering from a recent surgery may temporarily not be strong enough to care for themselves, but a patient with a major and permanent spinal cord injury will never regain full function.

There are many diseases and conditions that diminish the patient's ability to perform these activities. When a patient is unable to perform his or her basic ADLs, then help must be arranged. Family and friends are often able to assist, but if this is not possible, there are a number of agencies and facilities that will need to be evaluated to determine the best service for specific patient needs. This type of assessment is often performed by specially trained personnel (e.g., social workers, case managers, discharge planners) who are familiar with the various services available in the community. Chapter 2 presents information on some of the health care delivery systems available to assist patients to meet their health care needs.

VITAL SIGNS

The term **vital signs** refers to taking a patient's temperature, pulse, respiratory rate, and blood pressure. Taking the vital signs provides important information on the status of the patient. The temperature measures how much heat is in the body, and its elevation may indicate that an infection or other disease process is present. The pulse measures how fast the heart is beating. The respiratory rate measures how fast the patient is breathing. The blood pressure indicates how hard the heart is working to distribute blood to all parts of the body. When referring to the temperature, pulse, and respiratory rate of a patient, it is common to use the abbreviation TPR. The abbreviation for blood pressure is B/P.

Vital signs have normal ranges. Readings that fall below or above normal may indicate a problem that needs further assessment. Comparing new readings with previous readings can provide information about whether the patient is improving or not. It is necessary to follow specific procedures to obtain accurate results. Never estimate or assume that the readings are the same as before, because inaccurate results can cause the wrong health care decisions to be made, which can jeopardize the patient's health.

Temperature

The body functions to maintain its temperature within a range that is best for maintaining homeostasis. If the body gets too warm it will feel hot, begin to sweat, and cause a sense of thirst to be experienced. Sweating is a normal cooling system of the body. The intake of fluids will assist in the sweating process as well as in the replacement of lost fluids. If the body gets too cool, the skin will feel cool, and shivering will start as a way to increase metabolism through muscular activity. The normal average temperature will vary with the route used to obtain the temperature. The oral (mouth) and aural (ear) routes have the same range, but the rectal route normally runs a degree higher, and the axillary (under the arm) runs a degree lower (Procedure 20–1). Other factors that affect the temperature are age of the patient (temperature control in the younger patient is less stable and runs higher than in adulthood), time of day (early morning readings are typically the lowest), and pregnancy (higher). The temperature will also vary with the temperature of the room, amount of clothes being worn, and number of blankets used while in bed. There are also normal variations among patients. Always refer to the chart to review prior readings as a comparison.

Mercury, electronic, tympanic (aural), and chemical-dot are different types of thermometers available today (Figure 20–1a–c). When using a glass *mercury thermometer*, it must be shaken down so that the mercury descends into the bulb until it is below 96° F. It can be covered with a disposable plastic sheath that is discarded after each use. An *electronic thermometer* and *tympanic thermometer* will have a disposable plastic probe that is placed on the thermometer prior to use and discarded after each use. Follow the manufacturer's instructions for the proper use, care, and cleaning of this equipment. When using *chemical-dot thermometers*, do not remove them from their protective covers in advance because they will begin to react to the room temperature. Be sure to follow directions supplied by the manufacturer. Always remember to follow Standard Precautions and facility policies regarding cleaning of equipment when working with patients.

When the temperature is within the normal range, the patient is said to be **afebrile**. When it is elevated above the normal range, they are **febrile**. An *intermittent fever* means that the temperature rises and falls. It can become elevated and then return to normal or even below normal. A *continuous fever* stays elevated over a prolonged period of time.

A fever is a defense mechanism against microorganisms. In an effort to kill the invading microorganisms, the body triggers the muscles to shiver, which increases metabolic activity and further increases the temperature. When the febrile episode subsides it is accompanied by profuse sweating that acts as a cooling mechanism. When the sweating episodes occur at night, they are called *night sweats*. It is common for intermittent fevers to occur at night.

If the health care worker notes signs that may indicate that the temperature is rising, such as that the body feels warmer than normal to the touch or the patient is shivering, he or she should take the patient's temperature at this time. If the patient is sweating profusely, it means that the fever has broken and is coming back down to a lower temperature.

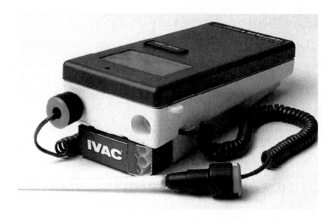

Figure 20–1b Electronic thermometers have a plastic probe that is placed on the thermometer and discarded after use. The temperature is read on a digital display. Photo courtesy of IVAC Corporation, San Diego, CA.

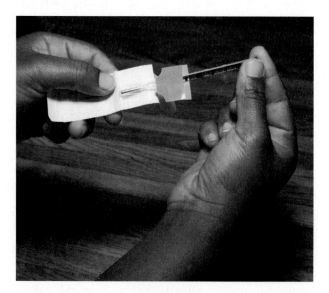

Figure 20–1a Glass mercury thermometers can be covered with a paper or plastic sheath that is discarded after each use.

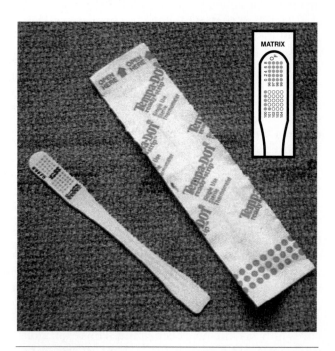

Figure 20–1c Chemical-dot thermometers change color in response to the temperature of the body.

PROCEDURE 20-1

How to Take a Temperature
*Observe Standard Precautions

ROUTE	PROCEDURE	NORMAL RANGE (ADULT)	PRECAUTIONS
Oral	1. You will need a clean thermometer (either glass or electronic), a watch, and something to record the results on.	97.6° F – 99.6° F 36.5° C – 37.5° C	Do not use this route if the patient is a mouth breather, unable to keep the mouth closed around the thermometer, had surgery or an injury to nose or mouth, is confused, unconscious, prone to seizures, has oxygen or a nasogastric tube, is too young, or is for any other reason unable or unwilling to follow directions.
	2. Verify that the patient has not taken any food or fluid by mouth, smoked, or chewed gum in the last 30 minutes.		This will result in an inaccurate reading.
	3. Shake down the thermometer to below 96° with sharp snaps of the wrist.		
	4. Ask the patient to open mouth.		
	5. Place the thermometer under the tongue on either side, as close to the midline as possible (Figure 20–2).		The thermometer must be placed close to the fleshy area where the tongue attaches in order to get an accurate reading. If it is placed too far to either side, it may result in an inaccurate reading (low).
	6. Instruct patient to close lips around thermometer, but not to bite down on it.		
	7. Leave it in place for 5 minutes if mercury thermometer (if electronic, follow the Manufacturer's Instructions).		
	8. Remove thermometer and read by holding horizontally and turning until the silver line of mercury is visible. If electronic, read digital display.		
	9. Immediately record your findings.		
	10. Clean thermometer or properly dispose of sheath.		

(continues)

PROCEDURE 20-1

(continued)

ROUTE	PROCEDURE	NORMAL RANGE (ADULT)	PRECAUTIONS
Axillary	1. You will need a thermometer, a watch, and something to record the results on.	96.6° F – 98.6° F 36° C – 37° C	This is the least accurate method, but is frequently used when the oral route is not appropriate.
	2. Shake down the thermometer to below 96° with sharp snaps of the wrist.		
	3. Remove clothing from patient's shoulder and arm.		
	4. Ensure that axillary area is dry, wiping with dry towel if necessary.		Moisture can cause an inaccurate reading.
	5. Place thermometer in the center of the armpit and place arm close to side of body (Figure 20–3).		
	6. Leave in place 10 minutes if mercury thermometer (if electronic, follow Manufacturer's Instructions).		
	7. Remove thermometer and read by holding horizontally and turning until the silver line of mercury is visible. If electronic, read the digital display.		
	8. Immediately record your findings.		
	9. Clean thermometer or properly dispose of sheath.		
Rectal	1. You will need a thermometer, a watch, and something to record the results on.	98.6° F – 100.6° F 37° C – 38° C	The rectal route is often inappropriate for infants and young children. Policies regarding its use vary among facilities.
	2. Position adults in a side lying position with top leg flexed forward.		
	3. Lubricate the thermometer.		Do not use this method if patient has diarrhea, recent surgery or injury to the rectum or prostate, or had a recent myocardial infarct (heart attack).
	4. Insert the thermometer into the rectum (i.e., 1 inch for children, and 1 ½ inches for adults).		Never force the thermometer into the colon.

(continues)

PROCEDURE 20-1

(continued)

ROUTE	PROCEDURE	NORMAL RANGE (ADULT)	PRECAUTIONS
	5. Leave in 3-5 minutes if mercury thermometer (if electronic, follow Manufacturer's Instructions).		
	6. Hold tip of thermometer while in place.		The thermometer must be held in place to prevent damage to rectal tissue or loss of thermometer into rectum.
	7. Remove thermometer and read by holding horizontally and turning until the silver line of mercury is visible. If electronic, read digital display.		
	8. Immediately record your findings.		
	9. Clean thermometer or properly dispose of sheath.		
Aural: (Tympanic)	1. You will need a thermometer, a watch, and something to record the results on.	97.6° F – 99.6° F 36.5° C – 37.5° C	
	2. Place disposable probe on the thermometer.		Follow Manufacturer's Instructions.
	3. Stabilize the patient's head.		
	4. In children less than 1 year, gently pull the ear straight back; in children over 1 year and adults, pull the ear back and up.		
	5. Insert the probe into ear canal until you obtain seal (Figure 20–4).		
	6. Press scan button. (Results obtained within seconds.)		
	7. Immediately record results.		
	8. Properly dispose of probe.		

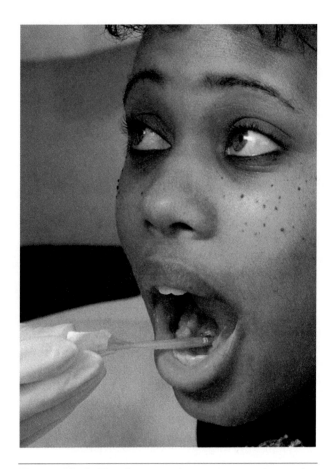

Figure 20–2 To take an oral temperature, insert the bulb of the thermometer under the tongue (sublingually). Have the patient close his or her lips and not talk until thermometer is removed.

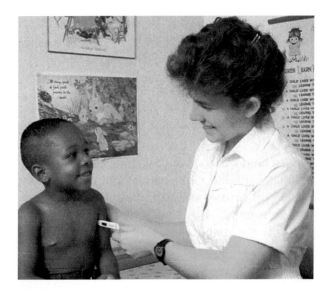

Figure 20–3 To take an axillary temperature, place the bulb of the thermometer into the center of the armpit and hold the arm close to body.

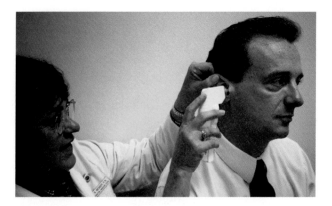

Figure 20–4 To take an aural temperature, insert the disposable covered probe into the ear canal until you obtain a seal.

Pulse

When the heart contracts and forces blood out of the heart and into the arteries, it creates a pulsing sensation that can be felt by the health care worker at

[Thinking it Through]

Mr. Hulchanski calls the physician's office and speaks with Becky Smith, the medical assistant. Mr. Hulchanski has had recent surgery and was instructed to call the office in 1 week to report how he is doing. Mr. Hulchanski reports that he is feeling fine and that the surgical incision looks like it is healing well. He says the only thing that he has noticed is that when he awakens in the morning, his pajamas and linens are soaked. Becky asks if he has been running a fever, and he states that he has routinely taken it several times during the day and it has been normal. In fact, he states that he is sure he is not having a fever because he actually feels chilled at times. Becky states that she is glad to hear that he is doing so well and to call back if any problems develop.

1. Has Becky done an adequate assessment?
2. Did Mr. Hulchanski report any variances from the norm?
3. What could possibly be happening to Mr. Hulchanski?

certain points in the body. There are a number of locations where an artery comes close enough to the surface of the skin and where it passes over a firm surface (e.g., bone) that it can be felt (Figure 20–5). These major **pulse points** are:

- Temporal: Located on either side of the forehead
- Carotid: Located on the front side of the neck on either side of the trachea (never massage this area or compress both carotids at the same time when taking a pulse; massages can trigger a sudden slowing of the heart rate, and compressing both carotids can decrease the blood flow to the brain)
- Brachial: Located in the inner side of the antecubital space (crease created when elbow is bent)
- Radial: Located in the wrist (thumb side); most frequently used site
- Femoral: Located in the inner aspect of the crease where the upper thigh joins the trunk of the body
- Popliteal: Located behind the knee
- Dorsalis pedis: Located on top of the foot arch

When taking a pulse (Procedure 20–2), there are three observations that are made:

1. Rate: The number of beats that occur in one minute
2. Rhythm: When the beats occur at even intervals, it is called a *regular rhythm.* If they do not occur at regular intervals, it is called an *irregular rhythm.* It is also possible to have a recurring pattern with an irregular rhythm. For example, there may be a beat missed every two beats, and this happens consistently. This pattern is called a *regular irregular rhythm.* If there is no pattern to the irregular rhythm, then it is called an *irregular irregular rhythm.*
3. Pulse volume (strength of the beat): This describes the character of the beat. It may be described as weak, strong, thready (very fine and scarcely perceptible), or bounding (higher intensity than normal, then disappears quickly).

Another method for taking the pulse is to take an *apical pulse.* This method requires the use of a stethoscope (Figure 20–6). A **stethoscope** is an instrument that amplifies sound and allows a health care worker to hear sounds from within the body. The stethoscope is placed over the apex of the heart, and the beats are counted as they are heard. The sound heard through the stethoscope will sound like "lub dub" and represents one beat (Procedure 20–3). The sounds heard as "lub dub" are actually the sounds of the various valves opening and closing as the blood flows through the heart's chambers. Sometimes the physician will order an apical pulse, but frequently it will not be specified, and it is left up to the judgment of the health care worker. An apical pulse should be done when there is an irregular rate, on cardiac patients, when the radial pulse is difficult to palpate, and with infants and young children.

When the pulse rate is abnormally low, it is called **bradycardia**. For example, with an adult patient, less than 60 beats per minute would be called bradycardia. When the pulse rate is abnormally high, it is called **tachycardia.** For example, with an adult patient, more than 100 beats per minute would be called tachycardia. The pulse rate is affected by many factors, including the age of the patient (Table 20–1), certain medications and disease conditions, physical activity, fever, and pregnancy.

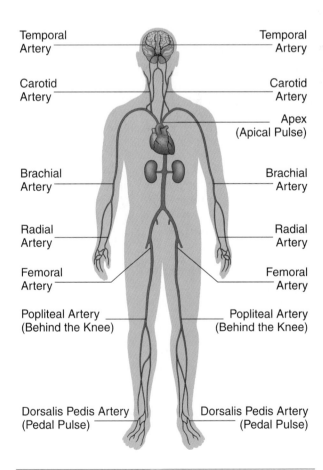

Figure 20–5 Location of pulse points that can be felt on the body.

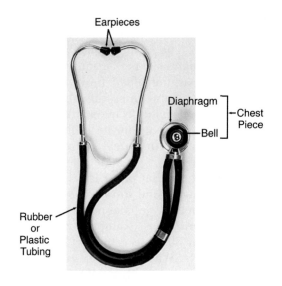

Figure 20–6 The parts of a stethoscope.

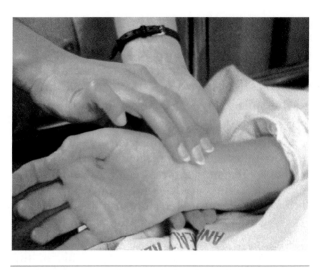

Figure 20–7 To take a radial pulse, place two or three fingers in an indented area on the thumb side of the wrist.

PROCEDURE 20-2

How to Take a Radial Pulse
*Observe Standard Precautions

STEPS	RATIONALE
1. You will need a watch with a second hand and something to record the results on.	As a health care worker, you should, at all times, have a watch with a second hand, a pen, and notepaper with you. A water-resistant watch with a large face for ease in reading is recommended.
2. Locate the radial pulse by gently but firmly pressing on the thumb side of the wrist, until an indented area is felt. This is where the pulse is located. Use two or three fingers to feel the pulse (Figure 20–7).	The health care worker always uses the fingers and never the thumb in taking a patient's pulse. The thumb has a pulse of its own, and if the thumb is used, the worker's own pulse may be mistaken for the patient's.
3. Place the patient's hand on his or her chest (Figure 20–8).	This makes it easier to count the respirations after the pulse is taken because the health care worker can feel the rise and fall of the chest.
4. Count the pulsations you feel in a 60 second period.	Counting the heart rate for a full minute increases the accuracy of the result. If the pulse is strong, regular, and within the normal range, you can count the pulsations for 30 seconds and multiply times two for the 1-minute reading.
5. When you complete the procedure, leave your fingers on the pulse, and count the respirations.	See Procedure 20–4.
6. Immediately record your findings.	Getting in the habit of writing down the actual numbers, instead of relying on your memory, will prevent errors.

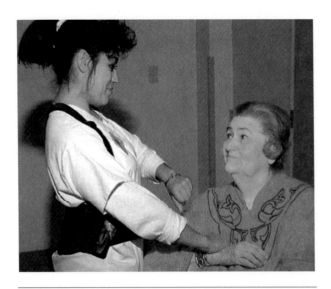

Figure 20–8 Positioning the patient's hand over the chest makes it easier to count the respirations without the patient's awareness.

Table 20–1 Pulse Rates at Various Ages

Age	Average Pulse	Normal Range
Newborn	140	120–160
Infant	110	80–140
Toddler	105	80–130
Preschool Children	100	74–120
School-Age Children	95	70–110
Adolescent–Adult	80	60–100

PROCEDURE 20-3

How to Take an Apical Pulse Using a Stethoscope
*Observe Standard Precautions

STEPS	RATIONALE
1. You will need a stethoscope, a watch with a second hand, and something to record the results on.	As a health care worker, you should, at all times, have a watch with a second hand, pen, and notepaper with you. A water-resistant watch with a large face for ease in reading is recommended.
2. Wipe the earpieces and diaphragm of stethoscope with alcohol wipes, and inspect the stethoscope prior to use.	If the earpieces have wax in them, remove wax prior to use, so the sound will not be diminished; do not use a stethoscope that has cracks or tears in the tubing because it may lead to inaccurate results.
3. Verify that the diaphragm side is where the sound will be heard.	The end of the stethoscope can be turned to switch between the diaphragm and the bell side (Refer back to Figure 20–6); some stethoscopes have only a diaphragm, and then no adjustment is needed.
4. If the diaphragm is cold to the touch, rub it against your clothing or hand until it is warm.	A cold instrument placed on the skin creates a very uncomfortable sensation for the patient.
5. Place earpieces into your ears, with the earpieces pointing forward.	This directs the sound into the ear canal at the correct angle.
6. Place the diaphragm of the stethoscope directly on the skin, over the apex of the heart and hold it with gentle, but firm pressure.	If placed over clothing, there are sounds caused by it rubbing on the clothing that may be misinterpreted as beats.

(continues)

PROCEDURE 20-3

(continued)

STEPS	RATIONALE
7. Count the beats you hear in a 60-second period.	Counting the heart rate for a full minute increases the accuracy of the result. If the pulse is strong, regular, and within the normal range, you can count the pulsations for 30 seconds and multiply times two for the 1-minute reading.
8. When you are done, leave the stethoscope in place and count the respirations.	See Procedure 20–4.
9. Immediately record your findings.	Getting in the habit of writing down the actual numbers, instead of relying on your memory, will prevent errors.

Another procedure that the health care worker may be asked to assist with is a pulse deficit assessment check. This requires two health care workers. One will take the pulse at one of the pulse points (usually radial), and the other will simultaneously take the apical pulse (Figure 20–9). This is always taken for a full minute and must be coordinated to start and stop at the same time. If there is a difference between the two readings, it is called the **pulse deficit**. For example, if the apical rate is 100 and the radial is 80, the apical-radial pulse deficit is 20 beats. The deficit represents the number of cardiac beats that do not reach the radial artery. Normally, there should be no pulse deficit.

An apical-radial deficit can be present in a number of cardiac conditions. For example, the heart may not contract with enough force for a pulse to reach the extremity, or the heart may be beating so rapidly that not enough blood can enter the heart on each beat. When doing an apical-radial pulse reading, the reading will be the same or the apical will be higher. It is not possible to get a radial pulse reading that is higher than the apical reading.

Respirations

Respiration refers to the process of moving air into and out of the lungs. When air is taken into the lungs it is called **inhalation** (inspiration), and there is a corresponding expansion of the chest as the lungs fill. When the air is expelled back out of the lungs, it is called **exhalation** (expiration), and there is a corresponding deflation of the chest cavity as the lungs

empty. One full cycle (inhalation and exhalation) is called one respiration. Normal breathing is called **eupnea** and should be within the normal range, unlabored, and have an even rhythm. If the respiratory rate is above the normal range, it is called **tachypnea**, and below normal it is **bradypnea**.

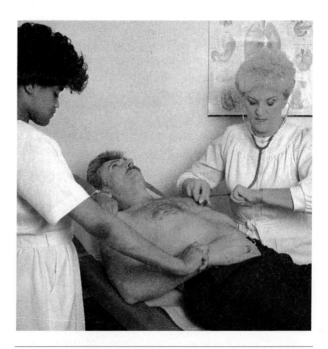

Figure 20–9 To determine a pulse deficit, one person counts the apical pulse while a second person counts the radial pulse.

When taking the respiratory rate (Procedure 20–4), there are three observations that are made:

1. Rate: The number of respiratory cycles that occur in one minute

2. Rhythm: Both the respirations and the intervals between them should be evenly spaced; when there is a temporary absence of respirations, it is call **apnea**, and the length of the interval should be timed. Report any periods of apnea to your supervisor. **Cheyne-Stokes** is a particular breathing pattern that has a period of apnea that can last for 10–60 seconds, and then is followed by a gradually increasing depth and frequency of respirations.

3. Respiratory effort: Breathing should occur through the nose, be unlabored, and be without sound; report to your supervisor if you note that the patient shows extra effort during breathing or if any sounds are heard (i.e., wheezing, gurgling, or other sounds). Also note the depth of the breathing, such as shallow, normal, or deep.

Many factors can affect the respiratory rate, but if the rate is outside of the normal range, has an irregular rhythm, or is labored, report it to your supervisor. Factors that can affect the rate are age (Table 20–2), illness, drugs, exercise, and emotions. Since the respiratory rate can be consciously altered, it is important that the patient not know when you are counting the respirations. The best approach is to place the patient's arm across his or her chest to take the pulse and then, when completed, leave your fingers on the radial pulse while counting the respirations. Do not tell the patient that you are now counting the respirations, or the rate may not be accurate. This is also an appropriate time to note the color of the nailbeds. They should be pink in color, and if they are cyanotic, report this to the supervisor immediately.

PROCEDURE 20-4

How to Count Respirations
*Observe Standard Precautions

STEPS	RATIONALE
1. You will need a watch with a second hand and something to record the results on.	As a health care worker, you should, at all times, have a watch with a second hand, pen, and notepaper with you. A water-resistant watch with a large face for ease in reading is recommended.
2. After you finish counting the pulse, leave your fingers in position (or the stethoscope on the chest), and count the respirations.	Since the respiratory rate can be consciously altered, it is important that the patient not know when you are counting the respirations. Do not tell the patient that you are now counting the respirations, or the rate may not be accurate. The health care worker can also feel the chest rise and fall by leaving the arm on the chest or the stethoscope in place.
3. Count the number of respirations taken in one full minute.	One respiration is a complete cycle that includes inhalation and exhalation.
4. Immediately record your findings.	Getting in the habit of writing down the actual numbers, instead of relying on your memory, will prevent errors.

Table 20–2 Respiratory Rates at Various Ages

Age	Normal Range
Infant	30–60
Toddler	20–40
Preschool Children	22–34
School-Age Children	18–24
Adolescent–Adult	16–20

Blood Pressure

The blood pressure (B/P) is written as two numbers separated by a slash. For example, 120/80 or 140/90. The first number is referred to as the *systolic pressure* and is the highest pressure in the cardiovascular system. The second number is the *diastolic pressure* and is the lowest pressure in the cardiovascular system. The average adult's blood pressure is 120/80, but a range for an adult between 90/60 to 140/90 is considered normal. If the patient's reading falls below this range, it is called **hypotension**. If the reading is above the range, it is called **hypertension**.

Another way of correlating the reading of the B/P is to think of a normal cardiac cycle. When listening to the heartbeat, there is a lub-dub sound. The lub sound occurs as the heart chambers are contracting at their maximum force to push the blood out of the heart and into the arteries. This is the systolic phase of the heart. The dub sound is when the heart relaxes and is refilling with blood. This is the diastolic phase of the heart.

The equipment needed to take a manual blood pressure is a stethoscope and sphygmomanometer. A **sphygmomanometer** is an instrument that records the blood pressure in millimeters (mm) of mercury (Hg). There are different types of recording devices (Figure 20–10a–c) that the health care worker may encounter. Some units show pressure with a column of mercury and others on a circular dial. Both the mercury column and the circular dial type of meters are calibrated so that each mark represents 2 mm of Hg (Figure 20–11a–b). The mercury type needs to be placed flat on a surface and read at eye level for accuracy. There are also electronic sphygmomanometers that take the blood pressure and pulse automatically and display the readings on a digital read out (once they are placed on the arm, the machine can be programmed to automatically take readings at specific intervals). It takes repeated practice to master the skills for taking an accurate manual blood pressure. See Procedure 20–5 for the steps in taking a blood pressure.

When working with a manual sphygmomanometer, it is necessary to close the screw to inflate the cuff and to loosen the screw to release the air. Some health care workers have difficulty remembering if turning the screw to the left or right will close or open the valve. It may be helpful to remember the saying "righty tighty, lefty loosey." This means that if you turn the screw to the *right* (as you look straight down at it) the valve will *tighten*, and the cuff can be inflated. Turning the screw to the *left*, *loosens* the screw, and air escapes.

The blood pressure cuff must fit correctly to get accurate results. Patients with very large or small upper arms may need a larger cuff or a pediatric cuff. An inflatable bladder is located within the outer covering of a cuff and should be long enough to cover 80% of the circumference of the arm (Figure 20–12). The width of the cuff should fit comfortably below the armpit and extends no further than 1–1½ inches above the antecubital space.

Blood pressure is affected by many factors, including the age of the patient (Table 20–3), certain medications and disease conditions, physical activity, the position of patient, and emotions. In fact, blood pressure is so variable in response to different factors that a diagnosis of hypertension is never made on just one reading. When patients visit the physician's office, they may feel anxious, and this causes the blood pressure reading to be higher than normal. Most physicians will want to see several high readings over a period of time, when the patient is lying down in a resting position, before they conclude that the patient has high blood pressure.

When a patient's cardiovascular system is unable to make rapid changes to accommodate changes in position, he or she will experience a condition call **orthostatic (postural) hypotension**. Normally, when a person rises to a standing position, the blood vessels in the lower extremities constrict, and the blood pressure increases to maintain adequate flow of blood to the brain. When that does not occur, the blood pools in the lower extremities, and the blood pressure drops quickly, which results in a lack of oxygen to the brain. The patient will experience lightheadedness and may even pass out. This can also occur when someone has been

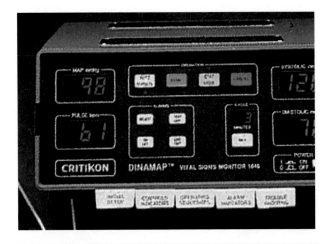

Figure 20–10c Electronic sphygmomanometer

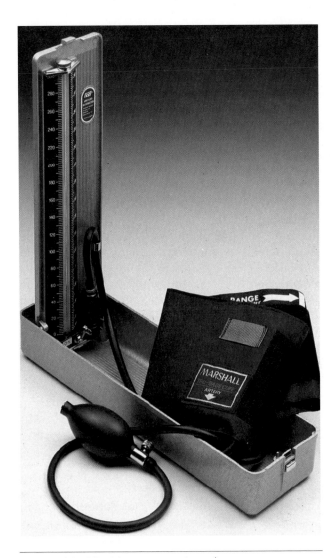

Figure 20–10a Mercury gravity sphygmomanometer

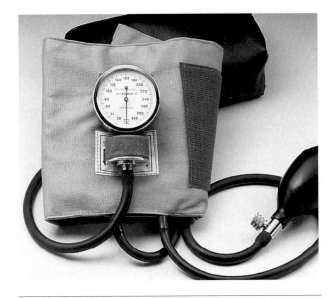

Figure 20–10b Dial (aneroid) sphygmomanometer

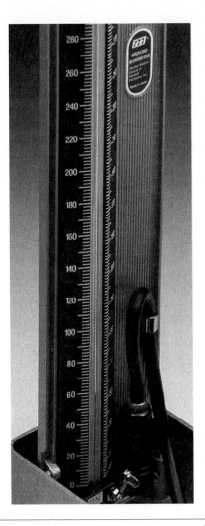

Figure 20–11a The gauge on a mercury sphygmomanometer has a column of mercury. Record the number at the top of the column when you take the systolic and diastolic readings. Readings are recorded as even numbers. Keep the unit flat and read it at eye level.

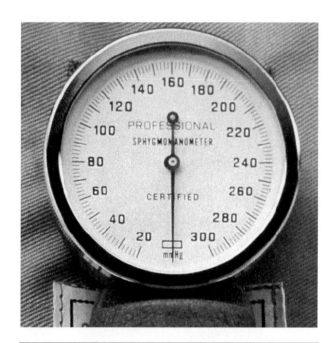

Figure 20–11b The gauge of a dial (aneroid) sphygmomanometer. Systolic and diastolic readings are recorded as even numbers.

repeated for the standing position. Check your facilities' policies on this procedure because some specify the exact timing required between the subsequent blood pressures while performing this procedure. Also remember to ensure the patient's safety at the time of the test to prevent injury if they get dizzy or pass out.

There are certain times when the arm cannot be used for blood pressure readings. Do not use the arm if there was surgery performed on it, if there is an intravenous infusion running into the arm (fluids running through a tube into a needle placed in a vein). Patients who have a shunt for the purpose of dialysis can never have blood pressures done on that arm. If neither arm is available for taking a blood pressure (e.g., burns to both arms), the popliteal artery can be used. A large blood pressure cuff will be required that fits around the thigh. Follow the same blood pressure procedure as with the brachial artery, only place the stethoscope behind the knee to use the popliteal artery.

on bedrest and is getting up for the first time, recently had surgery, or is on certain medications. Patients with low blood pressure or low pulse rates are also prone to this problem. When working with patients, always be on the alert to ensure their safety. Have the patients get up slowly to allow more time for their cardiovascular system to adjust to the change in position. To assist the physician in diagnosing this problem, the health care worker may be asked to check a lying, sitting, and standing B/P. To do this, the health care worker takes a blood pressure with the patient lying down, then leaves the blood pressure cuff in place and instructs the patient to sit up, and then rechecks the blood pressure. Then the same routine is

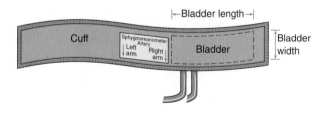

Figure 20–12 The blood pressure cuff must fit correctly to get accurate results. The bladder should cover 80% of the circumference of the patient's arm. Position the arrows on the cuff over the brachial artery.

[Thinking it Through]

Ms. Sanchez is a nursing assistant at an acute hospital in her hometown. Her supervisor has requested that she take Mr. Jordan's vital signs in Room 303B. When she enters the room, she introduces herself to Mr. Jordan and informs him that she will be taking his vital signs. He asks what she means by vital signs. He also tells her that he was hospitalized after having a myocardial infarct two days ago. She notes that he is receiving oxygen and has an IV in his left arm.

1. What are vital signs?
2. Which arm should be used to take the blood pressure? Why?
3. What route should be used to take the temperature? Why?
4. Should the pulse be taken radially or apically? Why?
5. What three observations should be made when taking the pulse?
6. What three observations should be made when taking the respiratory rate?

PROCEDURE 20-5

How to Take a Manual Blood Pressure
*Observe Standard Precautions

STEP	RATIONALE
1. You will need a stethoscope, a sphygmomanometer, and something to record the results on.	To verify that the sphygmomanometer is calibrated correctly, check that the mercury level or that the dial is resting at zero prior to use.
2. Verify that the cuff is the correct size for the patient and that the valve is closed to allow for inflation of bladder.	The bladder in cuff needs to cover at least 80% of the circumference of the arm and clear the antecubital space by 1–1½ inches to give accurate results.
3. Place the patient in a relaxed lying or sitting position, remove the clothing from the arm, and position the arm at heart level. Instruct the patient not to talk during the procedure.	Rolled up sleeves can constrict the arm and alter the results; talking can interfere with hearing the readings correctly (it may also be necessary to turn off the television or radio).
4. Locate the pulse of the brachial artery in the inner aspect of the antecubital space and place the arrows on cuff over this area.	Placing the stethoscope directly over the brachial artery will give the strongest sound.
5. Place your fingers on the radial artery and inflate the cuff until you can no longer feel the pulse. Note the reading and add 30 to it. For example, if the dial reads 120 when the radial pulsation ceases, add 30 to equal 150.	To get an accurate reading, it is necessary to pump the cuff to 30 mm Hg higher than the anticipated systolic pressure. This is the amount of inflation you will use when the blood pressure is taken.
6. Deflate the cuff by opening the screw. Wait at least 30 seconds.	Repeated inflation on the same arm in rapid succession will give inaccurate results.
7. Place the stethoscope in your ears and place the diaphragm over the brachial artery. Press gently.	The stethoscope diaphragm should be in full contact with the skin surface, but not be pressed too hard.
8. Close the screw and inflate the cuff to the predetermined amount (from example above, this would be 150 mm of Hg).	Never guess how high to inflate the cuff based on previous readings; check each time.
9. Slowly release the screw so the cuff deflates evenly and listen for the first sound of the pulse returning to the brachial artery. Make a mental note of the reading.	If the cuff is deflated too rapidly, the health care worker may not hear the first beat until a lower number is reached; the first sound of the brachial artery is called the systolic pressure.
10. Continue allowing the cuff to deflate until you no longer hear any further sounds from the brachial artery.	The health care worker will continue to hear a pulsing sound until it ceases, which is the reading for the diastolic pressure.
11. Continue to listen for any return of sounds from the brachial artery for an additional 20–30 mm Hg.	Some patients have what is called an auscultatory gap where the beat of the brachial artery will again be heard. Note the new beginning and ending beats and chart the findings. For example, if you first heard beats at 170, the beats ceased at 120, then resumed at 100, then ceased again at 60, you would chart B/P 170/60 with auscultatory gap between 120 and 100.

(continues)

PROCEDURE 20-5

(continued)

STEP	RATIONALE
12. Open the screw completely and let the cuff deflate rapidly.	The procedure is completed, and many patients do not like the tightness created by the cuff being inflated.
13. Remove the stethoscope from your ears and the cuff from the patient's arm and immediately record your results.	Getting in the habit of writing down the actual numbers, instead of relying on your memory, will prevent errors.
14. If you are unsure of the blood pressure readings and want to recheck it, use the other arm or wait several minutes before using the same arm.	Repeated blood pressure attempts can cause inaccurate results.

HEIGHT AND WEIGHT

Height and weight measurements are routinely taken as part of the patient's assessment when he or she visits the doctor's office or is admitted to a health care facility. The height measurement for an adult does not need to be repeated once it is recorded in the patient's chart, because it will not vary. An exception to this may be elderly patients with severe osteoporosis. When this condition is present, the height will actually decrease as they age. For younger patients, it is important to take both the height and weight. There are growth charts used to record the measurements that show the normal ranges for various ages. When the readings fall outside the normal ranges, it will alert the physician to potential problems requiring further evaluation. Refer back to the Suggested Learning Activities in Chapter 8 for the Web site that contains growth charts.

The weight will vary with a change in the patient's condition. How frequently the patient is to be weighed is ordered by the physician or may be determined by your supervisor. Weight loss or gain may indicate a loss or gain of fat, muscle, or fluid. Patients with kidney or cardiac conditions frequently have problems with fluid balance and are weighed to determine the effectiveness of their medical regime. When a patient starts to retain fluid, it will be seen on the scale long before it is visible on the body in the form of edema (swelling caused by excess fluid in the tissues of the body).

Table 20–3 Blood Pressure at Various Ages

Age	Average B/P	Normal Range
Infant	94/64	40/20–80/56
Toddler	100/64	80/60–100/64
Preschool Children	100/64	84/50–110/60
School-Age Children	110/72	90/56–112/60
Adolescent–Adult	120/80	90/60–140/90

[Fascinating Facts]

- The Centers for Disease Control and Prevention, National Center for Health statistics, report that as many as 50 million Americans have hypertension. The prevalence of hypertension is 17% among white women, 26% among white men, 37% among black women, and 44% among black men, 35–45 years of age. In persons over age 65, the incidence of high blood pressure is almost the same among men and women. In this age group, about 63% of whites and 76% of blacks will develop hypertension.

- Hypertension is called the silent killer because there are few, if any symptoms, but if left untreated, it can lead to a heart attack, stroke, embolism, and kidney failure.

- In 90–95% of the cases, hypertension has no known cause. This type of high blood pressure is known as essential hypertension. In rarer cases, high blood pressure can result from other illnesses such as kidney or adrenal gland problems. That type of high blood pressure is called secondary hypertension.

When a patient has edema or *ascites* (fluid accumulation in the peritoneal cavity), additional measurements may be indicated. Measuring the ankles or abdominal girth (around the abdomen) gives objective data on the patient's condition, when results are compared to previous readings.

There are a variety of scales available for taking the weight. Some of the most common are:

- Standing Balance Scale: Scale must be balanced prior to use, and the patient must be able to stand upright in a steady position without holding onto anything or anyone. The weights on the bars are then moved until the bar balances at the center point. The height can be obtained at the same time by extending the height bar. See Figures 20–13 a-c.

- Chair and wheelchair scales: Some chairs come equipped with a scale so the patient can sit while the weight is being taken. Another method is to place the patient in a wheelchair and then push it onto a scale, but in this case the wheelchair needs to be weighed while it is empty and its weight subtracted from the total weight of the patient in the chair to get the actual weight of the patient. See Figure 20–14.

- Mechanical lift scales (Figure 20–15 a & b): Patients unable to move on their own can have a sling positioned under them and then be lifted off the bed to obtain their weight.

- Bed scales: Some hospital beds now come equipped with a scale. The advantage is that the patient does not have to be moved to take a weight. The patient lies in bed, and the scale is activated while a digital display shows the weight. Remove any excess items from the bed before weighing the patient.

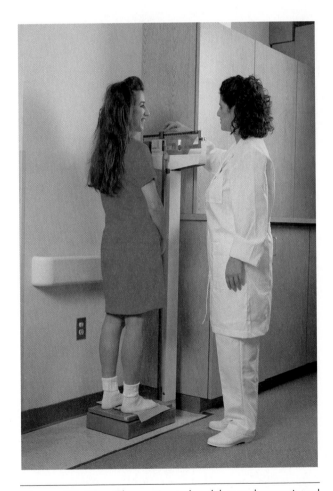

Figure 20–13a The patient should stand unassisted on the scale, with the feet centered on the platform and slightly apart.

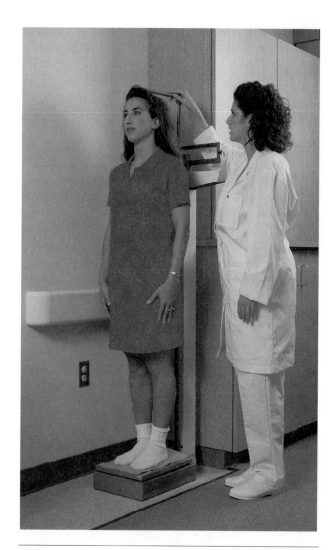

Figure 20–13b The patient should stand as erect as possible while height is being measured.

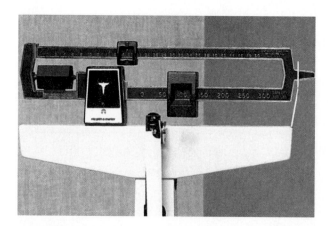

Figure 20–13c Adjust the weights on the balance bar until the bar balances at the center point. The combined total of the top and bottom bars is the weight of the patient.

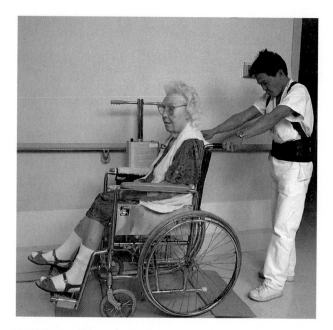

Figure 20–14 Subtract the weight of the wheelchair from the total weight of the patient sitting in the wheelchair.

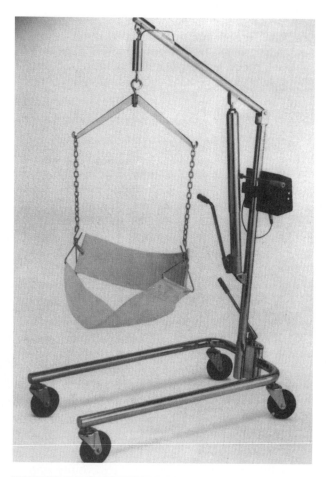

Figure 20–15a Chair-style mechanical lift with scale.

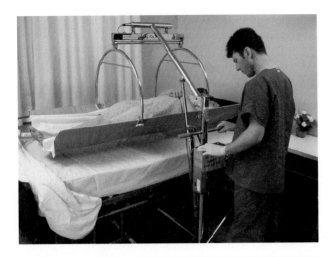

Figure 20–15b Bed-style mechanical lift with scale.

Following certain guidelines when weighing patients will ensure more accurate results. These guidelines are listed in Box 20–1.

If a patient is unable to stand for a height measurement, the measurement will need to be done when the patient is lying down. Place the patient flat on the bed or examining table in a straight aligned position. Then place a mark at the top of the head and one at the bottom of the heels. Measure the distance between the marks and record it as the height. This method is also used with infants, and children who are unable to stand.

Box 20–1   Guidelines for Weighing Patients

- Weigh patients at the same time every day; the recommendation is to weigh patients first thing in the morning, after they empty their bladder and before they eat or drink.

- Use the same scale each time.

- Balance the scale before use, if indicated.

- Have the same amount of clothes on the patient each time and remove the shoes (place a paper towel on the scale for the patient to stand on).

- Maintain the safety of the patient at all times by monitoring and assessing him or her for signs of unsteadiness that could result in a fall.

SUGGESTED LEARNING ACTIVITIES

1. Identify the information included in a History and Physical for yourself, a family member, or a friend, and write the information down in a chronological and organized manner.

2. Perform a head-to-toe assessment on yourself and write the results down in a narrative documentation format (refer back to Chapter 19).

3. Next time you experience pain (e.g., headache, stub your toe), assess your level of pain on a scale of 1–10. Then note how this level changes over time, until it is completely gone (level zero).

4. It will take time to develop the ability to feel a pulse, to hear the apical heartbeat, and to hear the blood pressure. Practice on yourself and your family to assist you in developing the needed sensitivity in your fingertips and to hear the sounds with a stethoscope. Closing your eyes to help focus all of your attention on your fingertips or ears may be a helpful technique to use when practicing.

5. Find all the pulse points on your body.

REVIEW QUESTIONS

1. State the components that comprise a History and Physical.

2. What does the phrase "noting variances from the norm" mean?

3. Why is it a critical function for the health care worker to be able to discriminate between normal and abnormal conditions and situations?

4. What are sample questions to be asked to evaluate each of the body's systems?

5. What does it mean to use a pain assessment scale?

6. What are Activities of Daily Living (ADLs)?

7. What are the different types of equipment for taking a temperature?

8. What is an apical-radial deficit?

9. How do the vital signs vary over the life span?

10. What are the steps in taking an accurate TPR and B/P?

11. What problems may be indicated by a rapid weight gain in a patient?

APPLICATION EXERCISES

1. Refer back to The Case of the Missed Assessment and answer these questions.

   a. What variances from the normal was Mrs. Becker displaying?

   b. What are the possible outcomes of the patient losing consciousness and falling?

   c. How could Carrie have handled the situation differently?

2. Mr. Hussar, a 76-year-old patient, walks into the physician's office for his regular checkup. Mr. Hussar seems to be limping slightly as he approaches the desk to sign in for his appointment. Mrs. Jacobs, the receptionist, inquires how he is doing, to which he replies, "Fine." Mrs. Jacobs always looks forward to seeing Mr. Hussar because he is usually so cheerful and talkative, but she is disappointed when he just takes a chair in the waiting room to wait for the doctor. She notes that Mr. Hussar also isn't as neatly dressed or as well-groomed as usual.

   a. Is there an alteration in the patient's gait?

   b. What does "noting variances from normal" mean? What knowledge is needed to be able to determine a variance from the normal?

   c. Are there any physical variances? If so, what are they?

   d. Are there any psychosocial variances? If so, what are they?

SUGGESTED READINGS AND RESOURCES

Bickley, L. S. & Hoekelman, R. A. (1998). *Bate's guide to physical examination and history taking.* Philadelphia: Lippincott Williams & Wilkins Publishers.

Estes, M. E. Z. (2002). *Health assessment & physical examination.* Albany, NY: Delmar.

CHAPTER

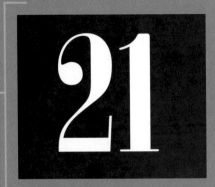

EMERGENCY PROCEDURES

OBJECTIVES

Studying and applying the material in this chapter will help you to:

- Explain when first aid should be administered.

- Discuss how the Good Samaritan Act protects the rescuer.

- State the Golden Rule of first aid.

- Understand the seven steps to follow when an emergency occurs that will protect both the victim and rescuer.

- Identify when CPR should be performed.

- Identify illnesses and injuries that may require first aid, including their signs and symptoms and treatment.

- Demonstrate the proper application of slings, and spiral, figure-eight, and finger wraps.

KEY TERMS

anaphylactic shock

cardiopulmonary resusitation (CPR)

closed fracture

external bleeding

first aid

frostbite

Golden Rule

Good Samaritan Act

hemorrhage

hyperthermia

hypothermia

internal bleeding

joint dislocation

Medic Alert

open fracture

rescue breathing

rescuer

sprain

strain (muscle)

sucking wound

victim

wound

The Case of

the Out-of-Control Party

Josephine Robbins is a nurse at a local hospital. She lives in a nearby apartment complex and is trying to tune out loud noises coming from a party in the next complex. The noise seems to escalate, then she hears someone shout, "Oh my God, he stabbed him," and then there is silence. She calls 9-1-1, gets dressed, and goes to see if it is safe to offer assistance. After deeming it safe to enter, she enters and sees the victim lying on the couch, unconscious. His respirations are shallow and rapid, his skin is pale and cold to the touch, and his lips, earlobes and fingertips have a bluish tinge. The victim has a 2-inch cut on the left side of his chest where a knife is still inserted, but it is currently not bleeding. There is, however, a great deal of blood in the kitchen area, on the living room carpet, and on the victim's clothing. Josephine does her assessment, gives first aid, and monitors the victim's condition until the paramedics arrive. When the paramedics arrive, she introduces herself and gives them a report of observations and care given. The paramedics continue the care and transport the victim to the hospital. In this chapter, you will learn how to approach emergency situations and how to give appropriate first aid measures to assist victims.

EMERGENCY SITUATIONS

First aid refers to providing emergency care to an accident victim or to someone who has suddenly become ill. The goal of first aid is to provide care to minimize the effects of the injury or illness until the victim can be treated by a physician.

The American Red Cross recommends that all persons take a First Aid and Safety Course. The course covers what to do in an emergency, how to give first aid, and how to prevent accidents and injuries. The American Red Cross (ARC) and the American Heart Association (AHA) recommend that everyone be trained in giving cardiopulmonary resuscitation (CPR). CPR is administered when someone is not breathing and does not have a pulse. The ARC and AHA believe that many lives would be saved if more people were trained to give emergency care. More people trained in emergency care increases the chance that an injured person can start to receive immediate care rather than it being delayed until medical help arrives.

To encourage individuals to get involved in helping victims during an emergency, a law has

been passed by most states called the **Good Samaritan Act**. This protects individuals from liability when they stop to assist someone who has been hurt or is ill. This protection covers acts that are within the ability of the person to provide as long as there is no gross negligence or willful intent to harm the victim. The Good Samaritan laws vary somewhat between states. Specific information should be requested from the local police department, the library, or an attorney (Box 21–1).

The **Golden Rule** in providing first aid is to "do no further HARM." When a person goes into health care as a career, it is because of a desire to help others. When an emergency situation arises, it is natural to want to do anything and everything possible to assist the victim. The best way to be ready for this situation is to learn as much as possible about first aid and CPR. But it is also just as critical not to attempt anything you do not have the skills to perform. If the procedure needed is beyond your skill level, then immediately seek help. Getting the appropriate help for the victim can save a life.

Many people fantasize about having the ability to assist someone in an emergency. The thoughts

Box 21–1   Example of Good Samaritan Law as Written for the State of Arizona

Good Samaritan Act—Article 4 ARS.#32-1471

Health care providers and other persons administering emergency aid are not liable. Any health care provider licensed or certified to practice as such in this state or elsewhere or any other person who renders emergency care at a public gathering or at a scene of an emergency occurrence gratuitously and in good faith, shall not be liable for any civil or other damages as the result of any act or omission by which person rendering the emergency care, or as the result of any act or failure to act to provide or arrange for further medical treatment or care for the injured persons, unless such person, while rendering such care, is guilty of gross negligence.

Internet Site: Good Samaritan Links: http://www.ci.phoenix.az.us/FIRE/cpr.html

are that the intervention performed saved a life, they are declared a hero or heroine, and the victim recovers and is very grateful. This indeed may be the situation, but another reality can also occur. Perhaps there is little that can be done to help, the victim is uncooperative, or all attempts at first aid fail, and the victim dies. Some accident sites can be extremely upsetting, and the images and sounds can continue to emotionally upset the Good Samaritan for some time after the event. If the outcome of assisting someone is less than ideal, then enjoy the satisfaction of knowing that you did the best you could to assist in a very difficult situation.

When an Emergency Occurs

When approaching an injured or ill person there are certain steps to follow. These steps include actions that will protect the **rescuer** (person giving care) as well as well as the **victim** (person requiring care).

Assess the Environment

Before approaching the victim, assess the situation to determine if it is safe to approach. If there are loose electrical wires, the potential for a sudden fire or explosion, the smell of gas, or any other hazards that would put the Good Samaritan at risk, the appropriate course of action is to not approach, but to call for help immediately. If the victim is

conscious, inform him or her that you are going to call for assistance and then will return to be with them until help arrives. Most states have Emergency Medical Services (EMS) that are reached by dialing 9-1-1 on a telephone. The person answering has been specially trained and will ask questions that should be answered as accurately as possible. They will want to know the name and location of the victim, what the nature of the emergency is, and what, if any, treatment has been given. The EMS personnel will send services as deemed appropriate, such as an ambulance, a fire engine, and the police. They may also be able to advise you on what to do to further assist the victim. Remember that your first priority is to keep yourself safe. If you take a risk and become a victim too, then there is no one to call EMS. Assessing a situation is not done only once; the situation must be repeatedly monitored. For example, if there is smoke in the immediate area, is the amount increasing?

Obtain Consent to Treat

When approaching a stranger, identify yourself and your intent to give assistance. If the victim is conscious, permission must be obtained prior to administering care. If the victim is a child, determine if a parent or guardian is present, to obtain consent for care. If the victim is unconscious, consent is implied and first aid can be administered. Remember that victims have the right to refuse care, and this request must be respected. If consent for care is not given and it is obvious that care is required, immediately call EMS.

Try to Determine What Happened

Do not assume what might have occurred. If the victim is conscious, ask for information. Look around the environment for any clues that would assist in determining what care is needed. For example, if there is an empty bottle of pills or chemicals that may have been ingested, note what they are and inform EMS because they may be able to give you directions on how to treat the victim immediately. Many people with specific medical conditions wear necklaces or bracelets or carry cards with them that contain specific information that will assist you in determining what care to consider and also in informing the EMS on what type of help to send. This form of identification is called **Medic Alert** and may specify if the victim is diabetic, epileptic, or has specific heart problems. There may also be information about specific allergies that will be helpful for the personnel from EMS to know before administering medications. Another thing to determine is if there are other victims. Perhaps someone was thrown from the car or is located in a different area than where you are located.

Follow Standard Precautions

Following Standard Precautions is essential in all situations that may result in the rescuer coming into contact with body fluids. Carry disposable gloves that can be put on prior to contact. Another valuable item to carry at all times is a barrier device for giving mouth-to-mouth resuscitation. These resuscitation devices have a mouth piece with a one-way valve attached to a plastic shield that prevents the rescuer from getting saliva, blood, or vomit into their mouth (Figure 21–1). Some of these devices are small enough to fold into a small pouch that is attached to a key chain. Information about the contents of a first aid kit can be obtained from the American Red Cross. A first aid kit can be kept in the home, car, or office for ready access when needed.

Enlist the Help of Bystanders

Determine if there are others in the area who can assist in the care of the victim. If you are the most experienced person, then stay with the victim and instruct someone else to leave to call EMS. Instruct those willing to help to do other tasks, such as rerouting traffic, keeping onlookers away from the scene, looking for clues as to what happened, or tending to other victims.

Never Move a Victim

A neck or back injury can be made worse or result in permanent paralysis if the victim is moved. The only exception to this rule is if the victim's life is in immediate danger if he or she is not moved. When it is absolutely necessary to move the victim, make every attempt to keep the spine in straight alignment. When turning a victim with a neck or back injury, turn the body as a unit to prevent spinal cord injury. If you move an injured extremity, support it during the move to prevent further vessel or nerve damage.

Stay Calm

A calm, reassuring manner in treating victims will decrease the stress of the situation for the victim, others in the area, and you. Many people who feel they cannot handle certain situations are quite surprised to discover how effectively they can think and act in an emergency situation. If the scene is more than the rescuer can handle, the best thing to do is to call EMS immediately.

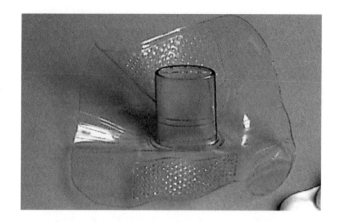

Figure 21–1 Portable barrier device to protect rescuer during resuscitation.

CARDIOPULMONARY RESUSCITATION (CPR)

An expectation of most health care employers is that all health care workers will attend classes to maintain a current certification for performing **Cardiopulmonary Resuscitation (CPR)**. These classes provide theory and hands-on practice on how to assist a victim in the following situations:

- Obstructed airway: Perform the Heimlich Maneuver, a method that uses pressure to expel material that is stuck in the throat preventing the victim from being able to inhale air.
- Not breathing: Perform **rescue breathing** which is a technique in which the rescuer breathes for the victim.
- Not breathing and has no pulse: Perform CPR, which includes rescue breathing and doing compressions to the chest to stimulate cardiac blood flow for the victim.

Since the specific guidelines for CPR may be revised annually and the best approach to learning this material is to receive training from a CPR-certified instructor, the specific procedures will not be presented in this text. It is highly recommended that every person be certified in CPR. It is of particular importance that all health care workers and students obtain and maintain CPR certification.

FIRST AID PROCEDURES

When approaching any victim to administer first aid, the first step is always to determine that the victim is breathing and has a pulse. If not, CPR should be started.

CPR is always the first priority in an emergency. If the victim does not require CPR, then the next step is to assess the victim for any other problems that may need attention. Implementing proper first aid procedures can prevent further injury and assist in the recovery of the injured person. Discussed in the following sections are a variety of first aid procedures that are commonly used in medical emergencies.

Allergic Reactions

Allergic reactions can range from mild to life threatening. The reaction is the result of the body's defense mechanism being triggered by a normally harmless substance. An allergic reaction can be triggered by skin contact (e.g., lotions, poison ivy), ingestion (e.g., certain foods and drugs), inhalation (e.g., sprays and pollen), or injection (e.g., venom from insect and snakebites). Once an allergy has developed, it will frequently become more severe with each reexposure. In the most extreme case a condition called anaphylaxis occurs where the respiratory system swells to such an extent that air is prevented from entering the lungs. This is called **anaphylactic shock** and if it occurs, death will follow if it's not treated immediately.

See Procedure 21–1 for first aid related to allergic reactions.

PROCEDURE 21-1

First Aid for Allergic Reactions
*Observe Standard Precautions

CONDITION AND SIGNS AND SYMPTOMS	PROCEDURE	RATIONALE
Mild to Moderate Reaction *S/S*: Itching, hives, and flushed face. Swelling may involve the eyes, face, or tongue. The victim may be weak and dizzy and have nausea and vomiting.	• Be calm and reassuring in approach to victim. • If there is an itchy rash, apply anti-itch lotion (e.g., calamine lotion) and cool compresses. • Try to determine the source of the allergic reaction. • A physician may recommend an over-the-counter medication (e.g., Benadryl). • Call EMS if the condition worsens.	• Anxiety increases the allergic reaction. • Soothing the itch makes it less likely that the victim will scratch the area which not only increases the intensity of the rash, but may also cause an infection. • The victim can avoid it in the future. • Taking an antihistamine can decrease the effect of an allergic reaction. • It may advance to a severe reaction.
Severe Reaction *S/S*: The above reactions may be present, but more severe. In the worst cases that lead to anaphylaxis, there will be difficulty breathing, wheezing, and tightness of the chest. The victim may have difficulty swallowing and become unconscious. Untreated anaphylaxis can lead to death.	• Call EMS. • If the victim has emergency allergy medication, help him or her administer it. • Do not give the victim anything by mouth if he or she is having difficulty breathing. • Do not place a pillow under the victim's head.	• Severe reactions can lead to anaphylactic shock. • Victims with known severe allergies may carry a kit for administering an injection to stop a reaction. • It may enter the lungs and cause further breathing difficulties. • Elevating the head may close off the airway.

(continues)

PROCEDURE 21-1

(continued)

CONDITION AND SIGNS AND SYMPTOMS	PROCEDURE	RATIONALE
Bites and Stings (e.g., insects, spiders, scorpions, and snakes) *S/S*: Localized reaction to bite or sting may be seen, such as redness, pain, and swelling. There may be an obvious bite mark. An allergic reaction may occur as noted in the section on allergic reactions.	• Try to identify what bit or stung the victim. • Kill it if there is no risk to the rescuer and keep it for identification. • If there is a stinger (e.g., honey bee), remove it by scraping it with your fingernail or a credit card. • Do not forcibly remove a tick, instead suffocate it by covering it with a heavy oil (e.g., Vaseline, mineral oil), wait 30 minutes, then carefully remove it with tweezers, placing them as close to the mouth parts as possible (if all parts are not removed, seek medical attention). • Call EMS immediately if a poisonous spider, scorpion, or snake has bitten the victim. • If an allergic reaction occurs, treat it as noted above under allergic reactions. • Stay with the victim for at least an hour. • Clean the area with soap and water and apply antiseptic ointment. • Remove any confining clothing or jewelry. • Apply a cold compress. • Have the victim lie still and keep the bite area below heart level. • Do not apply a tourniquet.	• Will assist EMS personnel to treat victim. • The rescuer's safety comes first, or there will be two victims and no one to call EMS. • Do not use a tweezers because it may force more venom into victim. • Decreases the chance of mouth parts remaining in the victim. • So they can receive the appropriate injection of antivenom without delay. • Same as for allergic reactions. • Sometimes reactions are delayed. • Helps to prevent infection. • Clothing and jewelry act as a constricting band if swelling occurs. • Decreases pain, swelling, and the spread of venom. • Slows the rate at which the venom spreads. • Cuts off blood to the extremity and may result in damage to tissues and could result in the need for an amputation.

(continues)

PROCEDURE 21-1

(continued)

CONDITION AND SIGNS AND SYMPTOMS	PROCEDURE	RATIONALE
Bites and Stings (continued)	• Consult with a physician to determine if any additional preventive measures should be taken. • Instruct the victim to observe for infection (e.g., increased pain, redness, or swelling, discharge from the site, swollen glands, fever, flu-like symptoms, or red streaks coming from site) and get to medical help immediately if symptoms occur.	• The victim may need additional treatment to prevent disease that may have been contracted through the bite or sting (e.g., tetanus, lyme disease). • Infections require follow-up care and treatment by a physician.

Bleeding and Wounds

Bleeding occurs when a blood vessel is damaged. If there is heavy bleeding, it is called a **hemorrhage**. When there is damage to the soft tissue of the body from violence or trauma, it is called a **wound**. It is called **external bleeding** when blood drains to the outside of the body through a break in the skin. If there is bleeding that occurs inside the body, it is called **internal bleeding** and is more difficult to detect. Suspect internal bleeding if the victim has a broken bone or been hit forcibly (e.g., car accident where victim hits the dashboard or steering wheel, is struck by an object, or receives other types of trauma to the head or body). If internal bleeding is suspected, the victim must have a medical evaluation.

When giving first aid to a victim who has a wound, the rescuer must clean the wound and protect it from further damage. If there is external bleeding that does not stop spontaneously, first aid will be required to stop the bleeding, before the victim loses too much blood.

Bleeding can occur from a vein or an artery. *Arterial bleeding* is a brighter red and comes out in spurts with each heartbeat. This is a life-threatening situation and must be stopped as soon as possible. *Venous bleeding* flows evenly and can also result in a great deal of blood loss. Remember to follow Standard Precautions when caring for victims with wounds and bleeding.

See Procedure 21–2 for first aid related to bleeding and wounds.

[Fascinating Facts]

The National Center for Environmental Health (NCEH), which is part of the CDC, reports the following statistics:

- Accidents are the fourth leading cause of death among the total population and the leading cause of death for ages 1 through 37.
- Accidents cost over $43 billion a year—in the form of time away from work and a loss in productivity, medical expenses, administrative costs, and property loss.
- Medical attention is required by over 15 million persons injured each year in home accidents.
- One-third of all nonfatal accidental injuries and more than one-fourth of all fatal injuries occur in and around the home.
- An estimated 22 million persons (or one out of every nine Americans) were injured in the home environment last year. Disabling injuries numbered 4,100,000 including 110,000 with some degree of permanent impairment.

Source: www.cdc.gov/nceh/publications/books/housing/cha9.htm

PROCEDURE 21-2

First Aid for Bleeding and Wounds
*Observe Standard Precautions

CONDITION AND SIGNS AND SYMPTOMS	PROCEDURE	RATIONALE
External Bleeding *S/S*: Blood coming from a wound. Weakness, confusion, and/or a decreasing level of consciousness may indicate excessive blood loss. Loss of function distal to the wound indicates damage to tendons or muscles. Loss of sensation distal to the wound indicates damage to the nerves.	• Call EMS if you suspect internal bleeding or if there is heavy external bleeding or other serious injuries. • Apply cold compresses to bruised areas. • If bleeding from the leg or arm, elevate it above heart level (unless contraindicated by neck or back injury, or discomfort). • Do not use a tourniquet. • To stop bleeding, apply direct pressure with a clean cloth or sterile dressing over the area (Figure 21–2). If the rescuer needs his or her hands free to do additional first aid, a pressure dressing can be applied to decrease the bleeding (Figure 21–3a–e). • When the dressing becomes soaked with blood, do not remove it, instead place the new dressing on top. • Also, do not look under the dressing to see if the bleeding has stopped. • Do not apply pressure over an embedded object, the eye, or on a head injury if a skull fracture is suspected. • If bleeding from an arm or leg does not stop after 15 minutes of direct pressure, then use pressure point bleeding control (Figure 21–4a–b).	• Will require medical evaluation and intervention. • Bruising can be decreased as the cold constricts the blood vessels. • Elevation of the extremity will decrease the pressure in the vascular system of the arm or leg and thus decrease bleeding. • Cuts off blood to the extremity, resulting in damage to tissues and the possible need for an amputation. • Slows the blood flow so body can use its natural clotting mechanism. • Removing the dressing may reinitiate bleeding. • Lifting the dressing may reinitiate bleeding. • This may cause further damage. • Will decrease the flow of blood to the affected area.
Internal Bleeding Abdominal injuries can cause internal bleeding.	• Call EMS.	• Must be evaluated and treated by medical personnel.

(continues)

PROCEDURE 21-2

(continued)

CONDITION AND SIGNS AND SYMPTOMS	PROCEDURE	RATIONALE
Internal Bleeding (continued) *S/S*: Blood in the vomit, urine, stool, or from the vagina. Distended abdomen, nausea, abdominal tenderness, signs and symptoms of shock. See shock under Other Conditions. Weakness, confusion, and/or a decreasing level of consciousness may indicate bleeding inside the skull that is causing pressure on the brain.	• Do not give the victim anything to eat or drink. • Place the victim on his or her back and elevate the knees with a pillow or blanket, if there is abdominal discomfort. • Keep the victim still and treat him or her for shock as needed. • Stay with victim until medical assistance arrives.	• The victim may need surgical intervention; may cause vomiting. • Relaxes the abdominal muscles and decreases pain. • To prevent further injury. • Give rescue breathing or CPR as needed.
Wounds *S/S*: Tear or open area anywhere on the body.	• Do not try to clean a large wound or remove any embedded objects. • Remove any obvious loose debris from the wound. • If an object is protruding from the body, do not remove it (Figure 21–5).	• Can increase the bleeding and cause additional damage. • Decreases contamination of wound. • May cause further damage or initiate bleeding.
Sucking Wounds *S/S*: Bubbling from any wound of the neck or chest; difficulty breathing.	• If the chest or neck has been punctured or if there is an object protruding from the chest or neck, note if there is any bubbling from the wound. If so, this is called a **sucking wound**, and it needs to be sealed as soon as possible. • With a sucking wound, apply an airtight dressing (e.g., saran wrap, tin foil, plastic bag or other nonporous material) over the site. If you do not have non-porous material, you can use a regular gauze pad or clean cloth coated with petroleum jelly (i.e., Vaseline). • When applying an airtight dressing leave one edge uptaped or unsealed. • Do not move the patient unless absolutely necessary. • Do not give them anything by mouth.	• Bubbling is caused by air passing through a wound that has penetrated the respiratory system. The victim will be experiencing difficulty with breathing because air is escaping as he or she breathes. • An airtight dressing prevents the escape of air from the respiratory system. • This allows trapped air to escape. • May cause further injury. • Surgery may be required.

(continues)

PROCEDURE 21-2

(continued)

CONDITION AND SIGNS AND SYMPTOMS	PROCEDURE	RATIONALE
Amputations *S/S*: Part of the body severed from its attachment (e.g., all or part of an arm, leg, nose, or ear).	• If an amputation of a body part occurs, save the severed part. • After giving the appropriate first aid to the victim, try to locate the part if it is not in the immediate area. • Once the body part is found, rinse it off, wrap it in a moistened cloth, and place in a plastic bag or other container. • If ice is available, place the bag in a container with ice and water. Do not place the part directly on ice. • Write the name of the patient and the time of the accident on the container with the body part. • Make sure the amputated body part remains with the victim when he or she is transported to the hospital.	• It may be possible to reattach the amputated part on reaching the hospital • First aid for the victim is the first priority. • A clean moist body part is more apt to be successfully reattached. • Lowering the temperature of the body part will extend the amount of time for successful reattachment. Direct contact with the ice will cause freezing and damage the tissue. • Assists medical personnel at the hospital who will decide if reattachment is possible. • Prevents unnecessary delays in locating the part.

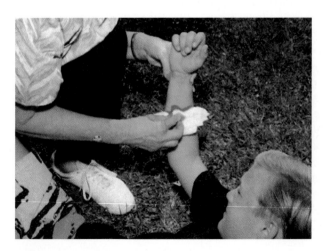

Figure 21–2 By using direct pressure and elevation, most severe bleeding can be controlled.

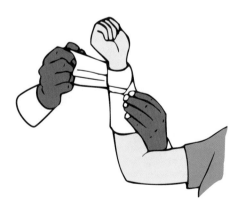

Figure 21–3a Maintain direct pressure and elevation when applying a pressure dressing. Do not remove previous dressing, but apply the pressure dressing over the previous dressing.

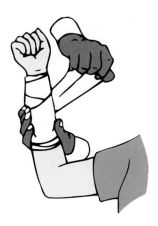

Figure 21–3b Wrap the roller bandage or long strip of cloth firmly around the wound. Overlap each rotation partially over the previous one to hold it securely in place.

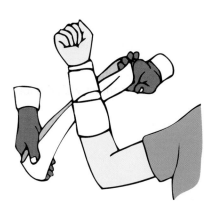

Figure 21–3c Split the end of the bandage into two strips.

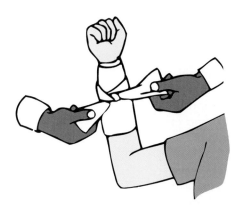

Figure 21–3d Tie the ends tightly into a knot right over the wound.

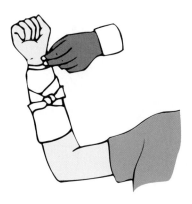

Figure 21–3e Check for circulation to verify that the dressing is not too tight. If there is no pulse or the fingers are turning bluish, loosen the dressing and rewrap it.

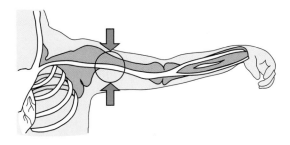

Figure 21–4a For an arm wound, the pressure point is on the brachial artery. It is located between the large muscles (biceps and triceps) on the inside of the arm. Press firmly with your fingers, until you no longer feel a pulse.

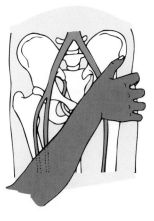

Figure 21–4b For a leg wound, the pressure point is on the femoral artery. It is located in the groin at the bend of the leg. Press firmly with the palm of your hand (or use both hands for more pressure) against the pelvic bone, until you no longer feel a pulse.

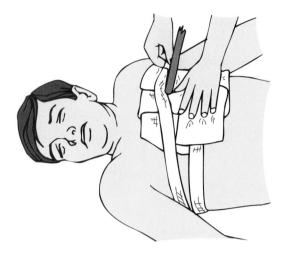

Figure 21–5 Never remove an object protruding from the body. Immobilize the object by placing dressings around the object and taping the dressing in place.

Bone, Joint, and Muscle Injuries

When a bone is broken it is called a fracture. An **open fracture** is when the broken bone protrudes through the skin. A **closed fracture** is a broken bone that does not break the skin. When a joint becomes disconnected from its socket, it is called a **joint dislocation**.

Marlow Barrons is a nurse on vacation in Alaska. After fishing all day, she and her friends are unloading their boat when an emergency call comes in to the Coast Guard. She overhears them discussing a professional fisherman who has amputated his arm in the gears of his boat. She tells them she is a nurse and offers assistance.

1. What signs and symptoms can Marlow anticipate seeing, based on the report of the accident?
2. What type of first aid should she anticipate that the victim will need?
3. Are there special considerations regarding the amputated arm?

Strains result from the sudden tearing of muscle fibers during exertion and are frequently referred to as pulled muscles. **Sprains** are torn ligament fibers that result in a loosening of the joint.

See Procedure 21–3 for first aid related to bones, joints, and muscle injuries.

PROCEDURE 21-3

First Aid for Bone, Joint, and Muscle Injuries
*Observe Standard Precautions

CONDITION AND SIGNS AND SYMPTOMS	PROCEDURE	RATIONALE
Fractures and Joint Dislocations *S/S*: Pain, swelling, and loss of function. In an open fracture, there is a bone protruding through the skin, creating a wound. If the joint is dislocated, the joint will appear deformed. Deformity may also occur with fractures.	• Immobilize the broken bone or dislocated joint using a splint (Figure 21–6a–c). Do not move the victim until it is immobilized unless there is no other option. If no medical supplies are available, look around for items that will work as an alternate splint (e.g., a thick twig or board could be used on each side of a leg or arm and attached with strips of cloth, a sweater could be used to make a sling for the arm).	• This prevents further injury.

(continues)

PROCEDURE 21-3

(continued)

CONDITION AND SIGNS AND SYMPTOMS	PROCEDURE	RATIONALE
Fractures and Joint Dislocations (continued)	• Do not attempt to realign a misshapen bone or joint. Do not test for function.	• This may cause further injury to the tissues. For example, it could cause hemorrhage, nerve damage, or embolus (a mass that travels through the body and can cause damage elsewhere by obstructing blood flow).
	• Do not give anything by mouth.	• May require surgical repair of the bone.
	• If there is an open fracture, cover it with a dressing prior to immobilizing the area. Do not wash or attempt to remove anything from the area.	• The dressing prevents further contamination of the wound. Washing or removing anything from the area can result in further damage.
	• When immobilizing an area, leave it in the position you found it and make sure that the area above and below is supported, so the injured area is immobilized.	• This prevents further injury.
	• Check for circulation below the injury to ensure that the splint is not too tight.	• Lack of circulation can result in damage to and death of the tissues.
Muscle Strain (Pulled Muscle) *S/S:* Sudden tearing sensation felt during exertion, followed by pain and swelling.	• Remove any constricting clothing or jewelry.	• Clothing and jewelry act as a constricting band if swelling occurs.
	• Apply cold compresses as soon as possible and repeat every 3–4 hours for 15–20 minutes.	• This decreases swelling.
	• Do not place ice directly on the skin.	• Freezing the skin causes tissue damage.
	• Elevate the limb.	• This decreases swelling.
	• Contact a physician if the pain is severe, if there is loss of function or impairment of circulation below injury, or if the area is misshapen.	• The injury will need medical evaluation and treatment.
	• A physician may also recommend an over-the-counter anti-inflammatory medication.	• This decreases inflammation and swelling.

(continues)

PROCEDURE 21-3

(continued)

CONDITION AND SIGNS AND SYMPTOMS	PROCEDURE	RATIONALE
Muscle Strain (pulled muscle) (continued)	• Rest the injured area for at least 24 hours. Do not use the injured area if pain occurs with movement.	• Allows the injury to heal and prevents further injury.
	• If there is no improvement, seek medical assistance.	• The injured area needs further evaluation.
Sprain *S/S:* Pain and swelling; loosening of the joint. Unless there is a complete tear, the joint will still function.	• Same as for muscle strain.	• Same as for muscle strain.

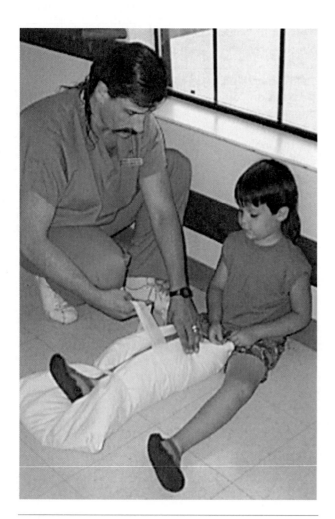

Figure 21–6a Splints should be long enough to immobilize the joint above and below the injured area.

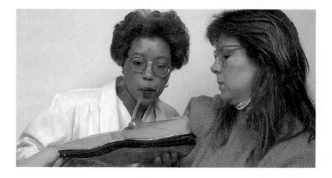

Figure 21–6b Some air splints are inflated by blowing into a nozzle. Care must be taken to avoid over-inflating any split. Always check for a pulse.

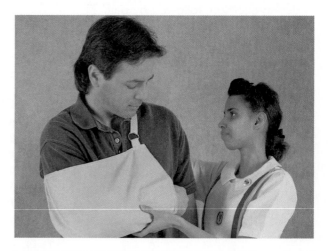

Figure 21–6c Commercial slings usually have a series of straps that extend around the neck and the trunk of the body.

Injuries to Facial Structures

Injuries to the eyes, ears, and nose are common. Any eye injury should always be taken very seriously because it can involve the loss of vision. A blow to the ear can cause loss of hearing.

See Procedure 21–4 for first aid related to injuries of the facial structures.

P R O C E D U R E 21-4

First Aid for Facial Injuries
***Observe Standard Precautions**

CONDITION AND SIGNS AND SYMPTOMS	PROCEDURE	RATIONALE
Eye Injuries *S/S*: Tearing, redness, stinging, burning, or pain in or around eye, sensitivity to light, and rapid blinking. Blows to the eye can cause internal bleeding and damage to the tissues.	• Do not press on the eye or allow the victim to rub the eyes. • If a foreign object is irritating the eye, flush the eye with a large amount of water. • Do not use cotton swabs (e.g., Q-Tips) or any instruments (tweezers) to try and remove objects from eye. • If the object is not flushed out and is embedded, do not attempt to remove it, instead cover both eyes with a dressing and await medical assistance. • If there has been a blow to the eye, lay victim flat, cover both eyes, and call for medical assistance. • If a "black eye" is forming, apply cold compress to area.	• This prevents further injury. • Loose particles will wash away in the water. • Cotton sheds fibers that will get in the eye. Sharp instruments can cause further damage. • Trying to remove the object can create more damage. Covering both eyes decreases movement of injured eye. • Laying the victim flat decreases loss of fluid from the eye. Covering both eyes decreases movement of the eyes. • Decreases bleeding by causing vasoconstriction (constriction of blood vessels).
Ear Injuries *S/S*: Bleeding or drainage from the ear, loss of hearing, earache, redness, bruising, or swelling around ear. Ruptured eardrum causes severe pain.	• Do not block bleeding or drainage from the ear. If possible, lay the victim on his or her side with the injured ear down. • Do not attempt to clean inside the ear. • If an object is in the ear and clearly visible, place the victim's injured ear downward and gently wiggle the object with a tweezers.	• Promoting drainage will prevent build up of pressure in ear that can cause more damage. • This prevents further injury and contamination. • This may dislodge the object, and it will fall out as a result of gravity.

(continues)

PROCEDURE 21-4

(continued)

CONDITION AND SIGNS AND SYMPTOMS	PROCEDURE	RATIONALE
Ear Injuries (continued)	• Do not attempt to remove an object that is not visible. Seek medical assistance. • If ruptured eardrum is suspected, place a dressing over ear. Seek medical assistance. • If an insect is in the ear, do not allow the victim to poke a finger into ear. Have the victim hold his or her head with the ear pointing up. If medical assistance is not immediately available, the victim is very uncomfortable, and that you are sure it is only an insect, place several drops of room-temperature oil into the ear (e.g., cooking oil, baby oil, mineral oil). Seek medical assistance.	• This may push the object further into the ear canal. • This prevents contamination of ear. • Putting an object in the ear may cause an insect to bite or sting. The insect may climb out on its own if given an opportunity. Oil will drown the insect, but can dangerously expand other objects that may be in the ear.
Nose Injuries Most nose bleeds (epitaxis) stop on their own, but if not, first aid may be needed. *S/S*: Blood coming from the nostrils or running down the back of the throat. If the bleeding is from the back of the nose, there may be a feeling of fullness in the ears, coughing up blood, gagging, or choking due to blood in the back of the throat. A broken nose may look crooked.	• If there is an object lodged in the nostril, attempt to remove it by having the victim hold the other nostril and blow out the nostril with the object, or have the victim sniff some pepper to induce a sneeze. If this does not work, get medical help. • Do not put anything into the nostril to try and grab hold of the object. • Instruct the victim to breathe through the mouth and not inhale through the nostril. • If the nose may be broken, have the victim sit down, lean forward, and apply a cold compress. • Do not attempt to straighten a broken nose, but seek medical assistance.	• This increases pressure behind the object to propel it out. • This may push the object in further. • This decreases the risk of blood entering into lungs. • Leaning forward helps prevent blood from running down the back of the throat. A cold compress decreases bleeding by constricting blood vessels. • This may cause further damage.

(continues)

PROCEDURE 21-4

(continued)

CONDITION AND SIGNS AND SYMPTOMS	PROCEDURE	RATIONALE
Nose Injuries (continued)	• If the nose is not broken, attempt to stop the bleeding by instructing the victim to sit down and lean forward while applying pressure on the soft part of the nose. Maintain the pressure for at least 15 minutes, then release. If there's still bleeding, repeat the procedure for 15 more minutes. Then, if it has not stopped, seek medical assistance.	• Leaning forward helps prevent blood from running down the back of throat. Applying pressure decreases the blood flow and encourages clotting. If you cannot stop the bleeding, medical evaluation and treatment is needed.

Burns

Burns can occur from heat, radiation, chemicals, or electrical current. The severity of the burn is determined by the size, depth, and location of the burn. Minor burns are referred to as *superficial* or *first degree burns* because only the top layer of skin (epidermis) is involved. If the burn continues and extends beyond the superficial layer to the dermis, it is a *partial thickness* or *second-degree burn* (Figure 21–7). If the burn continues even deeper, it is a *full thickness* or *third degree burn* (Figure 21–8). The amount of pain the victim reports does not necessarily reflect the severity of the burn as the deeper burns can destroy nerve endings and be painless (Figure 21–9).

When caring for burns, remember the following three steps:

1. Stop the burning.
2. Cool the burned area.
3. Cover the burned area with clean, dry dressings (apply loosely).

See Procedure 21–5 for first aid related to the various sources of burns.

When treating burn victims, always assess them for the possibility of damage to the respiratory system through inhalation of smoke or fumes from chemicals. The damage to the respiratory system can cause swelling that will prevent the

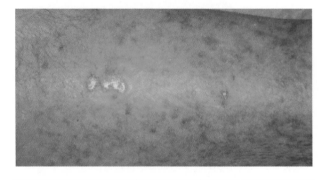

Figure 21–7 Second-degree or partial thickness burn: The skin is wet, red, swollen, painful, and blistered. (Courtesy of the Phoenix Society of Burn Survivors, Inc.)

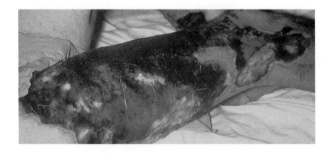

Figure 21–8 Third-degree or full thickness burn: All layers of the skin, plus the fat, muscles, bone and nerve tissues may be destroyed. (Courtesy of the Phoenix Society of Burn Survivors, Inc.)

victim from breathing properly. Look for discoloration around the nostrils or mouth as a possible indication. If it is likely the victim has inhaled smoke or fumes (was in a smoky room, exposed to chemical fumes, or has discolored nostrils) but is not experiencing difficulty in breathing, do not dismiss the problem because the effects can be delayed for up to 24 hours.

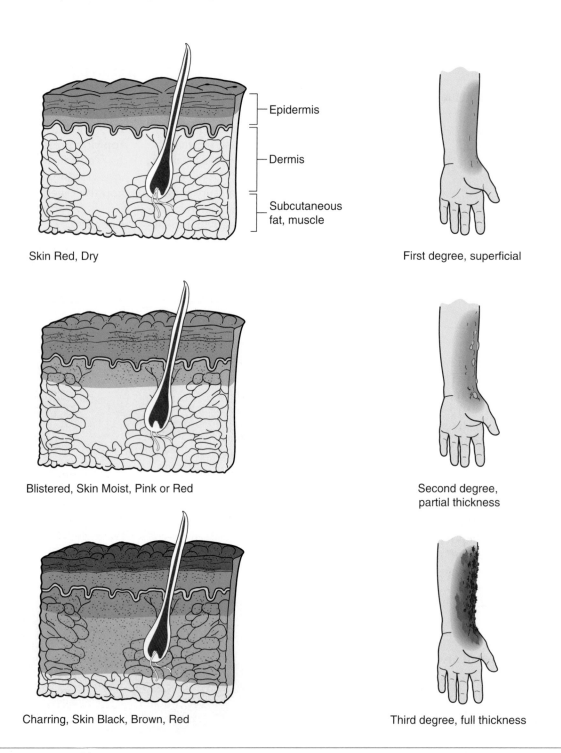

Epidermis

Dermis

Subcutaneous fat, muscle

Skin Red, Dry

First degree, superficial

Blistered, Skin Moist, Pink or Red

Second degree, partial thickness

Charring, Skin Black, Brown, Red

Third degree, full thickness

Figure 21–9 Types of burns.

PROCEDURE 21-5

First Aid for Burns
*Observe Standard Precautions

CONDITION	PROCEDURE	RATIONALE
Heat (e.g., flames, hot liquids, or grease)	• Extinguish the fire (i.e., if the victim's clothing is on fire).	• This stops the burning.
	• Move the victim to a well-ventilated area, if smoke is present. Move accident victims only when it is necessary to protect them.	• This protects victim from damage to respiratory tract due to smoke inhalation.
	• When moving victims, maintain their body alignment.	• This prevents further damage in the event they may have a neck or back injury.
	• Run cool water over the burn area for several minutes or immerse the area in cool water (use a cool, wet cloth on areas that cannot be immersed and rewet as necessary by pouring additional cool water onto the cloth).	• This cools the burned area. Cooling should not be done if a burn is major or covers an extensive area, because it can dangerously lower the body temperature.
	• Do not apply ice except on a minor burn, such as a finger burnt on the stove.	• This can freeze tissue and cause further damage.
	• Remove clothing from the burn area if possible, but if it's stuck to the burn, do not use force.	• It will increase damage to tissues if clothing is forcibly removed.
	• Do not break blisters.	• Blisters form a natural sterile protection to area.
	• Cover the burn with a clean, dry cloth (use sterile, non-adhesive dressings if available).	• Cover the burned area to prevent contamination.
	• Do not apply any ointments to a severe burn.	• Ointments can hold the heat in, increasing the severity of the burn.
	• Apply a bandage loosely.	• This prevents pressure on the burn.
	• Do not use cotton as a dressing.	• Cotton adheres and leaves small fibers embedded in the wound.
	• Prevent chilling.	• Chilling is common with burns.

(continues)

PROCEDURE 21-5

(continued)

CONDITION	PROCEDURE	RATIONALE
Radiation (e.g., sunburn)	• Move the victim so he or she is no longer exposed to the sun.	• This stops the burning.
	• Cool the burn as discussed above.	• Same as above
	• Apply a dressing as discussed above.	• Same as above
	• Prevent chilling.	• Same as above
Chemicals (numerous household and environmental products cause burns when in contact with skin)	• Prevent any further contact of the victim with the chemical.	• If any chemical remains on the victim's clothing, it will continue to burn the victim; if possible, remove any clothing and jewelry exposed to the chemical.
	• Move the victim to a well-ventilated area if fumes are present. Move accident victims only when it is necessary to protect them.	• Protects victim from damage to the respiratory tract due to inhalation of fumes.
	• When moving victims, maintain their body alignment.	• Same as above
	• Flush the burn with large amounts of cool water and continue to do so until EMS arrive.	• This cools the burn.
	• Always flush away from the body.	• This prevents the chemical-laden water from touching unexposed areas of the skin.
	• If there is any chemical in the eyes, flush them continuously with cool water.	• Eyes are very sensitive to chemical burns, and vision may be lost if chemicals are not completely removed.
	• If only one eye is affected, flush from the inner aspect of the eye to the outer (Figure 21–10).	• Prevents the chemical from getting into the other eye.
Electrical Current (electrical cords or lines and lightning)	• Do not touch the victim if he or she is still in contact with a live electrical wire (have the power turned off first).	• As the rescuer, you must protect yourself first. If you are unable to touch the victim, call EMS.

(continues)

PROCEDURE 21-5

(continued)

CONDITION	PROCEDURE	RATIONALE
Electrical Current (continued)	• Do not cool the burn. • Apply a clean dry dressing. • Prevent chilling and do not move victim if possible, because other injuries may be present.	• Burns are not on the surface. • This prevents contamination. • There will usually be only a small burn area noted on the surface, but extensive internal damage can be present, caused by the current as it traveled through the body (look for an exit burn also).

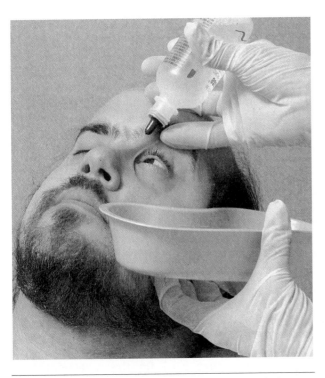

Figure 21–10 To flush an eye, hold the eyelid open and run the water from the inner part of the eye toward the outer part.

Drug Abuse

Drug abuse refers to the misuse or overuse of any drug. These drugs may be legal or illegal, prescription or over the counter, and include any substance that alters how the body functions. For example, prescription and over-the-counter medications, caffeine, alcohol, nicotine, or any illegal drug preparation can cause life-threatening situations.

Another condition that can cause the need for medical intervention is when an addictive drug is taken and the body develops a craving for more of the drug. If the drug is not continued, the body will go through a process of withdrawal that can also create life-threatening situations.

See Procedure 21–6 for first aid related to drug overdose and withdrawal.

Poisoning

Poisoning most frequently occurs through ingestion and inhalation. Poisons that come in contact with the skin are treated similarly to burns that occur when caustic chemicals come into contact with skin. The procedure is to perform lots of flushing to remove the poison, while taking care not to get it on the victim's uncontaminated areas or on the rescuer's skin.

If you suspect poisoning, do not wait for signs and symptoms to develop, instead seek medical assistance immediately. Do not rely on the label's directions, because they may be incorrect. Instead call the Poison Control Center or EMS because they can supply you with the information needed to immediately and most effectively treat the poison victim.

PROCEDURE 21-6

First Aid for Drug-Related Problems
*Observe Standard Precautions

CONDITION AND SIGNS AND SYMPTOMS	PROCEDURE	RATIONALE
Drug Overdose *S/S:* Behavioral changes, such as over-excitation, hallucinations, and agitation. There may be difficulty breathing, drowsiness, tremors, and excessive sweating. The size of the pupil is frequently smaller or larger than normal. Nausea and vomiting may occur. Seizures and unconsciousness may develop.	• Call EMS. • Try to determine what was taken, when, how much, and which route (e.g. oral, inhalation, injection). Be aware that it may have been more than one type or also combined with alcohol or other substances. • If possible, collect samples of the drug and of any vomit for analysis.	• Needs medical evaluation and intervention. • Assists in determination of treatment. • Can be analyzed to assist in determination of treatment.
Withdrawal From Addictive Drug *S/S:* Behavioral changes, such as extreme restlessness, hallucinations, depression, anxiety, and agitation. Tremors and cold sweats may occur. Nausea and vomiting may occur. Seizures may develop. The main focus of the victim may be to find some of the drug he or she is withdrawing from in order to alleviate the discomfort.	• Call EMS. • Try to determine what drug the victim has been taking. • Keep the victim safe and comfortable until medical assistance arrives.	• Same as above • Same as above • The victim may harm himself or herself when experiencing severe behavioral changes or if seizures occur.

Identifying the source of the poison is important in determining the proper treatment for the victim. If the victim is unable to give any information (is a child, unconscious, or confused), look around for any clues as to the source of the poison (e.g., empty bottle or other container, source of fumes, traces of powders or liquids in area, poisonous plants, and bystander information).

The most critical component of poisoning first aid is prevention. Since young children are the frequent victims of accidental poisoning, it is essential to keep all harmful substances locked in cabinets or out of the reach of children. Remember that children can be quite inventive in using furniture to climb up to reach desired objects, so using a locked cabinet is the preferred approach.

Poisoning by ingestion can be caused by many common products found around the home such as cleaning agents, yard care products, cosmetics, medications, paints, plants, car fluids, personal care items, and spoiled food or contaminated water. Inhalation dangers include sources of poisonous fumes, such as gas leaks, automobile exhaust, and chemical fumes.

See Procedure 21–7 for first aid related to poisoning.

Temperature-Related Illness

Exposure to excessive cold can cause cold-related injuries. If the skin begins to freeze, it is called **frostbite**. Frostbite occurs most frequently on the extremities or exposed areas, such as fingers, toes, nose, cheeks, and earlobes. If the body

PROCEDURE 21-7

First Aid for Poisonings
*Observe Standard Precautions

CONDITION AND SIGNS AND SYMPTOMS	PROCEDURE	RATIONALE
Ingestion (swallowing) *S/S:* Vary widely depending on the substance ingested and how it affects the various systems. For example GI symptoms may include nausea, vomiting, diarrhea, abdominal pain, or loss of appetite. The skin may be pale, and the victim may feel dizzy, weak, irritable, or drowsy. There may be pain on swallowing or burns or residue around the mouth. There may be seizures or complete loss of consciousness.	• The goal of immediate treatment is to get the poison out of the body, but do not administer any food, fluids, or home remedies, or induce vomiting unless directed to do so by medical personnel. • If the victim does vomit, make sure the vomit is cleared from the mouth. • Save any vomit. • Keep the patient safe and comfortable until help can arrive.	• Getting the poison out of the body will prevent further absorption of the poison, but inducing vomiting for a substance that burned the GI system on the way down, will also burn it on the way up. • This prevents it from blocking the airway and from entering the lungs. • It can be analyzed to identify the source of the poisoning. • This prevents further injury and decreases anxiety.
Inhalation (breathing) *S/S:* Vary depending on the substance inhaled. May be similar to the above listed S&S.	• The goal of immediate treatment is to get the victim into fresh air. • Before entering an environment where poisonous gases may be present, apply protective breathing gear. If no protective breathing gear is available, place a wet cloth over your nose and mouth, and then take several deep breaths of fresh air before entering to remove the victim. • If there is a visible cloud of fumes, keep your head above or below it. • If possible, open windows and doors and turn off any source of fumes. • Do not light any flames or flip any switches. • When the victim is in fresh air, the Poison Control Center or EMS can be called. • The victim should be kept safe and comfortable until help arrives.	• Prevents further inhalation of poisonous gas. • The rescuer must protect himself or herself against becoming the second victim of the fumes. • The cloud will contain the highest concentration of fumes. • This decreases the concentration of fumes in area. • Fumes may ignite. • You will need further directions on care and the victim may need medical intervention. • Prevents further injury and decreases anxiety.

temperature drops below normal, it is **hypothermia**. Hypothermia can occur inside and outside of the home, depending on a number of conditions. Conditions that contribute to hypothermia are extreme cold, wet clothes, and being immersed in cold water. Newborns, the elderly, and those in poor health can become hypothermic in an underheated room.

Exposure to excessive heat can cause heat-related injuries. Being outside in high temperatures and humidity can cause the body temperature to increase above normal (**hyperthermia**),

and a loss of body fluids by excessive perspiration can result in the loss of salt and subsequent dehydration. Certain medications and medical conditions can aggravate the problem. Newborns, the elderly, and those in poor health can become hyperthermic in an overheated room with poor ventilation. Other contributing factors are obesity, excessive exercise, and ingestion of alcohol. The heat-related illnesses from least to most severe are heat cramps, heat exhaustion, and heat stroke.

See Procedure 21–8 for first aid for temperature-related illnesses.

PROCEDURE 21-8

First Aid for Temperature-Related Illnesses
*Observe Standard Precautions

CONDITION AND SIGNS AND SYMPTOMS	PROCEDURE	RATIONALE
Frostbite *S/S*: Initially the skin is red and painful, then as the skin begins to freeze, it loses feeling (numbness), then becomes hard and white and blisters. In severe frostbite, the blood vessels freeze, and the skin becomes black due to the death of tissues from lack of oxygen.	• Do not thaw out the area unless it can be kept thawed. • Do not massage the area. • Do not use direct heat to thaw the area. • Remove any constricting clothes or jewelry. • To thaw the frozen area, place it in warm water or apply a warm cloth; keep water or cloth warm (not hot) until area softens, and color and sensation return; as the area thaws, pain and swelling can be expected. • After thawing, apply a sterile, dry dressing. • If fingers or toes are frostbitten, place a dressing between them. • Move the thawed area as little as possible. • Discourage smoking or drinking alcohol.	• Refreezing will increase damage. • This increases damage to tissues • This thaws the area too quickly. • This increases circulation. • This thaws the area slowly. • This prevents contamination. • This keeps them separated. • This minimizes damage to tissue. • Both constrict the blood vessels and decrease circulation to the affected area.

(continues)

PROCEDURE 21-8

(continued)

CONDITION AND SIGNS AND SYMPTOMS	PROCEDURE	RATIONALE
Hypothermia *S/S*: In mild cases there is shivering, skin is cold to the touch, and there is confusion and lack of coordination. In severe cases the shivering stops; coordination problems increase, along with slurred speech and problems with vision; the heart rate slows; and the victim becomes drowsy and just wants to be left alone. The victim can become irrational and uncooperative. If untreated, the victim will progress to coma and death.	• If frostbite and hypothermia are present, treat the hypothermia first. • If respirations are below 6/minute, begin rescue breathing. • If possible, gently move the victim to a shelter. • Remove wet clothes and replace them with dry ones. • Remove constricting clothes and jewelry. • Do not use direct heat. • Apply warm packs (towels or linens) to the neck, chest, and groin. • If the victim is able to drink, give him or her warm, sweet fluids. • Wrap the victim in a space blanket (contains an insulating material that prevents heat from escaping) or aluminum foil, including the neck and head; the rescuer can also place his or her own body next to the victim to warm him or her.	• Hypothermia is the most life-threatening. • This supplies victim with needed oxygen. • This removes victim from further exposure. • Wet clothes increase the cooling of the body. • This increases circulation. • It may burn victim. • Warms the body. • This warms the body internally and supplies some calories. • Assists in rewarming the victim.
HEAT-RELATED CONDITIONS: **Heat Cramps** *S/S*: Muscle cramps in the abdomen and legs, lightheadedness, and weakness may occur when excess salt and fluid is lost from the body (heavy perspiration). If the problem progresses to heat exhaustion, the skin may appear pale or red, cool to the touch, and moist; the victim may complain of headache, thirst, weakness, and dizziness; the pupils will be dilated (larger than normal), and nausea and vomiting may occur; behavior may be irrational or victim may be unconscious.	• Do not give liquids that contain alcohol or caffeine. • Do not give any medication used to lower the temperature (e.g., aspirin or Tylenol). • Do not give salt tablets, instead use a salt and water solution or an electrolyte drink (e.g., Gatorade or Pedialyte).	• The victim needs water and electrolytes to replenish their loss. • This does not treat the underlying problem. • Salt and water solutions replenish fluid and electrolytes.

(continues)

PROCEDURE 21-8

(continued)

CONDITION AND SIGNS AND SYMPTOMS	PROCEDURE	RATIONALE
Heat Cramps (continued)	• Move the victim to the shade or a cooled room and elevate the feet if not prohibited (e.g., causes difficulty breathing; there's a head, neck, spine or leg injury; or it makes the victim uncomfortable).	• It is important to begin the cooling process immediately.
	• Apply cool water to their body (do not use alcohol rub); wrap the victim in cool towels and turn on fan.	• This aids in cooling by increasing the evaporative process.
	• Apply cold towels to the back of the neck, on the groin, and under the arms.	• This cools the major areas where blood vessels are close to the surface.
	• When the temperature lowers to 100 degrees F, the cooling effort can be stopped, but monitor victim closely for the next 2–4 hours.	• This victim may relapse even after apparent recovery.
Heat Stroke The skin will be dry, hot, and red; confusion, weakness, and seizures may occur; pupils will be constricted (smaller than normal), pulse rapid and weak, and breathing rapid and shallow; the body temperature will be markedly increased (above 102 degrees F); the victim may be unconscious.	• Call EMS.	• This condition is life-threatening.
	• Do not give liquids to a victim with heat stroke.	• Fluids may enter lungs. EMS will start an IV when they arrive.
	• If EMS are not immediately available, immerse victim in cold water, but monitor his or her alertness, pulse and respirations closely.	• This starts the cooling process.

Other Conditions

There are a number of other conditions that frequently occur that may require the assistance of someone trained in first aid. Some of them may be seen in conjunction with other conditions discussed in the last section, such as shock, fainting, and seizures. Knowledge of these conditions will prepare the rescuer to take the appropriate actions when they occur. See Procedure 21–9 for first aid related to these conditions.

PROCEDURE 21-9

First Aid for Other Common Conditions
*Observe Standard Precautions

CONDITION AND SIGNS AND SYMPTOMS	PROCEDURE	RATIONALE
Breathing Difficulty Problems with breathing can be caused by many sudden illnesses, injuries, or worsening medical conditions. *S/S*: Shortness of breath, coughing, audible sounds (wheezing, gurgling, whistling) coming from respiratory system, and exaggerated use of chest muscles to breath. If victim is not getting enough oxygen, the mouth and fingertips may be pale or bluish in color.	• Do not place a pillow under the victim's head. • Loosen any constricting clothing and assist the victim into the most comfortable position, unless neck or back injury is suspected. • Ask the victim if there is any medication he or she takes for the problem (i.e., an asthmatic may have an inhaler with them). • Call EMS and keep the victim safe and comfortable until help arrives.	• This may close off the airway. • Constricting clothing may prevent the victim from breathing deeply. • Symptoms may be alleviated with their medication. • The victim may need evaluation and treatment.
Hyperventilation Rapid breathing that causes the carbon dioxide level in the blood to fall too low. The most common cause is anxiety, but it may also be caused by illness, injury, or certain medications. *S/S*: Fast, shallow respiratory rate, followed by the sensation of numbness around mouth and in the hands and feet. The blood pressure may fall and fainting can occur.	• Have the victim breath into a paper bag, hold one nostril closed (make sure the mouth is closed) while breathing, or have them cup their hands over their mouth and nose while breathing. • Victim will need a calm and reassuring approach. Encouraging the victim to talk is often helpful.	• These techniques are effective in returning the carbon dioxide level in the blood stream to normal. • Condition is often caused by or worsened with anxiety.
Chest pain (angina) Chest pain associated with a lack of oxygen getting to the heart muscle. Damage to the heart muscle from a lack of oxygen is called a heart attack or myocardial infarction. *S/S*: Pain is described as dull or crushing (victim may state that "it feels like an elephant is sitting on my chest"). The pain may radiate to the shoulder, arm or jaw. There may be difficulty breathing and heart palpitations. Frequently, the victim will perspire heavily, feel nauseated and anxious, and skin will be pale or bluish and moist.	• Always call EMS immediately.	• Many victims deny that they are having a heart attack and instead explain it as indigestion. They may be correct, but any chest pain needs to be evaluated medically to determine if the victim had a heart attack.

(continues)

PROCEDURE 21-9

(continued)

CONDITION AND SIGNS AND SYMPTOMS	PROCEDURE	RATIONALE
Chest pain (angina) (continued)	• Have the victim stop any activity they were doing. • If the victim has medication for angina, assist him or her in taking it. • Do not give the victim anything to eat or drink. • Loosen any constricting clothing and keep the victim warm. • Stay with the victim until help arrives. • Start rescue breathing if he or she stops breathing or give full CPR if the heart stops.	• This decreases the demand on the heart. • Many people with recurring chest pain have a medication called nitroglycerine that is placed under the tongue. • This increases demand on the heart and the victim may develop nausea and vomiting. • This encourages full deep breathing and circulation. • If the condition worsens they may need rescue breathing or CPR. • Brain damage occurs in as little as 3–5 minutes when the brain is deprived of oxygen.
Diabetes Lack of adequate insulin production results in an elevated blood sugar; if too much medication is taken to correct this condition, the blood sugar may become too low. *S/S: High blood sugar* (hyperglycemia) develops gradually and is characterized by excessive thirst, hunger, and urination. There may be vomiting, flushed skin, rapid breathing, and a fruity smell to the breath. The victim may be confused and resist your attempt to assist. If left untreated, the victim will go into a diabetic coma. *S/S: Low blood sugar* (hypoglycemia) develops more rapidly and is characterized by sweating, hunger, confusion, pale skin, and poor coordination. This is referred to as an insulin reaction and if left untreated will result in coma and death.	• If the victim states that his or her blood sugar is too high and he or she needs to have an insulin injection, assist the patient with the administration of the medication. • Get medical help and stay with the victim to monitor his or her condition. • If the victim is conscious, give him or her unsweetened liquids. • If the victim states their blood sugar is too low, immediately give them something sweet (e.g. fruit juice, sugar in water, candy). If this is the problem, they should improve within 5–15 minutes after administration of the sweet.	• Many diabetics are very familiar with the signs and symptoms and know how to treat it. • The condition may worsen and further assistance will be needed. • Liquids with sugar will make the problem worse. Unsweetened liquids will combat the dehydration that occurs with hyperglycemia. • Many diabetics are very familiar with the signs and symptoms and know how to treat it. Sweetened items increase the blood sugar.

(continues)

PROCEDURE 21-9

(continued)

CONDITION AND SIGNS AND SYMPTOMS	PROCEDURE	RATIONALE
Diabetes (continued)	• When recovered, the victim should eat some protein and carbohydrates (e.g. crackers and cheese or peanut butter and bread). • If the victim does not recover or is unconscious, call EMS. • If in doubt as to whether it is high or low blood sugar treat it with something sweet.	• This prevents further insulin reaction because the quick acting sweets are digested and eliminated quickly. • The victim needs further evaluation and treatment. • If it is low blood sugar, the victim should recover quickly, and if high blood sugar, the additional sweet will not significantly affect the problem.
Fainting (syncope) *S/S*: Brief loss of consciousness that comes on quickly perhaps due to low blood sugar, standing too long, or low blood pressure when arising too rapidly from a lying or sitting position. Sometimes there are warning signs (dizziness, nausea, weakness, and blurred vision), but not always. A loss of consciousness after a head injury is not fainting, but a concussion.	• If you're present when victim is falling, assist him or her gently to the floor. • Place the victim on his or her back and elevate the legs 8–12 inches. • Do not place a pillow under the head. • Loosen any constricting clothing. • Do not attempt to awaken the victim by throwing water on him or her, shaking, or slapping the face. • If vomiting occurs turn the head to the side. • Call EMS if the victim is not alert within approximately 5 minutes, is elderly, or other signs and symptoms are noted that may indicate another problem.	• This prevents injury from the fall. • This increases blood circulation to the brain. • This may obstruct airway. • This allows for deeper breathing and better circulation. • This is not an effective technique and may injure victim. • This prevents vomit from obstructing airway and entering the lungs. • The victim needs further evaluation and treatment.

(continues)

PROCEDURE 21-9

(continued)

CONDITION AND SIGNS AND SYMPTOMS	PROCEDURE	RATIONALE
Fever (hyperthermia) *S/S*: An increase in body temperature. Is usually caused by the body's attempt to combat infection (for elevated temperature related to exposure to heat, see hyperthermia under Temperature-Related Illnesses). Children are particularly susceptible to high fevers when an infection is present. The fever can rise quickly and result in seizures. The younger the child, the more sensitive he or she is to an increase in temperature.	• Remove excess clothing and blankets. • Gently cool the child by sponging him or her with lukewarm water. • Call the physician at once for further instructions, such as giving medication to bring the fever down (e.g., aspirin or Tylenol). • Even lower fevers that persist over 24 hours need to be evaluated. • Call EMS if child is having difficulty breathing, has unusual skin color, a stiff neck, or appears ill.	• Excess coverings can increase body temperature. • This lowers the body temperature. • Fevers can rise very quickly in children, even to the point of causing brain damage. • The cause needs to be determined. • This may indicate a serious underlying condition requiring immediate treatment.
Drowning Unconsciousness and death results from the lack of oxygen to the body as water enters the respiratory tract. Drowning can occur in only a few inches of water if the victim is a child or an injured victim. The most common causes are accidents, sudden illness, cramping, alcohol consumption, and getting into areas where the person is not a strong enough swimmer to return to safety. *S/S*: Skin cold and pale. Lips, earlobes, and fingernails are a bluish color. The victim may not be breathing.	• Be on the alert for irregular swimming strokes, only the head is above the water, and if the person is fully dressed. • Call EMS. • Rescue the drowning victim if you can without endangering yourself. It is best not to enter the water, but to extend a stick, life preserver, or some other object for the victim to grab and then pull him or her to safety. • Do rescue breathing and treat the victim for hypothermia as needed. Do full CPR if no pulse is present.	• Drowning victims usually cannot call for help. • The victim will need evaluation and treatment. • If the rescuer enters the water he or she may become hypothermic, or the victim may panic and pull them under too. • If the water is quite cold, the victim may still be able to be revived, even if submerged for longer than 3–5 minutes.

(continues)

PROCEDURE 21-9

(continued)

CONDITION AND SIGNS AND SYMPTOMS	PROCEDURE	RATIONALE
Seizures (convulsions) Seizures are caused by irregular brain activity such as that seen in someone with epilepsy or they can be caused by a sudden change in a medical condition. Many of the other first aid emergencies discussed in this chapter can result in seizures. *S/S:* Sudden falling and loss of consciousness with drooling or frothing from the mouth. There may be loss of bowel or bladder control. Grunting or groaning may be heard. There are three common types of seizures: 1. Petit mal—brief unconsciousness, followed by confusion 2. Focal—localized twitching in one part of the body (e.g., face or arm) 3. Grand mal—generalized strong muscle spasms of entire body	• If the victim is falling, support the victim as he or she falls. • Remove any sharp objects in the area. • Loosen tight clothing. • Do not place anything into the mouth, try to restrain the victim, move the victim (unless in danger), or perform rescue breathing during a seizure. • Do not try to keep the victim awake, but place him or her on the stomach or side (if you suspect neck or back injury, roll the body as a unit to a side-lying position, while keeping the spine in straight alignment). Protect the airway if vomiting occurs. • Call EMS.	• This prevents injury to victim as he or she falls to the floor. • This protects the victim from injury. • This eases the ability to breathe. • Most seizures last less than a minute, and the main role of the rescuer is to keep the victim safe from harm. • After the seizure, the victim may go into a deep sleep after regaining consciousness momentarily and will probably be confused. • The victim may need further evaluation or treatment.
Shock Occurs when there is a disruption in the flow of blood to the cells throughout the body. Any medical emergency can cause shock. *S/S:* The victim may feel weak, dizzy, restless, or confused. The skin is pale, cold, and clammy. Lips, earlobes, and fingertips may be bluish in color. The respirations are shallow and rapid. Nausea, vomiting, and chest pain may be present. The victim may experience numbness and paralysis or be unconscious.	• Call EMS. • Place the victim in shock position if there is no neck or back injury (Figure 21–11). • Turn the victim's head to the side if there is vomiting or drooling. • Do not elevate the head. • Loosen restricting clothes and keep the victim warm. • Do not give the victim any liquids or food. • Give first aid for any under-lying illness or injury. • Do not use the shock position if it is uncomfortable.	• The victim needs further evaluation and treatment. • Elevating the lower extremities increases blood flow to the brain. • This prevents blockage of airway. • You want maximum flow of blood to brain to prevent brain damage. • This eases breathing and maintains blood flow. • The victim may vomit and block airway. • Shock is normally secondary to another problem. • The victim may have another injury or illness.

(continues)

PROCEDURE 21-9

(continued)

CONDITION AND SIGNS AND SYMPTOMS	PROCEDURE	RATIONALE
Shock (continued)	• Do not use the shock position if the victim has a sting or bite in the lower limbs. • Stay with patient and assist as needed until medical help arrives.	• This increases the release of venom into the system. • If the condition worsens, the victim may need rescue breathing or CPR performed.
Stroke or cerebrovascular accident (CVA) Caused by a ruptured or clogged artery in the brain resulting in death to the affected brain cells. *S/S:* Sudden onset of weakness, dizziness, headache, and unsteady coordination, followed by weakness or paralysis of face, arm, and leg or one side of the face. There may be slurred, garbled, or no speech, and the vision may be affected. If the signs and symptoms are temporary and disappear within 24 hours, it was not a stroke, but a condition called a transient ischemic attack (TIA). A TIA is a temporary lack of oxygen to brain cells and is completely reversible, but is a warning sign of a future potential stroke.	• Call EMS. • Help the victim get into a comfortable position. • Give no liquids or food by mouth. • Stay with patient and assist as needed until medical help arrives.	• The victim needs evaluation and treatment. • This eases breathing and anxiety. • The victim may vomit and block the airway. • If the condition worsens, the victim may need rescue breathing or CPR performed.
Unconsciousness Any medical emergency can result in the victim losing alertness and awareness of the surroundings. This state can range from a brief period, such as fainting to a prolonged coma. *S/S:* The victim may drift in and out of consciousness, varying from feeling drowsy, restless and unable to orient himself or herself or make sense when speaking to not moving or speaking at all.	• Call EMS if the victim does not quickly regain consciousness (i.e., fainting) or if illness or injury is evident. • The goal of the treatment of the unconscious victim is to maintain the airway. • Do not give anything by mouth. • Keep the victim warm.	• The victim needs medical evaluation and treatment. • The victim is unable to cough, clear the throat, or turn the head to drain vomit or drool from the mouth when the airway becomes obstructed. • The victim may choke on fluids or vomit and obstruct the airway. • This maintains good circulation.

(continues)

PROCEDURE 21-9

(continued)

CONDITION AND SIGNS AND SYMPTOMS	PROCEDURE	RATIONALE
Unconsciousness (continued)	• If there is no neck or back injury, place the victim in the recovery position by turning the head to the side, or turn the entire body to the side or onto the abdomen.	• This prevents obstruction of the airway if the victim vomits.
	• Gently tilt the victim's head back.	• This maintains the airway.
	• If neck or back injury is suspected leave the victim in the position you find him or her unless he or she is having difficulty breathing. If there is difficulty in breathing, choking, or vomiting, roll the entire body as a unit to a side-lying position while keeping the spine in straight alignment.	• This prevents further injury to neck or back.
	• Enlist the assistance of bystanders, if possible, when moving the victim to ensure the head, neck, and back stay in a straight line.	• It is easier to maintain body alignment when there are more people for turning in unison.
	• Give first aid for any underlying illness or injury.	• Unconsciousness is usually a result of another illness or condition.
	• If the victim becomes restless, you may have to gently restrain him or her.	• Prevents the victim from injuring himself or herself.
	• Stay with victim until medical assistance arrives.	• If the condition worsens, the victim may need rescue breathing or CPR performed.

Bandaging

Knowing how to apply slings and wraps can be very useful when working with a variety of injuries requiring first aid. The following types of slings and wraps are frequently used with musculoskeletal injuries.

Applying a Sling

A sling can be made from a large triangular cloth, a sweater, pillowcase, or other materials that can be cut to the appropriate size. It is used to support an injured shoulder, collarbone, or arm. If the arm is broken, apply the splint first to immobilize the broken bone, and then place it in the sling.

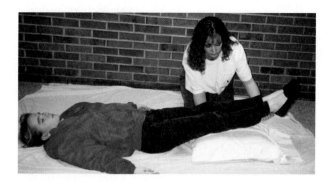

Figure 21–11 Place emergency victims in the shock position, unless they have neck, back, or lower limb injuries. Do not use the position if it is uncomfortable for the victim or if they have breathing difficulty.

Always check for circulation when applying splints and slings. Always support the injured arm when applying a sling. See Figure 21–12a–c for the steps to follow when applying a triangular sling.

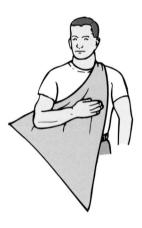

Figure 21–12a Support the injured part and slide the sling under the arm on the victim's injured side. Place top corner over the victim's non-injured shoulder.

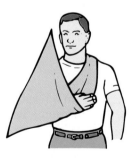

Figure 21–12b Pull the bottom corner of the sling up past the victim's chin and over the shoulder on the injured side. Leave the fingers showing.

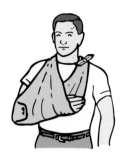

Figure 21–12c Tie the sling around the victim's neck, placing it a little to one side so the knot does not press on the back of the neck. Fold over the extra cloth at the victim's elbow and secure it with a safety pin.

Applying a Spiral Wrap

A spiral wrap can be used on arms, legs, and the trunk of the body. If you're using a wrap on the trunk, make sure that it is not so tight as to restrict chest movement during respirations. Also verify circulation in the fingers and toes if it's used on the arm or leg. See Figure 21–13a–b for the steps to follow when applying a spiral wrap.

Thinking it Through

John Street is a health care student and is feeling the need to get away from the stresses and routine of studying. He decides to take a hike in the local mountains with his friends. As they ascend the mountain it gets cooler and begins to rain. One of the hikers, Paul, starts to lag behind. Paul has always been a slower climber so they continue on. A little while later, John turns around to see how Paul is doing and can no longer see him. John backtracks and finds Paul sitting beside the trail. He is shivering and his skin is cold to the touch. Paul says he is just very tired and needs to rest for awhile and that he will catch up later.

1. Should John leave Paul to rest by himself?
2. What may be happening to Paul?
3. What first aid, if any, should be given to Paul?

Applying a Figure-Eight Wrap

A figure-eight wrap can be used to bandage a joint, such as an ankle, an elbow, or a wrist because it secures both sides of the joint. Using a spiral wrap is not effective for wrapping joints, because the wrap tends to slip off easily. Always verify circulation distal to the wrap to make sure the bandage is not too tight and cutting off circulation. See Figure 21–14a–b for the steps to follow when applying a figure-eight wrap.

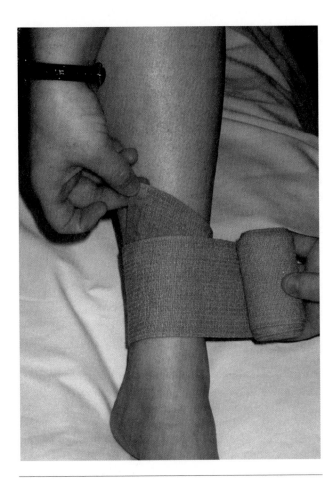

Figure 21–13a Always start wrap at distal end. Anchor the bandage by leaving a corner exposed. The corner is then folded down and covered when the bandage is circled around the limb. Overlap each rotation partially over the previous one to hold it securely in place.

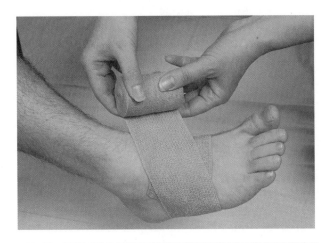

Figure 21–14a Anchor the bandage at the instep and secure it by wrapping it several times around the instep. Then bring the wrap up diagonally over the foot.

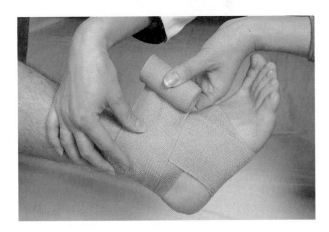

Figure 21–14b Bring it around back of the ankle and then down over the top of the foot and back under the instep. This creates a figure-eight pattern. Continue this process moving the wrap out in both directions (up the leg and toward the toes) with each repeat of pattern. Partially overlap each layer over the previous one to hold it securely in place.

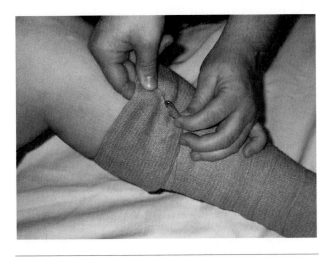

Figure 21–13b Place your hand between the bandage and the victim's skin while inserting pin.

Applying a Bandage to a Finger

A wrap for a finger can be made from a thin strip of gauze or cloth. It is used to support the finger and decrease movement. If the finger is broken, apply the splint first, using small twigs, pencils, or popsicle sticks on both sides, then wrap the finger. See Figure 21–15a–d for the steps to follow when applying a bandage to a finger.

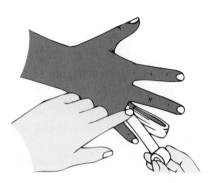

Figure 21–15a Place the end of the wrap at the bottom of one side of the finger and fold it over the tip of the finger and down to the bottom of the other side of the finger. Repeat this three to four times.

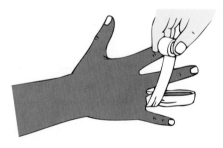

Figure 21–15b Start at the bottom of the finger and spiral the wrap up and down finger to hold it securely in place.

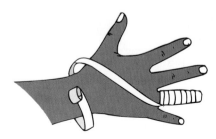

Figure 21–15c Secure the wrap by doing several figure-eight wraps around the wrist.

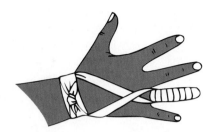

Figure 21–15d When the figure-eight wrap is complete, circle the wrist several times. Split the wrap and tie it in a knot or secure it with tape or a safety pin.

SUGGESTED LEARNING ACTIVITIES

1. If you do not already have a CPR certification, arrange to attend a class for certification. Classes can be located by calling your local health facilities, community colleges, the American Red Cross, or the American Heart Association.

2. Contact the American Red Cross and plan to attend their next first aid and safety class, if it is not part of your program of study.

3. Go to the Web site listed in the Fascinating Facts and learn more about home safety.

4. Evaluate your home environment for potential hazards and risks for injuries.

5. Practice the four types of slings and wraps on family, friends, or classmates.

REVIEW QUESTIONS

1. When should first aid be administered?
2. What is the Good Samaritan Act and how does it protect the rescuer?
3. What is the Golden Rule of first aid?
4. What are the seven steps to follow when an emergency occurs that will protect both the victim and rescuer?
5. When does the rescuer start CPR on a victim?

6. What are the signs and symptoms, and treatment for an allergic reaction?

7. What are the signs and symptoms, and treatment for bleeding and wounds?

8. What are the signs and symptoms, and treatment for bone, joint, and muscle injuries?

9. What are the signs and symptoms, and treatment for burns?

10. What are the signs and symptoms, and treatment for drug related emergencies?

11. What are the signs and symptoms, and treatment for poisoning?

12. What are the signs and symptoms, and treatment for temperature-related illnesses?

13. What are the signs and symptoms, and treatment for other common conditions that require emergency care?

14. What are the four common types of slings and wraps used to treat musculoskeletal injuries?

APPLICATION EXERCISES

1. Refer back to The Case of the Out-of-Control Party:

   a. What would have been appropriate first aid measures for the stabbing victim?

   b. Should Josephine remove the knife from the chest? Why or why not?

c. If there is bubbling coming from the chest wound, what would this indicate? What additional first aid measures would be necessary?

d. Which organs are located in the left chest that may have been damaged by the knife?

2. One hot day William notices his neighbor John mowing the lawn. He notes that John looks flushed and is sweating profusely, but he is overweight and out of shape and it is awfully hot and humid out to be doing any yard work today. Thirty minutes later, John's wife frantically knocks on the door and says John is having chest pain and she is very frightened. She says he has a heart condition and that she has called 9-1-1.

   a. What is the most likely cause of John's chest pain?

   b. What actions can William take until EMS arrives?

SUGGESTED READINGS AND RESOURCES

American Heart Association:
   http://www.americanheart.org
American Red Cross:
   http://www.redcross.org
American Red Cross (1995). *First aid fast.* Boston, MA: Staywell.
Tuttle-Yoder J. A. and Fraser-Nobbe, S. A. (1996). *STAT! Medical office emergency manual.* Albany, NY: Delmar.

UNIT

BUSINESS OF CARING

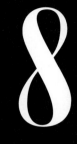
8

CHAPTER

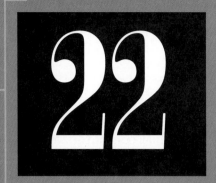

CONTROLLING HEALTH CARE COSTS

OBJECTIVES

Studying and applying the material in this chapter will help you to:

■ Describe how methods for paying medical costs have changed over the years.

■ Contrast fee-for-service and managed care reimbursement methods.

■ Explain the purpose of managed care systems and describe the methods used to control costs.

■ Define Medicare, Medicaid, and DRGs.

■ Identify the four major areas of expenditures incurred by a health care delivery system.

■ Define: accounts receivable, accounts payable, and the cost of money.

■ Explain ways that the health care worker can help control facility costs.

KEY TERMS

accounts payable

accounts receivable

capitation

copay

cost of money

diagnostic related group (DRG)

expenditures

fee-for-service

financing

gatekeeper

managed care

Medicare

Medicaid

negotiated fees

preauthorization

prepaid plans

premium

primary care provider (PCP)

profit

reimburse

The Case of

the Inefficient Office

Constance Madison has seen many changes in her career working in medical records. While computerization has helped organize recordkeeping, it has also brought feelings of disorder during periods of transition. Constance sometimes feels overwhelmed and frustrated with what seems to be endless paperwork, lack of support, duplication of effort, and insufficient time to do what needs to be done during the day. Her knowledge of the changes in health care delivery and the needs of the system keep her focused on doing her best to make a positive contribution during stressful times. She has made several suggestions to her supervisor that have been adopted by her department.

In this chapter you will gain an understanding of why there is a tremendous amount of change occurring in the health care environment and how you can look for ways to improve efficiency, rather than focusing on the problems. By learning how individual employees can contribute to the efficiency of the organization, you will be able to make a positive impact. Identifying areas of inefficiency and waste enables you to work toward their correction and the creation of a more enjoyable and productive work environment.

PAYING FOR HEALTH CARE

A major concern in the United States today is how to effectively control dramatically rising health care costs. As you recall from Chapter 2, the rise in health care costs has been attributed to technological advancements, specializations, aging population, and the number of diagnostic and treatment options available. More money is spent per person on health care in the United States than in any other country. One of the major focuses of the health care industry today is an attempt to control these costs. As a result, new ways of paying for health services are being developed.

In the past, patients paid the physician's asking price for services provided. For those who could not pay cash, payment might be fresh vegetables from the garden or a load of wood. As health care became more sophisticated and costly, insurance companies became the preferred method of covering costs. Patients paid the insurance company an agreed-upon amount, called a **premium**. When medical care was needed, patients would visit the physician of their choice and the physician would order tests, prescribe medications, admit the

patient to the hospital, or perform surgery. The physician determined what actions to take, and the insurance companies paid for the services. This was known as **fee-for-service**.

As costs rose in recent decades, insurance companies and other payers questioned the efficiency of fee-for-service as a pricing method. Rather than encouraging savings, they argued, it rewarded the providers who prescribed the most services, such as lab tests and diagnostic procedures. Payers believed that the providers of health care–physicians, hospitals, and other professionals and facilities–should be held accountable for costs. Duplication of services, unnecessarily long stays in hospitals, and expensive brand name drugs are examples of practices labeled as "wasteful."

Managed Care

One response to rising costs has been the development of **managed care** plans, which contain specific built-in cost controls. These plans incorporate business concepts designed to increase efficiency by giving health care providers incentives to cut costs. There are several variations of managed care plans in use today (Table 22–1). Simply stated, the goals of managed care are to:

- Provide health care that patients can afford.
- Ensure high-quality care.
- Discourage unnecessary costs.
- Eliminate duplication of procedures.
- Earn a **profit** (amount of money remaining after all costs of operating a business have been paid) for both health care providers and insurance companies. (Or, if nonprofit, ensure that income covers all costs.)

Managed care systems employ several methods in an effort to achieve these goals.

Prepaid Plans

One of the major attempts to reduce costs has been the development of **prepaid plans**. In these plans, health care providers are paid *before* rather than *after* services are performed. This payment method is based on the idea that providers can be motivated to be more efficient. Let's look at an example of how these plans work.

1. A health insurance company signs up 10,000 customers, known as enrollees.
2. Each of the 10,000 pays a monthly amount to the insurance company, known as a premium.
3. The insurance company contracts with a health care service group that agrees to provide medical services to the enrollees. The physicians are paid a set amount for each enrollee. This is the only payment they receive, regardless of the type or number of services provided to the patients. This method of payment is called **capitation**.
4. Enrollees must use the physicians who have contracted with the insurance company.

Depending on the plan, they may be required to pay a set amount for each visit to the health care provider. This is called a **copay**.

5. The goal is that costs will average out. Some patients will require more care than the set amount covers, while others will not seek any services.

While the practice of prepayment has been shown to increase efficiency in many cases, the method has opponents. Some argue that cost containment goals conflict with quality care goals. They worry that the number and quality of services will have to be sacrificed in order to increase profits. Several movements are underway at both the state and federal levels to pass laws to protect patient access to appropriate care.

Negotiated Fees

Another method for paying health care providers is by preagreed-upon amounts that are negotiated between health care providers and insurance companies, to pay for specific services. These are known as **negotiated fees**. They may cover all or only a percentage of the provider's actual charges. Depending on the type of plan, the patient pays the difference or the physicians accept as payment in full the amount paid by the insurance company.

Limitation of Access

Insurance coverage is based on the concept of spreading the risk. For example, the sellers of car insurance assume that not everyone who buys coverage will use it. There will be some accidents and stolen vehicles that must be paid for, but most people who are covered will never make a claim. Health insurance is based on the same principle. While some people will suffer serious health problems and

Table 22–1 Managed Care Systems

Health Maintenance Organization (HMO)	A prepaid medical group practice plan that provides a predetermined medical care benefit package. HMOs are both insurers and providers of health care.
Exclusive Provider Organization (EPO)	Similar to an HMO, but with greater flexibility for employers to create a benefits package specific to their company's needs.
Preferred Provider Organization (PPO)	A group of hospitals and physicians who contract on a fee-for-service basis with employers, insurance plans, or other third-party administrators.

cost more than the amount of their premiums, others will use much less. In order for this system to work, health insurance companies try to reduce the number of people who require expensive care. This can be accomplished in several ways:

- Requiring applicants for insurance to pass physical exams
- Not selling insurance to people who have certain preexisting conditions, such as heart disease
- Selling policies to people with preexisting conditions, but not covering the costs related to these conditions

While these methods help insurance companies earn enough money to cover their costs, it leaves many people who are most in need of health care without coverage. This challenge is one that has prompted calls for a system of national health care that would provide coverage for everyone, regardless of health condition or economic status.

Restriction of Usage

In addition to limiting access to coverage, several methods have been devised to reduce the overuse of services by patients.

Primary Care Providers

One of the most important control mechanisms is the use of **primary care providers (PCP)**, also known as **gatekeepers** (Williams, 2001). These are health care professionals, often physicians, who serve as the patient's first contact when entering the health care system. The PCP evaluates patient complaints and determines the appropriate level of care. Diagnostic procedures and treatment plans must be approved by PCPs in order to be covered by insurance. They provide the referrals that patients must have before seeing specialists. An advantage of the use of PCPs is that they provide consistency in patient care. They have a global picture of their patients' history and overall health care needs. A disadvantage is that patients must go through them when they may already know that they need to see a specialist. It adds time and expense to the process of receiving necessary care. For example, Dan O'Riley has been seeing a dermatologist for the past five years for treatment of a chronic skin condition. His employer changes insurance companies, and Dan enrolls in the new HMO. He discovers that he must choose and visit a primary care physician in order to get a referral to see his dermatologist in order for the insurance company to pay for his skin treatments.

Review of Services

As discussed in Chapter 2, many insurance companies use review procedures to determine which costs they will cover. Diagnostic tests, treatments, hospitalizations, and so forth are reviewed to determine medical necessity and cost-effectiveness. Insurance companies will not pay for certain nonessential medical services and referrals to specialists that have not been preapproved. Securing these approvals is known as **preauthorization**, and it is essential that health care workers know when preauthorizations are necessary.

Government Programs

The federal government has become a major payer of health care costs through the provision of **Medicare**. This program, established by Congress in 1965, is part of the Social Security Administration and provides health insurance for people aged 65 and older and others, such as the severely disabled, who qualify for Social Security. Administered by the Health Care Financing Administration (HCFA), it consists of two parts. Part A provides funding to cover most hospitalization, home care, and hospice. Part B covers part of the cost of outpatient services, such as physicians' fees, diagnostic tests, and physical and occupational therapy.

Medicaid is a cost assistance program to help pay the medical costs for low income and disabled persons. Funded by the federal government, it is operated at the state level by Departments of Human Services. The exact eligibility and payment procedures vary by state.

By providing funding, the government has assumed a leading role in regulating both the costs and quality of health care provided under Medicare and Medicaid. A major move to control costs was the development of **diagnostic related groups** (DRGs) by Congress in 1983. The typical, expected hospital costs of all common diagnoses were determined. Providers of care for Medicare patients receive that amount, regardless of the actual cost of care. For example, every hospital in the country that performs hip replacement surgery on a Medicare patient is **reimbursed** (paid) the same amount. Hospitals that can do the procedure for less than the amount reimbursed are allowed to keep the extra money. Hospitals that spend more must make up the difference themselves. Exceptions to this policy are made when there are documented complications or additional diagnosed problems.

Thinking it Through

Josephine Copley arrives at work late, having had little sleep the night before. She hopes she can get caught up on some of her personal calls and still get the insurance forms sent out on time to meet the deadlines for submitting claims for reimbursement. She is working intently when approached by a patient who is very confused by her Medicare Claim Statements. The patient has questions on some of the supplies she was charged for. She does not know what they were used for or why.

Josephine is feeling quite stressed and is curt with her, saying, "I am sure all the charges are correct. Besides, Medicare doesn't pay like they used to anyway, so it doesn't matter. I'm just too busy to deal with this right now. It seems that patients want more and Medicare wants to pay less."

1. What are the possible consequences of Josephine's comments?

2. Was it appropriate that Josephine make negative comments about the patient's health care plan?

3. How could she have handled this situation differently?

4. What external circumstances may have contributed to Josephine's behavior?

Medicare guidelines also limit which drugs can be prescribed. Less expensive generics (those not protected by a company's trademark) may be required instead of brand names.

Fascinating Facts

In 1995, the United States spent 988.5 *billion* dollars on health care. This represents $3621.00 for every man, woman, and child in the country. In the year 1940, it was only $30.00 per person!

Restrictions on the length of hospital stays has resulted in an increased demand for health care in the home. The result was an explosion in the number of home health agencies. It soon became evident that the cost of health care was still out of control. Expenses had simply been transferred to another care area. The administrators of Medicare then proceeded to develop guidelines for home health agencies to increase their accountability for the number of visits and length of time patients could receive home health services.

In addition to cost control measures, the government is involved in maintaining minimum standards of care. The following two examples represent major attempts in this area:

- Regulation of facilities: Health care facilities that bill Medicare or Medicaid for reimbursement of costs related to the care of a patient who is covered by one of these programs must be certified prior to incurring costs, in order to receive compensation. Many private health insurance plans also state that the facility must maintain Medicare and Medicaid reimbursement status for their plans, too.

- Regulation of training: Nursing and geriatric assistants have a significant role in providing care for the elderly. The Omnibus Budget Reconciliation Act of 1987 (OBRA) includes specific requirements for the training and certification of these workers. They must attend state-approved training programs that include a minimum number of classroom and clinical hours as well as the study of specific subjects. Additional requirements include passing a state-approved exam and earning certain numbers of continuing education credits.

These government actions have had a significant impact on the health care system, because Medicare patients make up a large portion of the patient population. Health care workers who provide services for Medicare and Medicaid patients must understand and follow all regulations and requirements in order to ensure compliance and reimbursement.

CONTROLLING ORGANIZATIONAL COSTS

The effects of managed care, insurance restrictions, and government regulations have greatly affected all types of health care organizations. Facilities must focus on controlling expenditures.

Expenditures refer to any money that is spent in the process of doing business. The expenditures are the cost of resources required to maintain a health care delivery system. These costs occur in four major areas (Williams, 1999). See Figure 22–1.

1. Financing
2. Technology and Supplies (pharmaceuticals and equipment)
3. Facilities
4. Personnel

Financing refers to the source of money used to run a business. Financing resources for a health care facility come primarily from a variety of health insurance companies (federal or private). Each of these insurance plans has its own set of rules, procedures, and paperwork to be completed before payment for patient services is sent to the facility. The key factor here is to be as efficient as possible in completing the paperwork correctly and completely, so the payment can be received as soon as possible for services provided. When services have been given and the payment not received, the amount owed is recorded in what is called an **account receivable**. A sound business practice is to keep the accounts receivable as low as possible. Other financing resources may be individuals who pay for their own care or donations that individuals and corporations give to nonprofit facilities.

Keeping the accounts receivable low is an important part of financial management and relates to the cost of money. The **cost of money** refers to the value that could be earned on money if it were received by the facility and invested. For example, if a facility has 1 million dollars in accounts receivable and a 10% interest rate could be earned on that money, the facility is losing $274 for each day the payment is delayed ($1,000,000 × 10% ÷ by 365 days/year). The facility may also be paying interest on loans that it cannot pay off until the receivables are in the account. When money is owed to others for services, supplies, or equipment received, it is recorded as an **account payable**.

Technology and supplies refer to the cost of equipment and supplies that are used in the process of giving health care services to patients. For example, diagnostic equipment, medications, catheters, beds, and linens.

Facilities are the physical buildings and the land they stand on and the cost of maintaining them. For example, the painting, repairing, and

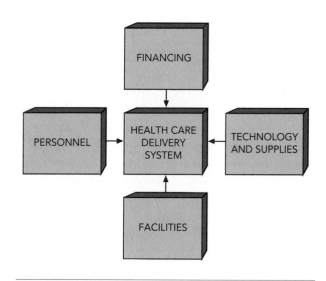

Figure 22–1 Resources required to maintain a health care delivery system.

remodeling of the buildings; landscaping; electricity; garbage removal; and maintenance of parking areas.

Personnel (labor costs) refers to the individuals who work in all areas associated with the functioning of the health care delivery system. They include both the direct care workers and those in support roles. Examples include nurses, physical and occupational therapists, medical assistants, x-ray and lab technicians, accountants, admissions staff, managers, pharmacists, dieticians, and maintenance workers. The total cost of the salaries of all the health care workers is frequently the largest cost incurred by a facility.

HEALTH CARE WORKERS' IMPACT ON COSTS

The career success of the health care worker will depend, to a great degree, on his or her ability to contribute to the control of rising costs. Every health care worker must take fiscal (financial) responsibility for his or her performance. The need for efficiency and accountability on the part of everyone in the system cannot be overemphasized. The question that must be asked is, "How can I help reduce unnecessary costs?" It is easy to dismiss the consequences of one person's impact on the finances of a health care facility. But when totaled up over a period of time and multiplied by the number of workers who are not concerned with efficiency, the costs can be quite significant.

There are many ways health care workers can contribute to the efficient and cost-effective functioning of the facility:

- Personal efficiency: This refers to the health care worker's performance and how each worker contributes to overall efficiency. For example, when workers arrive late or take excessive breaks, it affects their coworkers' work loads and their ability to perform their duties efficiently. This results in a decrease in patient satisfaction. The costs of poor-quality care are frequently related to the following problems (DeLaune, 1998):
    - Duplicated work between departments
    - Loss of time due to inefficient task performance
    - Loss of staff due to job dissatisfaction
    - Recruitment and training of new employees
    - Expenditure of energy and time in the investigation of complaints
    - Law suits (litigation) and malpractice settlements
    - Employees repeatedly making the same errors in tasks, despite instruction
    - Time wasted reporting and correcting errors
    - Expenses related to over utilization of diagnostic tests to avoid malpractice
- Focusing on the job: When at work, 100% of the health care worker's attention must be focused on the duties at hand. The needs of patients and the organization/employer must have top priority.
- Careful use of supplies or equipment: Damage or loss of supplies and equipment can add significantly to the cost of operations. Always use supplies only as needed and avoid waste by taking only that which is needed to complete the task. Handle equipment carefully and follow the manufacturer's instructions on the proper use and care of all equipment.
- Billing and coding correctly and not misplacing charges: Coding refers to the assignment of standardized numbers that designate diagnoses and procedures performed. It provides the information on which payment of insurance claims are based. Codes are classified by procedures and diagnoses and are contained in the following reference books: *Current Procedural Terminology* (*CPT*) and *Classification of Diseases, 9th Revision, Clinical Modification* (*ICD-9-CM*). Health care workers who have responsibility for coding must learn to properly use these references. Coding is very specific to the particular diagnosis or procedure (Box 22–1). Improper coding can lead to various problems, ranging from a loss of income for the provider to charges of fraud for overbilling. All health care workers need to be sure to note all supplies used and charges incurred in providing patient care. Not submitting charges can lead to not being reimbursed for care given or supplies used.

Box 22–1 Procedure (CPT) Code Examples

SAMPLE ANESTHESIA CODES

01200 Anesthesia for all closed procedures involving hip joint

01202 Anesthesia for arthroscopic procedures of hip joint

01210 Anesthesia for open procedures involving hip joint; not otherwise specified

01212 hip disarticulation

01214 total hip replacement or revision

Coding for procedures is very specific. It is important to read codes correctly to find the procedure performed.

SAMPLE SURGERY CODES

12001 Simple repair of superficial wounds of scalp, neck, axillae, external genitalia, trunk and/or extremities (including hands and feet): 2.5 cm or less

12002 2.6 cm to 7.5 cm

12004 7.6 cm to 12.5 cm

12005 12.6 cm to 20.0 cm

12006 20.1 cm to 30.0 cm

12007 over 30.0 cm

Notice that the size of the laceration (cut) to be sutured determines the code number to be used. Also note the use of the metric system to designate measurements.

- Maintaining inventory: Any item purchased by the health care facility belongs to the facility and cannot be taken for personal use without authorization. Even small items, such as pens and paper, should be used only for business purposes. If the health care worker accidentally takes some item home in a pocket, it is important to return it as soon as possible. The cost of items taken by employees is staggering and adds to the overall cost of goods and services in the United States.

- Educating patients: Promote the practice of healthy lifestyles to reduce the need for medical services. Encourage the use of preventive measures, such as immunizations and prenatal care, to reduce the need for more expensive care later. Clearly explain patient self-care practices to prevent unnecessary office visits.

- Being willing to cross-train: Cross-training means learning skills outside those traditionally expected in a given occupation. Health care workers who have a variety of skills and can perform many tasks are more cost effective than employees who have a limited number of skills. Cross-trained workers can fill in as needed, eliminating downtime and delays in delivering patient care or completing department tasks. Examples include respiratory therapists who learn to draw blood, and transcriptionists who can perform insurance coding and billing. Being willing to acquire additional skills, learned and practiced under proper supervision, can significantly increase the health care worker's value to an employer and create career opportunities.

Personal Efficiency

Employees who have difficulty performing efficiently on the job often have poor organizational skills, are confused about their priorities (what is most important), and may be slow in making decisions. Efforts to make personal changes may be necessary. Each individual must do a self-evaluation to identify areas that need improvement.

There are numerous books that help with personal assessment by presenting principles to follow in the process of change. Browsing the business and self-improvement sections in a bookstore may assist you to identify an author that relates the material in a manner that addresses your particular concerns and can assist you in your efforts to improve.

Thinking it Through

James deMelendez has been a respiratory therapist for 22 years. He enjoys working with patients and administering therapies. While James keeps up with the continuing educational requirements of his profession, he is resistant to learning skills that he considers to be outside the practice of respiratory therapy. James wants to move to a small town and applies for a position in a town's only hospital. He is surprised when he is not hired. When he follows up with the supervisor who interviewed him, he is told that due to cost control measures, the hospital is focusing on hiring multiskilled professionals who can perform duties in various departments.

1. How has James failed to keep up with trends in health care delivery?

2. What can he do to improve his future employment opportunities?

3. What are the implications for your future career?

The drive for personal effectiveness is a lifelong pursuit, but if developed can lead to tremendous improvements in the life of anyone struggling with ineffectiveness. There are certain behaviors that form a foundation for such improvement and some are listed below:

1. Use the problem-solving process identified in Chapter 1 to assist you in determining what areas in your life, if improved, would create the most dramatic changes for the positive. This is where the greatest effort and time should be spent.

2. Assume responsibility for your life and your decisions. Remember, not making a decision is a decision. Procrastination is a decision too—the decision to postpone the issue.

3. Don't just let life pass you by as you passively look at the world. Take action, make decisions, and initiate changes after a sound evaluation of what is needed. Be willing to accept the consequences of any actions you do or do not take.

4. Don't allow yourself to get sidetracked with the minutiae (trivia) of life. The details of daily life and the related interruptions can

seem compelling, but don't forget to focus on the big picture of what you have identified as central to your well-being.

5. Expect setbacks in your progress, but do not use this as an excuse not to continue.

6. If you feel you do not have enough time, monitor how your time is spent and then evaluate and eliminate the unimportant time wasters.

7. Communicate clearly and honestly with others when a conflict arises. Look for solutions that will satisfy all involved (this may require creative decision-making). Make sure you understand what the other person is truly saying and not just argue your side. If you are truly listening empathetically, you will not be planning what you will say next when the other person is speaking.

8. Look at your life from a holistic perspective. You and those around you have physical, social, emotional, and spiritual needs. Individuals who address all these areas function better.

If the health care worker is unable to find personal satisfaction, there is a greater likelihood of also having a dissatisfying professional life. Achieving maximum personal effectiveness enables the health care worker to make contributions that lead to an efficient and high quality organization.

Acting with Thought

The importance of thinking has been emphasized throughout this text. In order to control costs, all health care personnel must pay attention to their actions. The question presented earlier in this chapter, "How can I help reduce unnecessary costs?" should prompt additional questions, the answers to which will guide one's work:

1. What are the facts?

2. What is the best course of action?

3. What is the right thing to do?

4. What is the probable impact of my actions?

Applying the problem-solving model introduced in Chapter 1 will assist the health care worker to carefully review situations, gather necessary information, and make sound decisions.

SUGGESTED LEARNING ACTIVITIES

1. Consider your own financial situation and determine if there are any accounts receivable (any money due to be paid to you: money you have lent; a paycheck for the last two weeks' work; payments you have made in advance for services, such as newspaper or magazine delivery). Do you have any accounts payable (do you owe money)? How do these compare?

2. If you have worked or currently work, identify ways in which your performance has affected the cost of doing business. Review the areas listed under the section "Health Care Workers' Impact on Costs."

3. Look for articles in news magazines about the rising cost of health care. Are any solutions offered? Do you agree or disagree with the solutions proposed? Explain why.

REVIEW QUESTIONS

1. How have methods for paying medical costs changed over the years?

2. What is the difference between fee-for-service and managed care?

3. What is the purpose of managed care? What are three methods used to control costs?

4. Who is covered by Medicare? What services are covered?

5. What is Medicaid?

6. Explain the meaning of DRGs.

7. What are the four major areas of expenditures incurred by a health care delivery system?

8. What is the difference between accounts payable and accounts receivable?

9. What is the meaning of "the cost of money"?

10. What are five ways that the health care worker can assist in controlling facility costs?

APPLICATION EXERCISES

1. Refer to The Case of the Inefficient Office at the beginning of the chapter. What suggestions would you offer to your supervisor if you were in Constance's position?

2. It is a particularly busy day for Aubrey Casein as she rushes to assist several physicians as they perform patient procedures. It seems to her that the requests for supplies are coming in faster than she can meet the demand. She knows that the inventory tags on each of the items must be placed in the appropriate location for the charge to be billed to the correct patient's insurance. But today she decides to perform this task later when it slows down and places the inventory tags in her pocket. The day continues at the same fast pace, and Aubrey arrives home to discover numerous charge tags still in her pocket.

   a. What are the possible financial implications of Aubrey's actions?

   b. What are ways she can use to identify which inventory tag goes with which patient?

   c. What are the possible consequences if she charges the wrong supplies to a patient?

SUGGESTED READINGS AND RESOURCES

Campbell, C., Schmitz, H. and Waller, L. (1998). *Financial management in a managed care environment.* Albany, NY: Delmar.

Department of Health and Human Services Health Care Financing Administration: http://www.hcfa.gov

Rowell, J. (1998). *Understanding health insurance: A guide to professional billing* (4th ed.). Albany, NY: Delmar.

Williams, S. J. and Torrens, P. R. (1999). *Introduction to health services* (5th ed.). Albany, NY: Delmar.

CHAPTER

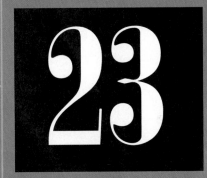

PERFORMANCE IMPROVEMENT AND CUSTOMER SERVICE

OBJECTIVES

Studying and applying the material in this chapter will help you to:

■ Understand the components used in determining quality of care.

■ Explain what is meant by quality assurance, continuous quality improvement, and total quality management.

■ Identify the internal and external customers in a health care setting.

■ Describe the steps in working with dissatisfied customers.

■ Describe the characteristics of constructive criticism.

■ Discuss how a health care worker can view destructive criticism in a constructive manner.

KEY TERMS

constructive criticism

continuous quality
   improvement (CQI)

external customer

internal customer

quality assurance (QA)

quality improvement

total quality management
   (TQM)

The Case of

the Angry Patient

Mr. Ramirez has been hospitalized for the last 6 days following orthopedic surgery. He is experiencing discomfort and is anxious about not being able to go home and be with his family. When Carolina Mims, physical therapy assistant, enters his room to assist him with his exercises, he lets her know how unhappy he is about how he is being treated. The food is bad, it took "forever" for the nurse to respond to his call button, and the portable urinal has not been emptied. "It's disgusting," he tells Carolina and then asks, "Who's in charge here, anyway?" The fact is, there have been numerous complaints about the quality of the food, and, unfortunately, the nursing staff is shorthanded because two nurses have called in sick. Carolina takes a few minutes to listen to Mr. Ramirez, demonstrates empathy for his discomfort, and tells him that she will report his complaints to the nursing supervisor. She is then able to proceed with the exercise session.

Knowing how to effectively handle complaints and work to make improvements in the system can make the difference between a high-quality patient care delivery system and one that fails. Understanding the principles of patient satisfaction will help you resolve problems that can lead to complaints and lawsuits.

QUALITY OF CARE

Finding the balance between maintaining high-quality patient care and controlling costs is a major struggle for modern providers of health care. High cost does not necessarily guarantee the highest level of care. As pointed out in Chapter 2, the United States ranks 14th among industrialized nations in infant mortality. And while Japan spends fewer health care dollars per person, the life expectancy for a Japanese female born in 1993 is just over 83 years, compared with an American female at just over 79 years.

Patient satisfaction does not seem to be directly related to amount spent. Eighty-nine percent of Americans believe major changes are needed. In contrast, only 43% of Canadians and 48% of Germans surveyed voiced major dissatisfaction with their health care systems (Campbell, 1998).

Discussions about improving the quality of care and raising patient satisfaction begin with two very difficult questions:

1. What is quality of care?
2. How can quality of care be measured?

Quality of care speaks to the excellence of the health care received. If this is measured by patient satisfaction, then the areas to look at for measurement would be based on patient concerns. Patients are concerned with the following:

- Easily accessible and available services
- Timely and safe delivery of care
- Coordination between services and continuity of care
- Effectiveness of services, that is, the delivery and outcome of care (DeLaune, 1998)

Unfortunately, if these concerns are addressed without regard to costs, they would lead to prohibitive health care costs. Others have tried to use the lowest costs as a measure of the effectiveness of health care facilities. This is obviously an inadequate tool because it means that those providing the least care are rated as the best.

Patient outcomes (how well the patients recover or manage their ailments) may seem an obvious choice for measuring the success of a health care experience. Did the patient recover to the prior state of health? This method also has its limitations because it ignores the value of the time spent in the health care system and only focuses on the end result. For example, if a patient received no education about an upcoming surgery prior to the procedure, but recovered and returned to an active and normal life, is this really quality of care? Perhaps the patient stayed in the hospital a few days longer because of not being prepared for the care requirements needed to return home earlier. Could this be classified as a positive outcome?

Another challenge in comparing patient outcomes is the tremendous number of variables that exists among patients with similar procedures. For example, if two patients go in for the same surgical procedure and have no complications, should they both be expected to be discharged from the hospital within the same time frame? On the surface, the answer may be yes, but other factors must be considered. What if one patient is 30-years-old and the other is 90-years-old? What if one has a preexisting condition (e.g., diabetes or heart disease) and the other does not? What if one lives alone and the other has family and friends willing to come in and assist with the care?

If the patient outcomes for one health care facility are compared to another as a measurement of quality, another concern arises in this approach. What if one hospital shows a much higher death rate than another? Is this an indication that one is giving better care than the other? Perhaps one hospital is located where there is a large elderly population and the other in a neighborhood with many young families. How would this affect the statistics?

Currently, there are no absolute answers when discussing such complex issues. These issues are far from being resolved and will continue to be central to health care in the foreseeable future. The focus of this text is not on solving these complex issues facing health care, but on assisting the health care worker in developing the skills and behaviors needed to perform at the highest level and deliver the highest possible quality of care. Health care workers must ask themselves what they can do to best meet the needs of the organization, their coworkers, and patients.

In health care the goal is 100% correct care with no errors, because any less can have serious consequences for both patients and health care workers. This may seem unrealistic, but review the examples in Box 23–1 to see how a 0.1% error rate can affect others when viewed from a broad perspective. Everyone must continually strive to provide competent, conscientious, and appropriate care.

Box 23–1 The Consequences of Performing 99.9% Versus 100% Correctly

A one-tenth percent (0.1%) error rate results in the following:

- 2 million documents will be lost by the Internal Revenue Service (IRS) in a year.

- 22,000 checks will be deducted from the wrong bank accounts in the next 60 minutes.

- 12 babies will be given to the wrong parents each day.

- 107 incorrect medical procedures will be performed within the next 24 hours.

- 18,322 pieces of mail will be mishandled in the next hour.

Data from Implementing total quality management: How to make TQM work in your organization, *V. Harnish, (1994). Boulder, CO: Career Track.*

QUALITY IMPROVEMENT

In the past the belief was that if more was done, the result would be an increase in quality of care. The examples at the beginning of this chapter demonstrate that this is not the case, and this approach is no longer used. When the Health Care Financing Administration (HCFA) and the Department of Health and Human Services (DHHS) implemented their regulations in connection with Medicare and Medicaid, they promoted the development of internal monitoring (within the health care organizations) and evaluation processes. These were designed to identify the changes needed to decrease costs while still *maintaining* quality. It is now believed that the focus can be on both *improving* quality of care and on cost containment. The processes used to find ways to preserve or improve quality of care while decreasing costs is called **quality improvement**.

Other terms that are frequently used in health care today and related to quality improvement are:

- **Quality assurance (QA):** Designed to meet external regulatory requirements. Problems are identified by the health care facility (e.g., a seemingly high rate of urinary infections in patients with a Foley catheter). These problems are called key indicators of quality care and are quantified (e.g., a chart review is done to determine how many patients with a

Foley catheter have developed a urinary infection during a specified care timeframe). The result is compared to industry standards to see if it exceeds the expected rate of such problems. If it is determined to be a problem area, education or other interventions are done to correct the identified problem. Then the study is repeated for subsequent time periods (usually on a quarterly basis) to determine if improvements have occurred or not as a result of the intervention. The results are used as measurements to determine if the quality of care is improving or declining. The focus is on individual performance, deviation from standards, and problem solving (Figure 23–1).

■ **Continuous quality improvement (CQI):** Designed by the health care facility to meet its internal needs. The assumption is that all areas can be improved (Box 23–2) and that this improvement will result in a higher quality of care and cost efficiency. This approach is based on data and uses a scientific approach to collect and analyze information and processes. The focus is on long-term system improvements.

■ **Total quality management (TQM):** Management philosophy of commitment to CQI to make organizational decisions. For CQI to work, the entire organization must be committed to this approach. TQM fosters a system that supports customer needs, empowers employees to work as teams, emphasizes self-development, and requires a leadership style in which employees are viewed as valuable resources who can make unique contributions to the organization.

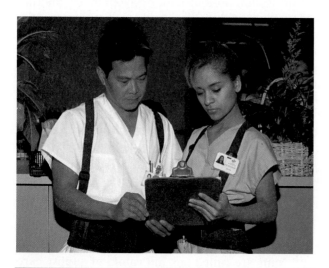

Figure 23–1 Quality assurance issues are identified by conducting studies of facility performance.

> ### Box 23–2   Three Primary Areas to Examine When Evaluating a Health Care Facility for Quality Improvement.
>
> 1. Organizational structure: How is the facility structured? What is the management style? How is communication encouraged? What changes would increase efficiency and accessibility?
>
> 2. Health care workers: How do the health care workers function as a team? What processes could be changed to increase efficiency and employee satisfaction?
>
> 3. Patient outcomes: Is the patient satisfied with the care? Was the outcome of his or her health care problem resolved in an efficient and appropriate manner with minimal suffering and confusion? Was the care provided in a coordinated manner to decrease duplication of services and minimize confusion?

There is some overlap in QA and CQI, but they can be used together effectively. QA can identify a problem. The CQI system approach can be used to analyze and make changes in the system to resolve the identified problem.

CQI can be a very effective process when the entire organization from top management on down is involved in and committed to making the changes that are identified by the process. If the top managers do not support CQI, then it is unlikely to succeed. Change must be possible throughout the organization and employees entrusted to do what is necessary at their level. Effective problem-solving is best done at the same level where the problem occurs. This requires that management approve resources needed by the group to resolve the situation. For example, materials and personnel may be needed to supply education, meeting time, the collection of data or accessing of data from other departments, and/or supplies and equipment (Campbell, 1998).

The following examples demonstrate how the quality of care can be improved while costs are decreased at the same time. Note that both are based on the scientific, data-driven approach used in CQI.

■ Prescribing broad-spectrum antibiotics: Past practice when prescribing antibiotics for a patient was to order a broad-spectrum antibiotic. The philosophy was that it would "get whatever was there." But as more was learned about the development of resistance when unnecessary antibiotics are prescribed, it was determined that performing a culture (a test to see what bacteria is present) and using a more specific antibiotic was the best treatment choice for the patient. This had the advantage of decreasing the risk of resistance developing and rendering the drug ineffective when it was really needed. The cost advantage in this case is that the more specific antibiotics are frequently less expensive than the broad-spectrum antibiotics (Campbell, 1998).

■ Ordering disposable bibs: The health care workers in a hospital would frequently use a towel as a bib when feeding patients to prevent the gown from being soiled. The administration conducted a study that demonstrated that the cost of sending the towels to the laundry was more than that of purchasing disposable bibs. The disposable bibs were purchased, and much to the delight of the staff, were more effective for their intended purpose, as well as costing less.

CUSTOMER SERVICE

Satisfactory customer service is essential to the successful health care business in today's competitive market. When the term customer is used, it refers to both internal and external customers.

Thinking it Through

Dr. Arthur has maintained a successful orthopedic practice in Midtown for many years. He has a good reputation for providing caring service. In recent months his medical assistant, Nathan Alberts, has received an increasing number of complaints about having to wait to see Dr. Arthur when they arrive for their appointments.

1. How should Nathan respond when patients complain about the delays?

2. According to the principles of CQI, what steps would you recommend Nathan take in order to resolve this problem?

Internal customers are those who work in the health care industry. For example, health care workers from other offices, outside suppliers of medical and pharmaceutical supplies, and coworkers are internal customers who are affected by the behavior of those they work with on a day-to-day basis. **External customers** are those who come to the health care provider for services. They may be referred to as customers, patients, or clients.

Patients come to health care providers for a variety of reasons. They may have a specific problem they hope to have cured and their prior level of health restored (Box 23-3). The visit may involve a request for a routine evaluation to confirm the patient's level of health or to obtain information on preventive measures that will help to avoid future problems. Or a sudden illness or emergency situation may develop that requires immediate attention. Whatever the reason for patients' contact with the health care facility, there is always the expectation that high-quality, professional service will be delivered (Figure 23-2).

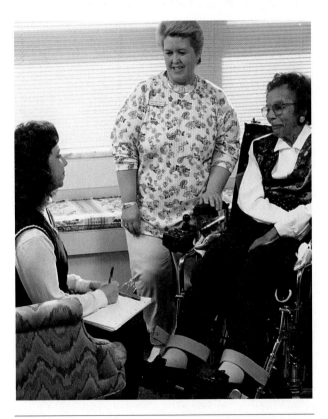

Figure 23-2 Patients expect high-quality care. Their satisfaction must be one of the goals of every health care worker.

Box 23–3　Services Sought by Patients Through the Health Care System

1. Prevention

   • Education: E.g. nutrition and exercise, prevention of heart disease, stop smoking programs, how to manage diabetes

   • Routine physical exams

   • Screening tests: E.g. mammogram, colonoscopy, Pap smear, blood pressure check, cholesterol and lipids blood tests

2. Emergency and Urgent Care Services

   • Illnesses and injuries that need immediate attention

3. Inpatient Services

   • Surgery

   • Illnesses and injuries requiring continuous care

   • Specialized treatments

   • Rehabilitation

4. Long-Term Care

   • Nursing homes

   • Assisted living

5. In-Home Care

   • Nursing

   • Therapy

   • Homemaking

6. Psychological/Psychiatric Services

   • Counseling

   • Medication

7. Dental Services

   • Preventive care

   • Treatment and restoration

8. Pharmaceuticals and Medical Supplies and Equipment

   • Medications and other items needed to restore and/or maintain health

When a patient evaluates the service received, it is not just the outcome that is important, but the entire experience. For example, two patients can have the same diagnosis, receive the same treatment, and return to their prior level of health within the same time frame, but one may be satisfied and the other very upset with the care received. It is necessary to review more than simply the medical problem that was presented. All aspects of contact with the patient must be examined when checking for quality. Examples of questions to ask about patient service include:

■ If the initial contact was made by telephone, how was the patient treated? Was he or she placed on hold? Disconnected? Was the health care worker courteous and did he or she express interest and concern?

■ When the patient arrived for the appointment, how long did he or she wait before being seen by the health care worker? Was the patient kept informed of any delays?

■ Was the patient required to wait for procedures and tests once they were scheduled?

■ Was he or she given clear instructions and were all questions answered? Was the patient given information about how to have future questions answered?

■ Were all procedures explained and consent obtained?

■ Were all personnel courteous and compassionate when delivering care? Or was the care rough and abrupt, and not considerate of the patient's needs?

■ If the patient was in the hospital, what was the temperature and quality of the food? Was it quiet at night so he or she could sleep with a minimum of interruptions? Was he or she able to get prompt assistance when needed?

As health care workers, it is sometimes easy to slip into a routine of just doing the job and forgetting that this may be a very frightening or stressful experience for the patient. When working with patients, use the time to learn more about their thoughts, concerns, and learning needs. This is not the time for the health care worker to share the exciting weekend trip or the fun date from the night before. Avoid engaging in social conversation with other health care workers and ignoring the patients. They are there for service, and the focus must be concentrated on their needs. Social interactions with coworkers should be saved for breaks or after-work hours.

Most people are surprised to learn that lawsuits brought by patients are more closely related to whether the patient does or does not like the health care workers than to any other factor. In the past, it was common to have lifelong relationships with physicians, based on mutual trust and respect. Today it is more common for patients to be treated by strangers. Changes in health care plans may require that new health care providers be chosen. If a referral to a specialist is required, the referring physician may have to be chosen from a list of approved specialists. Health care workers must take advantage of every patient contact to create positive relationships and provide the highest quality care possible.

It is a common belief that if a lawsuit is filed, there must be good cause. Someone must have made a mistake. This is not necessarily true. Lawsuits may be filed as a result of emotional responses to perceived wrongs. Or they may concern matters of little importance, known as frivolous lawsuits. Keep in mind though, that any lawsuit filed, whether it seems legitimate or not, will cause a great deal of stress for everyone involved. The amount of time and money spent in addressing a lawsuit can be overwhelming. Many lawsuits can be avoided by working to ensure that all patients are satisfied customers.

Customer Satisfaction

One approach that many health care businesses use to determine how satisfied their customers are is to conduct customer surveys. These can be done in two ways:

1. Mailing out questions that customers answer and return by mail

2. Calling customers and asking them to respond to questions over the telephone

Some health care facilities maintain a log listing all complaints, what was done to address the complaint, and if the resolution was satisfactory. If the results are made available to staff, it is worth the health care worker's time to review the comments. The areas of concern may be very different from what is expected and can lead to changes in performance that will create greater customer satisfaction.

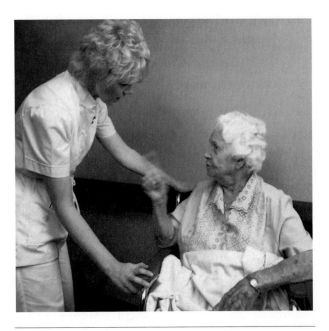

Figure 23–3 Good listening skills are essential when handling a patient complaint.

When working with dissatisfied customers, it is critical to fully understand their view of the situation (Figure 23–3). To accomplish this it is necessary to listen without interrupting and not to display signs of defensiveness. The guidelines in Table 23–1 will assist in handling this type of interaction.

[Fascinating Facts]

Cooperative Concepts Web site

a. A business only hears from 4% of its dissatisfied customers. The other 96% go elsewhere for service.

b. Sixty-eight percent of the dissatisfied customers leave because of an attitude of indifference towards them.

c. The average dissatisfied customer tells 8–10 others about the poor service.

d. It takes 12 positive service incidents to make up for one negative incident.

e. Seventy percent of complaining customers will do business with you again if you resolve the complaint in their favor. This increases to 95% if the complaint is resolved on the spot.

Table 23–1 Working with Dissatisfied Customers (Internal and External)

Steps	Comments
1. Identify the problem	• Listen to the complaint with an open mind. • Try to completely understand their side of the situation. • Ask questions to clarify as needed, but do not interrupt needlessly. • Do not display verbal or nonverbal defensiveness. • Thank them for the information, because the goal is to always obtain customer satisfaction.
2. Seek resolution	• If the problem is with you personally, it is appropriate to apologize, thank them for the feedback, and assure them you will do your best not to repeat the error. • If you need more information before the problem can be resolved, let the patient know when you will get back to him or her. • Provide information that the customer may be lacking. Make sure the customer is open to hearing what will be said and that it is phrased in a nondefensive manner. For example, if a customer complains about having had to pay for parking on the last visit, this could be addressed in a defensive or nondefensive manner. A defensive approach usually is an attempt to place blame on the patient, whereas, a nondefensive approach does not. Consider these statements: Defensive—"Well if you had just asked about it, we would have validated the ticket for you." Nondefensive—"I am sorry, we should have informed you that we validate parking tickets for patients. Do you have your ticket with you so we can validate it for you today?" • If you do not have the authority to deal with the problem, refer the patient to the proper person or ask the person with the authority to contact the patient.
3. Verify satisfaction	Does the patient feel the problem has been resolved satisfactorily?

Remember that each health care worker is responsible for patient satisfaction. The cost of an unhappy patient is much more than the loss of that one patient because they will probably tell their family, friends, and coworkers.

It is also important to recognize that satisfaction is a subjective perception. Therefore, a health care worker must listen carefully and constantly to determine if the patient has any concerns. The patient may have a positive outcome to their medical treatment, but may be dissatisfied with the experience due to a cold food tray, a delay in answering a call light, waiting for tests, delayed treatments, an unemptied bedpan, or delayed pain medications (DeLaune, 1998).

Internal Customers

It is just as important to maintain good relationships with internal customers as with external ones. One of the common mistakes made when working with coworkers is to quickly point out errors, but not take the time to stress what they do well. Praising coworkers for a job well done, a courtesy extended, or a quick response to a situation can build trusting and mutually satisfying working relationships. Everyone wants to do well on the job, to contribute to the effectiveness of the office or facility, and to have a sense of self-satisfaction with their contributions. When people take pride in their work, they will work harder and more cooperatively than they will if they feel that others are being overly critical.

Good relationships also require that criticism be given when appropriate. **Constructive criticism** is based on optimism. The intended message is that setbacks or failures are due to circumstances that can be changed for the better. It holds out the hope of improvement and suggests the beginning of a plan for doing so (Figure 23–4). On the other hand, *destructive criticism* has the effect of creating helplessness, anger, and rebellion. The person is immediately put on the defensive and may no longer be receptive to suggestions for improvement. When individuals are led to believe that their failures are due to personal faults that cannot be changed, they lose hope and stop trying. For example, a medical assistant is just starting a new job. In her haste to try to manage too many duties in order to make a good first impression, she inadvertently forgets to log two patient appointments. The result is that three patients are scheduled for the same time with the same nurse practitioner.

The medical assistant's supervisor addresses the situation: Constructively: "While I know how overwhelming all the duties you have to accomplish are, it is important that you accurately accomplish each duty. Until you feel more comfortable with all your duties, try to concentrate on one duty at a time (i.e., answer one phone call; finish the scheduling of a patient's appointment prior to answering another phone). Destructively: "You messed up! The nurse practitioner will not have a chance for a break, and the whole day's schedule is behind."

Box 23–4 contains effective guidelines for giving constructive criticism.

It is difficult hearing criticism, especially if it is not presented as constructive criticism. When receiving destructive criticism from someone, the health care worker can change it into a positive experience by implementing the suggestions in Box 23–5.

Box 23–4   How To Give Constructive Criticism

Be concise and clear during conversations. If the other person does not understand exactly what you mean, it increases the chances of misunderstandings. Giving specific examples that illustrate the issue is a great way to increase clarity.

Never use vague, general, or harsh terms. It is frustrating to hear that you are doing something wrong or not performing well and not understand exactly what can be done to correct the situation.

Include positive comments of what the other person is doing well. Using positive and negative comments is sometimes referred to as the "sandwich technique." Start and end the conversation with positive feedback and then incorporate (sandwich in) the area(s) that need improvement.

If the problem directly affects you, state how it makes you feel. For example, if a coworker is not completing his or her tasks before leaving the workplace, state that you feel taken advantage of and rushed by having to complete the extra tasks.

Show a respectful attitude toward the other person. Always strive to preserve the other person's self-respect. Everyone makes mistakes or has areas that need improvement.

Demonstrate a cooperative attitude. Give ample opportunity for the other person to ask questions and seek clarification about what is being stated. Offer positive suggestions for improvement.

Be sensitive that this may be difficult for the other person to hear. No one likes to confront their faults. If the reaction is defensive, do not respond defensively in turn. Acknowledge the reaction and attempt to redirect to a more positive exchange.

Provide time for face-to-face communication that is done in private. It is uncomfortable giving a criticism, but distancing oneself by using impersonal messages or memos creates greater discomfort and prevents the opportunity for the other person to respond or seek clarification.

Use empathy when communicating. Stay aware of the impact on the person of what you say and how you say it.

Never complain to others about the performance of a coworker. Communicate directly with him or her privately and confidentially.

Box 23–5   Responding to Destructive Criticism

Look for the "kernel of truth" in the statement.

Be aware of your emotional response and set it aside in an effort to benefit from the exchange.

Do not attack the other person. You may feel that you have information about his or her own performance, attitude, or practices, but now is not the time to share these thoughts.

If the situation becomes too emotional, ask to take a break and negotiate a time to resume the conversation later. This gives you an opportunity to put things in perspective.

Even if you do not agree with what is being said, be open to trying to understand it from the other person's point of view.

If the feedback is valid, take responsibility and initiate the needed changes in behavior.

Look at the experience as an opportunity to develop stronger team relationships with coworkers and to improve communications. Work with the person giving the criticism to solve the perceived problem.

Ask for specific examples if you are unclear about what is being said.

Ask for suggestions about how you might improve.

Positive relationships with coworkers provide the foundation for making efforts as an organization to offer high quality service to all customers. *Employee satisfaction leads to customer satisfaction.*

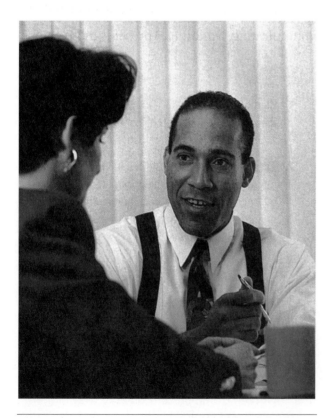

Figure 23–4 The goals of constructive criticism are to encourage improvement and to resolve problems.

Thinking it Through

Carstyn Franklin is an occupational therapy assistant (COTA) working in a busy hand therapy clinic. She and the other two assistants work with patients, make splints, and teach the use of adaptive devices so that patients can learn to perform homemaking and self-care practices as independently as possible. Brandon Williams, one of the other assistants, has the habit of leaving equipment, tools, and supplies wherever he last uses them instead of putting them away. This results in delays for the other assistants because they must locate needed items before they can do their own work.

1. Describe in detail how Carstyn can speak with Brandon about his work habits.
   - What is the goal of her communication?
   - How can she present the problem in order to increase the chances of resolution?
   - How can she respond if Brandon reacts defensively?

SUGGESTED LEARNING ACTIVITIES

1. Use the general periodical and business indexes in the library to look for articles about CQI, QA, and TQM. How are they being applied in various kinds of businesses?

2. Identify a problem in your family or personal life that could benefit from a CQI approach. Put together a plan using CQI principles to seek improvement or a resolution.

3. Watch for examples of good customer service. Describe what you believe makes them good.

4. Spend some time thinking about how you would want to be treated as a patient. What would be most important to you?

5. Survey friends and family members about their health care experiences. Were they positive or negative, and why? What did they want from health care workers? Did they receive it?

6. Try using the suggested critique methods the next time you need to confront someone about a problem or behavior. What methods did you use? What was the result?

7. Pay attention to how you receive criticism. Do you generally find it to be a learning experience? A confrontation? A waste of time?

REVIEW QUESTIONS

1. What components determine quality of care?

2. What is quality assurance, continuous quality improvement, and total quality management, and how are they related?

3. Who are internal and external customers?

4. What are the steps in working with dissatisfied customers?

5. What are the characteristics of constructive criticism?

6. How can a health care worker view destructive criticism in a constructive manner?

APPLICATION EXERCISES

1. Refer to The Case of the Angry Patient at the beginning of this Chapter. a. How would Carolina respond to Mr. Ramirez's criticism constructively? b. Destructively?

2. Alicia has just about had it at work. As a respiratory therapist, she loves working with patients. She knows that breathing difficulties create great anxiety, and she likes knowing that her work helps patients resolve more than just their physical problems. But Alicia is distressed by the disorder in the hospital department where she works. Her schedule is often changed, sometimes with very little notice. This causes problems with her child care arrangements. Equipment is not always put away where it should be, and supply inventories are frequently depleted. Alicia decides to discuss the situation with her supervisor. She recently took a workshop on CQI and believes that the techniques she learned about might be applied to resolving her department's disorder.

   a. How can Alicia present her concerns in a positive way to her supervisor?

   b. What can she share about CQI that might be helpful?

   c. What kinds of processes might be put in place to help resolve the department's problems?

SUGGESTED READINGS AND RESOURCES

Covey, S. R. (1994). *First things first.* NY: Fireside.

Covey, S. R. (1999). *Living the 7 habits: The courage to change.* NY: Fireside.

Martin, W. B. (1993). *Quality customer service* (revised edition). Menlo Park, CA: Crisp Publications.

UNIT

SECURING AND MAINTAINING EMPLOYMENT

CHAPTER

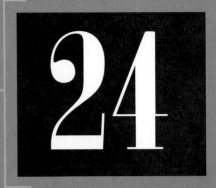

JOB LEADS AND THE RESUME

OBJECTIVES

Studying and applying the material in this chapter will help you to:

- Develop an inventory of your employment skills and personal traits that are of value to an employer.

- Identify your workplace preferences.

- Describe ways to get organized for the job search.

- List the most common sources of job leads and explain how to use each one effectively.

- Create a resume that highlights your qualifications and encourages employers to interview you.

- Write effective cover letters to accompany your resume.

KEY TERMS

career service center
chronological resume
cold calls
cover letter
functional resume
jobline
networking
objective
resume
traits

The Case of

the Unprepared Applicant

Jenny Nguyen recently passed her state exam to become a registered dental assistant and is seeking her first job. Jenny did well in her training but has not had very much experience applying for jobs. The career services counselor at Jenny's school calls her on Tuesday morning to tell her about a job opening with Dr. Chambers, a well-respected dentist in her area. A job in his dental clinic would be an excellent opportunity for a new dental assistant. Jenny is interested in the position but has put off completing her resume and needs a few more hours to finish it. She is also nervous about her interviewing skills and delays calling Dr. Chambers. When she finally calls on Friday afternoon, she learns that the job was filled that morning. In this chapter, you will learn how to be prepared for job opportunities and avoid experiencing disappointments like Jenny did.

OVERVIEW OF THE JOB SEARCH

The job search can be an exciting and challenging experience for the health care graduate. The purpose of this and Chapter 25 is to help students plan and carry out the activities necessary to secure satisfying employment.

It may surprise you to learn how much the job-seeking process is like a job in itself. You should plan to devote at least 20 hours each week to your job search. Some employment professionals even recommend that you spend up to 40 hours. That may sound like a lot, but think about it. Health care students spend a lot of time, money, and effort completing an education. Furthermore, a large percentage of waking hours are spent at work. It makes sense to devote the time necessary to find a job you like and that makes the best use of your education. Job satisfaction is an important factor in the quality of life. Investing time and effort in the job search will pay off in the future.

Developing a positive attitude will help make the job search more of an adventure than a chore. Almost everyone feels nervous or apprehensive about approaching potential employers in the hope of being hired. Job seekers often see themselves as powerless, but this is not true. You can increase your self-confidence if you understand that graduates who offer the skills and **traits** (personal characteristics) that employers need, and the positive, can-do attitude that they want, are a welcome addition to their staff. This is true for all types of health care occupations and all types of facilities such as hospitals, physicians' offices, insurance companies, and dental clinics.

Employers want to hire people who meet more than the position's minimum qualifications. They hope to find people who are pleasant, enthusiastic, and likeable. Graduates can project these qualities by approaching the job search positively and seeing it as an opportunity to make a contribution to the health care community.

What Do You Have to Offer?

A common problem for new graduates is that they don't realize how much they have to offer employers. Like many others, you may be concerned that your lack of health care experience will make it difficult for you to find a job. Students are often surprised to discover just how many qualifications they really have. The first step in a successful job search is to identify these qualifications. For example, your technical skills are up to date and fresh in your mind. This is a plus. However, these skills are only part of what makes an effective employee. The traits that will most likely determine your success in securing and maintaining employment include professionalism, enthusiasm, willingness to learn, a positive attitude, and reliability. In fact, many employers report that they prefer to hire an enthusiastic person who is willing to learn over someone with the best technical skills but who has a poor attitude (Source: Personal communication).

Spend some time developing an inventory of both your technical and nontechnical skills. The technical skills are the most obvious and can be collected by reviewing textbooks, class and lab materials, and clinical evaluations. Employers are also looking for applicants with strong nontechnical skills. Three of the most important are the ability to:

1. Communicate: Listen carefully to others. Organize thoughts and speak at a level appropriate for the listener.

2. Problem solve: Identify problems, gather necessary information, consider alternatives, and use good judgment when choosing a solution.

3. Work as a team member: Help others, work cooperatively, manage conflict (Source: Personal communication).

Other personal characteristics of value to health care employers include:

- Integrity: Be honest, maintain confidentiality, choose the right way rather than the easy way.
- Responsibility: Work without constant supervision, find tasks without being told, know when to ask for help.
- Dependability: Follow through on obligations without being reminded. Always be on time and rarely be absent.
- Organization: Be accurate and efficient. Use time well.
- Consideration: Be friendly, polite, empathetic and patient. Work with diverse populations.
- Willingness to learn: Ask questions, acquire new knowledge and skills, keep up to date in the field.

This list gives only a few suggestions. Students can add many more. Think about what you have learned in your roles as a parent, student, volunteer, group member, or employee. Life is rich with experiences to draw from.

Use your inventory to boost your self-confidence and prepare you to write an effective resume and present yourself well at interviews.

You have a strong foundation on which you can build a successful job search.

What Are Your Expectations?

Before starting the job search, it is important to identify your employment preferences. There are many types of working environments and finding the one in which you work best is an important factor in determining career success. Consider the following factors when thinking about the type of facility in which to work:

- Size of facility
- Work pace
- Amount of time spent working with others and working on your own
- Amount of supervision
- Hours of work
- Type of patient population
- Type of professional specialty
- Location

Identifying appropriate job leads is easier when you have thought about your preferences.

At the same time, remember that recent graduates are usually seeking entry-level positions. More job opportunities open up as experience is gained. A good career move may be to compromise some of your preferences in exchange for starting out with an employer who offers opportunities to learn and grow professionally.

It is also important to be aware of your financial needs. Track your current expenses for a few months and calculate the minimum amount needed to cover your cost of living. Be sure to consider the following basic expenses:

- Housing and associated costs: Rent or mortgage, insurance, utilities, telephone, repairs, cleaning supplies, day care
- Transportation: Vehicle, fees, insurance, gas, repairs
- Clothing and grooming supplies
- Health care, including insurance
- Food
- Entertainment

Organizing Your Time

Planning your time structures your job search and ensures that you focus on activities that are most likely to bring results. Decide how many hours you can devote to your search each week and make weekly and daily to-do lists of tasks. A typical list would include:

- Making phone calls
- Taking your resume to be printed
- Sending thank you letters
- Searching the Internet
- Following up on leads

Be prepared to take advantage of and follow up on every opportunity. If at the last minute you learn about a chance to attend an interview, you want to be ready. Have your resume, interview clothing, and reliable transportation available at all times during the job search process. Career services personnel report that many students lose job opportunities because they don't act fast enough on leads.

Organizing Your Space

A good way to keep yourself organized is to devote a specific area in your home to your job search. Keep all the supplies and materials you will need together so that they are easy to find. Don't take the chance of losing the phone number of a potential employer because you wrote it on a little scrap of paper in the kitchen. You will find the following items helpful in conducting an effective job search:

- Appointment calendar
- Notebook for recording information such as potential employers, the names and addresses of people who might provide assistance with the job search, and questions you want to ask potential employers
- Index cards for recording leads, contacts, and so on. Some people prefer these to a notebook.
- Good quality paper and matching envelopes for resumes, cover letters, and thank you notes. White is a good choice for the health care field.
- Computer supplies, if you have a home computer. Be sure to have an extra print cartridge on hand.
- Dictionary: Anything you send to a potential employer must be completely free of spelling errors.
- Yellow page telephone books
- Street maps of your area

Projecting a Professional Image

You will be receiving calls from your school, people who have contacts, or potential employers. Be sure that these calls are handled in a manner that reflects well on you. Review proper telephone manners and

message-taking with everyone who answers the telephone at your home. You don't want to miss a possible interview because you don't have the return telephone number or the caller was put off by rude manners. A family member who answers incoming calls with a hostile "Yeah?" may damage your efforts before you even have a chance to take the call. If you have an answering machine with a taped message, be sure that the message is not off-color or too cute. Remember that what the caller hears represents you as a potential employee.

Students who are rarely home during working hours or who don't have a telephone or an answering machine should arrange to have a dependable person take calls. The messages should be retrieved often so that potential appointments or information about jobs are not missed.

It is important that you look and act professional during all job search activities. Professionalism is a way of life, not behavior saved for "special occasions." For example, show courtesy and respect to receptionists when you call or go to an office for an interview. Their opinion may be valued by the people doing the hiring.

Always look your best. If you don't have an interview, but are running into an office to drop off a completed job application, it may be tempting to dress casually. *Don't do it.* You don't know who will see you and what authority they have in making hiring decisions. Think of the job search as a series of evaluations and be prepared for each one.

FINDING JOB LEADS

Finding an employer whose needs match your qualifications can take up most of the job search efforts. Knowing how and where to look can spell the difference between the success and failure of your efforts. There are many ways to locate job openings, and the chances of finding the right job are increased by using as many of these sources as possible.

Career Service Center

Some schools report that over 80% of their graduates find employment as a direct result of working with the staff in the **Career Service Center**. (This may have another name, such as "Placement," "Employment Assistance," etc.) This office provides students with job search assistance such as the following:

- Resume writing
- Interview practice

- Internet access
- Dressing for success hints
- Current information about local employers:
  - Major health care facilities
  - Directories of physicians and other health care professionals
  - Hiring practices
  - Who is most likely to hire recent graduates

While it is *your* responsibility to become employed, it is a mistake not to take advantage of the help that is available.

Many employers depend on schools to provide them with prequalified applicants for job openings. Schools may be notified before jobs are advertised. Work with the career service center to take advantage of these opportunities (Figure 24–1). Make a commitment to follow up on all leads and attend any interviews that are scheduled for you. An unhappy event for the school staff is to receive a call from an employer with the news that a student who was given a lead did not contact the employer or show up for the interview. Always follow up, even if the job does not seem to be exactly what you want. When students fail to show up, it damages the credibility of the school and may hurt its future relationship with the employment community. And the job may turn out to be the right one, after all. If not, it will provide practice for interviewing skills, and the employer may provide a connection to another job that is a match.

Keep the school informed of your job search progress and advise them of telephone and address changes. Many leads are lost because schools cannot locate students. Advise the school

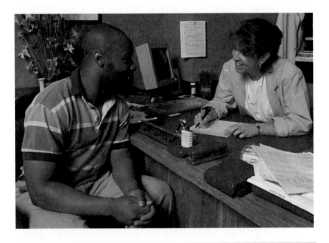

Figure 24–1 Seek the help of the employment personnel in your school.

Thinking it Through

Jasmine is feeling discouraged. She completed a nursing assistant program 2 months ago and still hasn't found a job. Joe Dorland from her school's placement office called this morning wanting to know if she had followed up on the job opening he gave her last week. She told him she hadn't, because the job was on the other side of the city, and it would take her at least 40 minutes to get there on the bus. Joe had called with other leads that she hadn't cared to follow up. They either sounded pretty boring, were in parts of town she didn't know, or the pay wasn't high enough. Jasmine really thinks that the school should help her more to get what she wants in a job.

1. Does Jasmine have realistic expectations about the job search?

2. Is she likely to continue receiving help from the school's placement office? Explain your answer.

3. What would you suggest that Jasmine do to increase her chances of finding a job?

when you accept a job. Some states require schools to report on the employment status of their graduates.

Networking

Networking means developing a group of contacts who might be helpful in meeting your professional goals. Ideally, you can return the help in some way. Networking is one of the most effective ways of securing employment.

There are two types of networking contacts, and both should be developed. The first consists of everyone you know. Tell as many people as possible that you are in the job market. A friend at church may know that his dentist is looking for an assistant. The pharmacist at the local drug store may have a colleague who needs a pharmacy tech. Be professional and project enthusiasm about starting a health care career.

The second type of networking contact is a health care professional or employer. In addition to being potential sources of job leads, they can provide general information about the field and tips on getting ahead. Professional networking contacts include the following:

- Instructors
- Other school staff
- Guest speakers
- Attendees at professional meetings, conferences, and workshops
- The supervisor and staff at your clinical site
- Professionals at job fairs
- Your personal physician, dentist, and so on

Don't be shy about approaching people who might be able to help. Smile, introduce yourself, and tell them that you are preparing to enter the health care field. In addition to being a source of job leads, professional contacts can provide valuable information (Figure 24–2). Here are some questions to ask:

- What skills are most important for succeeding in this career?
- What personal traits are most important?
- What qualities do employers look for when hiring for this occupation?
- What are the major duties?
- Which hospitals, facilities, companies, physicians, or dentists are good to work for and why?
- What is your best advice for someone who wants to work in this field?
- Can you recommend anyone else I can talk to about working in this field?

Keep accurate records of networking contacts. Create a section in your notebook or use index cards to keep track of names, titles, addresses and phone numbers, where met, and any planned follow-up action.

Send a thank you note to anyone who meets with you or provides information. The impact of this simple act of courtesy cannot be overemphasized. Let them know when you are hired and keep in touch. Networking should become a habit maintained throughout your career. It is a way to stay current in the field, develop friendships with other professionals, and add to the enjoyment of work.

Clinical Experience

Many students receive job offers as a result of their performance during their clinical experience (internship). This is *not*, however, the principal purpose of this part of your training and it is important that you *do not expect* to be offered a job. Do not ask, or even hint, about any expectations about being hired.

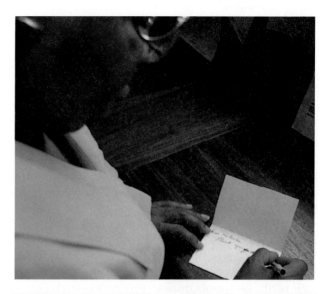

Figure 24–2 If you utilize networking, it is important to send a thank you note to anyone meets with you or helps you.

At the same time, conduct yourself at all times at your professional best. Facilities have created jobs for students who impress them with outstanding performance. Even if a job is not available, their recommendations are important.

Job Fairs and Orientations

There are many types of gatherings that employers attend to recruit employees. While interviews are not usually conducted nor job offers made, employers provide valuable information to job seekers and may collect resumes.

Take advantage of these activities. Dress professionally and take copies of your resume. Check your area for the following types of opportunities to meet employers:

- Career fairs sponsored by your school: The employers who attend these are sending the clear message that they hire recent graduates. Ask lots of questions and collect brochures, business cards, and any other handouts offered. Learn as much as you can. Organize the information collected. Write notes about who you met, application procedures, and who to contact for an interview. Keeping good records is especially important if it will be a while before you are ready to start the formal job search.
- Career fairs sponsored by Chambers of Commerce and government organizations: Look for announcements in the newspaper. These are commonly placed in the Help Wanted or Business section. Check the bulletin board in the career service center at school. Many job fairs are also listed on the Internet.

■ Career orientations and information meetings sponsored by employers: Some health care facilities conduct open meetings to recruit applicants and explain their hiring process. Contact the Human Resources Department at organizations in which you are interested.

■ Professional conventions and conferences: Some employers recruit at these meetings. Allied Health Opportunities Online, at www.gvpub.com, has a link to a list of health care organizations along with the cities and dates of their next meetings.

Help Wanted Ads

Newspapers list job openings alphabetically by job title or industry name in the Help Wanted (also called Employment) section of the classified ads (Figure 24–3). Sundays usually have the largest number of ads. Employers receive many responses, but applicants who meet their qualifications may be invited for an interview. Look under all job titles for which you might qualify. An ad for a laboratory technician can appear under "lab," "laboratory, "medical," "health," or "technician." Your education may qualify you for a variety of job titles. For example, the Patient Care Assistant program at a California school trains students for at least 16 job titles, including rehabilitation, physical therapy, occupational therapy, and mental health aide; patient care technician; and nursing assistant. It is important that you understand what similar titles mean and know for which positions you might apply. In some occupations, there is an important distinction made between the aide and assistant levels. For example, aide-level positions in physical and occupational therapy do not have specific educational requirements. Assistants, however, must have an associate's degree and pass standardized exams. Check with career services or your instructor if you are unsure if you qualify for an advertised position.

When responding to a newspaper ad, it is very important to follow the directions. Many employers today prefer that resumes be faxed or e-mailed. While it may be tempting to send a nicely printed copy on good quality paper, fax it anyway. A mailed resume may arrive too late for an interview to be scheduled. If the ad reads "no calls," doing so will not increase your chance of being hired. It will only show disregard for the employer's time. Employers want to hire people who can follow directions. If applicants refuse to follow them when applying for the job, why would employers expect them to do any better as employees?

Some employers are now including Web site addresses in their ads, and these should be

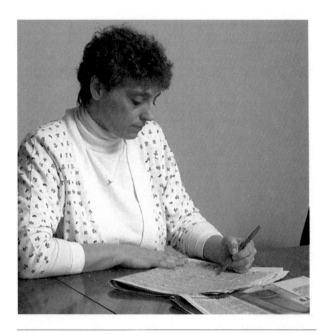

Figure 24–3 The help wanted ads are only one of many sources of job leads.

explored. They can be valuable sources of information and may include job postings and online application forms.

Cold Calls and Visits

Cold calling refers to calling or visiting employers to make the first contact. The purpose is to identify possible job openings and to inform the employer that you are looking for employment. Many jobs are not advertised, so this can be an excellent way to locate openings. Cold calling requires self-confidence and good communication skills. It is essential to be courteous and considerate when making contacts.

Use the Yellow Pages or professional directories available at the career services center, public library, or Chamber of Commerce. Cold calls can be a quick way of locating unadvertised openings and can be especially helpful for graduates who are relocating and want to identify leads before moving.

Personal, unscheduled visits to health care offices can be an effective way to find job openings. It is most efficient to visit buildings or complexes that have many offices. Be sure to dress professionally and take copies of your resume. Smile, introduce yourself, inquire about openings, and leave a resume. *Never* ask for an interview, however, when dropping in without an appointment. Whether calling or visiting in person, be brief, be appreciative, and be on your way.

Fascinating Facts

Published job openings represent only 15% of total available jobs at any given time. The remaining *85%* are never published anywhere. (Levitt, 1996.) The importance of networking and researching to find this "hidden" job market cannot be overemphasized.

Telephone Joblines

Large health care facilities often have **joblines**, taped recordings with information about current openings. The amount of information given varies, ranging from simply a list of job titles to more detailed information about applicant requirements. Jobline telephone numbers may be listed in Help Wanted ads. Some health care facilities feature joblines as a telephone menu option.

Internet

Computer technology is an exciting new way for job seekers and employers to connect. There are a growing number of ways to use the Internet in the job search:

- Learn job search techniques: There is excellent information available about using the Internet, search, resume writing, interviewing, and many other topics. A good place to start is at http://www.rileyguide.com, a large, but well-organized site that contains loads of information about using the Internet. It is linked to dozens of other useful sites. Other helpful sites are located at http://www.jobhuntersbible.com and http://jobstar.org (the second site says it is for California, but it contains lots of general information).

- Find job openings: Some sites collect Help Wanted ads from major newspapers across the country. Jobs are classified by category, and you can restrict your search to a specific geographic location. Example: http://www.careerpath.com. Other sites specialize in specific industries, such as health care, and contract with facilities to post their openings. Some of these sites have a limited number of postings, but they are likely to grow in the future. Example: http://www.medsearch.com.

- Get information about specific facilities: Many large health care providers, such as clinics and hospitals, have their own Web sites. These are excellent sources of general information and often contain job postings and information about how to apply. Some even include application or resume forms that you can fill out on the screen and submit electronically. Example: Scripps Clinic in San Diego, California at www.scrippsclinic.com. Search by name for facilities in your area.

- Check out professional organizations: In addition to general information about the profession, some have job banks available to members. An example is the American Health Information Management Association at http://www.ahima.org (Appendix 1).

- Post your resume: Some sites allow resumes to be placed online. Health care employers are beginning to review these sites when looking to fill positions. Some schools allow students to use the school's phone number as the contact so that inquiries can be screened. If you decide to put your resume online, be sure that it is perfect. Many people will see it. Example: http://www.job-hunt.org.

A valuable feature of the Internet is the ability to link sites. This allows sites to build links to others that contain related information. Most of the sites listed above have useful links. Making these connections is as easy as the click of a mouse button.

The number of Internet sites is growing daily. They tend to change names and addresses, discontinue operations, or merge with other sites. A few make unrealistic claims, such as having more job postings than they actually do. The Internet should not be your main source of job leads. Use it an as important, but not exclusive, tool in the job search.

For students who do not have experience using the Internet, this is an excellent time to learn. Many schools provide Internet access and classes on how to use it effectively. Consult the books and Web sites listed at the end of this chapter for more information about getting started.

THE RESUME

A **resume** is a written summary of professional qualifications. Its purpose is to convince employers to interview you. The resume must represent you well and convince employers that you are the kind of person they need.

Some students choose to have someone else, such as a professional resume preparer, write their resume. These students may be unsure about what to include or have weak word processing skills. It is a good idea to seek advice from employment professionals and essential to have someone qualified proofread your resume, but there are several important reasons why *you* should determine the content and organization:

- It must accurately represent your skills: It is essential to make sure that they are neither exaggerated nor minimized.

- It is important to include the personal traits identified earlier in this chapter: Only you know what these are.

- Canned resumes should be avoided: They tend to look insincere and give the impression that they were put together without much thought.

- You must know exactly what your resume says: It often serves as the basis for questions at interviews.

Resume Contents

Resumes contain several sections and each has a specific purpose. It is important that all contents be written accurately and completely.

1. Heading: This section includes your name, address, and phone number and is placed at the top of the resume. Make it easy for potential employers to contact you by listing a current telephone number, along with the area code. If necessary, include an alternate number where messages can be left. If you have an e-mail address and/or fax number, list these too. Do not be one of the people who loses opportunities because interested employers cannot find them. Center the heading at the top of the page and highlight your name by using capital letters. It is not necessary to use the label "Resume," because the content and format makes it easy to identify.

2. **Objective**: This is a statement of your job goal. It can be written as a simple job title or include additional information about your qualifications and preferences. Here are a few examples:

   Job title only: Position as a Medical Assistant

   More specific: Position as a Front-Office Medical Assistant

   Include information about your qualifications: Position as a Front-Office Medical Assistant in which I apply my computer skills and organizational ability.

   Include information about your preferences: Position as a Back-Office Medical Assistant in a pediatric office.

   Combination: Position as a Back-Office Medical Assistant in a busy pediatric office where I can apply my experience with children and ability to communicate with people of all ages.

   The more specific the objective, the more limited the choice of jobs. The student in the example must decide if she is willing to work anywhere other than a pediatric office in order to gain experience. Decisions will also be influenced by the current job market. How likely is it that she will find a pediatric position in a reasonable length of time?

   The best strategy is to write objectives that match each job for which you apply. This is easy if you have access to a word processor. Look for key words in ads and job descriptions that can be mirrored in the objective.

3. Qualifications: This is an optional section that highlights important skills and traits that relate directly to the objective and the jobs for which you are applying. Placed at the beginning of the resume, it informs employers immediately about why you are a good candidate. Items that are listed elsewhere in the resume should not be included. Review the qualifications section after completing the rest of the resume in order to avoid duplications. Here is a sample list of qualifications for a pediatric medical assistant applicant who has a background teaching in a preschool:

- 13 years experience working with children in a variety of settings

- 5 years experience teaching disabled children

- Bilingual, English-Spanish

- Certified medical assistant

- Up-to-date front- and back-office skills

- Ability to communicate with people of all ages

- Maintained perfect attendance while attending medical assisting program and working part-time

- Ability to work well under pressure and manage priorities

Notice how a variety of abilities and experiences are used to describe the applicant as a unique and well-qualified candidate. They do not have to be directly related to health care, but can come from previous work, school, or personal experience.

4. Education: This is an important section for graduates who are new to the health care field. Recently acquired skills are the major qualifications for employment. List the schools attended, starting with the most recent. Include high school only if graduation or a GED is a job requirement. List the dates attended or the date the certificate, diploma, or degree was awarded. The following items can also be added to this section:

   - Special training, such as CPR or computer classes, that are related to the job objective

   - Honors or awards earned

   - Cumulative GPA if it is 3.0 or higher

   - Special school projects that are related to the targeted job

   - Facts that demonstrate such traits as initiative, ability to manage time, and persistence

   - Summary of what you learned. List the courses taken or prepare a list of skills acquired. This is especially helpful for the employer if the program included an unusual variety of skills or if the occupational outcome is a relatively new job title. Here are two examples showing how to write the education section:

Example # 1:

Associate in Applied Science Degree, Medical Assisting, 1999

Healthcare College, Lincoln, NE

   - Completed CPR and first aid training
   - Honor Roll all semesters
   - Earned 3.7/4.0 GPA

Example # 2:

Diploma, Patient Care Assistant Program, 1998

BeWell School of Medical Careers

   - Received Perfect Attendance Award
   - Served as chairperson for annual, all-school diversity picnic
   - Completed program while working part-time and raising two young children
   - Knowledge and skills acquired include:
     - Medical terminology and body systems
     - Computer keyboarding and data entry
     - Medical and surgical asepsis
     - Nursing assistant skills
     - Home health aide skills
     - Rehabilitation aide skills
     - Unit clerk skills
     - Phlebotomy
     - EKGs

5. Certifications and licenses: Include this section only if they are not listed in another section.

Examples: Certified Medical Assistant

Licensed Vocational Nurse, California License # 1234568910

Current CPR certification

Registered Dental Assistant

6. Work Experience (also called Employment History): List your previous jobs starting with the most recent. Include the name and location of each employer, along with the dates worked and the titles of all positions held. Create a bulleted list of phrases, using active verbs, to describe your duties and achievements. Do not use complete sentences or the word "I." Think about how you contributed to the success of your previous employers. Were you extremely reliable? Did you increase sales? Develop a more efficient system for organizing the office?

Don't worry if your work history does not seem very impressive. Completing a health care educational program demonstrates the ability to set and meet new career goals.

It is appropriate to include clinical experience in either the work experience or education section. Give the name and location of the facility, as well as a list of the duties performed. Be sure to label these appropriately as "externship," "fieldwork experience," and so on. To imply that it was a paid position is dishonest.

Examples of work history section:

Example # 1:

Sales Associate   1996 to Present

Hercules Men's Store, Gary, IN

   - Assist customers
   - Increased sales by 17% first year employed
   - Consistently earn highest top-volume sales associate award each quarter
   - Close out cash register each night
   - Maintain perfect attendance

This job, while not related to health, demonstrates the ability to communicate, motivation to succeed, honesty, and reliability. Every employer is looking for these qualities.

Example # 2:

Medical Assistant Externship June 2001–September 2001

Caring Community Clinic, Charleston, SC

Perform back office duties under supervision of Dr. Emilio Jimenez

- Take medical histories
- Take vital signs
- Prepare patients for examinations and procedures
- Assist physician with procedures and minor surgeries
- Administer medications
- Apply principles of infection control
- Received highest ratings (5 on scale of 1–5) in all areas on final externship evaluation

The following are optional sections to include if they add important information not mentioned elsewhere.

9. Special Skills: Skills beyond what would normally be expected from your training. For example, a medical assistant applicant with the ability to troubleshoot and correct computer problems.

10. Languages: Languages other than English can be listed here or under special skills. It is customary to indicate the ability level. For example, Spanish: Speaking and comprehension good, writing ability fair.

11. Award and Honors: If applicable. List only those not already included in the education section. Provide brief explanations if it is not clear how they were earned.

12. Community Service and Volunteer Work: List the duties performed.

13. Memberships in Professional Organizations: These demonstrate commitment and interest in keeping up to date. Serving as an officer or member of a committee demonstrates willingness to accept responsibility, practice leadership, and take an active role in organizations.

14. Hobbies and Interests: List any that support your bid for the job. For example, sports such as swimming or tennis demonstrate that you value good health and recognize the importance of exercise.

Formatting the Resume

Formatting refers to the arrangement of the content in the resume. There are two commonly used formats, the chronological and the functional. The **chronological resume** features a work experience section in which the duties and accomplishments of previous jobs are listed. This type is a good choice for emphasizing education or to highlight jobs related to the current career objective. Figure 24–4 contains an example of a chronological resume.

The **functional resume** highlights clusters of skills and abilities gathered from a variety of experiences. Job titles are listed in the work experience section without detailing duties and accomplishments. Functional resumes are recommended for people who are changing careers and have a variety of skills and experiences that can be transferred to the new field. Three clusters are usually recommended. See Figure 24–5 for an example of a functional resume.

Resume content can be organized in a variety of ways. The fact is, there is no "best way" that everyone should use. The important thing is that the resume be reader-friendly and highlight the qualifications that best support the targeted job. These should be placed closest to the top of the page. For example, an applicant for a transcriptionist position with outstanding keyboarding speed and accuracy would list these under Qualifications. A bilingual medical assistant applicant in an area with a large Hispanic population could highlight the ability to speak Spanish in either the Objective or Qualifications section.

Thinking it Through

Greg Berglander recently graduated from a radiologic technician program and has passed his state's licensing exam. He's ready to begin applying for jobs. The only problem is that he doesn't have a resume prepared. While Greg can use a computer, he does not keyboard quickly and has poor word processing skills. He believes that the career services center at his school should be more helpful and put something together for him. After all, they know the courses he took and probably have access to his grades. And he can tell them anything else they need to know.

1. Do you agree with Greg? Why or why not?

2. What action would you recommend that he take?

LISA GRAZIANO
8407 Wentworth Ave.
Manchester, NH 03103
(603) 123-4567

OBJECTIVE

Position as a **Medical Transcriptionist** in a hospital

QUALIFICATIONS

9 years full-time experience working as a medical transcriptionist
Ability to prepare reports for all major specialties
Keyboarding speed of 97 wpm

WORK EXPERIENCE

Medical Transcriptionist   1995–Present
Chatsworth Medical Center, Manchester, NH
• Transcribe patient's medical reports as dictated by physicians
• Distribute reports to appropriate departments
• Obtain charts for physicians
• Received Employee of the Quarter award four times (based on reliability, cooperation, and efficiency)

Medical Transcriptionist   1993–1995
St. Claire Hospital, Boston, MA
• Transcribed daily reports for surgical department
• Copied records for billing
• Answered telephone and transfered calls

Administrative Assistant   1989–1993
Dr. Patrice Tibere, Boston, MA
• Word processed all correspondence and research reports
• Located and gathered reference materials as requested
• Handled mail, answered telephone, maintained Dr. Tibere's schedule, made travel arrangements

EDUCATION

AA Degree, Medical Transcription, 1993
Lawrence Medical College, Boston

Word Processing Certificate, 1989
Regal College, Boston

MEMBERSHIPS

American Association for Medical Transcription
Lawrence Medical College Advisory Board

Figure 24–4 Chronological resume.

KELLY CISNEROS
9125 Soledad Avenue
El Paso, TX 79907
(915) 123-4567

OBJECTIVE	Position as a **Back-Office Medical Assistant** in a busy pediatric office
EDUCATION	AS Degree, Medical Assistant, 2000 Caldwell Technical College, El Paso • Perfect Attendance Award three semesters out of four • Grade point average 3.8/4.0 • Externship at Valley Pediatric Center, El Paso • "Excellent Rating" for overall externship performance
EXPERIENCE WITH CHILDREN	6 years providing private daycare in home 3 years teaching disabled preschoolers Cub Scout leader Volunteer tutor at Sanchez Elementary School
ORGANIZATIONAL SKILLS	Maintained state-approved daycare facility Secretary of PTA at children's school Coordinate scheduling and activities for local junior soccer team
COMMUNICATION SKILLS	Make presentations to local organizations about child safety issues Write articles for Sanchez Elementary School parent newsletter 5 years experience as telephone receptionist in a busy insurance office Speak, read, and write Spanish fluently
WORK HISTORY	Cisneros Quality Daycare 1992–1998 Owner of home-based daycare for up to six children SpecialCare Preschool 1989–1992 Teacher Calderon Insurance Agency 1984–1989 Receptionist

Figure 24–5 Functional resume.

Important Resume Guidelines

While there are a variety of ways to organize the content, there are a few guidelines that should *always* be followed:

- Be accurate: Check for perfect spelling, correct grammar, and accurate dates. This is important for all professions, but especially when applying for a job in health care, which depends on accuracy for the well-being of both patients and workers.

- Be conservative: This is a characteristic of the medical field. Choose good quality paper in white or a very light gray or beige.

- Be neat: Have no corrections, smudges, or creases.

- Make it easy to read: Don't crowd the information; leave some white space. Margins should be at least 1-inch on all sides.

- Keep it professional: Don't include personal information such as marital status and number of children.

- Do not include information that is best discussed in person: This includes why you left previous jobs, salary information, or special conditions such as having a physical disability.

- Use proper spacing: Double-space between headings, then single-space within each section.

- Use special features for highlighting: Capitalize all major words in the headings. You may also want to bold all words in headings.

- Keep it concise: Limiting it to one page is highly recommended.

- Have someone qualified review and proofread your resume. This is the most important written document in your job search efforts, so keep working on it until it is error-free and represents you at your best.

Recent Resume Trends

- A common practice until recently was to state "References Available Upon Request" at the bottom of the resume. The current practice is to omit this statement. (But you *do* need to have at least three references listed on a separate piece of paper.)

- Internet posting: Some employers have standard resume forms that you can fill out on the screen and send electronically.

- Electronic scanning: Employers who receive large numbers of resumes and do not have time to review them all are using scanners to enter them into a computerized data bank. The computer looks for key words that match the words in job descriptions. When there is a job opening, all resumes matching its requirements are recalled for review. If an employer indicates that resumes will be scanned, it is important to include descriptive words in your objective and throughout the resume. Read ads and job descriptions carefully to identify key words. Avoid staples, folds, or special features, such as bolding or fancy fonts. These are difficult for the computer to read.

COVER LETTERS

Cover letters are sent with resumes as a way to introduce yourself and inform the employer why you are sending a resume. Customize your letters as needed for the following situations:

- When responding to an advertised opening: Refer to the ad in the letter and state that you are interested in the position. Explain briefly how you meet the requirements stated in the ad. Do not simply repeat the specific information listed on the resume, but refer the employer to it for more detailed information. Request an interview and thank the employer for his or her time and consideration. See Figure 24–6 for an example of a cover letter for responding to an advertised position.

- Sending the resume to be considered for an unadvertised position: State the purpose of the letter, who told you about the opening (be sure you have that person's permission), or simply say that you understand there is an opening for which you might qualify. Briefly state your qualifications, why you are interested in the job, and then close with a request for an interview and a thank you. See Figure 24–7 for an example of this type of letter.

- You are moving to a new location and sending letters of inquiry in advance: Inform the employer that you are relocating to the area. Explain the type of work you are seeking. Include a brief statement of your qualifications and when you will be available for an interview. Ask to be considered for any appropriate openings and state that you will follow up with a phone call. Conclude with a thank you. See Figure 24–8.

AD:

DENTAL ASSISTANT. Excellent verbal, scheduling and collection skills. Full-time. Front and back office as needed. Computer literate with good work ethic. Commitment to high-quality patient care.

1357 Keystone Drive
Chicago, IL 60606
July 23, 2001

Dr. Harold Mims
1842 Grand Avenue
Chicago, IL 60606

Dear Dr. Mims:

This letter is in response to your ad for a dental assistant. I recently graduated from Harrison Dental College and believe that I fulfill the requirements stated in your ad.

Providing **high-quality patient care** was emphasized throughout the dental assisting program at Harrison. I would welcome the opportunity to begin my dental assisting career in an environment where patients are the top priority.

The program at Harrison emphasized the need for good **verbal skills** in the workplace. We were given many opportunities to practice them. In the skills lab students were required to explain all procedures orally to "patients" before and during hands-on work. I also received grades of "A" in my communication courses, which included Oral Communication and Interpersonal Relations for the Health Care Worker.

I understand the need for a smooth-running **front office** and enjoyed the administrative and **computer training** portion of my training. Performing duties in both the **front and back office** would allow me to apply my organizational skills. My previous jobs, outlined in the enclosed resume, required me to be responsive to the needs of my employers.

My **strong work ethic** is demonstrated in my excellent attendance records, both at school and work, willingness to complete all assigned tasks, and commitment to doing my best at all times.

I would appreciate the opportunity to meet with you to further discuss how I might contribute to the success of your practice. I can be reached at (312) 123-4567.

Thank you for your consideration.

Sincerely,

Kelly Bosner

Kelly Bosner

Figure 24–6 Cover letter responding to an advertised position.

1357 Keystone Drive
Chicago, IL 60606
July 25, 2001

Ms. Tasha Jefferson, Office Manager
Compton Dental Clinic
6397 Flanders Street
Chicago, IL 60606

Dear Ms. Jefferson:

I am a recent graduate of Harrison Dental College. The Employment Coordinator at Harrison, Ms. Juanita Sanders, recommended that I contact you about a possible opening at Compton Dental Clinic. She believes you would be interested in an applicant with my excellent attendance record and academic achievements.

The dental assistant program at Harrison was rigorous and I feel well prepared to perform both front and back office skills. I developed good habits during my training as well as at my previous jobs, which are listed in my resume. In addition, I have excellent communication skills and am committed to becoming a successful member of a dental care team.

I would appreciate the opportunity to meet with you to further discuss the needs of Compton Dental Clinic and my qualifications. I can be reached at (312) 123-4567.

Thank you for your consideration.

Sincerely,

Kelly Bosner

Kelly Bosner

Figure 24–7 Cover letter responding to an unadvertised position.

900 Peach Blossom Lane
Atlanta, GA 30326
September 24, 2001

Sarah Masterson, RHIA
Director - Health Information Management Department
Blackwell Rehabilitation Hospital
2106 S.W. River Street
Portland, OR 97423

Dear Ms. Masterson:

The purpose of this letter is to inquire about possible openings for a Registered Health Information Technician at your facility. I graduated from Caprio Health Care Institute in Atlanta in June and am relocating to the Portland area in November.

My training at Caprio was comprehensive and I feel confident that my training has prepared me to work competently in the health information field. I work well with others, have strong computer skills, and look forward to contributing to the success of my future employer.

I will contact you the week of November 12 after my arrival in Portland. In the meantime I can be contacted at (404) 123-4567. Thank you for your consideration.

Sincerely,

Glenda Hayes

Glenda Hayes

Figure 24–8 Cover letter for a graduate moving to a new location.

Writing Good Cover Letters

Cover letters, like the resume, represent you and help determine if you will be invited for an interview. Here are some guidelines for writing winning letters:

- Word process or type them.
- Be sure that grammar and spelling are perfect.
- Use the same paper as for the resume.
- Address the letter, if possible, to a specific person. Call the facility and ask to whom it should be directed. Check for the correct spelling of the name.
- Send individualized letters for each employer or position, matching them to the targeted position.
- Do not write more than one page. Busy employers don't have time to read more than that.
- Use a standard business letter format. See Chapter 17.

SUGGESTED LEARNING ACTIVITIES

1. Talk with successfully employed friends and family members about how they got their jobs.
2. Review the newspaper regularly for articles about health care trends, facilities, and employment-related topics.
3. Learn to access the Internet, if you don't already know how. Check out the sites suggested in this chapter and use the links to see what information is available.
4. Visit your school's career service center and find out what resources are available. Introduce yourself to the people who work there, if you don't already know them.
5. Find a newspaper ad, Internet posting, or job description for a health care job in which you are interested.
   a. List the skills and traits that you think would be required.
   b. Write an objective that matches the position.
   c. Create an appropriate resume and cover letter to apply for the position.

REVIEW QUESTIONS

1. Why should you develop a personalized skill inventory as a first step in your job search?
2. What are eight factors that you should consider when identifying your workplace preferences?
3. How much time should you plan to spend each week on job search activities?
4. Describe why and how you should organize a workplace dedicated to your job search.
5. Select four sources of job leads and explain how to use each one.
6. What is the purpose of the resume?
7. What are the major sections of a resume?
8. What are 10 characteristics of a successful resume?
9. What is a cover letter and when is it used?
10. What are the characteristics of a good cover letter?

APPLICATION EXERCISES

1. Refer to The Case of the Unprepared Applicant at the beginning of the chapter. Describe what Jenny could have done differently to avoid missing the opportunity to interview with Dr. Chambers.
2. Omid Riazati is starting his last month of classes at PrepWell College. He will then have an 8-week externship before completing his medical laboratory technician program. He is not sure where he wants to work when he graduates, but wants to get started investigating employment possibilities and plan his job search activities. Create a job search to-do list and schedule for Omid to begin now and follow until he finds employment.

SUGGESTED READINGS AND RESOURCES

CareerBuilder: http://www.careerpath.com

Dikel, M. R., Roehm, F., & Oserman, S. (1998). *The guide to Internet job searching.* Lincolnwood, IL: VGM Career Horizons.

Ferrett, S. (1996). *Getting and keeping the job you want.* New York: Glencoe-McGraw Hill.

Jandt, F. E. & Nemnich, M. B. (1997). *Using the Internet and the world wide web in your job search: The complete guide to online job seeking and career information.* Indianapolis: JIST Works, Inc.

Job Hunters Bible: http://www.JobHuntersBible.com

JobStar: http://www.jobstar.org

Marino, K. (1993). *Resumes for health care professionals.* New York: John Wiley & Sons.

Monster Healthcare: http://www.medsearch.com

Perrin, C. & Dublin, P. (1994). *Successful resumes and interviews.* Albany, NY: Delmar.

Riley Guide: http://www.rileyguide.com

SoftSearch: http://www.job-hunt.com

CHAPTER

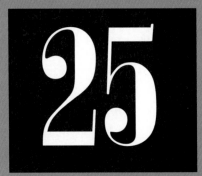

INTERVIEW, PORTFOLIO, AND APPLICATION

OBJECTIVES

Studying and applying the material in this chapter will help you to:

- Understand the importance of the job interview.

- Describe how to obtain background information about employers and health care organizations.

- Anticipate and prepare for questions that may be asked at interviews.

- Describe ways to handle illegal questions asked by employers.

- Create examples to illustrate your employment qualifications.

- Prepare appropriate questions to ask at interviews.

- Build a professional portfolio that provides evidence of your job skills and qualifications.

- Identify references who will support your job search efforts.

- Create a reference list to give to potential employers.

- Demonstrate successful interview behavior and appearance.

- Explain what actions to take after an interview to increase your chances of being hired.

- Fill out employment applications accurately and appropriately.

- Explain how to accept and reject job offers.

KEY TERMS

job interview

letters of recommendation

portfolio

reference

reference list

The Case of
the Modest Applicant

Sam Kingsley is seeking his first job as a phlebotomist. He has enjoyed his training and is eager to apply it in the workplace. While he went to school, Sam waited tables in a local family restaurant. Regular customers always liked to sit in Sam's section because of his friendly, helpful attitude. Many of the customers are elderly and especially liked Sam's respectful attitude toward them. Sam's first interview was at a medical laboratory which handles large numbers of walk-in patients. He felt that he handled the questions well by emphasizing his recent technical training. After all, he really didn't have anything else that related to work in phlebotomy. When Sam didn't get the job, he learned that the employer didn't believe he had really presented himself as a strong candidate. This chapter explains that students can draw on all kinds of experiences to best present themselves to potential employers.

THE JOB INTERVIEW

The **job interview** is a conversation between an applicant and a potential employer. It is an opportunity to present qualifications in person. Securing this interview has been the goal of all job search activity to this point. The purpose of this chapter is to help make interviewing as pleasant and productive as possible, resulting in an offer for the job you want.

Many job applicants are nervous about the idea of meeting face to face with an employer. The key to overcoming nerves is to prepare well and practice thoroughly. This helps ensure readiness for handling any interview situation and making a favorable impression.

Consider the interview as an opportunity for the applicant and employer to get to know each other and see if they fit each other's requirements. Keep in mind that interviews can be stressful for employers, too. A position must be filled, and the vacancy may be causing extra work. Inexperienced interviewers worry about their ability to choose the best-qualified applicant. They want to hire employees who can help solve problems, not create new ones.

The job interview is a two-way street and can be approached as a positive experience. Take advantage of this opportunity to evaluate the employer by observing and asking questions. The information gathered provides the basis on which to determine if the position fits your professional qualifications and personal preferences.

The Importance of Proper Preparation

Before attending a single interview, there are a number of things that must be done. Being prepared enables the applicant to focus on learning about the employer's needs and responding appropriately to all questions. Preparation prevents being caught off-guard and unable to think of an intelligent response. Answers to many of the most challenging interview questions will have been practiced in advance.

Not being prepared is the single best way to set yourself up for failure. Spend time developing interviewing skills and increase your chance for success.

Learn About the Employer

It is important to know something about the employer and the position being applied for in order to properly prepare for an interview. Having some background information will allow you to:

- Show the employer that you are motivated, interested in the job, and have self-initiative
- Create appropriate examples from your experience to demonstrate qualifications for the job
- Prepare your own questions about the facility and the job

Sources of information vary, based on the size of the facility. To learn about major organizations, check the Internet, as discussed in Chapter 24, or call the Personnel Office. Ask for written materials, announcements about job fairs or orientations, and other sources of information. Watch for information on a company in the local newspaper. Major employers are often the subject of articles, especially in the business and employment sections. With small employers, such as private medical or dental offices, it may be necessary to call or stop by to observe and ask a few questions. The receptionist is often a good source. The following are examples of appropriate questions to ask:

- How long has the facility or office been in business?
- What is the professional specialty?
- What are typical ages and types of patients served?
- What is the pace of the work?

Whether the employer is large or small, try to get a job description before the interview. Study it carefully and prepare specific examples that demonstrate your qualifications. If there are skills required that you do not have, but can learn, be prepared to explain to the employer how you plan to acquire them.

It is important for the applicant to demonstrate knowledge about the health care field in general. Keep informed about trends and issues of concern to employers. Newspapers and news magazines often contain articles about health care topics that affect health care careers. You should stay current on the ethical and legal issues facing health care providers. Employers want to hire people who can help them deal with the growing number of regulations and constant changes that affect the delivery of health care today.

Prepare to Demonstrate Your Qualifications

College employment professionals report that one of the main reasons students do not get hired is that they fail to sell themselves. Students fail to realize how much they have to offer an employer and do not explain fully how they can be of benefit. An essential part of interview preparation is to review your skills and create examples that illustrate mastery of them.

Start the review by looking at technical skills:

- What procedures and tests can you perform?
- Which ones are your best?
- On which ones have you received compliments from patients, classmates, or good evaluations from instructors, or supervisors?
- In which classes did you receive the highest grades?
- Which classes did you enjoy the most?
- Which skills and procedures did you practice most during your clinical experience?

Now recall some experiences that support your skills and think about ways to present them. Here are a few examples:

"I'm very efficient at performing blood draws. My classmates always want to work with me in the lab because. . . "

"I've worked hard to learn to do insurance coding accurately. I received top grades on all my assignments. The manager who supervised my externship allowed me to do more coding than externs are usually allowed to do because. . . "

"I enjoy word processing and reached a keyboarding speed of 83 words a minute. I also find medical terminology very interesting. Even more important for medical transcription, I'm very accurate. . . "

Next, review the personal inventory you developed in Chapter 24. The purpose of the inventory was not simply to build your self-confidence. It was to create a list of points to present at the interview to sell yourself as an applicant worth considering. Detailed examples will be needed to support these items, just as for technical skills:

"I'm good at calming people who are afraid of the dentist. For example, when I was on my externship, there was a woman who was really nervous and I helped her by . . . "

"My time management skills are strong. During the two years of my nursing program, I maintained part-time employment and still made sure that my three children and I arrived on time for school every day."

Prepare Your Questions

Asking questions shows that you are a motivated, thinking person who is sincerely interested in the job. The interview should also be an opportunity to find out about the employer and get the information needed to make an intelligent decision if a job offer is received. Here are some examples of appropriate questions to ask:

- What are the duties and responsibilities of this position?
- May I have a copy of the job description?

- I see on the job description that I would be required to _____. Will you tell me more about that?

- Could you describe a typical day for a person in this position?

- Is there a training program for new employees? How does it work?

- What equipment would I be working with?

- What do you think are the most important qualifications for a person to succeed in this position? What qualities in an employee are most important to you?

- Who would I be reporting to? Can you tell me about that person?

- How will I be evaluated?

- If I perform well, are there opportunities for advancement?

Be sure that the questions are appropriate for the situation. For example, a private physician's office with four employees is not likely to offer opportunities for promotion. To ask about them indicates a lack of knowledge about the employer. It may also give the impression that you will leave for a larger facility after acquiring a few months of experience.

Questions to Avoid

Showing more interest in personal gain than in contributions to the employer is one sure way to lose employment opportunities. The following questions should be avoided until late in the interview or when a job has been offered:

- How much is the pay?

- Do you provide medical insurance? Dental insurance?

- How many vacation days will I get?

- How long are the lunch hours and breaks?

- Can we leave early on Fridays?

- What are the paid holidays?

This information is needed, of course, before making a decision on whether to accept the job or not. First, however, concentrate on convincing the employer that you are the person for the job.

Anticipating an Employer's Questions

Certain kinds of questions are popular with interviewers everywhere. Avoid being caught off guard. Be prepared with answers for the following common questions. Create examples to support your answers.

General Employment Questions

- *Tell me about yourself.* OR *Describe yourself.* Give a brief personal history that concludes with why you want to work in health care. Include your education and any experiences that have reinforced your interest and qualifications for this job.

- *Why do you want to work here?* Explain how the facility matches your work goals and qualifications. Describe how you believe you can make a positive contribution. Explain why you are interested in the particular type of work being performed there.

- *Why do you think you are qualified for this job?* If you know the job requirements, explain how you meet them. If you don't, ask if the interviewer can explain them more fully. This will give you information on which to base your answer.

- *What are your strengths and weaknesses?* Give examples of strengths that relate to the job. Give a specific situation that illustrates the quality. Weaknesses can be handled in two ways. The first is to mention something that might actually be an advantage on the job. For example, if you are applying for a position in health information technology, a tendency to be a perfectionist could be interpreted as a weakness that is actually an advantage. You might explain that while it sometimes takes a little longer to complete a task, it is important to you that it be error-free. The second way is to name a skill, along with your plans for improving it. Do not, however, volunteer a weakness that is a major requirement for the job. You may decide on your own that you are not qualified for this particular job, but it is not necessary to disqualify yourself immediately. The only exception is if the interviewer asks you directly about your level of competency in specific areas. Do *not* claim a skill that you do not have or great expertise in something in which you are a beginner.

- *What did you like best about your last job? Least?* Again, try to focus on areas that are related to the job under discussion. Choose something you liked that is required on this job. Good answers, if they are true, to "liked least" would be that you did not have enough responsibility, the work was not challenging, and so forth. Avoid answers such as "there was too much work," or "the place was a mess." When answering this kind of question, *never* make negative remarks about previous employers. This will cause employers to wonder what you might say about *them* in the future.

- *Which classes did you like best? Least?* Be honest, but again, avoid saying that your least favorite class covered some of this job's major duties!

- *What are your short-term and long-term employment goals?* This can be a tricky question. You don't want to appear to lack professional goals or ambition. On the other hand, employers do not want employees who are only interested in staying for a short time to gain experience. Employers invest considerable time and money into hiring and training new employees. A stable staff also contributes to the quality of a facility. Let the employer know that you want to apply what you have learned in your program and welcome the opportunity to learn more. Your goal is to develop your skills and become an excellent and professional dental assistant, radiology technician, practical nurse, and so on.

- *How do you work under pressure?* Describe a situation in which you successfully coped with pressure. A workplace example is best, but it can also be taken from a personal or school-related experience.

- *How do you get along with others?* Again, be prepared with examples of how you work well with others. Good choices would include contributing to the successful completion of a group project, serving on a committee at school that achieved its goals, or working in a job in which you helped others.

- *How would you handle a conflict with a coworker? With a supervisor?* Choose an incident that had a positive outcome due to your efforts. Give examples of your ability to choose appropriate action based on the situation, apply effective communication skills, and seek a mutually satisfactory solution. Do *not* include negative remarks about the other person.

- *Describe a problem and how you handled it.* Choose a specific problem in which you applied the decision-making process.

- *How do you handle stress?* Describe what works best for you and how you keep stress from negatively affecting your work.

Health Care Questions

Questions may be asked that deal specifically with the job under consideration. These require a good understanding of the chosen occupation and might include examples like the following:

- What coping skills do you use during an emergency?

- What is the biggest issue facing nursing today?

- What would you do if you believed a coworker was stealing narcotic medications from the supply cabinet?

- How do you feel about the risk involved with radiation?

- What would you do if you had a stroke patient who was having difficulty getting dressed?

- Tell me what you know about the equipment you need to operate on this job.

- How would you deal with a mistake you made on a lab test that's already been reported?

- How do you deal with uncooperative patients? Suppose, for example, that you needed to draw blood twice in a sitting.

  (Adapted from *Resumes for the health care professional*, K. Marino, 1993, New York: John Wiley & Sons, Inc.)

Difficult Questions

Some questions are very difficult, especially if something in your history might be of concern to an employer. If it is necessary to explain past problems, stay calm and confident, be honest, and let the employer know that previous difficulties will not affect your ability to perform the job.

- *Have you ever been fired from a job?* If you have, be honest. Do *not* blame or badmouth a previous employer. You can say that you disagreed on issues. If you were in the right, explain the facts of the situation. ("I wasn't comfortable being asked to perform duties that were outside my scope of practice.") If you were at fault, explain how you have corrected the situation. ("I have improved my time management skills and have arrived at work on time every day for the past 18 months.")

- *Why have you changed jobs so often?* If the jobs were part-time or intended to be short-term while attending school, state this. If there were other reasons, try to show how this will no longer be a problem. For example, if previous jobs were boring, explain that this is what prompted you to become trained in health care. You have now found an area to which you can commit yourself.

Illegal Questions

It is illegal to use certain facts about an applicant when making hiring decisions. Questions that require the disclosure of information about these facts cannot be asked during the interview.

Listed below are examples of some commonly asked illegal questions:

- How old are you? What is your date of birth?
- Are you married?
- Do you have children?
- Have you ever been arrested?
- Where were you born?
- Do you own your home?
- Do you have a disability or handicap?
- Have you ever filed for workers' compensation insurance?

  (Adapted from *Job search: Career planning guide, book 2* (3rd ed.), by R. D. Lock, Pacific Grove, CA: Brooks/Cole Publishing Company)

These questions are often asked by employers who do not realize that they are illegal. Or they may be asked in an attempt to learn about characteristics such as the applicant's dependability and trustworthiness.

Applicants have the right to refuse to answer questions believed to be illegal. They may inform the employer that specific questions are illegal. If you want the job and believe the employer is not deliberately breaking the law, there are two strategies that may be more effective:

1. Ask how the questions relate to the job requirements. This allows you to directly respond to the employer's concern. For example, a question about where you live may be asked by an employer who has had difficulties with employee attendance. The issue is arriving on time, not financial status.

2. Incorporate answers to possible, but unasked questions. For example, if you are a female in the age range likely to have small children, explain how you have arranged reliable child care to ensure that you will not miss work.

On the rare occasion that questions are offensive, such as those that are sexual or racial in nature, it is appropriate to refuse to answer and leave the interview. An incident like this should be discussed with an instructor or school administrator.

Creating a Professional Appearance

The interviewer's first impression will be based on your appearance. If it is negative, chances for hire may be lost before the formal interview even starts. Give yourself every advantage by creating a look that says, "I'm a professional who will fit easily into a health care environment." In Chapter 13 the elements of a professional appearance for the

health care worker were discussed. The following summary highlights interview essentials:

- Make sure that everything about you is clean. This includes hair, fingernails, teeth, breath, clothing, and shoes. Bathe or shower and use a good deodorant.
- Demonstrate your knowledge of what is appropriate in the health care setting. Don't use products that have fragrances. Scents from perfumes, body lotions, hair spray, and other personal care products can be offensive when people are ill. Don't take the chance of clinging tobacco odors by smoking on the way to the interview. Remove nose, lip, tongue, and other visible rings that required piercing. Cover tattoos with long sleeves. Refrain from activities that result in hickeys being present at the time of the interview. (Health care employers have mentioned this as a problem with applicants.)
- Wear business attire. Women should choose a conservative dress, suit, blouse and skirt or

Thinking it Through

Cathy Nazerian is hoping that she will finally find an employer who understands what it's like to be a single mother. Before enrolling in the medical assistant program, she had to change jobs 6 times in the previous 14 months. Cathy found her employers to be very unsympathetic about things that really weren't her fault. She couldn't control her unreliable babysitter, old car, and the fact that working while caring for three children tired her out so much that she couldn't always make it to work. Fortunately, she was able to maintain good attendance while in school because her mother had just retired and agreed to help her out temporarily with the kids.

1. How should Cathy respond to employers who ask about her frequent job changes?

2. What changes, if any, should Cathy make in her attitude about employers?

3. What would you suggest she do to reduce the need to change jobs so frequently?

pantsuit. This means a simple style, not something that would be worn to a party. Avoid anything revealing or sexy in any way. Men should wear a suit or slacks and a white or light colored shirt.

- If you are unsure about what to wear, ask an instructor or career services for advice. If you are on a tight budget, ask if the school has interview clothes to lend students. Look in the yellow pages under "thrift shops." They often have very nice clothes at reasonable prices. Some cities now have special shops that provide job seekers with free clothing and accessories, along with good advice about how to dress appropriately.

- Avoid jeans, T-shirts, sunglasses, hats, athletic shoes, and anything symbolic of gangs, religious groups, or political organizations.

- Keep jewelry simple. Men should remove earrings and women should wear only one pair.

- Women should avoid heavy make up and colored nail polish. Long hair should be tied back or pinned up.

- Men with facial hair should trim it neatly. Men should tie long hair back. (These fashions are acceptable to employers in many parts of the country. Your area might be an exception.)

A professional appearance tells the employer that you take work seriously and consider the interview to be an important occasion (Figure 25–1).

Securing References

References are people who will vouch for your qualifications and character. They are willing to be contacted by potential employers to answer questions. References should not be family members, relatives, or friends. Good examples are former supervisors, instructors, clergy, or professionals who know you well.

Applicants should have between three and six references. Ask only those people whom you believe will give you a good recommendation. *Never* give anyone's name as a reference if he or she has not given permission in advance. Keep your references informed about the jobs for which you interview and tell them the name of the person who might call.

Create a **reference list** that can be given to prospective employers upon request. Use the same paper used for the resume. Label it "References" and put your own name, address, and telephone number centered at the top of the page. Then list

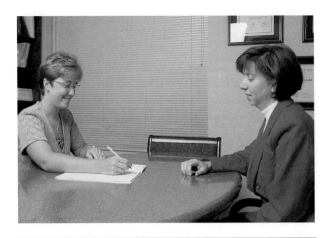

Figure 25–1 Make a strong, positive statement by dressing professionally.

the name, title, address, and phone number of each reference. It is also helpful to add the relationship you have with each person such as employee, coworker, or student. Be sure to give accurate phone numbers. People who are difficult to locate or have disconnected telephone numbers do not appear credible and may do you more harm than good.

Letters of recommendation are statements written on your behalf by former employers and other professionals who know your work. Ask for a letter from any job that you leave on satisfactory terms. Keep the original letter and make copies to give to potential employers.

Creating a Portfolio

A **portfolio** is an organized collection of written documents that can be shown to employers. Its purpose is to support claims about your qualifications. Employers in some parts of the country expect job applicants to have a portfolio. Check with your school or a professional contact to see if this is true for your area.

The following documents are examples of appropriate contents for health care graduates:

- Copy of your diploma or certificate of program completion

- Copy of your professional license, certification, or registration

- Certificates that demonstrate competencies: keyboarding speed, CPR, course completions, and so on

- Documentation of accomplishments and service: awards, letters of appreciation, and so on

- Positive evaluations from the clinical experience and previous employment

- Class assignments that demonstrate proficiency in the tasks related to the job target: completed insurance forms, business letters, charting samples, and documents created with medical management software. Be sure that anything included is absolutely perfect.

- A list of your technical skills and competencies. Organize them by work categories: administrative, clinical, patient care, computer, and so on

- Letters of recommendation from previous employers and others who can vouch for your character

To assemble the portfolio, group similar materials together and place them in a logical order. If there are many items, make a table of contents. Insert the papers in plastic page protectors and place them in a three-ring binder that has a nicely finished cover in a conservative color. A presentation binder containing page protectors can also be purchased.

Do not send the portfolio with the resume. Take it to interviews to demonstrate your competencies. For example, if the employer asks if you know CPT coding, an accurately completed coding assignment would be an appropriate exhibit. You may not have an opportunity to show the portfolio at every interview. Use it only when it can support responses to questions or if the employer asks to see it.

Start early in your educational program to collect items for a portfolio. Keep them neatly in one place so they can be found when needed. Focus on completing all class assignments correctly and neatly so that they not only fulfill class requirements, but can also serve you in the job search.

What to Take to an Interview

Demonstrate your organizational skills and ability to plan ahead by having everything that might be needed at the interview. This will also prevent you from feeling flustered when you can't find a pen to fill out an application. Use the following checklist as a guide:

- Extra resumes
- Application, if you filled it out at home
- Reference list
- List of important facts: driver's license and Social Security numbers, details about employers that are not listed on your resume that might be requested on an application
- Portfolio
- Letters of recommendation (if not in your portfolio)

- Licenses and certifications (if not in your portfolio)
- Pen and notepad
- Appointment calendar

Getting to interviews on time while fulfilling other responsibilities can be challenging. If you will be going directly from school or work, take along appropriate emergency supplies: extra pantyhose, breath mints, a clean shirt, and so on. Take steps to avoid feeling rushed and unprepared; this will help you be at your best.

Practice, Practice, Practice

Practice is the best way to perform well at every interview. Ask a friend, family member, or classmate to play the part of the employer. Practice smiling, introducing yourself, and shaking hands. You may feel silly practicing such simple actions, but the basics are important. A surprising number of job offers are lost because of lifeless handshakes and poor eye contact.

Give your "employer" the list of commonly asked questions and practice answering them. Practice your closing (described in the next section) and leaving the interview on a positive note.

Participate in any mock (pretend) interviews offered by your school. If possible, have your interview taped so that you can critique yourself. Listen and watch carefully. Did you:

- Maintain eye contact?
- Speak clearly using a pleasant voice?
- Avoid using meaningless words like "uh" and "you know?"
- Sit calmly with good posture?
- Answer questions fully, but without rambling on?
- Appear to be interested in the other person?

Practice as often as possible so that when it comes time for the real interview, you can be more relaxed. You would never think of performing a procedure on a patient without sufficient practice. Prepare for job interviews in the same way.

Starting off on the Right Foot

Do everything possible to avoid being late for an interview. Don't lose a job opportunity before even having the chance to present your qualifications. Plan to arrive about 15 minutes early. This gives you time to check your appearance in the restroom and fill out any necessary paperwork. If you are unfamiliar with the area where the facility is located, make a dry run before the day of the interview.

Attend job interviews alone. Bringing a friend or family member demonstrates a lack of self-confidence. Bringing your children, rather than arranging for childcare, demonstrates disorganization. If someone gives you a ride, have the person wait outside.

Be courteous and pleasant with *everyone* you meet, including the receptionist. Do not show impatience or comment negatively if you had trouble finding the location, must wait for the interviewer, or encounter other difficulties. Demonstrate the same professionalism that you will apply on the job. The interview is not just the time spent sitting with the employer in a formal setting. It starts with the first contact, whether that is a telephone call, a resume submitted, or a personal visit.

When you are introduced to the interviewer, smile, establish eye contact, and return the handshake firmly. Wait to sit down until you are offered a seat (Figure 25–2).

Here are some key points to help you do well during the discussion portion of the interview:

- Keep your purpose in mind: to sell yourself and your qualifications.
- *Listen* carefully to the employer (Figure 25–3). What are the employment needs and concerns or problems? What is he or she looking for in an employee?
- Answer questions in ways that show how you are qualified for the job.
- Answer questions fully, but don't talk too long or give out information that wasn't requested.

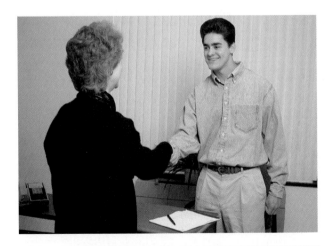

Figure 25–2 Greet the employer with a smile, eye contact, and a firm handshake.

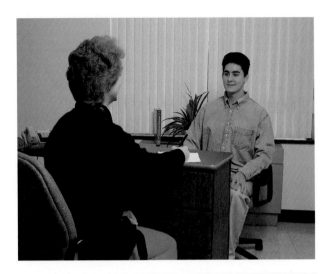

Figure 25–3 Listening carefully to the employer is essential for a successful interview.

- Show interest in the job by asking questions when invited to do so or when you have the opportunity.
- Balance warmth and friendliness with professionalism. *Employers hire people they like.*
- Never share gossip, negative remarks about previous employers or anyone else. Don't discuss your personal problems.
- Do not place anything on the employer's desk unless invited to do so. And *never* read papers or appear to be snooping in any way.
- Project positive nonverbal communication: sit up straight in the chair or lean forward slightly to show interest, maintain eye contact, speak clearly using good expression and enthusiasm. Do not chew gum, and avoid nervous habits such as twisting your hair or jiggling your leg.
- *Never* lie. You should be prepared to answer difficult questions honestly. If a lie is discovered after you are hired, it can be grounds for dismissal.

When the employer indicates that the interview is drawing to a close and you are unsure of the next step in the process, ask what it is. Is there anything you need to send to the employer? When will applicants be notified of a hiring decision? Don't be afraid to ask these questions. At the same time, don't take too much time if it is obvious the employer needs to end the interview promptly. Whether you are interested in the job or not, express appreciation for the opportunity to interview and leave courteously.

After the Interview

Think of the interview as a process that continues until the job is filled, either by you or someone else. Here are some follow-up activities that can tip the scale in your favor:

- *Send a thank you note.* This is one of the most overlooked ways to demonstrate consideration for the interviewer and interest in the job. It never fails to make a positive impression. Do it immediately after the interview, even if you decide that you are not qualified or interested in the job. This employer may have a more appropriate job in the future or may know another employer whose needs match your skills. If you want the job, restate your interest. If you have applicable qualifications you didn't discuss at the interview, mention them in your note (Figure 25–4).

- Send in any requested information, applications, or other items.

- Advise all references that they may be called.

- Review your impressions of the employer and facility. Be prepared to either accept or reject the position if it is offered.

- Place a follow-up telephone call if you do not hear by the date you were told you would be contacted. Let the employer know that you are still interested in the job and ask if a hiring decision has been made. If not, ask when it is expected to be made.

- Continue your job search activities, even if the interview went very well.

Additional Requirements

Many health care facilities are adding new requirements to the hiring process in response to social problems and public health concerns. The following may be encountered in the job search:

- Tests for the presence of illegal drugs

- Psychological tests to determine tendencies toward violence

- Immunizations, such as the hepatitis B vaccinations. (OSHA requires the employer to give these free of charge if the job involves exposure.)

- Health screening tests, such as those for tuberculosis

In addition to questions, some employers give written tests, ask applicants to complete a task, or

1357 Keystone Drive
Chicago, IL 60606
July 31, 2001

Ms. Tasha Jefferson, Office Manager
Compton Dental Clinic
6397 Flanders Street
Chicago, IL 60606

Dear Ms. Jefferson:

Thank you very much for giving me the opportunity to interview for the position of dental assistant at Compton Dental Clinic. I enjoyed talking with you and learning more about the needs of the clinic.

Compton impressed me as being committed to providing high-quality patient care and developing its patient education programs. I believe that my experience as a peer tutor during my studies at Harrison Dental College would help me contribute to your educational efforts. I may not have mentioned during the interview that I am proficient in desktop publishing software and enjoy creating informational materials.

I am very interested in the position and would be pleased to have the opportunity to join the Compton team. Thank you again for your consideration.

Sincerely,

Kelly Bosner

Kelly Bosner

Figure 25–4 Follow up every interview with a thank you letter.

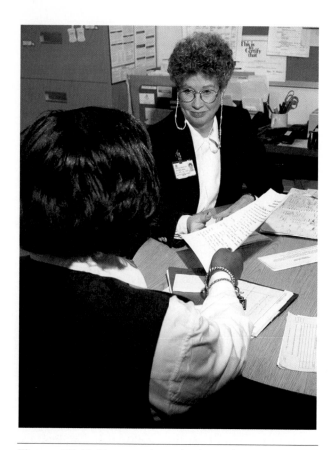

Figure 25–5 You may be asked to take a written test as part of the job-application process.

describe a scenario and ask how you would handle it. In these cases, draw on what you have learned, try to relax, and do your best (Figure 25–5).

ACCEPTING THE JOB

Congratulations! Your hard work and persistence have paid off, and you have received a job offer that you want to accept. If the offer is accepted verbally, such as over the telephone, follow up with a letter in which you express your thanks for the offer, the fact that you accept it, and a statement of what you understand to be the title, salary, and start date.

If you are not sure about whether to accept a position, ask the employer if you can respond in 1 or 2 days. Do not take longer than that. It may not be possible for the employer to extend the extra time if it is urgent that the vacancy be filled.

DECLINING THE JOB

Just as with the acceptance, respond in writing even if you decline the job in a telephone call. Thank the employer for the time spent and confidence in your abilities. State simply that you have decided not to accept the offer. It is not necessary to explain your decision. *Never* ignore a job offer. Remember that this employer may have an extensive network in the health care community. Lack of courtesy in rejecting an offer can damage your chances with other employers.

DEALING WITH REJECTION

All jobs are not meant for all people. If you are not offered a position, it can be for many reasons: you did not have all the required qualifications, someone with the "perfect" combination of skills and experience applied for the same job, or your preferred work style was not a fit. Not being selected for a job should not be taken as a personal rejection. Talking with someone supportive can help you deal with disappointments encountered during the job search.

If you find that you repeatedly fail to receive an offer, review your interviewing skills and ask career services or your instructor for advice. Some employment professionals recommend that you ask the employers with whom you have interviewed for feedback and suggestions. Do *not* approach them in a hostile manner, demanding to know why you didn't get the job. Explain that you want to improve your job-seeking skills and would appreciate their help. Some employers have a policy of not answering this kind of question, so don't insist if they are not willing to discuss the reason why you were not hired.

FILLING OUT APPLICATIONS

You may be asked to fill out an application at any time during the job search. Some facilities that don't have current openings will allow applicants to submit an application that is kept on file for future openings. Others have applicants fill them out at the time of the interview. Be sure to have all necessary information, including dates and locations regarding your education and previous employment. You also need the names and telephone numbers of all references. Regardless of when the application is completed, here are a few important guidelines:

- Read the entire application *before* filling it in. Then start back at the beginning and answer each question completely. In the employment section, do not say "See resume." If you are hired, your application can serve as a legal document, and it must be filled in completely to be valid.

- Type or print neatly using a black pen. The way you fill out an application tells the employer about your ability to follow directions and your attention to detail.
- Be sure that all your facts are accurate. Check that all dates and numbers are correct, especially your telephone number.
- Write "N/A" (not applicable) if a question does not pertain to you, so the reader will know that you did not miss the question.
- Write "negotiable" in the salary section, unless you have already been told what it is.
- Include your signature and the date.
- Review it for accuracy. Look at every item.

Make a copy of any applications you fill out at home. These will serve as a record of your job search as well as supply a convenient source of information for filling out future applications.

SUGGESTED LEARNING ACTIVITIES

1. Practice applying the listening skills described in Chapter 16 to everyday situations. It will pay off when it's time for interviews.
2. Start writing down ideas for answering common interview questions.
3. Make a list of people who might serve as your references.
4. Review your wardrobe for clothes that would be suitable for an interview.
5. Observe your own behavior. Do you make it a habit to be courteous? Do you speak clearly and in a pleasant tone?
6. Enlist the help of two friends, family members, or classmates and set up a practice interview. Choose a specific job to apply for. Give the "employer" questions from all the categories discussed in this chapter. Start the "interview" with the greeting and handshake, and complete it with an appropriate closing. Have the second person observe and critique your performance.

REVIEW QUESTIONS

1. Describe two methods for learning about employers.
2. What are 10 commonly asked general interview questions?
3. How should you handle interview questions about sensitive issues?
4. What are three possible responses to illegal questions asked by an employer?
5. What is the best way to support your qualifications during an interview?
6. What are five appropriate questions to ask a potential employer at the first interview?
7. What are five questions that you should not ask at the first interview?
8. Describe the ideal appearance of either a man or woman who is attending a health care job interview.
9. List eight documents that would be appropriate to include in the health care applicant's professional portfolio.
10. Give three examples of people who would be good references.
11. How can you show an employer you are interested in the job?
12. What are three ways you can show respect for the interviewer?
13. How can you project positive nonverbal messages during the interview?
14. What is the most important interview follow-up activity?
15. How can you ensure that your employment application represents you well?

APPLICATION EXERCISES

1. Refer to The Case of the Modest Applicant at the beginning of the chapter. Describe how Sam could have more effectively sold himself to the employer.

2. Carol-Ann LaRoche has completed her dental hygiene program. She is the first child in two generations to go to college, and her family is extremely proud of her. Carol-Ann did well in her courses. The most difficult part of her training was carrying on conversations with patients. She is very shy and feels unsure of herself socially. While she is looking forward to working as a hygienist, she is terrified at having to attend job interviews. She just knows she'll get tongue-tied and be unable to make a good impression. Recommend a step-by-step plan that Carol-Ann can use to prepare to interview successfully.

SUGGESTED READINGS AND RESOURCES

Drake, J. D. (1997). *The perfect interview: How to get the job you really want* (2nd ed.). New York: American Management Association.

CHAPTER

SUCCESSFUL EMPLOYMENT STRATEGIES

OBJECTIVES

Studying and applying the material in this chapter will help you to:

- Identify important information that new employees should learn about the facility in which they work.

- Explain the importance of understanding the facility's policies and procedures.

- Describe the purpose of the probationary period.

- Identify seven behaviors that contribute to professional success.

- List and explain the major laws that affect hiring and employment practices.

- Explain the meaning of a grievance and how it should be handled.

- Explain the meaning of sexual harassment and the actions to take if it occurs.

- Identify the steps to take when leaving a job voluntarily.

- Describe ways to cope with being fired from a job.

- List activities that promote professional development of the health care worker.

KEY TERMS

chain of command
employee handbook
grievance
integrity
job description
mentor
minimum wage
performance evaluation
policy
probationary period
procedure
professional development
reasonable accommodation
risk management
role model
sexual harassment
team

The Case of

the Irritating New Hire

Katie Cormack began her first job as a laboratory technician at Excelsior Medical Lab 5 weeks ago. She finds the work interesting and especially likes working with patients who come in to have blood drawn for various tests. Katie is surprised when the lab director, Gwen Hendricks, meets with her privately to let her know that other staff members have complained about the time they are having to spend answering Katie's questions. While they appreciate her enthusiasm and desire to do a good job, they are frustrated at having their work frequently interrupted to answer questions regarding common lab policies and procedures and the location of supplies and equipment. Ms. Hendricks explains to Katie that almost all of the information she needs appears in the laboratory manuals or was presented in the new-employee orientation that she received when she started her job. This chapter explains the importance of accepting responsibility for learning a new job and explains the major methods and resources that new employees can use.

GETTING OFF TO A GOOD START

Obtaining the first job after graduation is exciting for the new health care worker. Beginning a new job represents a very important time in the health care worker's career. Your professional reputation starts to be established during the first few months of employment. The habits and relationships developed at this time contribute to future success.

Learning About the Job

Succeeding at a new job requires understanding the basics of the workplace. When Aileen McConnor reported for her first day of work as a health information technician at South Bay Hospital, her supervisor, Stan Bergman, conducted an orientation that included the following components:

- Tour of the facility
  - The Medical Records Department
  - Aileen's desk and work area
  - Lunch room and rest rooms
  - Storage of supplies
  - Personal storage area

- Explanation of safety rules and security precautions
- Demonstration of how to use equipment
- Introduction to coworkers
- Review of her job description

Aileen was glad for the opportunity to ask detailed questions about some of the job duties that were discussed during her employment interview. It is important to clearly understand the duties that the health care worker is expected to perform. Aileen also wanted to make sure that she clearly understood the work schedule that was discussed at the time of the job offer. Misunderstandings about these important issues can lead to employment nightmares. Aileen knew that Mr. Bergman would use her job description as a basis for judging her work performance. **Job descriptions** include important information about a specific job. They serve as guides for the actions and performance of the employee. See Table 26–1 for a description of the contents of a typical health care job description.

Policies and Procedures

Policies are the rules established and followed by an organization. **Procedures** are the specific steps

Table 26–1 Components of the Job Description

Section Title	What It Contains	Examples
Job Title	Exact name of the position	• Medical Transcriptionist • Patient Care Assistant II • Ultrasound Technician
Minimum Requirements	Required knowledge, education, license or certification, and/or experience that must be demonstrated to qualify for the position	• Knowledge of medical terminology, A&P, and English grammar • State nursing assistant certification • Registration with ARDMS (American Registry of Diagnostic Medical Sonographers)
Working Conditions/Physical Requirements	Type of working environment Physical abilities needed to perform the job	• Primarily sedentary work with use of earphones • Able to lift up to 30 pounds • Requires standing during 80% of workday
Reports to	Title of the supervisor who directly oversees the position	• Director of Medical Records • Director of Health Services • Imaging Center Director
Responsibilities, Duties, and Tasks	Specific work to be performed	• Transcribe daily dictation for outpatient surgical center • Transport patients to and from dining room • Perform diagnostic ultrasound procedures for abdominal and OB/GYN patients

taken to perform a task. Every facility develops and records its policies and procedures in order to ensure the quality and consistency of operations. Many health care policies and procedures are required by legal and regulatory agencies. Most facilities assemble manuals that contain all policies and procedures. Employees are expected to know and follow them.

The **employee handbook** is another source of employment policies. It contains information specific to employment conditions such as:

■ Vacation policies

■ Rules regarding overtime

■ Paid holidays

■ How to request a leave of absence

- Benefits such as medical insurance
- Rules of conduct

If you are not shown these materials when you are hired, be sure to ask for them. Take time to study the sections that relate to your job. Ask questions about anything you do not understand. Manuals and handbooks serve as valuable references for both new and experienced staff members.

New employees sometimes do not understand the purpose of certain policies. Never refuse to follow policies with which you disagree. (The only, very rare, exception is if they involve illegal or unsafe activities.) Courteously ask to have the purpose of the policy explained. The reason for it may not be obvious. For example, some facilities prohibit the wearing of colored nail polish. This may seem like a silly rule, but it is founded on principles of good hygiene. Colored polish can hide dirt beneath the nails and around the cuticles. The edges of chipped polish trap germs. Once understood, policies are easier to follow. New employees who have suggestions for policy changes should wait until gaining some experience before suggesting "improvements."

Policies that deal with safety must be carefully followed by health care workers. **Risk management** refers to all the policies and procedures designed to ensure patient safety. Their purpose also includes protecting health care workers and the public from various risks. Many safety practices are mandated by law, and violating them can be cause for immediate dismissal. Be sure that you understand and follow all rules and regulations that apply to your job.

Probationary Period

Most jobs begin with a **probationary period** that typically lasts between 60 and 90 days. This time allows the employer and employee to determine if they have a "match." The employer can evaluate the new hire's performance and decide if continued employment is advisable. This is often accomplished through a formal review process, which evaluates how the new employee has performed in areas such as the following:

- Cooperation with supervisor and coworkers (Figure 26–1)
- Adequate skills to perform job tasks
- Ability to follow directions
- Willingness to learn
- Good attendance record
- Appearance

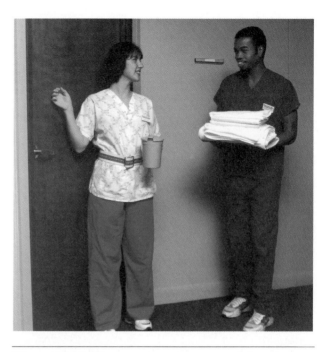

Figure 26–1 Cooperation among coworkers is an important factor in a high quality health care system.

The probationary period is extremely important. In most states, employees can be terminated for any reason during this time. Once the designated probationary period ends, termination is more difficult, and a formal step-by-step process must be followed.

At the same time, the employee can decide if the job is appropriate. Does it require the skills that were acquired in training? Are the duties compatible with the individual's personality and work preferences? While it is unreasonable to expect any job to be ideal, especially at the entry level, it is important that the new employee feel competent and experience satisfaction with the work performed.

GUIDELINES FOR WORKPLACE SUCCESS

There are certain basic guidelines that apply to all types of facilities and positions. Whether the health care worker works directly with patients, such as a nurse, or provides a support service, such as a health information technician, the following recommendations will help ensure long-term career success.

Act with Integrity

Having **integrity** means conducting oneself honestly and morally. It means doing the "right thing" even under difficult conditions. For example, admitting an error and facing the consequences is acting with integrity, or spending extra time to retype a report until it is perfect, without being asked to do so.

Demonstrate Loyalty

Loyalty to the employer and one's immediate supervisor is expected in all occupations. It is unacceptable to spend paid work time complaining about the supervisor or conditions of employment. This is especially true in a health care facility. It can cause serious problems. Patients who sense employee discontent or overhear negative comments may experience doubts about the quality of the facility. This can lead to a loss of confidence about their care. At best, patients feel uncomfortable. At worst, they sue for malpractice. All employees must realize that they represent the organization and dedicate their work efforts to contributing to its success. Learning to work for the good of the organization means expanding one's view from simply personal success to that of the entire organization and those that it serves.

Being loyal does not mean ignoring difficulties at work. On the contrary, these should be discussed directly and courteously with the supervisor. Problems that are not addressed do not disappear. They tend to become worse. Misunderstandings that could be cleared up in minutes can cause resentment and ruin working relationships. Give your supervisor the opportunity to work with you to create a positive working environment.

Employers appreciate employees who have thought through a problem and have ideas for solutions. This is a much more effective approach than simply presenting complaints.

When the health care worker finds it impossible to feel positive about the place of employment, it is best to seek another job. There is too much at risk to do otherwise.

Observe the Chain of Command

Health care facilities organize their personnel so that there is a clear **chain of command**. This means that each person reports to a supervisor who, in turn, reports to another supervisor at the next higher level. This arrangement provides coverage of all necessary tasks along with quality control of employee performance. See Figure 26–2 for a sample organizational chart.

It is important for the health care worker to observe the chain of command. As discussed in

Thinking it Through

Lack of information and failure to communicate are common causes of workplace conflict. Hank Stuart is experiencing a situation now that really has him upset. He is a physical therapist assistant at a busy sports medicine clinic. He also has an interest in computers and worked in a large computer retail store while he went to school. It didn't surprise Hank when one of the owners of the clinic, Kathy Chin, asked him to gather information about computer systems and software that could be used for patient management. Hank spent several hours of both work and personal time and gave his recommendation last week. It was then that he discovered that a system had already been purchased. The clinic's other owner had assigned the computer research task to another employee. Upset that his time and ideas were wasted, Hank has let everyone know just how disorganized and unfair his employers are. His coworkers are tired of hearing about it and wish Hank would just forget it.

1. Do you believe that Hank's reaction to the situation is appropriate? Why or why not?

2. How can he better deal with the situation?

3. What action would you recommend that he take?

the previous section, problems should be discussed with one's supervisor. Workplace problems should not be discussed with coworkers. Nor is it appropriate to go to the next higher level of management without first approaching the person directly involved. It is unfair to "report" your supervisor without giving him or her the opportunity to resolve the situation. It is also inefficient because it brings in another person who is not directly involved in the problem. (Exceptions to this are cases of serious improper behavior on the part of the supervisor, such as sexual harassment or intimidation. These should be reported immediately to the next level of management.)

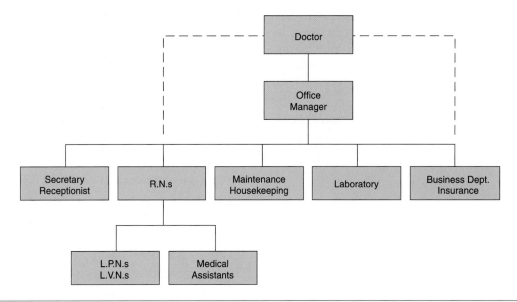

Figure 26–2 Sample organizational chart.

Give a Full Day's Work

Consistent attendance and punctuality are essential when working in health care. Patients depend on services being provided as promised or required. In turn, employers depend on their employees to be available as scheduled to provide these services. Set perfect attendance as a goal. Plan back-up child care and transportation. Maintain good health habits, as discussed in Chapter 12. If an illness or emergency does require an absence, notify your supervisor as far in advance as possible so that the work can be covered.

While at work, full attention should be focused on the job. Avoid personal telephone calls and excessive socializing with coworkers. Do not use work time to discuss personal problems. Patients are annoyed when they are required to wait while health care workers complete their personal business.

Respect the time limits for breaks and meals. If your own tasks are completed and there is extra time, find something productive to do: volunteer to help a busy coworker, reorganize the supply cabinet, or practice a new skill. Devote all efforts to your employer during work hours.

Effective time management increases productivity and efficiency, important in today's managed care environment. It also helps prevent frayed nerves and the panic brought on when tasks are not completed on schedule. The following tips promote the wise use of time at work:

- Write a to-do list when planning each work day.

- Prioritize tasks in order of importance.

- Complete the most important tasks first.

- Batch similar tasks. For example, do all the filing in one session.

- Learn to deal efficiently with interruptions and to quickly refocus on the task at hand.

- Develop time-saving habits. For example, learning to use all the features of a computer program can speed up data entry, word processing, or patient billing duties.

- Avoid procrastinating. If tasks seem overwhelming, break them into small steps and get started. See Chapter 12.

Emergencies will occur and schedules will be disrupted. Patient needs are unpredictable. Visits from regulatory agencies that check on facility quality and adherence to standards can take place on short notice. Health care workers must be willing to cover the necessary work. Effective time management will help keep avoidable emergencies to a minimum.

Become Part of the Team

The specialized and complex nature of health care work requires the participation of many people. Patient care today is accomplished by **teams**, groups of people working together in a coordinated effort to achieve a common goal or set of goals. A football team cannot win if only the quarterback plays the game. In the same way, the success of a health care facility cannot depend on the achievements of just one person. A team may consist of all members of a department, or it may be a small group assigned to work on a specific project. Team goals may be ongoing, such as consistently providing high-quality patient care, or they may be short-term and project-oriented, such as computerizing the office record-keeping system.

Teams that work well can often accomplish more than individuals working separately. There are many ways that teams increase the effectiveness of a facility:

- They provide opportunities for mutual support and encouragement.
- Many viewpoints and ideas are available for solving problems.
- The members contribute a variety of skills.
- Creativity is generated through discussion.
- Work can be coordinated to take advantage of the interests and abilities of the members.
- Duplication of work and wasted effort can be avoided.

The variety of viewpoints and work styles that make teams successful can also be the source of frustration. For example, members who are very creative can contribute good ideas during brainstorming sessions, but become bored during discussions about the details and schedules necessary for the implementation of these ideas. It is necessary to be patient and take advantage of the strengths that each person brings to the group. If the entire group consisted of idea-generators, there might be lots of discussion and little action.

New employees are expected to become contributing members of one or more teams. Making a commitment to the organization and to coworkers is the first step toward becoming a helpful team member. The needs of the group must be considered when making work-related decisions. Therefore, it is important to identify the goals of the team and to find out what is important to the team members as a group.

Here are suggestions for becoming a valued member of the team:

- Keep the group goals in mind.
- Listen actively to others.
- Be positive and productive.
- Contribute ideas.
- Do your fair share of the work.
- Follow through on promises.
- Know when to ask for help.
- Give credit to others for work well done.

- Be flexible and willing to adapt to changes.
- Discuss personal differences in private.

Staff meetings are a common way for team members to share ideas and information, plan work schedules, and keep up on issues of common interest. Workplace etiquette requires that employees arrive on time and be ready to participate. Respect others by paying attention. Avoid side conversations, reading, and other behavior that indicates a lack of interest.

Meetings are not a place to discuss personal problems or grievances. Conduct these conversations in private with the appropriate person. Concentrate on issues of importance to the group. See Box 26–1 for an illustration of the consequences when there is a lack of teamwork.

Go Beyond the Minimum

Achieving professional success requires more than meeting minimum job requirements. It means setting high personal standards and striving to meet them every day. Developing the following habits will help lead to both professional success and personal satisfaction:

- Be enthusiastic: Develop an interest in your job. Be passionate about what you do.
- Project a positive attitude: Focus on the positive aspects of your work. Motivate yourself and others with a can-do attitude. Keep in mind that what you do each day contributes to the welfare of others (Figure 26–3).
- Become a problem-solver: Use your energy to think of solutions instead of voicing complaints. Enjoying the challenge of solving daily problems is an essential ingredient for a successful work life.

Box 26–1 Lack of Teamwork

This is a story about people named Everybody, Somebody, Anybody and Nobody. There was an important job to be done and Everybody was sure that Somebody would do it. Anybody could have done it. Nobody did it.

Somebody got angry about that because it was Everybody's job. Everybody thought Anybody could do it, but Nobody realized that Everybody would not do it. It ended up that Everybody blamed Somebody when Nobody did what Anybody could have done. (Author unknown)

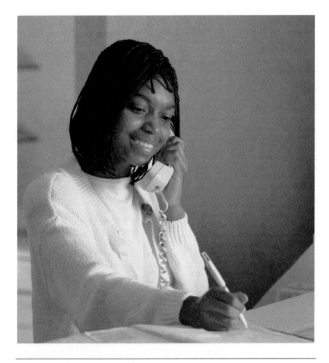

Figure 26–3 A positive attitude helps promote patient satisfaction.

- Do more than is expected: Be willing to work extra time, if requested, to finish a task. If you finish your own work, offer to help others. Pitch in and help with major projects.
- Practice quality control: Take the time to proofread your work. Memorize the abbreviations needed for charting. Practice procedures until you are proficient–on your own time, if necessary.
- Continue to learn: Add to your skills and knowledge. Participate in continuing education activities (Chapter 14).

See Box 26–2 for a summary of the characteristics of great employees.

Learn from Role Models and Mentors

A **role model** is a person who serves as a positive example. Role models demonstrate high levels of professionalism and competence. They strive to be their best and provide inspiration through their abilities, courage, and dedication. Following the example of appropriate role models is an excellent way for the new health care worker to continue the education received during formal training.

What are the qualities to look for when choosing roles models?

- Dedication to their profession
- Respectful of others

- High standards
- Confidence gained through experience
- High level of integrity
- Ability to work well with people
- Understanding of the health care field

A **mentor** is a combination coach and advisor. A mentor should also have the qualities of a role model. Having a good mentor is a tremendous career advantage. However, it does not happen automatically. Look for someone with professional experience, expertise, and an interest in helping others. This person might work in the same department or facility or be someone you meet at a professional meeting or through networking activities pursued during the job search.

The following are a few of the ways that a mentor can help the beginning health care worker:

- Offer suggestions and advice about career strategies
- Provide introductions to people in the field
- Pass on information about job openings
- Encourage you to be your best

EMPLOYMENT LAWS

Job applicants and employees are protected by a number of laws. Some of these laws guarantee access to jobs. This means that it is illegal for employers to refuse to consider an applicant because of characteristics such as race, religion, and gender. The laws do not guarantee that a person will be hired. That depends on the applicant's qualifications.

Other laws protect the health and safety of employees. These are especially important in health care work because employees are exposed to many potential risks. Table 26–2 contains a list of the most common laws that address the employer-employee relationship.

Box 26–2 Characteristics of a GREAT Employee

Compassionate

Competent

Considerate

Cooperative

Courteous

Table 26–2 Major Employment Laws

Law	Purpose	Example
Americans with Disabilities Act	Prevents employment discrimination against disabled applicants who are qualified to perform the job with **reasonable accommodations** (changes in equipment, special ramps for wheelchairs, etc.).	An applicant applying for a medical transcription position cannot be denied the job because the arms of the wheelchair don't fit under the desks in the medical transcription area. A reasonable accommodation would be for the employer to furnish a higher desk or table.
Civil Rights Act of 1964	Prevents hiring discrimination on the basis of race, color, religion, sex, age, or national origin.	A recently graduated nurse cannot be denied employment because she is 52 years old and the employer believes she will not follow directions as willingly as a younger person.
Title VII of 1964 Civil Rights Act	Prohibits sexual harassment, a form of sex discrimination.	It is illegal for a medical laboratory director to continue to ask a lab technician under his supervision for dates when she has clearly stated that she is not interested in dating him.
Equal Pay Act of 1963	Prevents wage discrimination for jobs that require equal skills, effort, and responsibility.	A female medical assistant in an urgent care center must be paid the same wage as a male medical assistant who does the same level of work and has comparable experience.
Family Medical Leave Act, 1993	Allows employees up to 12 months of unpaid leave to meet family needs. Same or equivalent job must be given upon return.	The father of a newborn infant cannot be dismissed for requesting 3 months to assist his wife in caring for their child.
Immigration Reform Act	Prevents employment of persons who do not have the right to work in the United States.	A home health agency that hires young women who do not have the legal right to work in the United States is subject to penalties under this law.
Occupational Safety and Health Act	Prevents unsafe working conditions.	It is illegal for an employer to refuse to pay for a hepatitis B vaccination for a newly hired nurse who provides direct patient care and is exposed to blood and other bodily fluids.

In addition, all states have laws that address **minimum wage** (the lowest hourly amount that an employee can be paid), overtime pay, and other issues regarding work conditions. These differ widely, so health care workers should become familiar with the laws in their area.

Grievances

A **grievance** is a complaint about a circumstance considered to be unfair or potentially harmful. Employees have the right to present grievances to their employer. Many organizations have formal grievance policies that outline the steps required to file a grievance. Look in the employee handbook or ask your supervisor for a copy of the policy.

It is always best to try to resolve workplace issues at the lowest level possible. This means first presenting a problem to your supervisor for discussion and resolution. If the issue is not resolved satisfactorily, then it is appropriate to contact the next level of management. Grievances should be filed only after working up the chain of command, described in an earlier section.

Sexual Harassment

Sexual harassment refers to unwelcome actions that are sexual in nature. It is a form of sex discrimination that is prohibited by Title VII of the Civil Rights Act of 1964. Sexual harassment can occur in a variety of circumstances.

- The victim as well as the harasser may be a woman or a man. The victim does not have to be of the opposite sex.
- The harasser can be the victim's supervisor, a supervisor in another area, a coworker, or a nonemployee.
- The victim does not have to be the person harassed but can be anyone affected by the offensive conduct.
  (Adapted from "Facts About Sexual Harassment," http://www.eeoc.gov/facts/fs-sex.html)

The following are examples of sexual harassment:

- A supervisor repeatedly asks an employee for a date after being turned down.
- A high-level manager promises promotional opportunities in exchange for sex.
- A coworker makes crude remarks about the body of a female coworker.
- A female employee tells dirty jokes in the presence of coworkers who have stated their objections to such stories.
- A male consultant hired by the facility touches a female employee inappropriately.

Mutual friendships and dating are not considered sexual harassment. Workplace romances, however, are not advised. If relationships end, working at the same facility can be uncomfortable and affect the quality of work performed by the people involved. For this reason, some facilities have policies that prohibit dating among employees who work in the same department.

The Equal Employment Opportunity Commission, a government agency that handles sexual harassment complaints that cannot be settled at the workplace, suggests that victims first speak directly to the harasser. Clearly identify the unwelcome behavior and state that it must stop. If the harassment continues, follow the facility's sexual harassment policy or grievance procedure to file a complaint ("Facts About Sexual Harassment," http://www.eeoc.gov/facts/fs-sex.html).

Health care workers can protect themselves against being accused of sexual harassment by avoiding the following behaviors:

- Discussing sexual matters that are not related to the job
- Telling "dirty" jokes
- Describing intimate details of their personal lives
- Joking around about sexual matters
- Touching coworkers and patients in suggestive ways

New employees should carefully observe and learn the level of formality that is customary in their workplace. Some workplaces are more casual than others. Behaviors that are acceptable in one may be considered unacceptable in others.

Employees who work together sometimes become friends and engage in playful conversation. The best way to prevent problems is to be aware of the reactions of others to your actions or conversation. If in doubt, ask them if they are uncomfortable, and immediately discontinue any conduct that they indicate is inappropriate.

TRACKING YOUR PROGRESS

Employees need to know how they are performing in order to grow professionally and improve their skills. If they are not meeting their employer's standards, evaluations provide an opportunity to learn about deficiencies and plan to make improvements.

Performance evaluations can be valuable learning experiences if approached with a positive attitude.

Most new employees are evaluated at the end of a probationary period, as discussed in an earlier section. When the mutual decision is to continue the employment, the evaluation meeting provides an excellent opportunity for the employee to ask questions that have come up during the probationary period. It is appropriate to ask for an honest appraisal of performance and suggestions for improvement. If there have been any misunderstandings about the employer's expectations and priorities, this is the time to clarify them. Employees have the right to know the employer's expectations and the standards used for judging their performance.

The annual **performance evaluation (review)** takes place about one year after the hire date. It typically consists of numerical ratings of the employee's performance of the duties outlined in the job description. It also includes ratings of important employee characteristics such as cooperation. Box 26–3 contains a list of items that commonly appear on performance evaluations. Not every item will appear on every form.

Performance evaluations may include a description of the employee's strengths, behaviors that require improvement, and goals to be met by the next evaluation.

This evaluation may or may not include a salary review. Some employers prefer to conduct the performance evaluation and salary review separately. They believe that this encourages a more honest appraisal of and open discussion about performance.

The evaluation is summarized in a written document that is placed in the employee's personnel file following its discussion in a meeting with the supervisor. More benefit can be gained from the evaluation if the employee conducts a self-appraisal in advance. In fact, some employers require this. Be honest about both your strengths and weaknesses. And be prepared to give examples that justify your "ratings." This is a good time to review the job description to see if there have been changes that need to be addressed. Employees should request copies of all documents that are to be placed in the file, including signed performance evaluations.

Do not react defensively or become angry if any low ratings are received. Ask for clarification and examples of how your work is below standard. Request suggestions for how to make improvements. Demonstrate a willingness to accept

Box 26–3 Common Components of Performance Evaluations

- **Accuracy:** Performs work without errors

- **Appearance:** Maintains appropriate, professional appearance for position held

- **Attendance and punctuality:** Consistently on time and on-duty during assigned hours

- **Communication:** Clear and effective oral and written communication, reports to supervisor as required

- **Cooperation:** Works well with others, contributes to team effort

- **Dependability:** Performs work without reminders

- **Effectiveness under stress:** Remains calm under demanding conditions and during emergencies

- **Flexibility:** Responds well to changing conditions, patient, and facility needs

- **Initiative:** Willing and able to problem-solve and make decisions

- **Operation and care of equipment:** Uses equipment safely and correctly, performs or requests maintenance as needed

- **Quality of work:** Performs task correctly, follows facility procedures

- **Quantity of work:** Completes tasks, meets deadlines, maintains work schedules

- **Safety practices:** Follows facility policies and Standard Precautions

responsibility for your work and an interest in achieving higher standards.

If a performance review is not scheduled within a few weeks after the first anniversary of hire, it is a good idea to remind the supervisor that it is due. These can be overlooked, and your interest in receiving a progress report is usually appreciated.

Employees have the right to see the contents of their personnel files at any time. This includes examining completed performance evaluations and any written warnings or disciplinary notices. Check your file periodically to remain aware of the contents.

MOVING ON

There are many reasons for leaving a job. It is important to do so for the right ones. No job is perfect and care should be taken to make sure that leaving is a good decision. Before resigning, conduct an honest self-assessment. Sometimes we are part of the problem without realizing it. If this is the case, leaving a job is not necessarily an effective solution. Seeking ways to improve the situation may be a better plan.

If the dissatisfaction is limited to one department, a transfer to another part of the facility might be a workable solution. Requesting a promotion, if earned, can add needed challenges and interest to work that has become routine.

When considering whether to leave a job, it helps to review the working conditions that are most important to you. Rank them in order of importance and use the list to compare present and potential opportunities. The following list contains common reasons for changing jobs; you may want to add others.

- More opportunities to learn and apply new skills

- Higher level of job security

- Wider variety of duties

- Distribution of duties better suited to the employee's personality

- More education or training benefits available

- Better work schedule

- Opportunity to work with experts in the field of interest

- Better salary and benefits

It is usually advisable to obtain a new job before leaving the old one. Take care, however, that time at the current job is not spent conducting job search activities. It is also unacceptable to use the current employer's supplies and equipment, such as paper and the copier for preparing resumes or the fax machine to send them out. If you must attend interviews during the workday, schedule them during meal times or use personal time. Prospective employers will respect your efforts to be considerate of your current employer. It is also possible that you will ask the current employer to serve as a future reference. "Don't burn any bridges" is excellent employment advice.

Plan to have adequate savings or financial support if the decision is made to leave the present job before finding a new position. This prevents having to accept the first position that is offered, whether it is satisfactory or not.

Resigning the "right way" helps maintain a positive reputation in the health care community. The following professional courtesies are recommended:

- Give adequate notice. Two to four weeks is customary.

- Submit a letter of resignation. See Figure 26–4 for a sample letter.

- Do not list complaints or grievances in the letter.

- Tell your supervisor before telling anyone else at work.

- Complete all tasks and assignments.

- Do not slack off during the last few days.

- Leave everything in order.

- Offer to help train your replacement.

Thank your employer for the opportunity to work and learn. Ask for a reference letter, even if you have been hired elsewhere. It may be needed in the future.

There are occasional employment situations that present legal and ethical problems. If you are reasonably certain that any of the conditions listed below exist, they must be reported to your supervisor immediately.

- You are required to perform duties that are clearly outside your scope of practice or for which you are not trained.

- Safe practices are not followed.

- Dishonest practices regarding insurance billing are being done.

- Other illegal or unethical activities are allowed or encouraged.

If no corrective actions are taken, then it is appropriate to go up the chain of command and report to the next levels as needed. If your concerns are still not addressed, then resignation may be the wisest alternative. Fortunately, these instances are rare. Most resignations serve as transitions to the next step in a successful career path.

IF YOU ARE FIRED

Being fired from a job is never a pleasant experience. It can be emotionally upsetting and create doubts about personal worth. Try to remain calm and avoid lashing out verbally in anger. If this action is unexpected, ask clarifying questions about the reasons for the dismissal. It is not helpful to argue, but if you feel that this is the result of a misunderstanding or misinformation, request an opportunity to explain your side.

2610 Flanders Court
Tampa, FL 33629
October 5, 2001

Grace Stonefield, Manager
Orthopedic Specialty Group
8884 Orange Parkway
Tampa, FL 33629

Dear Ms. Stonefield:

The purpose of this letter is to advise you of my decision to resign from my position as Radiologic Technician at OSP. I will be relocating to Nashville in November. My last day of work will be October 19, 2001.

I have enjoyed my work at OSP and especially appreciate being given many opportunities to learn and expand my skills. The dedication to patient care and high level of team cooperation made this an excellent choice for starting my professional career.

Your guidance was especially helpful. Having a supervisor who was willing to give me so many opportunities to learn and take on additional responsibilities was an exceptional benefit. I hope I have a chance in the future to help a new technician in the same way.

I wish you and the staff continued success serving the needs of patients.

Respectfully,

Tyler Adams

Tyler Adams

Figure 26–4 Sample letter of resignation.

Most employers dread having to dismiss an employee and try to conduct the firing as quickly as possible. They may state that the decision is final and that they are not willing to discuss it in detail. In this situation it is best to leave as graciously as possible.

Do not be offended if you are accompanied to your work area, observed as you pack your belongings, and escorted to the door. This is standard procedure that employers are advised to follow. They are usually as uncomfortable about it as the employee. It does not necessarily mean that you are suspected of being dishonest.

Being dismissed can be a learning experience that contributes to future job success. This requires taking a hard look at oneself. The following are common reasons for dismissal:

- Lack of skills needed to perform required tasks
- Refusal to cooperate with supervisor and/or coworkers
- Theft
- Repeated failure to practice safe techniques
- Breach of patient confidentiality
- Continual attendance problems
- Dishonesty
- Poor interpersonal skills

Be honest with yourself. Blaming others will not help. Only by accepting responsibility can a plan for positive change be developed. Taking charge and making needed changes is an empowering and positive experience. For example, if skills need improvement, contact your school to see if refresher training is available.

Feeling depressed after being fired is natural. Seek the support of friends and family. Talk over your feelings with someone you trust. Ask for their help as you conduct your self-assessment and make plans for the future.

PROFESSIONAL DEVELOPMENT

Professional development means continually striving to improve and be the best at your profession. It means finding satisfaction in your work and participating in professional activities beyond those required during the normal workday. Obtaining a job is only the first step on the career path. Professional development keeps the journey headed in the right direction.

Whether the health care worker spends an entire career at the same job or makes many changes, professional development is necessary for long-term professional success. All health care occupations are affected by rapidly occurring medical discoveries and technological advances. Continual learning is required to stay current and perform effectively. In many occupations, it is required to maintain a license or certification. Do not view professional education as a burden, but rather as an opportunity to expand your knowledge and opportunities.

In addition to the learning activities discussed in Chapter 14, there are other ways to grow professionally and maintain a lively interest in work:

- Set goals: Setting attainable goals and periodically reviewing progress are powerful motivators for growth. Well-planned goals serve as road maps toward a fulfilling future. Here are a few examples of professional goals:
  - Increase keyboarding speed to 85 wpm
  - Learn health-related conversational Spanish

Thinking it Through

Fran Nichols is angry. She can't believe what happened at work today and how unfairly she was treated by her supervisor, Dan Watson, RN. Dan's been on her case from the beginning, always criticizing her work. But she never thought he would actually fire her. After all, working an 8-hour shift as a nursing assistant is hard work, and it only makes sense to take some shortcuts to complete all the duties. The safety precautions that Dan insisted on were very time-consuming and really didn't seem necessary. After all, the patients she worked with didn't have AIDS or anything, so it didn't really make sense to go to so much trouble with gloves and special waste disposal and so on.

1. From the description, do you believe that Fran's dismissal was fair? Explain your answer.
2. What would you advise Fran if she wants to continue to pursue a career in health care?

- ▪ Earn certificate in echocardiography
- ▪ Be promoted to supervisory position at hospital within 5 years

- ▪ Join professional organizations: In addition to providing learning opportunities, these organizations are a place to share experiences with other health care workers. Friendship and mutual support increase career satisfaction. Active participation on committees or as an officer is an excellent way to practice teamwork and leadership skills. Professional organizations are also good sources for obtaining necessary continuing education credits. See Appendix 1 for a list of health care organizations.

- ▪ Network: Networking is not limited to the initial job search. Maintaining and expanding your networking contacts exposes you to new ideas and opportunities for advancement. Once employed, consider helping others start their careers by giving them information and encouragement. Networking goes in both directions and should be considered a career-long activity.

- ▪ Request additional responsibility: This is a way to both show interest and maintain interest in the job. Once you have mastered the basic duties and work routine, adding new responsibilities keeps the challenge alive.

- ▪ Stay in touch with your mentor: A good mentor keeps you motivated and aiming toward excellence by providing ongoing career advice.

A career in health care involves enormous responsibilities and tremendous rewards. Engaging in professional development activities can help maintain the balance and ensure a long and satisfying career in the service of others.

SUGGESTED LEARNING ACTIVITIES

1. Find out about the professional organization in an occupational area of interest. Using the list in Appendix 1, visit its Web site, call, or send for information. Are the characteristics needed for successful employment identified? What are they?

2. Conduct an Internet search to investigate a variety of health care occupations. Which ones have the most growth? Which are expected to have increasing staffing needs in the future? In which geographical areas is the fastest growth taking place? What are current salary ranges?

3. Identify friends, family, and acquaintances who are successful at their jobs. These can be other than health care. Ask them what they believe makes them successful.

4. Prepare a list of questions you would want to know when starting a new job.

5. Look for opportunities to work with others on teams. For example, volunteer for a committee with an organization you are interested in. Help on a project at your child's school. Participate fully on group assignments given in your classes.

REVIEW QUESTIONS

1. What are 5 important things a new employee should do and/or learn when starting a job?

2. What is the difference between a policy and a procedure?

3. How does the probationary period benefit both the employer and the health care worker?

4. What are 7 behaviors that contribute to professional success?

5. What is the purpose of each of the following laws: Title VII of the Civil Rights Act, Equal Pay Act, Family Medical Leave Act, and the Occupational Safety and Health Act?

6. What is a grievance? What action should an employee with a grievance take?

7. What is the definition of sexual harassment, and what steps should a victim take?

8. What actions should an employee take when leaving a job?

9. How can an employee who is fired learn from the experience?

10. Why are professional development activities important throughout the career of the health care worker?

APPLICATION EXERCISES

1. Refer back to The Case of The Irritating New Hire. Describe all the ways that Katie could have learned about her job to avoid burdening her coworkers with too many questions.

2. Ronnie Martinez, a medical assistant at a busy urgent care center, has an appointment with his supervisor, Dr. Barnes, in 2 weeks for his first annual performance review. His first review took place about 3 months after he was hired. At that time, Dr. Barnes indicated that Ronnie's overall performance was satisfactory. He did recommend that Ronnie spend some time working on his venipuncture skills and that he strive to always arrive at work on time, not a couple of minutes after 8 A.M. as sometimes happened. Ronnie feels that he has made progress in these areas. Describe how Ronnie should prepare for his performance evaluation meeting.

SUGGESTED READINGS AND RESOURCES

Americans with Disabilities:
    http://usdoj.gov/crt/ada/adahom1/htm
U.S. Department of Justice, Civil Rights Division:
    http:www.usdoj.gov/crt
U.S. Department of Labor Family Medical Leave Act:
    http://www.dol.gov/dol/esa/fmla.htm
U.S. Equal Employment Opportunity Commission:
    http://www.eeoc.gov/
Sexual harassment:
    http://www.eeoc.gov/facts/fs-sex.html

APPENDIX

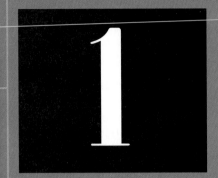

HEALTH CARE PROFESSIONAL ORGANIZATIONS

THERAPEUTIC AND TREATING OCCUPATIONS

Dental Occupations

American Association of Dental Schools
1625 Massachusetts Avenue, NW
Washington, DC 20036

American Dental Assistants' Association
666 N. Lake Shore Drive, Suite 1130
Chicago, IL 60611

American Dental Association
Council on Dental Education
Commission on Dental Accreditation
211 E. Chicago Avenue
Chicago, IL 60611
www.ada.org

American Dental Hygienists' Association
Division of Professional Development
444 N. Michigan Avenue, Suite 3400
Chicago, IL 60611
www.adha.org

Dental Assisting National Board, Inc.
676 N. St. Clair, Suite 1880
Chicago, IL 60611-9796

National Association of Dental Laboratories
National Board for Certification in Dental Laboratory
Technology
8201 Greensboro Drive, Suite 300
McLean, VA 22102
www.nadl.org

National Association of Health Career Schools
750 First Street NE, Suite 940
Washington, DC 20002

Emergency Medical Occupations

National Association of Emergency Medical
Technicians
408 Monroe Street
Clinton, MS 39056
www.naemt.org

National Registry of Emergency Medical
Technicians
P.O. Box 29233
Columbus, OH 43229
www.nremt.org

Society of Emergency Medical Physician
Assistants
950 N. Washington Street
Alexandria, VA 22314
www.sempa.org

Medical Office Occupations

American Academy of Physician Assistants
Association of Physician Assistant Programs
950 N. Washington Street
Alexandria, VA 22314
www.aapa.org

American Association of Medical Assistants
20 N. Wacker Drive, Suite 1575
Chicago, IL 60606
www.aama-ntl.org

American Medical Association
515 North State Street
Chicago, IL 60610
www.ama-assn.org

American Medical Technologists Association
710 Higgins Road
Park Ridge, IL 60068
www.amt1.com
(Medical assistant registration)

American Osteopathic Association
142 East Ontario Street
Chicago, IL 60611
www.am-osteo-assn.org

American Podiatric Medical Association
9312 Old Georgetown Road
Bethesda, MD 20814
www.apma.org

American Society of Podiatric Medical Assistants
2124 S. Austin Blvd.
Cicero, IL 60804

National Commission on Certification of
Physician Assistants, Inc.
6849-B2 Peachtree Dunwoody Road
Atlanta, GA 30328
www.nccpa.net

Mental Health Occupations

American Association of Psychiatric Technicians
336 Johnson Road, Suite 2
Michigan City, IN 46360

American Psychiatric Association
1400 K Street NW
Washington, DC 20005
www.psych.org

American Psychological Association
750 1st Street NE
Washington, DC 20002
www.apa.org

Center for Mental Health Services
Human Resource Planning and Development
Branch
Room 15C 18
Rockville, MD 20857

Nursing

American Association of Colleges of Nursing
1 Dupont Circle NW, Suite 530
Washington, DC 20036
www.aacn.nche.edu

American Health Care Association
1201 L Street NW
Washington, DC 20005
www.ahca.org
(Careers in long-term health care)

American Nurses' Association
600 Maryland Avenue SW, Suite 100 West
Washington, DC 20024
www.ana.org

National Association for Home Care
228 Seventh Street SE
Washington, DC 20003
www.nahc.org

National Association for Practical Nurse
Education and Service, Inc.
1400 Spring Street, Suite 330
Silver Springs, MD 20910
www.aoa.dhhs.gov/aoa/dir/130.html

National Association of Health Career Schools
750 First Street NE, Suite 940
Washington, DC 20002
(Careers as nursing aide)

National League for Nursing
350 Hudson Street
New York, NY 10014
www.nln.org

National Student Nurses' Association
555 W. 57th Street
New York, NY 10019
www.nsna.org/index.html

Occupational Therapy

American Occupational Therapy Association
4720 Montgomery Lane
P.O. Box 31220
Bethesda, MD 20824
www.aota.org

Pharmacy

American Association of Colleges of Pharmacy
1426 Prince Street
Alexandria, VA 22314
www.aacp.org

American Pharmaceutical Association
2215 Constitution Avenue NW
Washington, DC 20037
www.aphanet.org

Pharmacy Technician Certification Council
2215 Constitution Avenue NW
Washington, DC 20037
www.ptcb.org

Physical Therapy

American Physical Therapy Association
1111 North Fairfax Street
Alexandria, VA 22314
www.apta.org

Respiratory Therapy

American Association for Respiratory Care
11030 Ables Lane
Dallas, TX 75229
www.aarc.org

Joint Review Committee for Respiratory Therapy
Education
1701 West Euless Blvd., Suite 300
Euless, TX 76040

National Board for Respiratory Care
8310 Nieman Road
Lenexa, KS 66214
www.nbrc.org

Surgical

Association of Surgical Technologists
7108-C S. Alton Way
Englewood, CO 80112
www.ast.org

Liaison Council on Certification for the Surgical
Technologist
7790 E. Arapahoe Road, Suite 240
Englewood, CO 80112

Vision Care

American Optometric Association, Paraoptometric
Section
243 North Lindbergh Blvd.
St. Louis, MO 63141
www.aoanet.org

Association of Schools and Colleges of Optometry
6110 Executive Blvd., Suite 510
Rockville, MD 20852
www.opted.org

Commission on Opticianry Accreditation
7023 Little River Turnpike, Suite 207
Annandale, VA 22003
www.coaccreditation.com

Joint Commission on Allied Health Personnel in
Ophthalmology
2025 Woodlane Drive
St. Paul, MN 55125
www.jcahpo.org

National Association of Manufacturing Opticians
13140 Coit Road
Dallas, TX 75240

Opticians Association of America
10341 Democracy Lane
Fairfax, VA 22030
www.opticians.org

DIAGNOSTIC OCCUPATIONS

Biometrics

Alliance of Cardiovascular Professionals
910 Charles Street
Fredericksburg, VA 22401

American College of Cardiology
9111 Old Georgetown Road
Bethesda, MD 20814

American Society of Cardiovascular Professionals
120 Falcon Drive, Unit 3
Fredericksburg, VA 22408

American Society of Echocardiography
4101 Lake Boone Trail, Suite 201
Raleigh, NC 27607
www.asecho.org

Cardiovascular Credentialing International
4456 Corporation Lane, Suite 110
Virginia Beach, VA 23462

Joint Review Committee on Education in
Cardiovascular Technology
3525 Ellicott Mills Drive, Suite N
Ellicott City, MD 21043

The Society of Vascular Technology
4601 Presidents Drive, Suite 260
Lanham, MD 20706
www.svtnet.org

Medical Laboratory

American Medical Technologists Association
710 Higgins Road
Park Ridge, IL 60068
www.amt1.com

American Society for Clinical Laboratory Science
National Certification Agency for Medical
Laboratory Personnel
7910 Woodmont Avenue, Suite 530
Bethesda, MD 20814
www.ascls.org

Board of Registry
American Society of Clinical Pathologists
P.O. Box 12277
Chicago, IL 60612
www.ascp.org

International Society for Clinical Laboratory
Technology
917 Locust Street, Suite 1100
St. Louis, MO 63101

National Accrediting Agency for Clinical
Laboratory Sciences
8410 W. Bryn Mawr Avenue, Suite 670
Chicago, IL 60631
www.naacls.org

Radiology

American College of Radiology
1891 Preston White Drive
Reston, VA 20191
www.acr.org

American Registry of Diagnostic Medical
Sonographers
600 Jefferson Plaza, Suite 360
Rockville, MD 20852
http://aztec.asu.edu/medical/azse/ardms.html

The American Registry of Radiologic Technologists
1255 Northland Drive
St. Paul, MN 55120
(651) 687-0048
www.arrt.org

American Society of Radiologic Technologists
15000 Central Avenue SE
Albuquerque, NM 87123
www.asrt.org

The Joint Review Committee on Education in
Diagnostic Medical Sonography
7108 S. Alton Way, Building C
Englewood, CO 80112

Joint Review Committee on Education in
Radiologic Technology
20 North Wacker Drive, Suite 600
Chicago, IL 60606

Section for Magnetic Resonance Technologists
c/o International Society of Magnetic Resonance
in Medicine
2118 Milvia Street, Suite 201
Berkeley, CA 94704
www.ismrm.org

Society of Diagnostic Medical Sonographers
12770 Coit Road, Suite 708
Dallas, TX 75251

HEALTH INFORMATION MANAGEMENT OCCUPATIONS

American Academy of Procedural Coders
309 West 700 South
Salt Lake City, UT 84101
www.aapcnatl.org

American Association for Medical Transcription
3460 Oakdale Road, Suite M
Modesto, CA 95355
www.aamt.org

American Association of Medical Billers
642 South Sunset, Suite B
West Covina, CA 91790
www.billers.com

American Health Information Management
Association
919 N. Michigan Avenue, Suite 1400
Chicago, IL 60611
www.ahima.org

American Medical Association
Division of Allied Health Education and
Accreditation
515 State Street
Chicago, IL 60610
www.ama-assn.org

American Medical Billing Association
4297 Forrest Drive
Sulphur, OK 73086
www.webcom.com/medical/AMBA.htm

ENVIRONMENTAL OCCUPATIONS

Dietary Services

American Dietetic Association
216 West Jackson Boulevard, Suite 800
Chicago, IL 60606-6995
www.eatright.org

Biomedical Engineering

Association for the Advancement of Medical
Instrumentation
International Certification Commission
The Society for Biomedical Equipment
Technicians
3330 Washington Boulevard, Suite 400
Arlington, VA 22201
www.aami.org

Junior Engineering Technology Society
1420 King Street, Suite 405
Alexandria, VA 22314

APPENDIX

USEFUL SPANISH EXPRESSIONS FOR HEALTH CARE WORKERS

Hello, hi.	Hola. (OH-lah)
Good morning.	Buenos dias. (bway-nohs DEE-ahs)
Good afternoon.	Buenas tardes. (bway-nahs TAR-days)
Good evening, good night.	Buenas noches. (bway-nahs NO-chase)
Please.	Por favor. (por fah-VOR)
Thank you.	Gracias. (GRAH-see-us)
You're welcome.	De nada. (day NAH-dah)
Yes/No.	Sí/No (see/no)
My name is ____	Me llamo (may YAH-mo) ____ OR Mi nombre es (me NOM-bray es) ____
What is your name?	¿Cómo se llama usted? (CO-mo say YA-mah oo-sted)
Nice to meet you.	Mucho gusto. (MOO-choh GOO-stoh)
Do you speak English?	¿Habla usted inglés? (AH-blah oo-STED eeng-GLACE)
Do you understand English?	¿Comprende usted ingles? (comb-PREN-day oo-STED eeng-GLACE)
Do you understand me?	¿Me comprende usted? (may comb-PREN-day oo-STED)
Repeat, please.	Repita usted, por favor. (ray-PEE-tah oo-STED por fah-VOR)
I don't understand Spanish very well.	No comprendo el español muy bien. (no comb-PREN-doh el es-pahn-NYOL moo-ee bee-EN)

509

How do you feel?	¿Cómo se siente? (CO-mo say see-EN-tay)
Good.	Bien. (bee-EN)
Fair.	Así, así *or* Regular. (ah-SEE, ah-SEE *or* ray-goo-LAHR)
Bad.	Mal. (mahl)
Do you have pain?	¿Tiene usted dolor? (tee-EN-ay oo-STED do-LOR)
Where?	¿Donde? (DON-day)
Show me.	Enséñeme. (en-SEN-yeh-may)
Are you comfortable?	¿Está usted cómodo? (es-TAH oo-STED CO-mo-do)
What's the matter?	¿Qué pasa? (Kay PAH-sah)
Do you want something?	¿Desea usted algo? (de-SAY-ah oo-STED AHL-go)
It is important.	Es importante. (es eem-por-TAHN-tay)
Be calm, please.	Cálmese usted, por favor. (CALL-meh-say oo-STED, por fah-VOR)
Don't be frightened.	No tenga usted miedo. (no TANG-gah oo-STED mee-A-doh)
We are here to help you.	Estamos aquí para ayudarle. (eh-STAH-mos ah-KEY pah-rah ah-you-DAR-lay)

(Adapted from *Conversational Spanish for medical personnel* (2nd ed.), by R. Kelz, 1982, Albany, NY: Delmar; and *Textbook of basic nursing* (6th ed.), by C. B. Rosdahl, 1995, Philadelphia: Lippincott in *Lippincott's textbook for medical assistants* by J. Hosley, S. Jones, and E. Molle-Matthews, 1997, Philadelphia: Lippincott.)

GLOSSARY

Abdominal cavity Located in the abdomen; contains the stomach, intestines, liver, gallbladder, pancreas and spleen.

Accounts payable Amounts owed to other businesses for services, supplies, or equipment.

Accounts receivable Amounts due from customers for services, supplies, or equipment.

Adult Someone who is 18 years of age or older.

Advance directive Written documents that detail the patient's wishes regarding health care decisions; consists of the living will and the durable power of attorney.

Aerobic Mircroorganisms that require oxygen to live; a type of exercise that elevates the heart rate beyond normal resting rate.

Afebrile A temperature that is within the normal range.

Agenda A list of what is to take place at a meeting.

Agent Someone who has the authority to represent another person.

AIDS A disease that occurs when an HIV positive person develops signs and symptoms of a weakened immune system.

Anaerobic Does not require oxygen to live.

Anaphylactic shock A life-threatening severe allergic reaction resulting in swelling of the respiratory system that restricts breathing.

Anatomical position The body as viewed in a full upright position (standing), with the arms relaxed at the sides of the body, palms facing forward, feet pointed forward, and the eyes directed straight ahead.

Anatomy The study of the form and structure of an organism.

Angle The amount of variance from a reference plane expressed in degrees.

Anorexia nervosa A disease based on the distorted belief that one is overweight, even when severely underweight, and the cutting of calories below the number necessary to maintain health.

Anterior (ventral) Toward the front of body.

Anterior body cavity Consists of the thoracic, abdominal, and pelvic cavities; protects the internal organs; also called ventral body cavity.

Antibiotic Classification of medications capable of inhibiting the growth of or destroying microorganisms.

Antiseptics Chemical agents that prevent or inhibit growth of microorganisms.

Apex At the top (highest point).

Apnea Absence of respirations.

Apothecary system A measurement system that is used infrequently except for a measurement of weight (grain).

Application program A type of software that performs specialized tasks.

Asepsis or Aseptic technique Methods used to make the patient, the worker, and the environment as pathogen-free as possible.

Assault Any threatened or implied act, whether carried out or not; e.g., a patient feels threatened about receiving unwanted treatment, even if not performed.

Assertiveness The ability to express feelings freely in a nonthreatening manner.

Assessment Gathering information; a step in charting that is the health care professional's impression of what is wrong with the patient, based on the signs and symptoms.

Assisted living Residence facility that provides housing, meals, and personal care to individuals who need help with daily living activities, but do not need daily nursing care; may also be referred to as supportive housing, residential long-term care facilities, adult residential care facilities, board-and-care, and rest homes.

Attitude How one mentally views a situation.

Auditory learner A person who learns best by hearing new material.

Autonomy Self-determination.

Bacteria Microorganisms that are one-celled plants; can be either pathogenic or nonpathogenic.

Bacteriocidal A method or chemical that kills bacteria; also called germicidal.

Bacteriostatic A method or chemical that inhibits the growth of bacteria.

Barriers Blocks to communication.

Base At the bottom (lowest point).

Battery Unauthorized touching of another person.

Bias Opinion made before facts are known.

Binge eating The compulsive consumption of large quantities of food, beyond that needed to satisfy hunger.

Bioinformatics The organization of biological data into databases.

Block letter A format in which all lines are flush with the left margin except the date, closing, and signature.

Body mechanics The correct positioning of the body for a given task, such as lifting a heavy object or typing; when the correct muscles are used and the body is in alignment, good body mechanics are being demonstrated.

Body system Combination of two or more organs to provide a major body function.

Bradycardia A heart rate that is below the normal rate.

Bradypnea A respiratory rate that is below the normal range.

Breach of contract When one of the parties in a contract fails to fulfill their part of the agreement.

Browser Special software that allows the user to view Web pages and conduct searches for information.

Bulimia Condition characterized by compulsive eating of huge quantities of food, followed by self-induced vomiting and/or the use of large amounts of laxatives.

Burnout A form of physical and emotional exhaustion that is caused by a variety of personal and environmental stressors that are experienced over an extended period of time.

Calories Energy content of foods.

Capitation Payment of a fixed fee by an insurance company to a health care provider for each patient enrolled in a health care plan, regardless of services rendered to the patient.

Carbohydrate Food substances that are composed of units of sugar and provide the body with immediate energy.

Cardiopulmonary resusitation (CPR) Manually providing respiratory and cardiac support for a patient who is not breathing and whose heart has stopped beating.

Career ladders The various levels within an occupational area that require different amounts of education and training.

Career service center A department of a school or college that functions to assist students in their preparation and search for employment.

Caudal Closer to the coccyx (lower back).

CDC Abbreviation for the government agency titled Centers for Disease Control and Prevention.

Cell Smallest living structure of the body.

Centigrade (C) Measurement of temperature based on a freezing point of (0) degrees and a boiling point of 100 degrees.

Central processing unit Located inside the computer, functions to manage all operations, perform calculations, manipulate data, and store program instructions and data.

Cephalic (cranial) Closer to the head.

Certification The process of determining whether a person has met predetermined standards.

Chain of command The organization of employees in which each person reports to a supervisor who, in turn, reports to another supervisor at the next higher level.

Chain of infection Defines the six criteria that must be present for an infection to develop.

Charting Recording observations and information about patients.

Cheyne-Stokes A breathing pattern that has a period of apnea followed by a gradually increasing depth and frequency of respirations.

Chief complaint The patient's statement of the main reason he or she is seeking medical care.

Chiropractic Health care practice based on the belief that pressure on the nerves leaving the spinal column causes pain and/or dysfunction of the body part served by that nerve.

Cholesterol Fatty substances that can clog arteries.

Chronic illness Health problem of long duration in which the disease condition shows little change, or slowly gets progressively worse.

Chronological resume Employment resume that emphasizes work experience. Contains a section in which the duties and accomplishments of previous jobs are described.

Closed fracture When a bone is broken but does not protrude through the skin.

Closed-ended questions Inquiries that can be answered with a single word or a response of "yes" or "no."

Code of ethics Principles created by professional organizations to serve as a guide for the conduct of health care workers in that profession.

Cognitive The intellectual processes that include thought, awareness, and the ability to rationally comprehend the world and determine meaning.

Cold calls Calling or visiting employers to make the first contact.

Combining form A root word plus a vowel, in a medical term.

Combining vowel The letters a, e, i, o, or u when used to link the root word to the next element in a medical term.

Communicable disease A disease that can be transmitted either directly or indirectly from one individual to another.

Communication Process in which messages are exchanged between a sender and a receiver.

Compatibility The ability to be combined without unfavorable results.

Complementary therapies Health care practices that have not traditionally been performed in conventional medical offices.

Computer literacy Understanding how a computer functions, being able to perform basic operations, and having an awareness of the impact of technology on the quality of human life.

Confidentiality Preserving the legal right of a patient to privacy concerning his or her medical affairs.

Consent To give permission; permission that is given.

Consonant Any letter except a, e, i, o, and u.

Constructive criticism Appropriate feedback on performance of others, based on the belief that it can be improved.

Contaminated Infectious material is present.

Continuing care community Provides a variety of living arrangements that support lifestyles as they change from independent living to the need for regular medical and nursing care.

Continuing education Learning experiences beyond those needed to earn the initial certificate or degree to work in an occupation.

Continuing education unit (CEU) The credits granted for certain types of learning that take place after the completion of formal education; same as continuing professional education (CPE).

Continuing professional education (CPE) The credits granted for certain types of learning that take place after the completion of formal education; same as continuing education unit (CEU).

Continuous quality improvement (CQI) Process designed by the health care facility to improve quality of care and cost efficiency.

Contract Promise that is enforceable by law.

Contraction The combined form of two words; e.g., it is = it's.

Copay The set amount that the patient pays when medical services are received.

Cost of money The amount that is lost when money is not invested; often used to refer to money that is owed to a business but not collected in a timely way.

Cover letter A written document sent with resumes as a way to introduce oneself and inform the employer why the resume is being sent.

Cranial cavity Located in the skull; contains the brain.

Cross-training When health care employees are trained to perform tasks in addition to those traditionally performed by those with their job titles.

Culture The values, shared beliefs and attitudes, social organizations, family and personal relationships, language, everyday activities, religious practices, and concepts of time and space of a given group of people.

Damages Money to compensate for an injury or loss.

Database The organization of computerized information in a structured way that makes it easy to sort and access.

Decimal A linear arrangement of numbers based on units of 10, containing a point (decimal point) to separate the whole number from the fractional part of a number (e.g., 2.5).

Deep Farther from the body surface.

Defamation of character A legal charge for disclosing unauthorized information that could harm the reputation of another.

Defense mechanism Behaviors that are usually performed unconsciously in response to perceived threats to self-esteem in order to provide temporary relief from the mental discomfort and anxiety.

Degree Unit of measurement used in angles, temperature readings, and depth of burns.

Development The mental, emotional, and social growth of individuals as they progress through life stages.

Diagnosis Name of a disease or syndrome.

Diagnostic procedures Tests performed to determine the diagnosis.

Diagnostic related group (DRG) A classification system of patients based on their diagnoses to predetermine Medicare payments.

Discreet Being careful about what you say, preserving confidences, and respecting privacy.

Diseases Abnormal conditions created when the normal anatomy and physiology of the body is altered.

Disinfectants Agents or methods that destroy most bacteria and viruses.

Diskette Magnetic material enclosed in a flat hard plastic case and used to store computer data.

Distal Farther from the reference base point.

Dominant culture Refers to what are generally considered to be the foundational beliefs and ideal behavior of a society or country.

Download Transfer data from one computer to another.

Durable power of attorney The part of the advance directive that designates specific people to act on the patient's behalf if they are unable to make health care decisions.

Dyspnea Labored breathing or difficulty with breathing.

Electronic mail A means of creating and sending messages from one computer to another, using the Internet system of networks.

Electronic spreadsheet Software that permits the user to apply the computer's ability to perform high-speed calculations of numerical data.

Emancipated minor Someone under the age of 18 who is financially independent, married, or in the military.

Emergency disaster plan Policy and procedures to be followed when an event occurs that has the potential to kill or injure a group of people.

Empathy Understanding another person's thoughts, feelings, and behavior.

Employee handbook A source of employment policies.

Environmental safety The identification and correction of potential hazards that can cause accidents and injuries.

Ergonomics The science of designing and arranging things in the working and living environments for maximum efficiency and maximum health and safety; a good ergonomic environment maximizes the comfort level and efficiency of the person while limiting possible exposure to discomfort or potential injury.

Erikson's Stages of Psychosocial Development A theory based on the psychosocial challenges that are presented to individuals as they progress through life stages.

Estimating Expressing the approximate answer.

Ethical dilemma When the underlying principles of an ethical system appear to contradict each other and no clear answer emerges.

Ethics A system of principles (fundamental truths) a society develops to guide decision-making about what is right and wrong; it helps people deal with difficult and complex problems that lack easy answers.

Etiology Study of the causes of diseases.

Etiquette Manners, acceptable conduct.

Eupnea Breathing that is within the normal range, unlabored, and has an even rhythm.

Euthanasia Performing a deliberate action that results in a painless, easy death for individuals with an incurable disease; same as mercy killing.

Exhalation The part of the respiratory cycle when air is removed from the lungs.

Expanding consciousness A theory by Margaret Newman developed to assist patients in making their lives as meaningful as possible by focusing on their possibilities rather than their limitations.

Expenditures The money that must be spent in the process of doing business (e.g., the cost of resources required to maintain a health care delivery system).

Expert systems Computerized databases that are designed to assist health care professionals in diagnosing and treating specific conditions.

Express consent Permission that is given in writing.

Express contract Result of the parties discussing and agreeing on specific terms and conditions.

External bleeding When blood drains to the outside of the body through a break in the skin.

External customer People who come to the health care provider for services; they may be referred to as customers, patients, or clients.

Fahrenheit (F) Measurement of temperature based on a freezing point of 32 degrees and a boiling point of 212 degrees.

False imprisonment A legal claim patients can charge if they are held against their will, unless they are mentally incompetent or a danger to themselves.

Fat Food substances that contain fatty acids and provide the most concentrated form of energy for the body.

Febrile A temperature that is elevated above the normal range.

Feedback A way for the sender of a communication to check the understanding of the receiver.

Fee-for-service Method of payment in which patient pays health care provider an amount from an established schedule of fees.

Fiber A substance in food that cannot be fully digested.

Fiber optics Technology that uses hair-thin cables to transmit computer data.

Field Basic data category in a database.

File A group of related computer records.

Financing The source of money used to run a business.

First aid Emergency care provided to an accident victim or to someone who has become suddenly ill.

Flammable Easily set on fire; same as inflammable.

Food guide pyramid An eating plan developed by the United States Department of Agriculture that ensures the daily diet contains all the components necessary for good health.

Fraction A method used to express numbers that are not whole numbers; a fraction is read as parts (numerator) to a whole (denominator).

Fraud A form of dishonesty that involves cheating or trickery.

Frontal plane Divides the body vertically into front and back portions.

Frostbite Condition in which the skin begins to freeze.

Full block letter A format in which all lines are flush with the left margin.

Functional resume Employment resume that emphasizes professional qualifications.

Fungi (pl. of fungus) Microorganisms that represent a large group of simple plants; may be pathogenic or nonpathogenic.

Gatekeeper A health care provider, often a physician, who serves as the patient's first contact when entering the health care system; also known as primary care provider.

Germ theory States that specific microorganisms called bacteria are the cause of specific diseases in both humans and animals.

Golden Rule A primary principle when assisting others to "do no further harm."

Good Samaritan Act A law to protect individuals from liability when they stop to assist someone who has been hurt or is ill.

Grammar A set of rules that determines proper word order, sentence construction, punctuation, and capitalization.

Grievance A complaint about a circumstance considered to be unfair or potentially harmful.

Growth Refers to the physical changes that normally take place as the body matures.

Hard drive A storage device located inside the computer.

Hardware The physical components of the computer.

Hemorrhage Severe, heavy bleeding.

Hepatitis B A virus that causes a blood-borne infection. An occupational hazard for health care workers.

HIV positive The condition of being infected by the Human Immunodeficiency Virus.

Holistic medicine Health care practices based on the belief that the traditional view of medicine must be expanded and that all aspects of the individual— physical, mental, emotional, and spiritual—contribute to states of health and disease.

Homeopathy A health care practice that is based on the idea that "like cures like." Disorders are treated with very small amounts of the natural substances that cause symptoms of the disorder in healthy people.

Homeostasis Tendency of a cell or the whole organism to maintain a state of balance.

Hospice A facility or service that offers palliative (relieves but does not cure) care and support to dying patients and their families.

Host Living plants or animals from which microorganisms derive nourishment.

Household system A measurement system based on common household items used to measure length, volume, and weight.

Hypertension Blood pressure above the normal range.

Hyperthermia Condition in which the body temperature is above the normal range.

Hypotension Blood pressure below the normal range.

Hypothermia Condition in which the body temperature is below the normal range.

Illness A state experienced by the body when one or more of the control systems loses the ability to maintain homeostasis.

Immune response Defense used by the body to fight infection and disease by producing antibodies.

Implied consent Permission for procedures indicated by the patient's actions; e.g., showing up for a medical appointment, opening the mouth for the dentist to administer an injection, or participating in therapeutic exercises.

Implied contract When the actions of the parties create a contract without it being detailed in a written format.

Improper fraction A fraction that has a numerator that is larger than the denominator.

Incident report Written document that is filled out when any unexpected situation occurs that can cause harm to a patient, employee, or any other person.

Independent clause Part of a sentence that can stand on its own as a complete sentence.

Infection control Procedures to be followed to prevent the spread of infectious diseases.

Infectious disease Disease caused by growth of pathogens.

Inferior Below.

Inflammable Easily set on fire; same as flammable.

Informed consent To give permission for a procedure after it has been explained along with possible consequences.

Inhalation The part of the respiratory cycle when air enters the lungs.

Inpatient Patients who are treated within the hospital setting.

Integrity A personal characteristic reflected as honesty; choosing the right rather than the easy way; conducting oneself honestly and morally.

Intermediate care facility (ICF) A type of nursing home that provides personal care, social services, and regular nursing care for individuals who do not require 24-hour nursing, but are unable to care for themselves.

Internal bleeding When blood loss occurs inside the body.

Internal customer People who work within the healthcare industry, in other words, other health care workers.

Internet A vast global system of computer networks linked with other networks that allows instant communication and the sharing of information.

Invasive procedures Punctures or incisions of the skin or insertion of instruments or foreign material into the body.

Job description A list of duties, responsibilities, and other important information about a specific job.

Job interview A conversation between an applicant and a potential employer to determine if there is a match between the needs of the employer and the qualifications of the applicant.

Jobline Taped recordings with information about current job openings.

Joint dislocation When a joint becomes disconnected from its socket.

Justice Fairness.

Justified (text) A written format in which the text is lined up with the margins.

Kinesthetic learner A person who learns new material best through the performance of hands-on activities.

Lateral Away from center of body (toward the sides).

Leadership An approach to working with others that encourages people to work together to do their best to achieve common goals.

Leading questions Inquiries in which all or part of the answer is included in the wording of the question.

Learning objectives Educational goals or what students are to accomplish during a lesson.

Learning styles A theory that states that individuals learn in different ways; the most common categories are classified by the senses (sight, sound, and touch).

Legislation Laws.

Letters of recommendation Statements written on a job applicant's behalf by former employers and other professionals.

Libel A legal charge for defamation of character committed in a written form.

Licensure A designation that means a person has been granted permission to legally perform certain acts.

Life review Telling the events of one's life as a form of self-evaluation and closure as the end of life approaches.

Lifelong learning Refers to all purposeful learning activities, both formal and informal, that take place throughout our lives.

Living will The part of the advance directive that outlines the individual's wishes regarding the type and extent of care to be given.

Malpractice Professional negligence.

Managed care Promotion of cost-effective health care through the management and control of its delivery.

Manual dexterity Skill in working with the hands.

Maslow's Hierarchy of Needs A model that categorizes and ranks basic human needs into five areas in an effort to explain how human behavior is motivated by each individual's efforts to fulfill certain requirements for complete physical and mental well-being.

Massage therapy A method of rubbing or kneading the body to enable muscles to relax.

Math anxiety A strong negative reaction to math that interferes with the ability to concentrate, learn, and perform math calculations.

Medial Toward the midline or center of body.

Medic Alert An organization that provides bracelets or pendants for patients to wear that contain information or warnings about specific medical problems.

Medicaid Federally funded, but state-administered insurance plan for individuals who qualify due to low income.

Medical asepsis or clean technique Procedures to decrease the numbers and spread of pathogens in the environment.

Medical documentation Notes and documents that health care workers add to the medical record.

Medical history Data collected on a patient that includes personal, familial, and social information.

Medical record The collection of all documents that are filed together and form a complete chronological health history of a particular patient.

Medical terminology A language used by health care workers that includes specialized terms and abbreviations.

Medicare Federally funded insurance program for individuals who qualify for Social Security benefits.

Meditation A process for quieting the mind by clearing it of thoughts.

Mentor A combination of coach and advisor.

Mercy killing Performing a deliberate action that results in a painless, easy death in individuals with an incurable disease; same as euthanasia.

Metric system A measurement system based on tens; basic units are length (meter), volume (liter), and weight (gram).

Microbes Term used for microorganisms that are pathogenic.

Microbiology Scientific study of microorganisms.

Microorganisms Small, usually one-celled, living plants or animals.

Microscope Instrument fitted with a powerful magnifying lens.

Midsagittal plane Passes through the midline and divides the body vertically into equal right and left portions.

Military time A method of telling time that is based on a 24-hour clock.

Minimum wage The lowest hourly amount that an employee can legally be paid.

Modem A device that converts outgoing messages from a computer to a form that can be sent over telephone lines.

Modified block letter A format similar to the block letter except that paragraphs are indented five spaces.

Negligence Failure to meet the standard of care that can be reasonably expected from a person with certain training and experiences.

Negotiated fees Amount negotiated between insurance companies and health care groups for the cost of services; depending on the plan, the patient either pays the difference in actual cost of service or the health care group accepts the negotiated amount as payment in full.

Network Computers that are linked by cables or telephone lines that enable them to communicate and share data.

Networking Developing a group of individuals who might help you meet your professional goals.

Nomenclature Method of naming.

Nonverbal communication Meaning conveyed by tone of voice, body language, gestures, facial expressions, touch, and physical appearance.

Normal flora Microorganisms that commonly reside in a particular environment on or in the body.

Nosocomial infection Infection that occurs while the patient is receiving health care.

Objective Approaching situations from a factual rather than an emotional perspective; statement of your job goal.

Objective data Direct observations made by the health care worker to evaluate a patient's condition.

Open fracture When a broken bone protrudes through the skin.

Open-ended questions Inquiries that require more than a one-word response and are used to encourage patients to provide more detailed information or explanations.

Opinion Beliefs that are not based on certainty and/or are made without researching the facts.

Opportunistic infections Infection that occurs due to the weakened physiological state of the body.

Organ The combination of two or more types of tissues that work together to perform a specific body function.

Orthopnea When a patient has difficulty breathing unless in a sitting or standing position.

Orthostatic (postural) hypotension Rapid lowering of the blood pressure as a result of changing positions.

OSHA Abbreviation for the government agency titled Occupational Safety and Health Administration.

Osteopathy Health care practices based on the belief that the body can protect itself against disease if the musculoskeletal system, especially the spine, is in good order.

Outpatient services Health care services that do not require hospitalization; also referred to as ambulatory services.

Pantomime Using body movement to convey ideas or actions.

Paraphrasing A method for obtaining feedback by restating the sender's message in his or her own words and asking the sender for confirmation.

Parasite Organism that nourishes itself at the expense of other living things and causes them damage.

PASS Acronym for proper use of a portable fire extinguisher (**P**ull the pin, **A**im the nozzle at the base of the fire, **S**queeze the handle, **S**weep back and forth along the base of the fire).

Pathogens Disease-causing microorganisms.

Pathophysiology The study of why diseases occur and how the body reacts to them (changes in function caused by disease).

Pelvic cavity Located in the lower abdomen; contains the urinary bladder, rectum, and reproductive organs.

Percentage A method used to express a whole or part of a whole. The whole is written as 100%.

Performance evaluation An evaluation and rating of an employee's performance; also referred to as a performance review.

Peripheral Anatomical term meaning away from the center; computer term for equipment that allows the user to interact with the CPU.

Personal space The distance at which people feel comfortable when carrying on a conversation.

Philosophy of Individual Worth A view based on the belief that every human being, regardless of personal circumstances or personal qualities, has worth.

Physical Refers to the growth of the body, including motor sensory adaptation.

Physiological needs Level 1 in Maslow's Hierarchy of Needs that must be satisfied in order to maintain life; these necessities include oxygen, water, and food.

Physiology The study of the functions (how and why something works) of an organism.

Plan A step in SOAP charting that documents the procedures, treatments, and patient instructions that make up the patient's care.

Point of care charting Entering information about patients into the computer from the patient's home or hospital bedside.

Policy A rule established and followed by an organization.

Portfolio An organized collection of written documents that can be shown to employers to support claims about an applicant's qualifications.

Posterior (dorsal) Toward the back of the body.

Posterior body cavity Consists of the cranial and spinal cavity; protects the structures of the nervous system; also called dorsal body cavity.

Preauthorization Approval from an insurance company prior to certain health care services, for the purposes of determining medical necessity and cost-effectiveness.

Prefix A word element that is attached to the beginning of roots and combining forms to add to or change their meaning.

Prejudice Negative feelings about a person because he or she belongs to a specific cultural or racial group.

Premium An agreed-upon amount paid to an insurance company for the benefit of having the company pay for a specified amount of future health care costs.

Prepaid plans A contracted type of insurance plan in which health care providers are paid a specific amount to provide certain health benefits.

Prevention (of disease) Behaviors that promote health and prevent disease.

Primary care provider (PCP) Health care providers, often physicians, who serve as the patient's first contact when entering the health care system; also known as gatekeepers.

Principles Fundamental truths.

Prioritize Ranking items that need to be done in order of importance.

Probation period Typically the first 60 to 90 days of employment that provide an opportunity for the employer and employee to determine if they have a "match."

Probing questions Inquiries that request additional information or clarification.

Problem-solving process A sequence of organized steps that is followed to assist in making good decisions.

Procedure Specific steps taken to perform a task.

Professional development Continually striving to improve and be the best possible at your profession.

Professional distance Refers to a healthy balance in the worker-patient relationship that involves demonstrating a caring attitude toward patients without the goal of becoming their friends.

Professionalism A set of characteristics and behaviors that enables one to do the best job possible to provide and maintain high quality service to patients and employers.

Profit Amount of money remaining after all costs of operating a business have been paid.

Prognosis Prediction of the possible outcome of a disease and the potential for recovery.

Progress notes Written chronological statements about a patient's care.

Proportion A mathematical statement of equality between two ratios.

Protein Food substances that contain amino acids which are necessary for both building and maintaining the structural components of the body.

Protocols Standard methods of perform-ing tasks.

Protozoa Microorganisms that are classified as animals.

Proximal Closer to the reference point.

Psychiatric hospital A facility that offers treatment to individuals with psychiatric and behavioral disorders, including assistance with crises, medication management, counseling, and monitoring of activities of daily living.

Psychosocial Refers to the emotions, attitudes, and other aspects of the mind, in addition to the individual's interactions and relationships with other members of society.

Psychosomatic Disorders caused by mental and/or emotional factors.

Pulse deficit The rate difference between a pulse point and an apical rate that are taken simultaneously.

Pulse points Specific sites on the body where arterial pulsations can be felt.

Quality assurance (QA) Process designed to meet external regulatory requirements by identifying problems, quantifying occurrences, and comparing results to industry standards.

Quality improvement Processes used to find ways to preserve or improve quality of care while decreasing costs.

Quotation Words written exactly as spoken.

RACE Acronym for responding to fires (**R**emove patients, sound the **A**larm, **C**ontain the fire, and **E**xtinguish the fire or **E**vacuate the area).

RAM An internal computer workspace that stores data only while the computer is on.

Ratio A method used to express the strength of a solution; it represents how many parts of one element are added in relationship to the parts of another element.

Reasonable accommodation A legal requirement to supply or make changes in equipment or other aspects of the environment if necessary, to accommodate a disabled applicant who is qualified to perform the job.

Receiver The person to whom the sender directs the message; also called the listener.

Reciprocal A fraction that has been "turned upside-down" during the process of dividing fractions.

Record A collection of related computer data.

Reference People who will vouch for your qualifications and character.

Reference list A written list that can be given to prospective employers upon request that includes contact information for people who will vouch for your qualifications and character.

Reference plane A real or imaginary flat surface from which an angle is measured.

Reflecting A method of obtaining feedback by prompting the receiver to either complete or add more detail to the original message.

Registration Being placed on an official list after meeting the educational and testing requirements for a specific profession.

Reimburse To pay back.

Relaxation Refers to techniques used to reduce stress by releasing tension in the muscles in order to improve blood circulation.

Reliable Trustworthy.

Repetitive motion injury (RMI) Injury resulting from a repeated movement that causes damage to a nerve, ligament, tendon or muscle.

Rescue breathing A technique in which the rescuer breathes for the victim.

Rescuer Person giving care during an emergency.

Respiration The process of taking air into and removing air from the lungs; one respiration includes one full cycle of inhalation and exhalation.

Respondeat superior Individual, such as an employer, who is legally responsible for the behavior and actions of his or her employees.

Resume Written summary of professional qualifications.

Rickettsia A microorganism that is smaller than bacteria and has rod or spherical shapes.

Risk management Refers to all the policies and procedures designed to ensure patient safety.

Role model A person who serves as a positive example.

Roman numerals A numbering system based on I (1), V (5), X (10), L (50), C (100), D (500), and M (1000).

Root word The part of the medical term that gives the main meaning to the word; often refers to the structure and function of the body.

Rounding numbers Rules that determine whether a number is changed to zero, increased, or remains the same when digits are dropped from the right side.

Salutation Greeting.

Scope of practice A description or list of skills that a specific occupational title is legally allowed to perform.

Self-actualization Level 5 of Maslow's Hierarchy of Needs defined as the achievement of one's greatest potential.

Self-directed learning Refers to all activities that you plan and participate in to increase your knowledge and skills.

Self-esteem An individual's opinion of himself or herself.

Sender The person who creates and delivers a message; also called the speaker.

Sexual harassment Refers to unwelcome actions that are sexual in nature.

Signs Objective evidence observed by health care workers regarding the patient's condition.

Signs and symptoms The objective evidence (signs) observed by the health care worker and the subjective data (symptoms) reported by patients about their condition.

Site license Permission granting the installation of software on more than one computer.

Skilled nursing facility (SNF) A type of nursing home that provides nursing and rehabilitation services on a 24-hour basis; includes regular medical care for patients with long-term illnesses or those recovering from illness, injury, or surgery.

Slander A legal charge for defamation of character committed in a spoken form.

SOAP A format for charting that uses a problem-oriented approach.

Software Computer programs that contain instructions that enable computers to function.

Sphygmomanometer An instrument that records the blood pressure.

Spinal cavity Located within the spinal column; contains the spinal cord.

Sprain Torn ligament fibers that result in a loosening of the joint.

Stages of dying Stages that dying persons may experience as they face the fact of their own death. The five stages are denial, anger, bargaining, depression, and acceptance.

Standard precautions Practices designed to reduce the risk of transmission of microorganisms from both recognized and unrecognized sources of infection in health care settings.

Sterile field Area designated to be free of microorganisms.

Sterilization Agents or methods that totally destroy all microorganisms, including viruses and spores.

Stethoscope An instrument that amplifies sounds so they can be heard from within the body.

Strain (muscle) Result of sudden tearing of muscle fibers during exertion; also referred to as pulled muscle.

Stress Physiological changes that occur in the body as it responds to danger, either real or imagined.

Stressor Any cause of stress to the individual.

Subjective data Information the patient tells the health care worker about his or her condition that cannot be directly observed.

Sucking wound A puncture into the respiratory system resulting in loss of air as the patient breathes.

Suffix A word element that is attached to the end of roots and combining forms to add to or change their meaning; any word ending.

Superficial Near or close to the body surface.

Superior Above.

Surgical asepsis or sterile technique Procedures to completely eliminate the presence of pathogens from objects and areas.

Syllable Part of a word that has a single spoken sound.

Symptoms Subjective data reported to the health care provider by the patient.

Syndrome Not a precise disease but a group of related signs and symptoms.

Tachycardia A heart rate that is above the normal range.

Tachypnea A respiratory rate that is above the normal range.

Team Groups of people working together in a coordinated effort to achieve a common goal or set of goals.

Telemedicine The practice of medicine over telephone lines.

Terminal illness An illness in which the patient is expected to die because there is no known cure.

Thoracic cavity Located in the chest; contains the heart, lungs, and major blood vessels.

Tissue Groups of cells with a similar function.

Total quality management (TQM) Organizational philosophy of commitment to continuous quality improvement as a process to make organizational decisions.

Toxic Poisonous.

Traits Personal characteristics.

Transmission-based precautions Includes three types of isolation procedures (airborne, droplet, and contact precautions) required for specific infections.

Transverse plane Divides the body horizontally into top and bottom portions.

Treatment Medications or procedures used to control or cure a disease or injury.

Triage system Guidelines to determine which patients to send where and what treatment will be given during an emergency.

Tuberculosis A disease caused by the contagious, airborne pathogen *Mycobacterium tuberculosis*.

Values Standards that provide the foundation for making decisions and guiding behavior.

Victim Person requiring care during an emergency.

Virtual communities Groups of individuals who use the Internet to communicate and share information.

Viruses Smallest of the microbes; cannot be seen under normal light; in computers, refers to programs that contain instructions to perform destructive operations.

Visual learner A person who learns best by seeing new material.

Vital signs Refers to measuring the blood pressure, temperature, pulse, and respiration to give some indication of how the body is functioning.

Vital statistics Tracking the number of occurrences related to a specific event (i.e. births and deaths) for purposes of reporting.

Vowel The letters a, e, i, o, and u.

Wellness Promotion of health through preventive measures and the practice of good health habits; when the body is in a state of homeostasis.

Whole numbers The traditional numbers we use to count (1, 2, 3...).

Word processing A software program for creating written documents on a computer.

Wound Damage to the soft tissue of the body as a result of violence or trauma.

REFERENCES

Acello, B. (1998). *Patient care: Basic skills for the health care provider.* Albany, NY: Delmar.

Alexander Graham Bell Association. (1996). *Communicating with people who have a hearing loss.* [Brochure]. Washington, DC: Author.

American Association for Respiratory Care. (1999). *Guide for members.* Dallas, TX: Author.

Anderson, S. (1992). *Computer literacy for health care professionals.* Albany, NY: Delmar.

Anderson, S. A. & Smith, K. J. (1997). *Delmar's handbook for health information careers.* Albany, NY: Delmar.

Benjamin-Chung, M. (1999). *Math principles & practices: Preparing for health career success.* Upper Saddle River, NJ: Prentice-Hall.

Borgstadt, M. (1995). *Understanding & caring for human diseases.* Albany, NY: Delmar.

Burke, L. & Weill, B. (2000). *Information technology for the health professions.* Upper Saddle River, NJ: Brady/Prentice Hall Health.

California State Department of Finance, Demographic Research Unit. Retrieved September 20, 2000 from the World Wide Web: http://www.dof.ca.gov/html/Demograp/Proj_age.htm

Campbell, C., Schmitz, H., & Waller, L. (1998). *Financial management in a managed care environment.* Albany, NY: Delmar.

CDC–Centers for Disease Control and Prevention, Division of Tuberculosis Elimination. Status of the tuberculosis epidemic in the United States. Retrieved August 27, 1999 from the World Wide Web: http://www.cdc.gov/nchstp/tb/pubs/tbstatus/tbstatus.htm

Colbert, B. J., Ankney, J., Wilson, J., & Havrilla, J. (1997). *An integrated approach to health sciences: Anatomy and physiology, math, physics, and chemistry.* Albany, NY: Delmar.

Collins, M. (1983). *Communication in health care: The human condition in the life cycle.* St. Louis, MO: Mosby.

Cooperative Concepts Customer Service Statistics. Retrieved September 8, 2000 from the World Wide Web: http://cooperativeconcepts.com/articles/custservstat.html

Cross, K. P. (1981). *Adults as learners: Increasing participation and facilitating learning.* San Francisco, CA: Jossey-Bass Publishers.

Danis, Susanne J. The impaired nurse. Retrieved September 27, 2000 from the World Wide Web: http://nsweb.nursingspectrum.com/ce/ce153.html.

DeLaune, S. & Ladner, P. (1998). *Fundamentals of nursing: Standards & practice.* Albany, NY: Delmar.

Edge, R. & Groves, J. R. (1999). *Ethics of health care.* Albany, NY: Delmar.

Ehrlich, A. (1997). *Medical terminology for health professions* (3rd ed.). Albany, NY: Delmar.

Erikson, Erik H. (1982). *The life cycle completed.* New York, NY: W. W. Norton & Company.

Estes, M. E. Z. (1998). *Health assessment & physical examination.* Albany, NY: Delmar.

Equal Employment Opportunity Commission. Facts about sexual harassment. Retrieved November 2, 1999 from the World Wide Web: http://www.eeoc.gov/facts/fs-sex.html

Flight, M. (1998). *Law, liability, and ethics for health care professionals* (3rd ed.). Albany, NY: Delmar.

Fong, E., Grover-Lakomia, L., & Ferris, E. (1994). *Microbiology for health careers* (5th ed.). Albany, NY: Delmar.

Fremgen, B. (1998). *Essentials of medical assisting: Administrative and clinical competencies.* Upper Saddle River, NJ: Brady Prentice Hall.

Gardner, J. S. (1996) The Hospital Infection Control Advisory Committee–guidelines and recommendations on standard precautions and transmission-based precautions. Retrieved from the World Wide Web: http://wonder.cdc.gov

Griffin, A. D. (1998). *Directory of internet sources for health professionals.* Albany, NY: Delmar.

Guyton, A. C. & Hall, J. (1995). *Textbook of medical physiology* (9th ed.). Philadelphia, PA: W. B. Saunders Company.

Haddad, A. M. (1992). Ethical problems in home healthcare. *Journal of Nursing Administration* 22 (3), 46–51.

Handel, K. (1992). *The American Red Cross: First aid & safety handbook.* Boston, MA: Little, Brown & Company.

Harnish, V. (1994). *Implementing total quality management: How to make TQM work in your organization.* Boulder, CO: Career Track.

Harteker, L. (1998). *The pharmacy technician companion.* Washington, DC: American Pharmaceutical Association.

Hegner, B., Caldwell, E., & Needham, J. (1999). *Nursing assistant: A nursing process approach* (8th ed.). Albany, NY: Delmar.

Hispanic Association on Corporate Responsibility. Retrieved June 1999 from the World Wide Web: http://www.aacc.nche.edu/hacr/demongrahics/population.html

Hosley, J., Jones, S., & Molle-Matthews, E. (1997). *Lippincott's textbook for medical assistants.* Philadelphia, PA: Lippincott.

Jondreau, F. (1998). American Sign Language Institute. Retrieved June 1999 from the World Wide Web: http://www.asli.com

Jones, B. D. (1999). *Delmar's comprehensive medical terminology: A competency-based approach.* Albany, NY: Delmar.

Kee, J. L. & Marshall, S. M. (1996). *Clinical calculations with applications to general and specialty areas* (3rd ed.). Philadelphia, PA: W. B. Saunders Company.

Keir, L., Wise, B., & Krebs, C. (1998). *Medical assisting: Administrative and clinical competencies* (4th ed.). Albany, NY: Delmar.

Kelz, R. (1982). *Conversational Spanish for medical personnel* (2nd ed.). Albany, NY: Delmar.

Kogelman, S. & Warren, J. (1978). *Mind over math: Put yourself on the road to success by freeing yourself from math anxiety.* New York, NY: McGraw-Hill.

Kouzes, J. M. & Posner, B. Z. (1995). *The leadership challenge.* San Francisco, CA: Jossey-Bass Publishers.

Kreps, G. & Kunimoto, E. (1994). *Effective communication in multicultural health care settings.* Thousand Oaks, CA: Sage Publications.

Kübler-Ross, Elisabeth (1975). *Death: The final stage of growth.* Englewood Cliffs, NJ: Prentice-Hall.

Kübler-Ross, Elisabeth (1977). *On death and dying.* New York, NY: Macmillan.

Leshin, C. (1998). *Student resource guide to the Internet.* Upper Saddle River, NJ: Prentice-Hall.

Levitt, J. G. (1996). *Your career: How to make it happen* (3rd ed.). Cincinnati, OH: South-Western Educational Publishing.

Lindh, W., Pooler, M., Tamparo, C., & Cerrato, J. (1998). *Delmar's comprehensive medical assisting: Administrative and clinical competencies.* Albany, NY: Delmar.

Lock, R. D. (1996). *Job search: Career planning guide, book 2* (3rd ed.). Pacific Grove, CA: Brooks/Cole.

Marino, K. (1993). *Resumes for the health care professional.* New York, NY: John Wiley & Sons.

Martini, F. H. & Bartholomew, E. F. (1997). *Essentials of anatomy and physiology.* Upper Saddle River, NJ: Prentice-Hall.

Marx, G. & Grauer, R. (1996). *Essentials of the Internet.* Upper Saddle River, NJ: Prentice-Hall.

McCutcheon, M. (1998). *Exploring health careers* (2nd ed.). Albany, NY: Delmar.

McGraw, Phillip (1999). *Life strategies: Doing what works, doing what matters.* New York, NY: Hyperion.

Miller-Keane encyclopedia & dictionary of medicine, nursing, & allied health (5th ed.). (1992). Philadelphia, PA: W. B. Saunders Company.

Miller-Keane encyclopedia & dictionary of medicine, nursing, & allied health (6th ed.). (1997). Philadelphia, PA: W. B. Saunders Company.

Milliken, M. E. (1998). *Understanding human behavior* (6th ed.). Albany, NY: Delmar.

National Institutes of Health. (1998). Federal obesity clinical guidelines. Retrieved September 6, 2000 from the World Wide Web: www.coloradohealthnet.org/ obesity/obs_stats.html

OSHA−Occupational Safety & Health Administration, U. S. Department of Labor. Retrieved from the World Wide Web: http://www.osha.gov.html

OSHA preambles−bloodborne pathogens 29 CFR 1910.1030. Retrieved August 27, 1999 from the World Wide Web: http://www.osha-slc.gov/ preamble/blood_data/blood4.html

OSHA Standards Interpretation and Compliant Letters. (1998, April 6). Prevention of back injuries and use of back belts. Retrieved April 3, 2000 from the World Wide Web: http://www.osha-slc.gov/oshdoc/ interp_data/ 119980406A.html

Perrin, C. & Dublin, P. (1994). *Successful resumes and interviews.* Albany, NY: Delmar.

Purtilo, R. & Haddad A. (1997). *Health professional and patient interaction* (5th ed.). Philadelphia, PA: W. B. Saunders Company.

Richardson, J. K. & Richardson, L. I. (1994). *The mathematics of drugs and solutions with clinical applications* (5th ed.). St. Louis, MO: Mosby-Year Book.

Rice, J. (1998). *Medications & mathematics for the nurse* (8th ed.). Albany, NY: Delmar.

Schimeld, L. A. (1999). *Essentials of diagnostic microbiology.* Albany, NY: Delmar.

Scott, A. S. & Fong, E. (1998). *Body structures & functions* (9th ed.). Albany, NY: Delmar.

Simmers, Louise. (2001). *Diversified health occupations* (5th ed.). Albany, NY: Delmar.

Sormunen, C. & Moisio, M. (1995). *Terminology for allied health professionals.* Albany, NY: Delmar.

Spangler, Z. Culture care of Philippine and Anglo-American nurses in a hospital context. In: Leininger, M. L. (Ed.). (1991). *Culture care diversity and universality: A theory of nursing.* New York, NY: National League for Nursing Press.

Steefel, Lorraine. (2000). Nursing in the face of diversity. Nursing Spectrum Career Fitness Online. Retrieved September 19, 2000 from the World Wide Web: http:// nsweb.nursingspectrum.com/Articles/ NursingFaceDiversityCF.htm

Stence, P. & Kegler, A. (1995). *Age specific self learning module.* Sharp HealthCare.

Swanson, B. (1994). *Careers in health care.* Lincolnwood, IL: VGM Career Horizons.

Tamparo, C. D. & Lewis, M. A. (1995). *Diseases of the human body* (2nd ed.). Philadelphia, PA: F.A. Davis Company.

Taylor, C., Lillis, C., & LeMone, P. (1997). *Fundamentals of nursing: The art and science of nursing care* (3rd ed.). Philadelphia, PA: Lippincott-Raven Publishers.

Thomas, C. L. (1989). *Taber's cyclopedic medical dictionary* (16th ed.). Philadelphia, PA: F. A. Davis Company.

Tuttle-Yoder, J. & Fraser-Nobbe, S. (1996). *STAT! Medical office emergency manual.* Albany, NY: Delmar.

U. S. Census Bureau. (1995). Statistical brief. Retrieved January 2001 from the World Wide Web: http://www.census.gov/socdemo/ www/agebrief.html

U. S. Department of Labor. (2000). *Occupational outlook handbook.* Indianapolis, IN: JIST Works.

Williams, S. J. (2001). *Essentials of health services.* Albany, NY: Delmar.

Williams, S. J. & Torrens, P. R. (1999). *Introduction to health services* (5th ed.). Albany, NY: Delmar.

Wilner, T. (Ed.). (1995). *Ethnic diversity and hospice care.* Sacramento, CA: California Association for Health Service at Home−Hospice Section Steering Committee.

Yena, D. J. (1997). *Career directions.* Chicago, IL: Irwin.

Yuma Regional Medical Center. (1999). *Orientation core competencies: Age specific resource.* Yuma, AZ: Author.